SECOND   EDITION

Therapeutic Choices

EDITOR-IN-CHIEF
JEAN GRAY, MD, FRCPC

ASSOCIATE EDITORS
JEAN CUSSON, MD, PhD, FRCPC

ANNE M. GILLIS, MD, FRCPC

GORDON E. JOHNSON, PhD

JEFFREY A. JOHNSON, PhD

STUART M. MacLEOD
MD, PhD(Pharmacol), FRCPC

JAMES McCORMACK, BSc(Pharm), PharmD

WILLIAM McLEAN, PharmD, FASHP, FCCP

CHRISTOPHER PATTERSON
MD, FRCPC, FACP

ROBERT E. RANGNO, BSc, MSc, MD, FRCPC

MICHAEL J. RIEDER, MD, PhD, FRCPC

Canadian Pharmacists Association
Association des pharmaciens du Canada

©1998 Canadian Pharmacists Association

Canadian Cataloguing in Publication Data

Main entry under title:

Therapeutic choices

2nd ed.
Includes index.
ISBN 0-919115-77-2

1. Therapeutics—Handbooks, manuals, etc.
I. Gray, Jean (Jean Dorothy), 1942– II. Canadian
Pharmacists Association.

RM121.5.T44 1998   615.5   C98-900341-8

Editorial Board

Editor-in-Chief

Jean Gray, MD, FRCPC
Professor of Medicine and Pharmacology
Dalhousie University
Halifax, N.S.

Associate Editors

Jean Cusson, MD, PhD, FRCPC
Chief, Internal Medicine Division, C.H.U.M.
Associate Researcher, Pharmacology
Université de Montréal
Montréal, P.Q.

Anne M. Gillis, MD, FRCPC
Professor of Medicine
University of Calgary
Calgary, Alta.

Gordon E. Johnson, PhD
Director, Saskatchewan Drug Research Institute
University of Saskatchewan
Saskatoon, Sask.

Jeffrey A. Johnson, PhD
Assistant Professor
Faculty of Pharmacy and Pharmaceutical Sciences
University of Alberta
Project Leader, Institute of Pharmaco-Economics
Edmonton, Alta.

Stuart M. MacLeod, MD, PhD(Pharmacol), FRCPC
Professor, Departments of Clinical Epidemiology and
    Biostatistics, Medicine and Pediatrics
Faculty of Health Sciences, McMaster University
Director, Father Sean O'Sullivan Research Centre
St. Joseph's Hospital
Hamilton, Ont.

James McCormack, BSc(Pharm), PharmD
Associate Professor
Faculty of Pharmaceutical Sciences
University of British Columbia
Vancouver, B.C.

Practitioner Review Board

Contributors

S.K. Afridi
Saskatoon, Sask.

Sueda Akkor
Vancouver, B.C.

Upton Allen
Toronto, Ont.

Fred Y. Aoki
Winnipeg, Man.

S.A. Awad
Halifax, N.S.

Tony R. Bai
Vancouver, B.C.

Frederic Bass
Vancouver, B.C.

Mary Bell
Toronto, Ont.

Shlomit Ben-David
Toronto, Ont.

C. Laird Birmingham
Vancouver, B.C.

David B. Boyd
London, Ont.

Glen R. Brown
Vancouver, B.C.

Donald B. Calne
Vancouver, B.C.

Bruce Carleton
Vancouver, B.C.

S. George Carruthers
London, Ont.

Andrew Chalmers
Vancouver, B.C.

Hugh Chaun
Vancouver, B.C.

Anthony W. Chow
Vancouver, B.C.

John Collins
Hamilton, Ont.

Janet Cooper
Ottawa, Ont.

Robert Côté
Montreal, P.Q.

Orna Diav-Citrin
Toronto, Ont.

Simon Dobson
Vancouver, B.C.

Paul Dorian
Toronto, Ont.

R.B. Dunlop
Hamilton, Ont.

Jean Ethier
Montreal, P.Q.

Ernest L. Fallen
Hamilton, Ont.

Brian G. Feagan
London, Ont.

Richard N. Fedorak
Edmonton, Alta.

William Feldman
Toronto, Ont.

Louis A. Fernandez
Halifax, N.S.

Laura A. Finlayson
Halifax, N.S.

Jonathan A.E.
  Fleming
Vancouver, B.C.

A. Mervyn Fox
London, Ont.

Jane Garland
Vancouver, B.C.

Glenn H. Gill
Halifax, N.S.

Anne M. Gillis
Calgary, Alta.

Jane E. Gloor
London, Ont.

Ronald Gold
Toronto, Ont.

Elliot M. Goldner
Vancouver, B.C.

Gillian Graves
Halifax, N.S.

Daniel B. Gregson
London, Ont.

Lyn Guenther
London, Ont.

David A. Hanley
Calgary, Alta.

Jenny Heathcote
Toronto, Ont.

David J. Hirsch
Halifax, N.S.

Vincent C. Ho
Vancouver, B.C.

John P. Hooge
Vancouver, B.C.

Richard H. Hunt
Hamilton, Ont.

Jeffrey A. Johnson
Edmonton, Alta.

Gary I. Joubert
London, Ont.

C. Joyce
St. John's, Nfld.

Sidney H. Kennedy
Toronto, Ont.

J.S. Keystone
Toronto, Ont.

James Kissick
Kanata, Ont.

Gideon Koren
Toronto, Ont.

Gunnar Kraag
Ottawa, Ont.

Suzann R. Kronovic
Toronto, Ont.

Elizabeth J. Latimer
Hamilton, Ont.

Raymond P. LeBlanc
Halifax, N.S.

Robert S. Lester
Toronto, Ont.

Lionel A. Mandell
Hamilton, Ont.

Thomas J. Marrie
Halifax, N.S.

David G. McCormack
London, Ont.

James McCormack
Vancouver, B.C.

W. Alastair McLeod
Vancouver, B.C.

Max Michalon
Halifax, N.S.

Rob Miller
Halifax, N.S.

Julio S.G. Montaner
Vancouver, B.C.

Valentina Montessori
Vancouver, B.C.

Mark Montgomery
Calgary, Alta.

D. William Moote
London, Ont.

Lynne Nakashima
Vancouver, B.C.

Claudio A. Naranjo
Toronto, Ont.

Lindsay E. Nicolle
Winnipeg, Man.

Richard W. Norman
Halifax, N.S.

Richard I. Ogilvie
Toronto, Ont.

Jake Onrot
Vancouver, B.C.

Sagar V. Parikh
Toronto, Ont.

John D. Parker
Toronto, Ont.

John O. Parker
Kingston, Ont.

Thomas W. Paton
Toronto, Ont.

Paul M. Peloso
Saskatoon, Sask.

Ross A. Pennie
Hamilton, Ont.

R.G. Peterson
Ottawa, Ont.

R. Allan Purdy
Halifax, N.S.

Harvey R. Rabin
Calgary, Alta.

Anita R. Rachlis
Toronto, Ont.

Paul Rafuse
Halifax, N.S.

Michael J. Rieder
London, Ont.

Kenneth Rockwood
Halifax, N.S.

Ghislaine O. Roederer
Montreal, P.Q.

Donald Rosenthal
Hamilton, Ont.

J. Barrie Ross
Halifax, N.S.

Jean L. Rouleau
Montreal, P.Q.

André Roussin
Montreal, P.Q.

R.D. Schwarz
Halifax, N.S.

John W. Sellors
Hamilton, Ont.

Eldon A. Shaffer
Calgary, Alta.

Neil H. Shear
Toronto, Ont.

Michael B.H. Smith
Halifax, N.S.

David P. Speert
Vancouver, B.C.

Mark G. Swain
Calgary, Alta.

R.P. Swinson
Toronto, Ont.

Sandra A.N. Tailor
Toronto, Ont.

Milton Tenenbein
Winnipeg, Man.

Robert D.L. Tremaine
Halifax, N.S.

Eldon Tunks
Hamilton, Ont.

Alexander G.G. Turpie
Hamilton, Ont.

Adrian R.M. Upton
Hamilton, Ont.

Stewart H. Van Vliet
Saskatoon, Sask.

Hillar Vellend
Toronto, Ont.

David Warren
London, Ont.

C. Peter N. Watson
Etobicoke, Ont.

Sharon Whiting
Ottawa, Ont.

N. Blair Whittemore
Montreal, P.Q.

W.L. Wobeser
Kingston, Ont.

Donna M.M. Woloschuk
Winnipeg, Man.

James M. Wright
Vancouver, B.C.

John R. Wright
Toronto, Ont.

D. George Wyse
Calgary, Alta.

Samuel E. York
Halifax, N.S.

Stanley Zlotkin
Toronto, Ont.

Canadian Pharmacists Association

President: *Tom Healy, PhC*
Executive Director: *Leroy Fevang, BScPharm, MBA*
Publisher: *Leesa D. Bruce*

Editor-in-Chief: *M. Claire Gillis, BSc(Pharm)*
Managing Editor: *Frances Hachborn, BScPhm*
Clinical Editor: *Carol Repchinsky, BSP*
Assistant Editor: *Dianne Baxter*

Manager, Book Production: *Darquise Leblanc*
Desktop Publisher: *Lucienne Prévost*

We are grateful for the editorial assistance of Diane Bergeron, BPharm, Marline Cormier-Boyd, BSc(Pharm), Barbara Jovaisas, BSc(Pharm), Lise Lafoley, BPharm, Sandra Pagotto, BSP, and Louise Welbanks, BScPhm.

We also wish to thank Murielle Danis, Ghislaine Laporte, Julie Lévesque, Rose MacGregor and Scott Sawler for their assistance.

Original Design: *Purich Design Studio*
Indexing: *Editor's Ink*
Printing: *Webcom Limited*

Table of Contents

Foreword

Soon after the release of the premier edition of *Therapeutic Choices,* the editorial board met to consider the content of the second edition. We realized that there was a need for more evidence-based recommendations, a reasonable turn-over of authors to reflect different perspectives, and new topics, as requested by the Practitioner Review Board. Hence, readers of the second edition will find that about 10% of the authors are new, all chapters have been revised (some extensively), and eleven new topics have been added, including Chronic Fatigue Syndrome, Drug Withdrawal Syndromes, HIV Infection, Herpesvirus Infections, Adverse Drug Reactions, Burns, Atopic Dermatitis, Headache in Children, Neuralgia, Croup, and Management of Overdose. We hope that readers will continue to make CPhA aware of other topics that should be included in subsequent editions.

The Editorial Board recognized that cost-effective use of drugs means a lot more than the acquisition cost of the medication, and invited Dr. Jeffrey Johnson to join the Editorial Board for this edition. Dr. Johnson has provided pharmacoeconomic analyses to the chapters for which such information is available.

I would like to express my personal gratitude to the staff at CPhA, particularly Claire Gillis, for her overall guidance in the production of this second edition; Frances Hachborn and Carol Repchinsky, who reviewed and edited each chapter and coordinated the efforts of the associate editors and authors; Dianne Baxter, whose eye for detail contributed to the high quality of the finished product; and Lucienne Prévost, who painstakingly managed the graphic design and layout. I am also indebted to the Associate Editors for their hard work and to those on the Practitioner Review Board for their ideas.

Once again my thanks go to Carmen Krogh, whose vision inspired the premier edition of *Therapeutic Choices.*

Jean Gray

How to Use *Therapeutic Choices*

The second edition of *Therapeutic Choices* consists of 107 chapters and 4 appendices. Each topic presents essential therapeutic information in easily readable algorithms and tables. Because of size constraints, each chapter contains a suggested reading list. Readers wishing more detailed references may contact the Canadian Pharmacists Association, 1785 Alta Vista Dr., Ottawa, ON K1G 3Y6.

Drug therapy is discussed using generic drug names. Brand name inclusion in the chapters is not intended as an endorsement of that brand name. Many Canadian brand names are listed in the tables to the chapters. These are not all inclusive and are not listed in any order of preference.

The true cost of a specific therapy involves a number of elements including the manufacturers' list price, the mark-up and the dispensing fee, the length of drug therapy and costs related to drug administration. Prices used to determine cost of therapy in this book are the acquisition costs in Ottawa at the time of writing. The drug costs in the tables do not involve a dispensing fee or mark-up.

Costs shown are relative and are indicated by the "$" symbol; actual costs are shown occasionally. For most conditions, calculations were made with the cost of the lowest priced product at the dosage specified by the author for a given period. The treatment period selected for most chronic conditions is 30 days. However, treatment periods vary, and the legend accompanying each table should be consulted.

Readers of *Therapeutic Choices* requiring more detailed information on pediatric therapy should consult specialized texts.

Ten chapters include pharmacoeconomic considerations written by a pharmacoeconomist. They appear in a shaded box at the end of each of these chapters. General principles of pharmacoeconomics are discussed in Appendix II.

An appendix of drugs requiring dosage adjustment in patients with compromised renal function is provided (Appendix I). In the tables, a small icon (❥) appears after the drug name if dosage adjustment should be considered.

Description and Limitations of Information

Therapeutic Choices contains selected information representing the opinions and experience of individual authors. The authors, editors and publishers have tried to ensure the accuracy of the information at the time of publication. Users of *Therapeutic Choices* should be aware that the text may contain information, statements and dosages for drugs different from those approved by the Therapeutic Products Programme, Health Canada. The manufacturers' approval has not been requested for such information. Users are advised that the information presented in *Therapeutic Choices* is not intended to be all inclusive. Consequently, health care professionals are encouraged to seek additional and confirmatory information to meet their practice requirements and standards as well as the information needs of the patient.

CHAPTER 1

The Acutely Agitated Patient

Max Michalon, MD, FRCPC

Goals of Therapy

- To prevent harm to patients and caregivers (safety first)
- To sedate the patient with as few adverse reactions as possible
- To diagnose quickly and treat all underlying causes (medical, surgical, psychiatric)
- Whenever possible, to protect patients' rights

Investigations

- Physical examination. Look for physical illnesses presenting as psychiatric disorders, paying particular attention to:
  - vital functions
  - neurological anomalies (seizures, head trauma, brain tumors/abscess, encephalopathies, stroke)
  - metabolic dysfunction (hypoxia/hypercarbia, electrolyte imbalance, vitamin deficiencies, e.g., B_1, B_{12}, hypoglycemia)
  - drug toxicity (anticholinergics, digitalis, sympathomimetics, alcohol, psychostimulants, opiates) or drug withdrawal
  - cardiovascular pathologies (myocardial infarction, congestive heart failure, arrhythmias, hypotension)
  - infections (septicemia, meningitis, encephalitis, pneumonia, urinary tract infection)
- Mental status examination
- Whenever possible, consent to treatment should be obtained

Therapeutic Choices (Figure 1)

Safety Measures

- Prevent harm to both the patient and the staff.
- When faced with overt violence, try verbal control first; if this fails, do not persist but call for help.
- Ensure adequate manpower; a strong patient may require five or more people.
- Designate a leader to assign the different tasks.
- Consider rapid neuroleptization (Tables 1 and 2), along with human intervention (mechanical restraints/isolation are good alternatives).

Figure 1: **Management of the Acutely Agitated Patient**

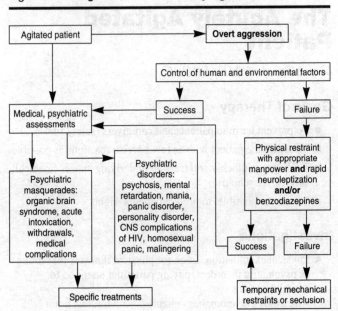

Nonpharmacologic Choices

Psychological interventions. Offer reassurance, clarification of misunderstandings/misconceptions and supportive (nonpaternalistic) psychotherapy.

Underlying medical causes. Correct infections, electrolyte imbalance, vitamin deficiencies, intoxications, etc., as soon as possible.

Pharmacologic Choices
General Measures

Short-acting benzodiazepines without active metabolites are good *temporary* measures as long as they do not affect the patient's alertness and respiratory function. **Lorazepam, oxazepam** and **temazepam** are metabolized by glucuronidation and are relatively safe for the elderly or patients with compromised liver function. Lorazepam may be given IM, PO, SL or IV. Oxazepam, which is predominantly anxiolytic with slow oral absorption, is a good temporary choice for the elderly.

Specific Situations
☐ The Demented Agitated Elderly

The most common causes of agitation in this population are:
- **catastrophic reaction:** explosive emotional response to stress and task failure

- **sundowning:** agitation as night approaches
- **pseudobulbar affect:** exaggerated emotions incongruous with mood
- **persecutory delusions and/or hallucinations:** may lead to violence

Neuroleptics have moderate to poor efficacy in treating the demented agitated elderly patient. A small dose of **high-potency** neuroleptic (HPN) (e.g., haloperidol 0.5 to 2.5 mg PO daily or BID plus occasional PRNs for extreme agitation) may be helpful. HPNs may induce intense extrapyramidal symptoms, parkinsonism in particular.

Low-potency neuroleptics (LPN) (e.g., chlorpromazine or thioridazine 10 to 25 mg PO daily) may cause hypotension or orthostatic hypotension, tachycardia and anticholinergic side effects (with worsening of dementia). These drugs are best avoided.

Middle-potency neuroleptics (e.g., loxapine 10 to 20 mg PO daily) may offer better tolerance and be more effective for agitation/aggression.[1]

Table 1: **Rapid Neuroleptization**

Rule out true allergies to neuroleptics (dystonias are often called allergies by patients).

Whenever possible, choose a high-potency neuroleptic (HPN) (Table 2); low-potency neuroleptics are not recommended for rapid neuroleptization.

Most clinicians prefer combining an HPN with a potent benzodiazepine (haloperidol 5–10 mg IM plus lorazepam 1–2 mg IM, half dosages or less for fragile patients or elderly. Repeat Q15–30 min until sedation), but closely monitor vital signs and be vigilant.

The most serious complication of this procedure is **neuroleptic malignant syndrome**; its frequency is higher in debilitated or dehydrated patients. Other side effects seen with HPN are dystonias, akathisia and pseudoparkinsonism.

Table 2: **Drugs* Used for Rapid Neuroleptization**

Drug	Young Adults	Older Patients
Haloperidol – Haldol, generics	5–10 mg IM/IV[†]	2.5–5 mg IM/IV[†]
Perphenazine – Trilafon	5–10 mg IM	2.5–5 mg IM
Fluphenazine HCl – Moditen	5–10 mg IM	2.5–5 mg IM
Trifluoperazine – Stelazine	2–3 mg IM	2–3 mg IM
Loxapine – Loxapac	25–50 mg IM	12.5 mg IM

* For adverse effects and drug interactions of neuroleptics, see Chapter 8.

[†] Neuroleptics are not officially indicated for IV use, but haloperidol IV is commonly and safely used in ICU settings.[2]

[1] Int Clin Psychopharmacol 1993;8:103–108.
[2] Hosp Commun Psychiatry 1992;43:215.

NB: Elderly people on neuroleptics are at a higher risk of tardive dyskinesia. Neuroleptics should be discontinued as soon as possible.

Alternatives to neuroleptics include:

- **Benzodiazepines** (see *General Measures*) – carry the risks of excessive sedation, ataxia and falls. Aggravation of cognitive impairment and depression may occur.
  Clonazepam (0.25 to 2 mg daily) may be prescribed alone or with a neuroleptic.

- **Trazodone**[3] (50 to 100 mg QHS) – sedative and serotonin modulator.

- **Buspirone**[4] (5 mg TID or 10 mg BID) – a partial serotonin agonist. If it is not effective, consider first decreasing, rather than increasing, the dosage.

- **Beta-blockers**[5] – propranolol and pindolol in small doses are the most commonly prescribed. Bradycardia, asthma and hypoglycemia are some contraindications.

- **Lithium** and **carbamazepine** – only rarely used.

Behavioral modification programs can complement pharmacologic interventions.

□ *Alcohol Withdrawal and Delirium (see also Chapter 9)*

Moderate withdrawal – observation and supportive care.

Moderate or *severe withdrawal*, with no withdrawal delirium, may be managed by oral **diazepam** loading: 20 mg PO Q1–2H until withdrawal is under control (mean dose 60 to 120 mg over 8 to 10 hours). Diazepam's active metabolites and long half-life offer a gradual pharmacokinetic tapering following initial loading (prevents drug-seeking behavior/dependency). Withdrawal seizures are less likely.

- Avoid alcohol plus diazepam (risk of respiratory depression).
- Always provide supportive care/psychotherapy.

Withdrawal delirium (delirium tremens [DTs]) occurs 2 to 3 days after discontinuation of prolonged/heavy drinking; confusion, illusions, hallucinations, agitation and autonomic hyperactivity are present.

- Nonspecific treatment of DTs and other deliria:
  – reduce environmental stimulation
  – 24 hours of dim light
  – reassurance/reorientation
  – prevent passive harm (falls)
  – diagnose/correct underlying causes

---

[3] *Am J Psychiatry 1988;145:1295–1296.*
[4] *Am J Geriatr Psychiatry 1993;1:249–253.*
[5] *J Clin Psychopharmacol 1984;4:282–285.*

- Specific treatment of DTs:
  - close monitoring of vital signs and electrolytes (ICU setting is preferable)
  - **thiamine** 100 mg IM/IV daily for 3 days followed by oral **B complex/folate** until normal nutritional intake is established
  - **glucose/saline** PO/IV *after* first thiamine dose (avoid overhydration)
  - high-dose oral **diazepam** (20 mg Q30–60 min) in the early stage only; most commonly slow bolus IV diazepam is required (5 to 10 mg repeated Q30–60 min until sedation)
  - always be prepared for respiratory resuscitation
  - in patients with marked agitation and/or compromised liver function, repeated doses of **lorazepam** (1 to 2 mg IM/IV Q30–60 min) may be preferable to diazepam
  - after sedation is achieved, maintain benzodiazepines for 1 to 2 weeks and taper gradually
- The mortality rate for DTs is high; be energetic in treatment.
- Poor response to initial treatment usually signals underlying complications (e.g., infection, subdural hematoma, meningitis, vitamin deficiency, hypo- or hypernatremia, hypomagnesemia, hypoglycemia).

❑ Benzodiazepine (BDZ) Intoxication

BDZ intoxication is usually part of a multiple drug overdose and/or often with alcohol. Diagnosis is usually made on clinical grounds (i.e., history of intake/overdose, sedation, respiratory depression, delirium, etc.) Standard urine drug screen assays may not detect commonly prescribed BDZs.

- Discontinue offending drug, provide physical supportive measures with particular attention to respiratory status.
- In case of coma, a trial of **flumazenil** 2 mg IV may temporarily reverse the syndrome. Caution: withdrawal seizures may be precipitated, and respiratory depression is not always reversed.
- Once the patient is improved, resuming a moderate dose of a long-acting BDZ (e.g., diazepam, chlordiazepoxide) may prevent withdrawal symptoms, especially when the offending drug has a short half-life and no active metabolites.

❑ Street-Drug-Induced Agitation/Intoxication

Psychiatric-like manifestations/psychomotor agitation are commonly induced by illicit drugs. Table 3 gives two examples that illustrate the seriousness of the emergencies faced by clinicians.

Table 3: **Treatment of Agitation Due to Drugs of Abuse**

Effects of Abuse	Treatment of Drug-Induced Agitation
Cocaine abuse causes intense euphoria, delusions/delirium, psychomotor agitation, tactile hallucinations, etc. Users are at risk of stroke, MI, heart failure (from IV crack) and status epilepticus	General life support with control of temperature/blood pressure Reassurance and observation Pharmacotherapy PRN; consider **diazepam** first **Haloperidol** PO/IM may be the next step, but **chlorpromazine** should be avoided When withdrawal symptoms are pronounced, consider desipramine, bromocriptine or amantadine. See chapter 9.
Phencyclidine (PCP) is an especially dangerous drug of abuse Effects are dose-related: ↓ response to pain, nystagmus, synesthesia, psychomotor agitation, ↑ BP and extreme paranoid ideation; assaults are common	Isolation is more effective than psychotherapy Continuous gastric suction **Ascorbic acid** 1 g PO QID **OR** **Ammonium chloride** 2.75 mmol/kg IV (as 1–2% solution in saline). When urine pH has reached 5.0, give **furosemide** 20-40 mg IV **Diazepam** to control seizures or for sedation **Haloperidol** if absolutely necessary; never use **chlorpromazine** (anticholinergic toxicity)

Psychiatric Disorders with Agitation

Begin treatment of acute or chronic psychosis with low doses of neuroleptics whenever possible[6] (Chapter 8).

- Rapid neuroleptization may be necessary if acute psychoses/mania with marked agitation are present (Tables 1 and 2).

- After sedation is achieved, start specific treatment for the underlying illness as soon as possible (e.g., lithium for mania, electroconvulsive therapy).

In extreme emergencies (e.g., patients with mental retardation or paranoid delusion with overt violent behavior), consider using a benzodiazepine with a rapid onset of action, good tolerance and absorption (PO/IM/IV) and rapid excretion (i.e., fast and brief action). **Lorazepam** (1 to 2 mg IV PRN) is commonly used. Neuroleptics (e.g., haloperidol) may be co-administered with lorazepam but should be avoided in catatonic patients (increased risk of extrapyramidal effects and neuroleptic malignant syndrome).[7] Benzodiazepines, usually lorazepam, may assist in clarifying the underlying diagnosis and in treating the condition in catatonic patients.

---

[6] *Arch Gen Psychiatry 1988;45:79–91.*

[7] *J Clin Psychiatry 1990;51:357–362.*

Therapeutic Tips

- Do not be a hero in the face of serious threats (guns or knives); isolate the patient and call for security/police.
- Staff are often injured when moving the patient after physical control has been established.
- A patient should not receive an injection without an attempt at explanation.
- The best predictor of violence is a history of violence.
- To prevent aspiration pneumonia and vascular or neurologic complications to limbs, restrained patients should never be left unattended.
- Never compromise your ability to escape a dangerous situation.
- Always fully document the seriousness of the situation and indicate the rationale for your interventions.

Suggested Reading List

Ancill RJ, Embury GD, MacEwan GW, et al. The use and misuse of psychotropic prescribing for elderly psychiatric patients. *Can J Psychiatry* 1988;33:585–589.

Corrigan PW, Yudofsky SC, Silver JM. Pharmacological and behavioral treatments of aggressive psychiatric inpatients. *Hosp Commun Psychiatry* 1993;44:125–133.

Michalon M. Cocaine use: distinguishing between fact and myth. *Can J Diagn* 1990;7:49–64.

Salzman C, Solomon D, Miyawaki E, et al. Parenteral lorazepam versus parenteral haloperidol for the control of psychotic disruptive behavior. *J Clin Psychiatry* 1991;52:177–180.

Winokur G, Clayton PJ, eds. *The medical basis of psychiatry.* 2nd ed. Philadelphia: W.B. Saunders, 1994.

CHAPTER 2

Anxiety Disorders

R.P. Swinson, MD, FRCPsy, FRCPC

Goals of Therapy

- To decrease symptomatic anxiety
- To decrease anxiety-based disability
- To prevent recurrence
- To treat comorbid conditions

Classification of Anxiety Disorders*

Panic disorder with or without agoraphobia
Agoraphobia without history of panic disorder
Social phobia
Specific phobia
Obsessive–compulsive disorder
Post-traumatic stress disorder
Acute stress disorder
Generalized anxiety disorder
Anxiety disorder due to a general medical condition
Substance-induced anxiety disorder
Anxiety disorder not otherwise specified

* As per DSM-IV-R (1994).

Investigations

- Thorough history with attention to:
  – nature of symptoms and onset
  – nature and extent of disability
  – presence of physical and psychological comorbid
    conditions

NB: Comorbid mood disorders, especially depression, should
be treated as the primary condition.

- Interview questions (Table 1) assist in obtaining an accurate
  diagnosis
- Physical examination to exclude endocrine or cardiac
  disorders and to look for signs of substance use
- Laboratory tests:
  – CBC, liver function tests, gamma-glutamyl transpeptidase
    (GGT), thyroid indices (supersensitive TSH), ECG

NB: Physical disorders should be treated before one makes a
definitive diagnosis of an anxiety disorder.

Figure 1: **Management of Anxiety Disorders**

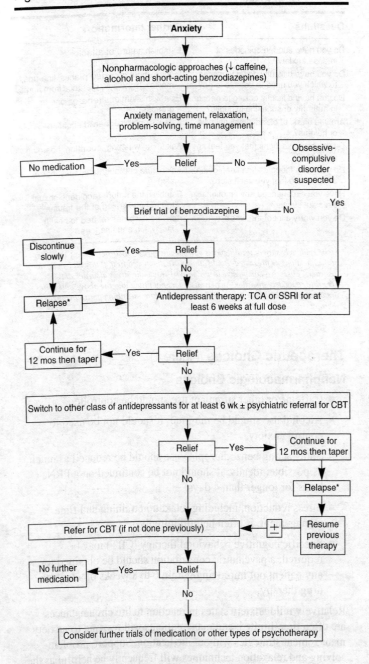

If patient has relapsed twice, long-term therapy is indicated.
Abbreviations: TCA = tricyclic antidepressant; SSRI = selective serotonin reuptake inhibitor; CBT = cognitive behavioral therapy.

Table 1: Interview Questions to Establish Specific Anxiety Diagnosis*

Questions	Further Information
Do you have sudden episodes of intense anxiety?	Establish nature of attack.
Do you have difficulty going to places to which you used to be able to go?	Inquire about crowded places, line-ups, movies, highways, distance from home.
Do you have difficulty talking to people in authority or speaking in public?	Establish situations (one-on-one or groups).
Are you afraid of blood, small animals or heights?	Establish precise feared situation.
Do you repeat actions that you feel are excessive?	Ask about washing, counting, hoarding.
Do you have thoughts that keep going in your mind that you can't stop?	Ask nature of thoughts (illness, harm, sex).
Have you experienced any emotionally stressful events?	Establish the nature (accident, sexual, torture) and timing of the trauma.
Do you worry a lot of the time?	Ask about worries related to health, family, job and finances.

* To be relatively sure of the diagnosis of a specific anxiety disorder, follow the order of the questions as presented. Panic attacks are diagnosed first, followed by phobic disorders, obsessive-compulsive disorder, post-traumatic stress disorder and generalized anxiety disorder. Anxiety disorders not fitting into the above categories are atypical. An accurate diagnosis is essential before instituting pharmacologic therapy.

Therapeutic Choices (Figure 1)

Nonpharmacologic Choices

- Caffeine or other stimulant use should be controlled.
- Alcohol use should be minimal; it should not be used to control anxiety.
- Short-acting benzodiazepine use should be reduced as much as possible; ideally, it should not be continued on a PRN basis for longer than 4 days.
- Stress reduction, including relaxation training and time management, is often helpful initially.
- Specific cognitive behavioral therapy (CBT) may be required; a psychiatric consultation should be obtained for any patient not improving within 6 to 8 weeks of adequate drug therapy.

Relatively mild anxiety states in reaction to life circumstances are often time-limited, and many patients will respond to anxiety management strategies without medication. Support, problem-solving and relaxation techniques will frequently be helpful as the environmental crisis resolves. However, specific anxiety or mood disorders may develop from the original reaction.

Pharmacologic Choices (Table 2)

The anxiety disorders respond differentially to the available medications.

Panic Disorder (PD)

◻ Benzodiazepines (BDZs)

Pharmacologic treatment of PD is determined by the acuity of the disorder at presentation. Low doses of high-potency BDZs (e.g., alprazolam, clonazepam) can be used to abort initial panic attacks and may control high-frequency panic attacks later in the development of the disorder. **Alprazolam** 0.25 mg TID or QID or **clonazepam** 0.25 to 0.5 mg BID will frequently make panic attacks more manageable.

Other BDZs (e.g., **lorazepam, diazepam**) may be used, but there are few data regarding their efficacy.

BDZs are best used short-term, but there is good evidence that long-term use does not lead to increasing dosage in most patients. Many patients remain on stable low doses for years.

◻ Antidepressants

The tricyclic antidepressants (TCAs) **imipramine, desipramine** and **clomipramine** have been shown to reduce the frequency and severity of panic attacks, as have the selective serotonin reuptake inhibitors (SSRIs) **fluoxetine**, **fluvoxamine, paroxetine** and **sertraline**. The older monoamine oxidase inhibitors (MAOIs) **phenelzine** and **tranylcypromine** are also effective.

The dose requirements and length of treatment are the same as for major depression (Chapter 5). The initial dose should be as low as possible (e.g., 10 mg daily of the TCAs or fluoxetine) and then raised, according to the patient's tolerance, to the usual anti-depressant dose range. If a higher starting dose is given, patients may become agitated and discontinue treatment abruptly. Determining the duration of drug treatment is a major difficulty; medication may be required for months or even years. There is evidence that a majority of patients suffer relapse after BDZs or antidepressants are discontinued.

Panic Disorder with Agoraphobia (PDA)

The drug treatment of PDA is the same as for PD. However, the disability in PDA arises from the avoidance behavior, not the panic attacks, and must be addressed behaviorally, even if medication reduces or eliminates panic attacks. Studies have shown that behavioral treatment can be more effective alone than when it is combined with medication; however, access to specialized behavioral treatment is often limited.

Social Phobia

This excessive fear of being criticized or negatively evaluated by others presents as shyness, avoidance of social contact or difficulty dealing with authority figures. It is particularly important to rule out major depression and alcohol use. CBT or other psychotherapy is usually necessary to deal with significant social phobia.

Drug treatment is not well defined. Simple stage fright or fear of public speaking may respond to low-dose **propranolol** (10 mg) taken 30 minutes before the event. Very low doses of **lorazepam** (0.5 to 1 mg) may also be used. More complex or pervasive social phobia can be treated with the same antidepressants used for PD. MAOIs may be the best drug treatment; **moclobemide** (in antidepressant doses) may be the best choice, given the safety of the reversible inhibitors of monoamine oxidase-A (RIMAs).

Specific Phobia

There is usually no indication for medication to treat the fear of heights, animals or blood. As few as 2 to 3 hours of behavioral treatment can be successful.

Obsessive–Compulsive Disorder (OCD)

A chronic disorder that often begins in childhood or adolescence, OCD can be extremely disabling. CBT is often helpful, but drug therapy is indicated for many patients. The most effective medications are **clomipramine** (a nonselective serotonin reuptake inhibitor) or the **SSRIs**, in the usual antidepressant range. It may take 6 to 8 weeks to produce any change in symptoms; an adequate trial at full dosages for at least 6 weeks is required. There is no evidence to suggest that SSRIs vary in efficacy, but patients may be able to tolerate one drug better than others in the same group. SSRIs may be better tolerated than clomipramine, but the initial agitation experienced with SSRIs may cause some patients to discontinue treatment. **Phenelzine** or **tranylcypromine** may be tried if SSRIs are not beneficial. Treatment, if successful, may continue for years.

Benzodiazepines alone are not helpful in treating OCD.

Post-traumatic Stress Disorder (PTSD)

There is no definitive treatment for PTSD, a mixture of anxiety, avoidance, mood change, insomnia and physical pain. Medication is one part of a multimodal treatment program that depends on the nature, severity and frequency of the trauma. Although **BDZs** are often used, there is little evidence of their efficacy. **Antidepressants** may help with mood, anxiety and pain complaints; selection is often based on the side effect profile. Amitriptyline, doxepin or clomipramine is given in low dosage for pain relief but must be given in full antidepressant dosage to affect mood changes.

Table 2: Drugs Used in the Management of Anxiety Disorders

Drug	Indication(s)*	Dosage	Adverse Effects	Comments	Cost†
Benzodiazepines	PD, PDA, GAD		Drowsiness (tolerance develops with continued therapy), dizziness, ↓ concentration, retrograde amnesia, physical dependence.	Discontinue gradually to avoid rebound anxiety.	
alprazolam Xanax, generics		*PD, PDA:* 0.25 mg TID–QID, up to 1 mg QID		Contraindicated in pregnancy and in patients with a known history of abuse.	$
clonazepam Rivotril		0.25–0.5 mg BID	Rarely, paradoxical anger or hostility.	Dose escalation is rare in patients taking BDZs for chronic anxiety. Use lower doses in elderly. Warn patients re: concomitant use of alcohol, other CNS depressants (↑ effect).	$
Tricyclic Antidepressants	PD, PDA, PTSD, GAD, SP		CNS effects (agitation on initiation of therapy, confusion, drowsiness, headache), anticholinergic effects (dry mouth, blurred vision, constipation, etc.), weight gain, nausea, cardiovascular effects (tachycardia, arrhythmias, orthostatic hypotension), anorgasmia.	May ↑ effect of anticholinergic drugs, CNS depressants, warfarin. Do not use MAOIs concurrently.	
clomipramine Anafranil, generics	OCD – clomipramine	75–225 mg/d		Other interactions include antiarrhythmics, lithium, levothyroxine.	$$–$$$
desipramine Norpramin, Pertofrane, generics		75–300 mg/d		May take 2–3 mos for maximum effect.	$–$$$$
imipramine Tofranil, generics		75–300 mg/d			$

(cont'd)

Table 2: Drugs Used in the Management of Anxiety Disorders *(cont'd)*

Drug	Indication(s)*	Dosage	Adverse Effects	Comments	Cost†
Selective Serotonin Reuptake Inhibitors	PD, PDA, OCD, PTSD, SP		**All:** Agitation (on initiation of therapy), nausea, anorgasmia.	Serotonergic syndrome with MAOIs (hypertension, tremor, agitation, hypomania).	
fluoxetine Prozac, generics		20–80 mg/d	Insomnia, headache, ↓ appetite, diarrhea.	Inhibition of cytochrome P450 enzymes results in many drug interactions.	$$–$$$$
fluvoxamine Luvox, generics		150–300 mg/d	Anticholinergic effects, sedation.	Avoid concurrent use of fluoxetine or fluvoxamine with astemizole and terfenadine.	$$$$–$$$$$
paroxetine Paxil		20–60 mg/d	Anticholinergic effects, sedation.		$$$–$$$$$
sertraline Zoloft		50–200 mg/d	Insomnia, diarrhea.		$$$–$$$$$
Monoamine Oxidase Inhibitors	PD, PDA, OCD (refractory)		Insomnia, dizziness, orthostatic hypotension, edema, sexual dysfunction.	Dietary restrictions (tyramine-containing foods) are necessary.	
phenelzine Nardil		45–90 mg/d		Sympathomimetics may ↑ BP; SSRIs, TCAs, levodopa may ↑ effects and side effects.	$$–$$$
tranylcypromine Parnate		20–60 mg/d		Do not use with meperidine (agitation, hyperpyrexia, circulatory collapse may occur).	$$–$$$
Reversible Inhibitors of Monoamine Oxidase-A	SP		Nausea, insomnia.	Do not use with meperidine, TCAs, SSRIs.	
moclobemide Manerix		300–600 mg/d			$$–$$$$

Azapirones *buspirone* Buspar, generics	GAD	5 mg BID–TID, up to 60 mg/d	Nausea, headache, dizziness, restlessness/insomnia.	Avoid use with MAOIs. Not as rapid an onset as with BDZs.	$$–$$$$$
Other *propranolol* Inderal, generics	SP (specific task anxiety)	10 mg, 30 min before task PRN	Hypotension.		$

* PD = panic disorder; PDA = panic disorder with agoraphobia; GAD = generalized anxiety disorder; OCD = obsessive–compulsive disorder; PTSD = post-traumatic stress disorder; SP = social phobia.

† Cost of 30-day supply – includes drug cost only.
Legend: $ < $20 $$ $20–40 $$$ $40–60 $$$$ $60–80 $$$$$ > $80

Generalized Anxiety Disorder (GAD)

A state of chronic worry that usually continues for years once it has begun, GAD tends to be diagnosed more often when there is little attention to the specific anxiety symptoms. Patients with GAD frequently exhibit mood change, social anxiety and obsessional traits that must be addressed; a combination of anxiety management and medication therapy is thus indicated.

Low-dose BDZs for several weeks at a time can be used for symptom relief. **Antidepressants** of all classes are helpful.

Buspirone (an azapirone) has low abuse potential and is less sedating. Like antidepressants, it is relatively slow to have effect; there is no cross-tolerance with BDZs. Care must be taken when switching from long-term BDZ therapy to buspirone to avoid precipitating BDZ withdrawal symptoms if the BDZ is discontinued abruptly.

Therapeutic Tips

- Short-term interventions may help.
- If BDZs are not quickly effective (within 2 weeks) at low doses, discontinue and switch to an antidepressant.
- If one antidepressant does not work in adequate dose and after adequate time, switch to one from another class.
- If the second antidepressant fails, refer the patient to a specialized anxiety or mood clinic.

Suggested Reading List

Antony MM, Swinson RP. *Anxiety disorders and their treatment: A critical review of the evidence-based literature.* Ottawa: Health Canada, 1996:1–101.

Antony MM, Swinson RP. *Anxiety disorders: Future directions for research and treatment.* Ottawa: Health Canada, 1996:1–37.

Last CG, ed. *Anxiety across the lifespan: a developmental perspective.* New York: Springer, 1993.

Salvador-Carulla L, Segui J, Fernandez-Cano P, Canet J. Costs and offset effect in panic disorders. *Br J Psychiatry* 1995:166 (suppl 27):23–28.

Steketee GS. *Treatment of obsessive compulsive disorder.* New York: Guilford, 1993.

Wardle J. Behavior therapy and benzodiazepines: Allies or antagonists? *Br J Psychiatry* 1990;156:163–168.

| **Azapirones** *buspirone* Buspar, generics | GAD | 5 mg BID–TID, up to 60 mg/d | Nausea, headache, dizziness, restlessness/insomnia. | Avoid use with MAOIs. Not as rapid an onset as with BDZs. | $$–$$$$$ |
| **Other** *propranolol* Inderal, generics | SP (specific task anxiety) | 10 mg, 30 min before task PRN | Hypotension. | | $ |

* PD = panic disorder; PDA = panic disorder with agoraphobia; GAD = generalized anxiety disorder; OCD = obsessive–compulsive disorder; PTSD = post-traumatic stress disorder; SP = social phobia.

† Cost of 30-day supply – includes drug cost only.
Legend: $ < $20 $$ $20–40 $$$ $40–60 $$$$ $60–80 $$$$$ > $80

Generalized Anxiety Disorder (GAD)

A state of chronic worry that usually continues for years once it has begun, GAD tends to be diagnosed more often when there is little attention to the specific anxiety symptoms. Patients with GAD frequently exhibit mood change, social anxiety and obsessional traits that must be addressed; a combination of anxiety management and medication therapy is thus indicated.

Low-dose BDZs for several weeks at a time can be used for symptom relief. **Antidepressants** of all classes are helpful.

Buspirone (an azapirone) has low abuse potential and is less sedating. Like antidepressants, it is relatively slow to have effect; there is no cross-tolerance with BDZs. Care must be taken when switching from long-term BDZ therapy to buspirone to avoid precipitating BDZ withdrawal symptoms if the BDZ is discontinued abruptly.

Therapeutic Tips

- Short-term interventions may help.
- If BDZs are not quickly effective (within 2 weeks) at low doses, discontinue and switch to an antidepressant.
- If one antidepressant does not work in adequate dose and after adequate time, switch to one from another class.
- If the second antidepressant fails, refer the patient to a specialized anxiety or mood clinic.

Suggested Reading List

Antony MM, Swinson RP. *Anxiety disorders and their treatment: A critical review of the evidence-based literature*. Ottawa: Health Canada, 1996:1–101.

Antony MM, Swinson RP. *Anxiety disorders: Future directions for research and treatment*. Ottawa: Health Canada, 1996:1–37.

Last CG, ed. *Anxiety across the lifespan: a developmental perspective*. New York: Springer, 1993.

Salvador-Carulla L, Segui J, Fernandez-Cano P, Canet J. Costs and offset effect in panic disorders. *Br J Psychiatry* 1995:166 (suppl 27):23–28.

Steketee GS. *Treatment of obsessive compulsive disorder*. New York: Guilford, 1993.

Wardle J. Behavior therapy and benzodiazepines: Allies or antagonists? *Br J Psychiatry* 1990;156:163–168.

CHAPTER 3

Attention Deficit Disorder

A. Mervyn Fox, MB, BS, FRCPC, DCH

Definition

Attention deficit disorder (ADD) is a lifelong behavioral syndrome characterized by poor organizational skills, poor listening, inattention to task, impulsivity, distractibility, fidgetiness and often inability to remain still. Only 50% of patients show hyperactivity. Daydreaming, dawdling, resistance to change and difficulties in school, especially in arithmetic, are characteristic. Sleep disorders are common. There is a strong familial tendency. Symptoms may reflect a variety of developmental, neurological and emotional disorders, as well as chaotic home environments, family dysfunction and child abuse. Most children with ADD have learning disabilities. Accurate diagnosis and successful therapy require time, since no universally accepted diagnostic test exists. Evidence of significant functional impairment in at least two settings such as home and school is now required for diagnosis.

Goals of Therapy

- To reduce symptoms
- To improve family functioning and child's self-esteem
- To improve child's academic attainments, especially in written assignments, spelling and arithmetic
- To improve child's ability to pay attention using behavior management, special education and social skills training

Investigations

- Comprehensive interview with special attention to:
  - age at onset and duration of symptoms
  - situations which elicit or reduce symptoms
  - family neurological, neuropsychiatric and educational history
  - symptoms of likely comorbid conditions
- Physical examination to:
  - screen for anemia, thyroid dysfunction, hearing loss and middle ear dysfunction, visual acuity, neurologic disorders
  - establish baselines for height and weight
- No routine laboratory, electrophysiological or neuroimaging investigations

- Obtain reports from school teachers, psychologists and special education consultants
- Medication history for drugs that may exacerbate symptoms (e.g., phenobarbital, tranquilizers, decongestants, antihistamines)

Therapeutic Choices

Pharmacologic **and** nonpharmacologic measures are usually used simultaneously (Figure 1). The child may not respond to nonpharmacologic adjuncts until medication has been initiated.

Nonpharmacologic Choices (Figure 1)

Foods that aggravate symptoms should be avoided.
NB: Going to school without breakfast is a common cause of classroom inattention.

The younger the child, the more important it is to recommend nonpharmacologic approaches first. Hyperactive behavior is commonplace in healthy toddlers aged 2 to 3 years and is often seen in gifted, curious and enquiring children. Side effects and treatment failures are more common in preschool children and may inhibit parental consent to medication in the school years, when the indications and benefits are clearer.

Pharmacologic Choices (Table 1)

First, decide on type of therapeutic trial and expected outcomes (shaded box below and Figure 1).

Patient Characteristics	Type of Trial
Questionable diagnosis Comorbidity present Unreliable family Multiple pre-existing "side effects"	Placebo trial Blind to family and school
Classroom symptoms predominate Few family concerns	Drug/placebo Blind to school
Pervasive symptoms Secure diagnosis	Titrate dose to response

Stimulants

Methylphenidate, **dextroamphetamine** or **pemoline** are each effective in over 70% of accurately diagnosed ADD; 97% of cases will respond to at least one stimulant. Methylphenidate is the first choice because its quick action and short half-life allow benefits to be recognized early and side effects to wear off quickly. Start with 5 to 10 mg with breakfast, increasing by no more than 10 mg weekly until benefit is no longer obtained,

Figure 1: **Management of Attention Deficit Disorder**

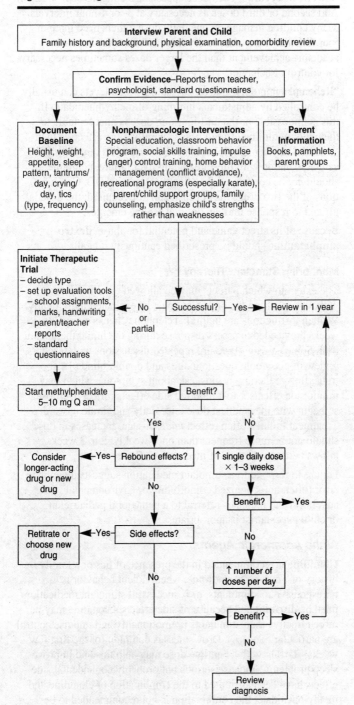

side effects occur, or each dose approaches 1 mg/kg body weight. Add second or third doses as necessary at 3- or 4-hour intervals. Many children manage on one daily dose, others need three or four. Smaller doses are usually more effective for improving academic achievement than the larger doses sometimes necessary for control of behavior.

"Rebound symptoms" due to fluctuating blood levels can usually be controlled by adjustments in timing of methylphenidate. If this is impossible or the mid-morning dose is unacceptable to the child, **pemoline** (1 mg/kg) is generally more effective than sustained action methylphenidate. Because of its rare but significant association with life-threatening liver failure, pemoline should *not* be considered first-line therapy for ADD. Combinations of the two drugs may occasionally be required; the dose is titrated to response until an optimal regime emerges.

Because of its street value and potential for abuse, **dextro-amphetamine** should be prescribed cautiously if at all.

Monitoring Stimulant Therapy

The extent to which parents may be allowed to adjust dosage without consulting the physician must be evaluated individually. Written instructions are helpful. Telephone checks every 2 to 3 weeks are needed to assess response during the initial therapeutic trial. Some cases will require repeated discussions with teachers, review of classroom questionnaires and double-blind placebo trials. Before therapy begins, ask about symptoms which may mimic side effects. Most reported side effects reflect *over*dosage, so begin with the smallest dose once daily and titrate upward. Treatment failures often reflect *under*dosage. Increases in dose should not be more frequent than once weekly; 2 to 3 weeks allows better evaluation of medication effects.

Failure to respond to a stimulant medication suggests diagnostic error (often unrecognized comorbidity or environmental adversity) and indicates referral to a behavioral pediatrician or child psychiatrist is appropriate.

Alpha Adrenergic Agents

Clonidine is recommended in the presence of tics or a family history of Tourette's syndrome, when violent behavior is unresponsive to stimulants, or if successful stimulant medication must be discontinued because of side effects. Clonidine may be more effective than stimulants if emotionality and impulse control are particular concerns. Drowsiness is common for the first few weeks; starting with a bedtime dose may help this and improve sleep problems. Because serious but probably coincidental side effects have been attributed to the combination of clonidine and methylphenidate, the combination is not recommended to be

Table 1: Drugs Used in Attention Deficit Disorder

Drug	Dosage	Adverse Effects	Comments	Cost*
Stimulants	Pharmacokinetics reflect wide individual variations; titrate dose against response.	Common, usually transient, continue trial: weepiness, headache, abdominal pain (if not taken with food), mild anorexia, mild insomnia.	First-line therapy: methylphenidate, dextroamphetamine.	
methylphenidate Ritalin, Ritalin SR, generics	**Methylphenidate** Usual: 0.3 mg/kg given once daily – TID Range: 0.15–1 mg/kg/dose	Transient, stop and re-evaluate: growth failure, psychotic reactions, insomnia, platelet changes, ↑ liver enzymes (pemoline).	Second-line therapy: pemoline. Avoid concurrent use of methylphenidate and dextroamphetamine with MAOIs.	10 mg/d $
		Overdose symptoms, stop and retitrate: weight loss, sedation, "glassy eyes", insomnia, hyperactivity.	Methylphenidate: uncertain effects on seizure disorders; discontinue if seizures occur. May ↑ plasma levels of phenytoin, TCAs.	
dextroamphetamine Dexedrine	**Dextroamphetamine** Usual: 0.15 mg/kg given once daily – TID Range: 0.15–0.3 mg/kg/dose	Significant, may be permanent, stop and re-evaluate: tics, neurologic symptoms, exacerbation of symptoms (may aggravate Tourette's syndrome).	Dextroamphetamine: do not use in cardiovascular disease.	5 mg/d $
pemoline ⬤ Cylert	**Pemoline** Usual: 1–2 mg/kg once daily Range: Up to 112.5 mg/d		Pemoline: contraindicated in renal failure. Fatal hepatotoxicity reported; monitor liver function.	37.5 mg/d $$$

(cont'd)

Table 1: Drugs Used in Attention Deficit Disorder (cont'd)

Drug	Dosage	Adverse Effects	Comments	Cost*
Antidepressants *imipramine* Tofranil, generics	**Imipramine** Usual: Up to 5 mg/kg/d once daily Range: 25–75 mg HS	Orthostatic hypotension, arrhythmias (potential for fatal arrhythmias in overdose), anticholinergic effects, drowsiness, tremor, weight gain.	Do ECG to exclude conduction defects before prescribing. Do not use with MAO inhibitors; may cause mania, excitation, hyperpyrexia.	$
desipramine Norpramin, Pertofrane, generics	**Desipramine** Usual: Up to 3.5 mg/kg/d, given once daily – TID Range: 25–50 mg/dose	Desipramine may be better tolerated.	Barbiturates, carbamazepine, rifampin may ↓ effect. Cimetidine, fluoxetine, neuroleptics may ↑ effect and toxicity.	$–$$
Alpha Adrenergic Agents *clonidine* ❢ Catapres, generics	Usual: 4–5 µg/kg/d, divided QID	Hypotension, sedation, dry mouth, could exacerbate depression.	Avoid concurrent use with amitriptyline, desipramine and imipramine. Safety in large numbers of patients unknown.	$
Neuroleptics *thioridazine* Mellaril, generics	Usual: 1–3 mg/kg/d, given once daily – TID	Sedation, anticholinergic effects, tardive and withdrawal dyskinesias, hypotension.	Use with caution in epileptic children or those with cardiovascular disease.	$

❢ Dosage adjustment may be required in renal impairment – see Appendix I.

* Cost of 30-day supply – includes drug cost only.
Legend: $ < $10 $$ $10–20 $$$ $20–30

prescribed by family physicians. Baseline blood pressure should be obtained and the patients warned of the possibility of hypertension if the drug is suddenly discontinued.

Antidepressants

Antidepressants are less successful than stimulants in improving cognitive aspects of ADD, but equally effective in reducing inappropriate behavior. Consider tricyclic antidepressants, **desipramine** or **imipramine** if stimulants fail or must be discontinued because of rebound symptoms or side effects (especially insomnia), or if there is a comorbid mood disorder. However, depressed patients with ADD respond at least as well to stimulants as to antidepressants.

Neuroleptics

There are no accepted criteria for the diagnosis of ADD in preschool children, in whom other developmental, temperamental and environmental factors are more likely to cause hyperactivity. Involvement in a good early childhood education program and improving parenting skills are recommended in preference to medication in all but extreme cases threatening family integrity. Neuroleptics may be considered when stimulant side effects are sufficient to discontinue therapy. However, neuroleptic use is recommended only for younger children in whom the diagnosis of ADD is somewhat speculative.

Therapeutic Tips

- Parents and teachers are exposed to much inaccurate information regarding diagnosis and management of ADD, especially the benefits and side effects of medication. Physicians should provide factual oral and written material, connect the family with knowledgeable support groups, and help parent and child to reach their own conclusions.

- Remember that every prescription of medication must be conducted as an individual therapeutic trial.

- It must be made clear that good and inappropriate behaviors remain the child's responsibility. Medication is neither a controlling straitjacket nor a magic wand.

- Drug holidays are unnecessary unless anorexia results in growth failure. Fluctuating behavioral competence may increase the child's sense of demoralization.

- Successful stimulant therapy should be continued as long as there is clear benefit, often into adult life. At least once a year medication should be withdrawn for 1 week to evaluate the need for prescription. Some children learn by experiencing normal attention and impulse control and manage well after 1 to 2 years.

Suggested Reading List

Cantwell DP. Attention deficit disorder: a review of the past 10 years. *J Am Acad Child Adolesc Psychiatry* 1996;35: 978–987.

Fox AM, Rieder MJ. Risks and benefits of drugs used in the management of the hyperactive child. *Drug Safety* 1993;9:38–50.

Spencer T, Biederman J, Wilens T, et al. Pharmacotherapy of attention-deficit disorder across the life cycle. *J Am Acad Child Adolesc Psychiatry* 1996;35:409–432.

Rostain AL. Attention deficit disorders in children. *Pediatr Clin North Am* 1991;38:607–635.

CHAPTER 4

Dementia

Kenneth Rockwood, MD, FRCPC

Dementia is a syndrome of acquired global impairment of cognitive function sufficient to interfere with normal activities. The most common causes are Alzheimer's disease, vascular dementia and a mixture of the two. Dementia with Lewy bodies, in which patients show dementia, marked fluctuations, early hallucinations, parkinsonism and sensitivity to neuroleptics, is also not uncommon.

Goals of Therapy

- To slow disease progression (chiefly Alzheimer's disease and vascular dementia)
- To treat concomitant depression
- To treat behavioral problems
- To alleviate caregiver burden

Investigations

Dementia

- History of memory impairment and potentially reversible causes. An estimation of cognitive impairment can be made using the Mini-Mental State Examination[1] (MMSE) and functional disability using the Functional Assessment Staging Tool[2]
- Physical examination to identify the cause and to look for potentially reversible causes
- Laboratory tests: CBC, electrolytes, kidney function, TSH, B_{12}, folate, calcium
- CT scan for young patients (< 60 years), new onset, rapid progression, post-head injury, focal or lateralizing signs

Behavioral Problems

Can be part of the illness or have medical and/or environmental precipitants:

- History of concomitant symptoms, environmental precipitants or medication changes

[1] *J Psychiatry Res 1975;12:185–189.*

[2] *Psychopharmacol Bull 1988;24:653–659.*

Figure 1: **Management of Elderly Patient with Behavioral Problems**

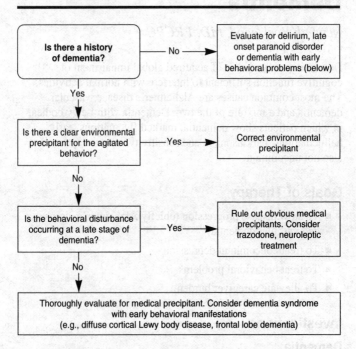

- Examination for focal or lateralizing signs or meningismus. Both sets of signs will usually be absent; thus toxic or metabolic causes should be evaluated, particularly signs of infection, congestive heart failure
- Laboratory tests: CBC, electrolytes, urea, creatinine, glucose, urinalysis, chest radiograph

Lack of **stage congruence** of the symptoms suggests a medical cause for behavior problems. In Alzheimer's disease, behavioral symptoms tend to occur in the later stages. If behavioral problems are seen early, a more aggressive medical investigation is warranted. Environmental precipitants should be sought (Figure 1). Hallucinations early in the course of dementia suggest Lewy body disease, or a focal lesion such as a stroke.

Therapeutic Choices

Nonpharmacologic Choices

- Before disease progression hampers competence, durable power of attorney and advance health care directives should be explored.

- Because individuals with dementia are at increased risk for accidents (falls, burns), environmental hazards should be removed.
- Patients should be counseled against driving after the initial stages of disease.

Pharmacologic Choices

Tacrine

Although approved for use in Alzheimer's disease in the United States, tacrine, a cholinesterase inhibitor, is not approved in Canada. Side effects are common, but some patients do well.[3,4] Several hundred Canadian patients have been treated with medication supplied on compassionate release from the manufacturer.[5]

Donepezil

This cholinesterase inhibitor has higher specificity for centrally active cholinesterases than tacrine. Improvement was shown after 12 weeks of donepezil 5 mg/day in patients with mild to moderate Alzheimer's disease (MMSE scores 10–26).[6] Side effects are cholinergic in nature, e.g., nausea, vomiting, diarrhea. Unlike tacrine, hepatic toxicity has not been reported. The dose range for donepezil is 5 to 10 mg. Until physicians achieve more familiarity with this drug, close attention to prescribing recommendations is advised.

Ergoloid Mesylates

Despite many trials, clinically significant beneficial effects in Alzheimer's disease have not been demonstrated.

Vitamin E

Vitamin E, in a dose of 2 000 IU per day of the alpha tocopherol form, has demonstrated evidence for very modest benefit in disease progression. Few side effects were apparent beyond an increased incidence of falls.[7]

Antidepressants

Many patients in the early stages of dementia suffer from depression; rarely, depression manifests as dementia. Anti-depressant therapy may be beneficial. Because most patients' symptoms tend to withdrawal and psychomotor retardation,

[3] *JAMA 1994;268:2546–2565.*

[4] *N Engl J Med 1992;327:1253–1259.*

[5] *Parke-Davis, 2200 Eglinton Ave. E., Scarborough, ON M1L 2N3.*

[6] *Dementia 1996;7:293–303.*

[7] *N Engl J Med 1997; 336:1216–1222.*

a more activating antidepressant is appropriate. **Selective serotonin reuptake inhibitors** are less likely than tricyclic antidepressants to cause anticholinergic side effects or to worsen orthostatic hypotension, which is common in this population. If used, a tricyclic with a low potential for anticholinergic effects, such as **desipramine**, should be chosen.

Trazodone for Behavioral Problems

To avoid iatrogenic problems, medical and environmental precipitants must be ruled out (Figure 1). Trazodone, a serotonergic agonist, is often used successfully to manage agitated behavior.[8] It is started with a low dose of 25 to 50 mg, usually first given at night and increased every few days until the desired effect is achieved (maximum dose of 400 mg per day).

Second-line Medications for Problem Behavior

❑ Benzodiazepines

Data on the efficacy of benzodiazepines for behavioral problems are conflicting. Although benzodiazepines can result in over-sedation and worsening cognition, their use is reasonable for severe agitation and sleep/wake cycle disruption. To manage severely agitated patients, **lorazepam** 0.5 mg can be mixed in the same syringe with **haloperidol** (0.5, 1 or 1.5 mg) and given IM every 8 hours. To alter a disrupted sleep/wake cycle, a short-acting benzodiazepine with no active metabolites, such as **oxazepam**, can be used short term.

❑ Neuroleptics

Non-neuroleptics have replaced neuroleptics as first-line treatment for agitated behavior in dementia. Good studies are lacking, but for many years, neuroleptics such as **thioridazine**, **loxapine**, or **haloperidol** have been used. As the elderly demented brain is exquisitely sensitive to neuroleptics, initial doses should be small (e.g., haloperidol 0.5, 1 or 1.5 mg BID to TID or the equivalent doses of other drugs).

Tips for using neuroleptics include:

- Start low, go slow.
- A designated treatment endpoint, usually an improvement in symptoms, should be chosen. When used **acutely**, to avoid pressure to increase the dose of a drug prematurely, only a 3-day supply should be prescribed, making clear that other measures during those 3 days must be nonpharmacologic.

---

[8] *Psychopharmacology.* New York: Raven, 1995:1427–1436.

■ Neuroleptic-induced akathisia (increased motor restlessness) may be misinterpreted as lack of drug effect. The dose then is increased, increasing motor restlessness. This cycle of worsening akathisia and increased neuroleptic use can result in extrapyramidal rigidity to the point of immobility.

❏ *Others*

Beta-blockers (particularly **pindolol**), **carbamazepine, lithium** and **buspirone** have also been used successfully in case reports, but better evidence is lacking.

Vascular Dementia: Slowing Disease Progression

Vascular risk factors should be modified, particularly to ensure good control of hypertension. **Acetylsalicylic acid** has been reported to slow progression of multi-infarct dementia.[9] There is very limited evidence for modest benefit from **pentoxifylline**.[10]

Prescribing for Other Dementias

Many of the previous comments apply. Because of the neuroleptic sensitivity syndrome in diffuse cortical Lewy body disease, neuroleptics should be avoided. These patients often present with hallucinations and early parkinsonism, which can be worsened by neuroleptics.[11]

Suggested Reading List

Raskind MA. Alzheimer's disease: treatment of noncognitive behavioural abnormalities. In: Bloom FE, Kupfer DY, eds. *Psychopharmacology*. New York: Raven, 1995.

---

[9] *J Am Geriatr Soc 1989;37:549–555.*
[10] *J Am Geriatr Soc 1992;40:237–244.*
[11] *Neurology 1996;47:1113–1124.*

CHAPTER 5

Depression

Sidney H. Kennedy, MD, FRCPC and
Sagar V. Parikh, MD, FRCPC

Goals of Therapy

- To relieve symptoms of depression
- To prevent suicide
- To restore optimal functioning
- To prevent recurrence

Classification (Tables 1 and 2)

Table 1: Criteria for a Major Depressive Episode*

Depressed mood and/or loss of interest or pleasure (irritability)
plus
At least four of the symptoms below for the same two week period
(must represent a change from previous functioning)

Physical	Psychological
Change in sleep	Feelings of worthlessness or guilt
Change in appetite or weight	Difficulty concentrating or making decisions
Fatigue	
Change in activity level (agitated or slowed down) observed by others	Recurrent thoughts of death or suicidal ideation
Not due to medical or drug induced conditions or normal bereavement	

*As defined by Diagnostic and Statistical Manual of Mental Disorders, fourth ed.
(DSM-IV). Washington, DC: American Psychiatric Association, 1994.*

Therapeutic Choices

Nonpharmacologic Choices

- Adherence to treatment and favorable response are strongly influenced by initial health education. One visit for "psycho-education" alone or with video and reading materials is strongly recommended. Five key points to stress: take medication daily; whom to call for questions about side effects or other issues; antidepressants must be taken for 2 to 4 weeks for a noticeable effect; continue to take medication even if feeling better; do not stop taking the antidepressant without checking with the physician.

- Both cognitive–behavioral and interpersonal psychotherapies are as effective as antidepressants in mild to moderate depression; antidepressants appear to be more effective in moderate to severe depression.

- All can be combined with antidepressant medications.

Table 2: **Common Depressive Syndromes**

Syndromes	Essential Features	Treatment Implications
Major Depression Typical	Depressed mood or loss of interest and four other depressive symptoms	Antidepressants and focused psychotherapies.
Atypical	Overeating/weight gain Oversleeping, reactive mood Rejection sensitivity	MAOIs, SSRIs are preferred; TCAs may be less effective.
"Anxious"	Prominent anxiety symptoms in addition to major depressive symptoms	Initial dose should be low, but may ultimately require a higher dose for longer duration. Consider paroxetine or sertraline for comorbid panic disorder.
Seasonal	Fall onset, spring offset Recurrent	Light therapy is optimal; SSRIs may be as effective.
Psychotic	Hallucinations Delusions	Electroconvulsive therapy or combination antidepressant (most evidence for TCAs) with neuroleptic therapy.
Dysthymia	Chronic depressive illness for two or more years, fewer and less severe symptoms than major depression	Antidepressants, but may be less effective than with major depression. Consider SSRIs (most evidence for fluoxetine and sertraline).
Bipolar Depression*	Prior history of mania or hypomania Mixed episodes may occur	Try to avoid antidepressants. Mood stabilizers preferred. Lithium, valproate, carbamazepine.

Can J Psychiatry 1997;42 Suppl 2: 675–1005.

Pharmacologic Choices (Table 3)
Selective Serotonin Reuptake Inhibitors (SSRIs)

Greater tolerability and **easy dosing** contributed to the rapid adoption of SSRIs as first-choice antidepressants. Although efficacy is considered comparable to established and novel antidepressants (4 to 6 weeks is still required for a therapeutic trial; about 65% of patients respond), the well-tolerated side effect profile greatly expands the population that may be treated

Table 3: Antidepressant Drugs

Drug	Dosage Adjustment			Adverse Effects	Drug Interactions	Cost[π]
	Starting*	Usual[†]	High[‡]			
SSRIs						
fluoxetine Prozac, generics	10–20 mg	20–40 mg	60–80 mg	Nausea, nervousness, anorexia, insomnia.	**For all SSRIs:** MAOIs may cause severe reaction – tremor, agitation, hypomania, hypertension. Drugs that inhibit cytochrome P-450 enzymes may ↑ SSRI levels. All SSRIs inhibit certain cytochrome P-450 isoenzymes involved in drug metabolism, resulting in many potential drug interactions.	\$\$–\$\$\$\$
fluvoxamine Luvox, generics	50–100 mg	150–200 mg	400 mg	Nausea, drowsiness, sweating, anorexia.		\$\$–\$\$\$
paroxetine Paxil	10–20 mg	20–40 mg	60 mg	Nausea, drowsiness, fatigue, sweating, dizziness.		\$\$\$–\$\$\$\$
sertraline Zoloft	25–50 mg	50–100 mg	150–200 mg	Nausea, tremors, diarrhea, dry mouth.		\$\$\$
MAOIs						
phenelzine Nardil	15–30 mg	30–75 mg	90–120 mg	**For both agents:** Edema, postural hypotension, insomnia, sexual dysfunction.	**For both agents:** Sympathomimetics may ↑ BP; meperidine may cause agitation, hyperpyrexia, circulatory collapse; TCAs, levodopa may ↑ effects and side effects; tyramine-containing food may cause hypertensive crisis. Avoid combination with SSRIs.	\$–\$\$\$
tranylcypromine Parnate	20–60 mg		60–80 mg			\$\$–\$\$\$

TCAs

amitriptyline Elavil, generics	25–50 mg	75–200 mg	250–300 mg	**For all TCAs:**	$
clomipramine Anafranil, generics	50–75 mg	100–250 mg	300–450 mg	Anticholinergic (dry mouth, blurred vision, constipation, urinary hesitancy, tachycardia, delirium), antihistaminergic (sedation, weight gain), orthostatic hypotension, lowered seizure threshold.	$–$$
desipramine Norpramin, Pertofrane, generics	50–75 mg	100–200 mg	300–450 mg		$$–$$$$
doxepin Sinequan, Triadapin, generics	50–75 mg	100–250 mg	300–450 mg		$–$$$
imipramine Tofranil, generics	50–75 mg	100–250 mg	300–450 mg		$
maprotiline	50–75 mg	100–250 mg	300–450 mg		$$–$$$
nortriptyline Aventyl	25–50 mg	75–150 mg	200 mg		$$–$$$
protriptyline Triptil	10–20 mg	30–60 mg	80–100 mg		$$–$$$$
trimipramine Surmontil, generics	50–75 mg	100–250 mg	300–450 mg		$–$$

For all TCAs:
Combination with MAOIs may result in mania, excitation, hyperpyrexia. Barbiturates, carbamazepine and rifampin may decrease effect. Cimetidine and neuroleptics may increase effect and toxicity.
Possible interaction with antiarrhythmics: may increase effect of either drug.
May decrease antihypertensive effect of clonidine. May augment hypotensive effect of thiazides.

(cont'd)

Table 3: Antidepressant Drugs *(cont'd)*

Drug	Dosage Adjustment Starting*	Dosage Adjustment Usual†	Dosage Adjustment High‡	Adverse Effects	Drug Interactions	Cost^π
Other						
nefazodone Serzone	100–200 mg	300–500 mg	600 mg	Dizziness, amblyopia, dry mouth, nausea, drowsiness.	May displace protein-bound drugs. May augment hypotensive effect of antihypertensives. May inhibit metabolism of triazolam, alprazolam, midazolam, cyclosporine, nifedipine, lidocaine, erythromycin.	$$–$$$$
venlafaxine Effexor	37.5–75 mg	112.5–225 mg	300–375 mg	Nausea, drowsiness, nervousness, dizziness, dry mouth, may ↑ BP if dose > 300 mg/d.	Drugs that inhibit cytochrome P-450 may ↑ venlafaxine levels. May interact with MAOIs.	$$$$–$$$$$
moclobemide Manerix	200–300 mg	450–600 mg	900 mg#	Nausea, insomnia, dizziness.	Avoid sympathomimetics, meperidine. Caution with opioids, antihypertensives, antipsychotics, SSRIs, selegiline, excessive tyramine, alcohol. Reduce dose with cimetidine.	$$$–$$$$
*bupropion** * Wellbutrin	75 mg	150–300 mg	375–450 mg	Agitation, insomnia, anorexia, contraindicated if history of seizures.		

*Lower starting dose indicated where previous side effect experience or polypharmacy; often applies to elderly patients.
†For SSRIs upper starting dose may be usual dose, e.g., fluoxetine 20 mg or sertraline 50 mg; otherwise increments every 5–7 days.
‡Higher doses often exceed manufacturer's recommended upper doses and usually result in more disabling side effects. These doses should be used with caution.
^π Cost of 30-day supply – includes drug cost only.
Legend: $ < $20 $$ $20–40 $$$ $40–60 $$$$ $60–100 $$$$$ > $100
#Exceeds manufacturer's recommended maximum dose of 600 mg.
**Sustained-release form likely to be available in Canada in 1998.

effectively. Sexual dysfunction (anorgasmia in women and delayed ejaculation in men) is more common with all SSRIs than was initially recognized.

Tricyclic Antidepressants (TCAs)

Long the mainstay of antidepressant pharmacotherapy, tricyclics are less favored now because of frequent side effects, especially cardiotoxicity, and lethality in overdose. However, they are equivalent to newer agents in efficacy, and prescription costs are often substantially lower.

Secondary amine TCAs include desipramine, nortriptyline and protriptyline. The severity of anticholinergic and anti-histaminergic side effects is less than with the **tertiary amines** (amitriptyline, imipramine, doxepin, clomipramine and trimipramine). Maprotiline is a related **tetracyclic** antidepressant with similar efficacy and side effects, although there is an increased risk of seizures at high doses (above 200 mg).

For most cyclic antidepressants, it is best to "start low and go slow." A usual starting dose is 50 mg given at night, building to 100 mg after 3 to 5 days and increasing weekly, depending on tolerability and antidepressant response. The average dose can be approximated by calculating 3 mg/kg body weight. In elderly, cachexic or medically ill patients, lower starting doses (10 to 25 mg) are more appropriate and can be gradually increased to 1.5 mg/kg body weight.

Classical Monoamine Oxidase Inhibitors (MAOIs)

Use of phenelzine and tranylcypromine is limited by concerns about hazardous drug–drug and food–drug interactions. However, many TCA nonresponders are responsive to MAOIs. Historically, phenelzine in doses of 30 to 90 mg per day has been the drug of choice in atypical depression. Tranylcypromine 20 to 60 mg per day may be superior to imipramine in treating bipolar depression. Because of the irreversible enzyme inhibition, food and drug cautions must be followed for 2 weeks after the last dose of MAOI.

Other Antidepressants

Reversible inhibitors of monoamine oxidase-A (RIMA) do not require dietary precautions and have less hazardous drug–drug interactions than MAOIs. The first RIMA available in Canada is **moclobemide**. In the treatment of outpatient depression, clinical trials suggest comparable efficacy to TCAs and SSRIs and a lower rate of adverse effects. Moclobemide is prescribed in divided doses between 300 and 600 mg daily, although higher doses have been used for partial responders when side effects are minimal or absent. Nausea may be an early but brief adverse effect; insomnia may persist.

Bupropion, soon to be available in Canada as a sustained-release form, acts on the norepinephrine and dopamine systems. It will likely be useful as a second-line agent for major depression and bipolar depression. An increased incidence of seizures at higher doses has been reported in patients with bulimia nervosa, head injury or a history of seizures.

Trazodone and **nefazodone** have serotonin reuptake inhibiting and $5HT_2$ receptor antagonism effects. Both may offer comparable efficacy to existing SSRIs. The role of trazodone is limited mainly because of excessive sedation at therapeutic doses; lower doses (50 to 100 mg) may provide a useful hypnotic effect in combination with other antidepressants. Both moclobemide and nefazodone have been reported to cause less sexual dysfunction than other antidepressants.

Venlafaxine inhibits serotonin and norepinephrine reuptake and may be effective in refractory patients. Preliminary suggestions that venlafaxine may be more effective than other antidepressants for inpatient depression deserve further study. Nausea is a common initial side effect.

Amoxapine is an older antidepressant that is metabolized to a loxapine-like antipsychotic compound; this has resulted in extrapyramidal side effects and tardive dyskinesia.

Several **augmentation** and **combination** therapies have been evaluated in refractory depression and are best carried out in consultation with specialized mood disorder clinics[1]: lithium carbonate, triiodothyronine (T_3), L-tryptophan, buspirone, pindolol or methylphenidate in combination with TCA, MAOI or SSRI drugs. Combination desipramine–fluoxetine has also been reported to be successful in previously unresponsive patients.

ECT is efficacious in 80 to 90% of depressed patients, superior to any single antidepressant drug therapy.

Duration of Antidepressant Treatment

Evidence supports the continuing use of antidepressant therapies beyond the conventional 4- to 6-month period, particularly when the intervals between depressive episodes become briefer and the disability associated with each depressive episode worsens. After one episode, treat for 1 year and after two or more episodes, treat for at least 2 years.

Therapeutic Tips

- Choose one or two agents from several antidepressant classes (SSRI, TCA, and other) and use them consistently.

---

[1] *Can J Psychiatry 1989;34:451–456.*

- Provide structured psychoeducation with initial prescription.
- Reinforce the importance of continuation and maintenance therapy.
- Although plasma drug levels are not useful with SSRI, MAOI, RIMA and other new antidepressants, there is a role for plasma monitoring with some TCAs, i.e., desipramine, imipramine, amitriptyline and nortriptyline.
- Switch or augment if no response at highest tolerable dose after 6 to 8 weeks.
- Review alcohol and drug abuse history in nonresponders.
- Refer for psychiatric consultation if there is psychotic symptoms, acute suicidal ideation or failure of 3 treatment trials.
- At the point of recovery and drug discontinuation, taper slowly over 1 to 2 months.

Suggested Reading List

Andrews JM, Nemeroff CB. Contemporary management of depression. *Am J Med* 1994;97 (Suppl 6A):24S–32S.

Paykel ES, Priest RG. Recognition and management of depression in general practice: consensus statement. *BMJ* 1992;305:1198–2002.

Rudorfer MV, Potter WZ. Antidepressants: a comparative review of the clinical pharmacology and therapeutic use of the "newer" versus "older" drugs. *Drugs* 1989;37:713–738.

CHAPTER 6

Eating Disorders

C. Laird Birmingham, MD, FRCPC and
Elliot M. Goldner, MD, FRCPC

A disturbance of perception of body image and weight is an essential feature of both anorexia nervosa and bulimia nervosa.

Anorexia nervosa is characterized by a refusal to maintain minimally normal body weight. The two subtypes, *restricting* and *binge-eating/purging* type, indicate the presence or absence of regular binge eating or purging during the current episode.

Bulimia nervosa is characterized by repeated episodes of binge eating followed by inappropriate compensatory behavior such as self-induced vomiting, misuse of laxatives, diuretics or other medications, fasting or excessive exercise. The two subtypes are *purging* and *nonpurging* (uses inappropriate compensatory behaviors, e.g., fasting or excessive exercise but has not regularly engaged in self-induced vomiting, misuse of laxatives, etc. during the current episode).

Goals of Therapy

- To assess and treat coexistent deficiencies
- To improve cognitive and emotional function
- To uncover and treat psychiatric comorbidity (e.g., anxiety, depression, family dysfunction, suicidal ideation)
- To develop healthy eating habits
- To treat binge and purge behavior (coexistent in 50% of patients with anorexia nervosa)
- For anorexia nervosa (in addition to above), to achieve a healthy weight (total body fat)

Investigations

- A thorough history with special attention to:
  - weight, eating habits, binge and purge behavior, menstruation, body image, use of vomiting, laxatives, suppositories, diuretics, ipecac, fasting, and overexercising
  - developmental and psychological history
  - depression, anxiety, suicidal ideation, family dysfunction and sexual abuse
  - symptoms of malnutrition including chest pain, palpitations, seizures, abdominal pain, muscle weakness and cramping
  - dietary history

Figure 1: **Management of Anorexia Nervosa**

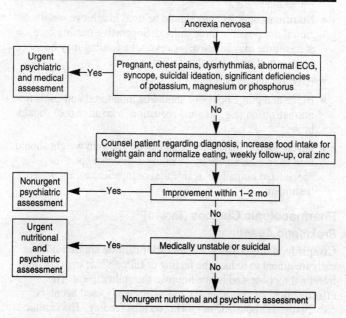

- Physical examination for parotid hypertrophy, edema, abnormal dentition; for anorexia nervosa (in addition to above), postural hypotension, heart rate, lanugo hair, hypercarotenemia, height, weight, measurements of body fat, Chvostek's and Trousseau's signs
- Laboratory tests:
  – sodium, potassium, chloride, bicarbonate, creatinine, magnesium, phosphorus, zinc, B_{12}, ferritin
  – for anorexia nervosa (in addition to above), ECG, hemoglobin, WBC count, urinalysis, folate, serum albumin, calcium
- For anorexia nervosa, a psychiatric and nutritional assessment if symptoms continue and weight does not normalize after weekly follow-up and counseling

Anorexia Nervosa

Therapeutic Choices (Figure 1)

Nonpharmacologic Choices

- A rapport and therapeutic alliance should be developed and maintained.
- The need for and role of family intervention and treatment should be considered.

- Nutrition should be normalized by setting and maintaining eating goals.
- Nutritional supplements should be used to achieve weight gain if not possible through food. Supportive nursing care at mealtime may improve success; tube feeding may be necessary if oral refeeding fails.
- Exercise should be limited.
- Binge and purge behavior should be monitored and goals for normalization (e.g., gradual reduction in laxative use) should be set.
- Psychological instability or an inability to gain weight should lead to an assessment by an eating disorders expert for specialized outpatient, residential or inpatient eating disorder treatment.

Pharmacologic Choices (Table 1)
Prokinetic Agents
Cisapride, domperidone and **metoclopramide** are useful in the early treatment to reduce the feeling of fullness due to decreased intestinal motility and hence improve the ability to eat. The effective dose of cisapride, the most commonly used agent, is 5 to 20 mg, 1/2 hour AC or Q6H if on tube feeding. The cardiac QT interval should be reassessed after starting cisapride.

Others
Anxiolytics (e.g., clonazepam) should be used for severe anxiety; their use should be minimized due to the potential for dependence. Initiate clonazepam at 0.5 to 1 mg BID and cautiously titrate upward to a maximum dose of 20 mg per day, no more than every 3 days.

Antidepressants should be used for coexistent depression (Chapter 5) or purge behavior only, and **only** when cardiac status is stable (no cardiac chest pain, dysrhythmia or abnormal ECG).

Cyproheptadine can be tried, particularly in chronic anorexia, to facilitate weight gain.

Oral **zinc supplementation**[1] improves the chance of weight gain irrespective of serum zinc level. Zinc gluconate 100 mg daily for 2 months should be tried.

Therapeutic Tips

- Normalization of body fat is necessary for psychological treatment to be effective and for cure.
- Treatment refusal is common. A careful reassessment of the treatment plan is necessary.

---

[1] *Int J Eat Disord 1994;3:251–255.*

Table 1: Drugs Used in Anorexia Nervosa

Drug	Dosage	Adverse Effects	Drug Interactions	Cost*
Prokinetic Agents				
cisapride Prepulsid	5–20 mg 1/2H AC (H): ↓ initial dose by 50%	Diarrhea (4%), abdominal discomfort (1%), hyperprolactinemia (with domperidone and metoclopramide).	Avoid use of cisapride with clarithromycin, erythromycin, fluconazole, itraconazole and ketoconazole (risk of ventricular arrhythmias).	$$–$$$$
metoclopramide ● Maxeran, Reglan, generics	5–20 mg 1/2H AC			$
domperidone Motilium, generic	10–30 mg 1/2H AC			$–$$
cyproheptadine Periactin, generic	4–16 mg QHS	Drowsiness (usual), dry mouth (common).	MAOIs; additive effect with other sedatives.	$–$$

● *Dosage adjustment may be required in renal impairment – see Appendix I.*
(H) Dosage adjustment in hepatic impairment.
Abbreviations: TCAs = tricyclic antidepressants; MAOIs = monoamine oxidase inhibitors; AC = before meals.

* *Cost of 30-day supply – includes drug cost only.*

Legend: $ < $25 $$ $25–50 $$$ $50–75 $$$$ $75–100

Figure 2: **Management of Bulimia Nervosa**

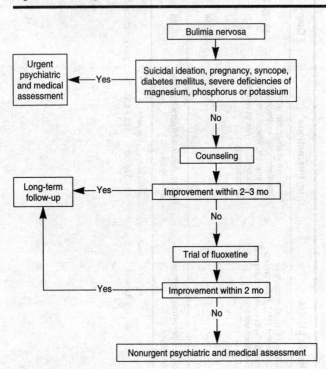

Bulimia Nervosa

Therapeutic Choices (Figure 2)

Nonpharmacologic Choices

- Counseling on normal eating behavior and cognitive and emotional issues should be provided and progress followed.
- Patients should be assessed for suicidal ideation and depression; these should be treated if present.
- Psychoeducational groups addressing nutritional and psychological issues can enhance individual therapy.

Pharmacologic Choices (Table 2)
Antidepressants

A number of antidepressants have shown some effectiveness in decreasing binge and purge behavior; the only agent currently approved as an antibulimic in Canada is **fluoxetine**.

Fluoxetine, imipramine, desipramine, phenelzine and **trazodone** all decrease binge and purge symptoms and may treat concurrent depression. Other SSRIs may be tried after failing

Table 2: Drugs Used in Bulimia Nervosa

Drug	Dosage	Adverse Effects	Drug Interactions	Cost*
fluoxetine Prozac, generics	20–60 mg daily (H): ↓ dose	Anxiety, GI discomfort (common). Fluoxetine – less anticholinergic effect than TCAs. Limited experience with fluoxetine overdose indicates that overdose symptoms are mild and usually well tolerated.	Avoid use with MAOIs, fenfluramine, L-tryptophan (serotonin syndrome); astemizole, terfenadine (ventricular arrhythmias).	$$–$$$$
desipramine ● Norpramin, Pertofrane, generics	50–250 mg daily (H): Use with caution	Anticholinergic effects (e.g., postural hypotension, dizziness, dry mouth, constipation, urinary retention). May prolong cardiac conduction and worsen cardiac dysrhythmias.	Avoid use with clonidine and sympathomimetics. Use extreme caution in combination with MAOIs.	$–$$$
imipramine ● Tofranil, generics	50–250 mg daily (H): Use with caution			$

(cont'd)

Table 2: Drugs Used in Bulimia Nervosa (cont'd)

Drug	Dosage	Adverse Effects	Drug Interactions	Cost*
trazodone Desyrel, generics	100–500 mg daily in single or divided doses (H): Use with caution	Sedation (common), anticholinergic adverse effects less common than with TCAs.	Avoid use with MAOIs.	$–$$$
phenelzine Nardil	15–75 mg daily in divided doses (H): ↓ dose	Orthostatic hypotension, common and sometimes severe, usually subsides by the fourth week of treatment. Hypertension is uncommon with usual doses and in the absence of drug–food interactions. Drowsiness, dizziness (common).	Avoid use with amphetamines, clomipramine, imipramine, levodopa, meperidine, sumatriptan, sympathomimetics, L-tryptophan.	$–$$

● *Dosage adjustment may be required in renal impairment – see Appendix I.*
(H) *Dosage adjustment in hepatic impairment.*
Abbreviations: TCAs = tricyclic antidepressants; MAOIs = monoamine oxidase inhibitors; AC = before meals.

* *Cost of 30-day supply – includes drug cost only.*
Legend: $ < $25 $$ $25–50 $$$ $50–75 $$$$ $75–100

one of these agents. Therapy should be maintained for at least 6 months; the usual recommendation is 1 year.

If symptoms persist after a trial of counseling and fluoxetine, treatment by a multidisciplinary team may be necessary.

Therapeutic Tips

- Antidepressants should be continued for 6 to 12 months if effective. If treatment with one antidepressant fails, another can be tried.

- Cotreatment with more than one antidepressant has no proven advantage and has the potential to increase adverse effects and cost.

- Often during psychological treatment or with significant life stress, a temporary worsening of binge and purge behavior occurs. This does not indicate a worsening in the patient's overall condition.

- Treatment of psychiatric comorbidity is necessary for long-term cure.

Suggested Reading List

Birmingham CL, Goldner EM, Bakan R. Controlled trial of zinc supplementation in anorexia nervosa. *Int J Eat Disord* 1994;3:251–255.

Birmingham CL, Alothman AF, Goldner EM. Anorexia nervosa: Refeeding and hypophosphatemia. *Int J Eat Disord* 1996;20(2):211–213.

Goldner EM, Birmingham CL. Anorexia nervosa: methods of treatment. In: Mott LA, Lumsden DB, eds. *Understanding eating disorders*. Washington: Taylor and Francis International Publishers, 1994:135–158.

Goldner EM, Birmingham CL, Smye V. Addressing treatment refusal in anorexia nervosa: Clinical, ethical and legal considerations. In: Garner, Garfinkel, eds. *Handbook of treatment for eating disorders*. New York: Guilford Publications, 1997:450–461.

Kim-Sing A, Birmingham CL. Clinical use of magnesium supplementation. *Can J Hosp Pharm* 1990;43(4):161–195.

Leung M, Birmingham CL. The management of anorexia nervosa and bulimia nervosa. *Pharmacy Practice* 1997;13:62–72.

CHAPTER 7

Insomnia

Jonathan A.E. Fleming, MB, FRCPC

Goals of Therapy

- To promote sound and restorative sleep when external (e.g., stress, noise, jet lag) or internal (e.g., pain, anxiety) factors disrupt natural sleep
- To reduce significant daytime impairment (dysphoria, fatigue, decreased alertness, etc.) associated with sleep loss
- To potentiate the effectiveness of behavioral interventions in managing patients with primary, chronic insomnia

Insomnia is a common symptom in a number of psychiatric, medical and sleep disorders. First determine if the complaint is primary (e.g., chronic psychophysiological insomnia), the focus of this chapter, or secondary (e.g., insomnia associated with a mood disorder or chronic pain). Secondary insomnia usually responds to treatment of the underlying disorder (e.g., a nocturnal dose of a sedating antidepressant).[1]

Investigations

- A complete sleep history (Table 1) is **essential**:
  - to quantify current sleep performance and daytime impairment (to measure the effects of any intervention)
  - to rule out other sleep pathologies including those where hypnotics are contraindicated and potentially lethal (e.g., obstructive sleep apnea)
- Psychiatric work-up to rule out associated mental disorders (especially mood and anxiety disorders, drug and alcohol use)
- Medical work-up to rule out associated medical disorders (especially those associated with nocturnal discomfort or pain)
- Medication and drug history (including caffeine, nicotine, alcohol and recreational drug use)
- Self-rating scales for depression and anxiety symptoms (e.g., Zung Depression Scale) are useful screening tools for evaluating the presence of depressive or anxiety disorders causing insomnia

---

[1] *For more information on secondary insomnia, refer to Principles and Practice of Sleep Medicine. 2nd ed. Toronto, W.B. Saunders, 1994.*

Figure 1: **Management of Primary Insomnia**

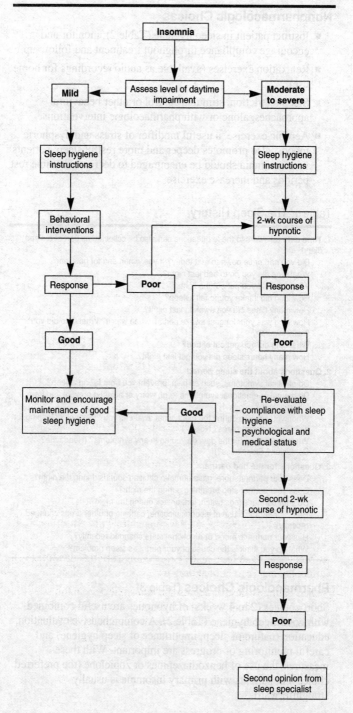

Therapeutic Choices (Figure 1)

Nonpharmacologic Choices

- Instruct patient in sleep hygiene (Table 2); monitor and encourage compliance throughout treatment and follow-up.
- Relaxation exercises (available as audio recordings for home use).
- Sleep restriction, stimulus control or other behavioral approaches, alone or with pharmacologic interventions.
- Aerobic exercise, a useful modifier of stress and dysphoric moods, also promotes deeper and more restful sleep; patients with insomnia should be encouraged to decrease daytime rest periods and increase exercise.

Table 1: The Sleep History

1. Time data (answers to these questions can also be collected as part of a sleep diary)

Did you nap or lie down to rest today? If yes, when and for how long?
What time did you go to bed last night?
What time did you put out the lights?
How long did it take you to fall asleep?
How many times did you awaken last night?
How long was your longest awake period; when was it? What time did you finally awaken?
What time did you get out of bed?
How many hours sleep did you get last night?

2. Questions about the sleep period

Do physical symptoms, such as pain, prevent you from falling asleep?
Do mental or emotional symptoms (e.g., worry or anxiety) prevent you from falling asleep?
When you awaken during the night, what awakens you? (Snoring? Gasping for air? Dreams/nightmares? Noise?)
When you get up for the day, do you have any symptoms? (Headache? Confusion? Sleepiness?)

3. Questions for the bed partner

Does your partner snore, gasp or make choking sounds during the night?
Does your partner stop breathing during the night?
Do your partner's legs twitch, jerk or kick during the night?
Has your partner's use of alcohol, nicotine, caffeine or other drugs changed recently?
Has your partner's mood or emotional state changed recently?
What do you think is the cause of your partner's sleep problem?

Pharmacologic Choices (Table 3)

Short courses (2 to 4 weeks) of hypnotics are useful combined with good sleep hygiene (Table 2). A comprehensive evaluation, education (nature of sleep, importance of sleep hygiene) and careful monitoring of progress are important. With these measures, the use of benzodiazepines or zopiclone (the preferred choices) in patients with primary insomnia is usually straightforward.

Table 2: **Sleep Hygiene Guidelines**

1. Keep a regular sleep–wake schedule, 7 days per week.
2. Restrict the sleep period to the average sleep time you have obtained each night over the preceding week.
3. Avoid lying in, extensive periods of horizontal rest or daytime napping; these activities usually affect the subsequent night's sleep.
4. Get regular exercise every day: about 40 minutes of an activity with sufficient intensity to cause sweating. If evening exercise prevents sleep, schedule the exercise earlier in the day.
5. Avoid caffeine, nicotine, alcohol and other recreational drugs, all of which disturb sleep. If you must smoke do not do so after 7:00 p.m.
6. Plan a quiet period before lights out; a warm bath may be helpful.
7. Avoid large meals late in the evening; a light carbohydrate snack (e.g., crackers and warm milk) before bedtime can be helpful.
8. Turn the clock face away and always use the alarm. Looking at the clock time on awakening can cause emotional arousal (performance anxiety or anger) that prevents return to sleep.
9. As much as possible, keep the bedroom dark and soundproofed. If you live in a noisy area, consider ear plugs.
10. Use the bedroom only for sleep and intimacy; using the bed as a reading place, office or media center conditions you to be alert in a place that should be associated with quiet and sleep. If you awaken during the night and are wide awake, get up, leave the bedroom and do something quiet until you feel drowsy-tired, then return to bed.

NB: Pharmacologic (or any) interventions will be less effective if these guidelines are not followed. In mild cases of insomnia, sleep hygiene guidelines, practised consistently and together, may be sufficient to reinstate a normal sleep pattern.

Benzodiazepines (BDZs)

All BDZs have sedative properties that allow their use as hypnotics, but they differ significantly in potency and pharmaco-kinetics. All may cause confusion and ataxia, especially in the elderly and in medically ill people. For pharmacodynamic and pharmacokinetic reasons, as well as the greater research and clinical experience with BDZ hypnotics in sleep-disturbed populations, they are preferred over BDZ anxiolytics. When insomnia is secondary to prominent anxiety symptoms, a long-acting BDZ given at night may promote sleep and manage daytime anxiety symptoms. It is inappropriate to use an anxiolytic BDZ during the day to manage anxiety and a hypnotic BDZ at night.

Temazepam is a good all-purpose hypnotic with a half-life sufficient to cover the whole sleep period without causing hangover effects. It has fewer rebound effects than more potent BDZs such as lorazepam.

Confidence in **triazolam**, once the most frequently used hypnotic in Canada, has been undermined by successive reductions in the recommended dose and widespread reports of rare but disturbing behavioral effects. Its pharmacokinetics make it more suitable for managing initial (first third of the night) rather than maintenance (last third of the night) insomnia. Short treatment courses (≤ 7 days) are recommended.

Although the number of comparative studies is relatively small, **oxazepam** is as effective as the hypnotic BDZs. Because of its slow absorption, it should be given 60 to 90 minutes before retiring. There are fewer studies (compared to other BDZ hypnotics) studying the effects of **lorazepam** on insomnia. As with other high-potency, short-acting BDZs, lorazepam may cause worse rebound effects on discontinuation than lower potency BDZs.

Estazolam offers no advantages over other benzodiazepines and is more costly.

Long-acting Benzodiazepines

Currently, **flurazepam** and **nitrazepam** are longer-acting BDZs marketed as hypnotics. Due to their long half-lives, they accumulate with repeated dosing and produce more hangover effects than short-acting BDZs. In the elderly, they cause higher cortical impairment resulting in confusion and falls. Their use, particularly in the elderly, is not recommended.

Zopiclone

Although not a BDZ, this drug acts at the BDZ receptor and so has similar therapeutic and side effects. However, higher cortical effects and significant interaction with low doses of alcohol are absent. Tolerance to the hypnotic effect may be delayed, and rebound insomnia may be reduced compared to BDZs. Zopiclone is preferred in those who must avoid cognitive and amnesic effects. The most common side effect is a bitter/metallic taste of the active drug secreted in saliva.

Chloral Hydrate

The toxicity and drug interaction profile of this drug make it less safe than BDZs. Tolerance to its hypnotic effect typically develops within 2 weeks. Its use is not recommended.

Barbiturates

The barbiturates are contraindicated in the management of insomnia due to their unacceptable safety profile.

L-Tryptophan

The Canadian supply of L-tryptophan has not been associated with the development of the eosinophilia–myalgia syndrome (a potentially lethal disorder) that has been described in the US. In high dosages (> 1 g), L-tryptophan has a hypnotic effect, but it is not as predictable as that seen with traditional hypnotics. It may be useful when one wishes to avoid BDZs.

Table 3: Drugs Used to Manage Primary Insomnia

Drug	Night-time Dose	Comments	Cost*
temazepam Restoril, generics	Starting 15 mg Maximum 30 mg	Good all-purpose hypnotic, but more expensive than other hypnotics. Does not accumulate.	$
triazolam Halcion, generics	Starting 0.125 mg Maximum 0.25 mg	Anterograde amnesia (especially with higher dosages, concurrent use of alcohol) and other potency and dose-related side effects (rebound insomnia, daytime anxiety) have limited its use. Useful for initiating sleep. Absence of hangover effects (does not affect daytime alertness) is a major advantage.	$
oxazepam Serax, generics	Starting 15 mg Maximum 30 mg	Slowly absorbed — onset of action is delayed; should be taken 60–90 min before retiring. No hangover effects.	$
lorazepam Ativan, generics	Starting 0.5 mg Maximum 1 mg	No hangover effects. May cause more rebound insomnia on withdrawal than temazepam or oxazepam. May cause amnesia with higher dosages.	$
zopiclone Imovane, generics	Starting 3.75 mg (geriatric) Usual adult 7.5 mg Maximum 7.5 mg	Does not accumulate. Free of cognitive effects; major adverse effect is bitter/metallic taste. May cause less rebound on withdrawal. Minimal additive effects with low doses of alcohol.	$$
L-tryptophan Tryptan, generics	1–3 g 20 min before bedtime	Alternative to benzodiazepines. May cause the serotonin syndrome (shivering, diaphoresis, hypomanic behavior and ataxia) alone or when combined with other medications, especially MAO inhibitors and serotonin reuptake inhibitors. Erratic response.	$$$$

* Cost of 14-day supply – includes drug cost only.
Legend: $ < $2 $$ $2–5 $$$ $5–10 $$$$ > $10

Melatonin

Melatonin is no longer available in health food stores in Canada but remains available in the United States. The use of pharmaceutical grade melatonin (1 to 5 mg) in primary insomnia remains controversial. It may be effective in a slow release format for the maintenance insomnia of middle and old age, but more studies are required. Patients should be discouraged from importing and using melatonin from the United States as its quality is uncontrolled.

Therapeutic Tips

- Sedative–hypnotics should always be started at the lowest dose and used for the shortest possible time. If after 2 courses of hypnotic therapy the patient continues to experience disrupted sleep and daytime impairment, the clinician should confirm compliance with sleep hygiene measures, carefully re-evaluate the patient's psychiatric and medical status and consider referral to a sleep specialist.
- Set realistic treatment goals with the patient, mainly to minimize daytime impairment; a chronic poor sleeper will not be turned into a good sleeper overnight.
- The degree of daytime impairment directs the intervention: if there is an acute change in daytime functioning, a short course of hypnotics may be indicated; if the daytime impairment is mild or chronic, a behavioral intervention (e.g., sleep restriction) should be tried first.
- Sleep diaries (Table 1) are often helpful in delineating the initial complaint, monitoring progress and facilitating withdrawal.
- It is inappropriate to use the sedative side effect of another medication (e.g., antihistamines, antidepressants) to avoid using a BDZ when the latter is the treatment of choice.
- Warn about combined effects when hypnotics are used with other CNS depressants (e.g., alcohol).
- If a short course of a hypnotic has been used, plan to withdraw it at a low-stress time (e.g., a weekend). Two nights before the planned withdrawal, the patient should shorten the sleep time (while staying on the medication) by 20 minutes. This modest degree of sleep deprivation will promote physiological sleepiness, which should counterbalance any sleep disruption associated with withdrawal. This shortened sleep period should be maintained for 1 week.

- Remain vigilant for the emergence of a mood disorder (which should always be treated with antidepressants rather than hypnotics alone) as protracted insomnia may be the prodrome of an affective illness. Furthermore, one year of continued sleep disturbance increases the risk of a mood disorder in the subsequent year.

Suggested Reading List

Gillin JC, Byerley WF. The diagnosis and management of insomnia. *N Engl J Med* 1990;322:239–248.

Kryger MH, Roth T, Dement WC. *Principles and practice of sleep medicine.* 2nd ed. Toronto: W.B. Saunders, 1994.

Kupfer DJ, Reynolds CF. Management of insomnia. *N Engl J Med* 1997;336:341–346.

Spielman AJ, Caruso LS, Glovinsky PB. A behavioral perspective on insomnia treatment. *Psychiatr Clin North Am* 1987;10:541–553.

Wooten V. Sleep disorders in geriatric patients. *Clin Geriatr Med* 1992;8:427–439.

CHAPTER 8

Psychoses

Jane Garland, MD, FRCPC

Goals of Therapy

- To control specific psychotic symptoms: hallucinations, delusions, disordered thinking
- To reduce agitation in acute psychosis
- To prevent relapse of chronic schizophrenic illness

Investigations

- Thorough history including longitudinal history of psychotic symptoms, drug abuse, drug sensitivities, medical conditions, mood symptoms, response to antipsychotics, including adverse effects
- Specific diagnosis:
  - differentiate acute delirium, organic psychotic disorder or mania from chronic schizophrenia or schizoaffective disorder
  - rule out drug withdrawal delirium and drug intoxication (hallucinogens, amphetamines, cocaine, anticholinergics)
- Physical examination:
  - to determine medical conditions that could produce or exacerbate an acute psychotic picture
  - to detect conditions such as parkinsonism and postural hypotension that may be exacerbated by antipsychotics
- Laboratory tests: baseline CBC and liver function tests; ECG in patients over 40

Therapeutic Choices (Figures 1 and 2)

Nonpharmacologic Choices

- Environmental stressors and stimulation should be reduced.
- Family and caregivers should be educated regarding symptoms and treatment.
- Adequate hydration, nutrition and safety should be ensured.
- Alcohol, psychoactive substances should be avoided.
- As patient improves, educational approaches to coping strategies, vocation and regularity of lifestyle should be introduced.
- Frequent, brief contacts with physician and other health care providers give support, increase compliance and enable early detection of psychotic relapse.

Figure 1: **Management of Acute Psychotic Symptoms**

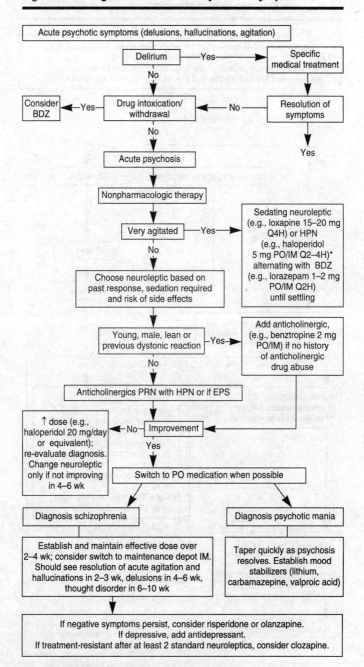

*Abbreviations: BDZ = benzodiazepine, HPN = high potency neuroleptic,
EPS = extrapyramidal symptoms.*
*In the frail, elderly patient, haloperidol 1 mg or equivalent should be used.

Figure 2: **Maintenance Treatment for Subacute Psychosis or Chronic Schizophrenia**

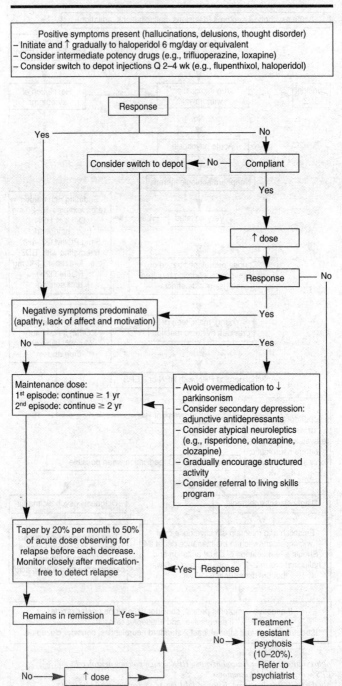

Pharmacologic Choices (Table 1)
Antipsychotics
Indications for Antipsychotics
Antipsychotics are indicated for:
- acute exacerbation of chronic schizophrenia
- acute psychotic symptoms in bipolar disorder and depression
- acute agitation and psychosis in delirium
- maintenance treatment of chronic schizophrenia

Choice of Drug

All traditional antipsychotics are of equal efficacy in controlling psychotic symptoms but vary in potency, receptor specificity, side effects and cost. Individual patients may respond more effectively to a particular medication. Choice of drug should be based on history of response, requirement for sedation, risk of motor side effects and side effect profile. Compliance is most important in determining practical effectiveness; patient acceptance of side effects, dosage schedule, convenience and cost should be considered. Informed consent, regarding tardive dyskinesia (TD), must be documented as soon as the patient is rendered competent.

Typical Antipsychotics

Typical antipsychotics (e.g., chlorpromazine, thioridazine, haloperidol) are thought to produce their primary therapeutic effect and extrapyramidal side effects by blocking dopamine receptors. They also block other receptors (serotonergic, cholinergic, adrenergic and histaminic) to varying degrees, producing sedation, and autonomic and cardiovascular side effects, especially orthostatic hypotension and tachycardia.

"Positive symptoms" of schizophrenia (i.e., hallucinations, delusions, thought disorders, paranoia) are more responsive to typical neuroleptics than the negative symptoms (i.e., amotivational state, apathy, poor self-care, social withdrawal, poverty of speech).

Atypical Antipsychotics

Clozapine, olanzapine and risperidone selectively block dopamine and serotonin receptors. Clozapine is effective in treatment-resistant psychosis. All improve negative symptoms, have fewer extrapyramidal side effects and a lower long-term risk of TD than typical agents. Due to its high risk of agranulocytosis (1 to 2%) and seizures (5%), high cost and the requirement for weekly WBC monitoring, clozapine is reserved for treatment-resistant patients. Some experts recommend risperidone or

Table 1: Drugs Used in Psychosis

Drug	CPZ Equivalence*	Potency†	Notable Adverse Effects	Drug Interactions	Comments	Cost‡
Typical Antipsychotics						
chlorpromazine Largactil, generics	100 mg	Low	Sedation, autonomic and cardiovascular effects, especially orthostatic	Serum level of anti-psychotics may be ↑ by TCAs.	Whenever possible, neuro-leptic dosage should be reduced, or a lower potency drug should be considered to reduce EPS.	$
thioridazine Mellaril, generics	90–100 mg	Low	hypotension, tachycardia (↑ with LPN). Tardive dyskinesia. Seizures (1%).	Serum level of anti-psychotics ↓ by carbamazepine (↑ liver metabolism), antacids (↓ absorption).		$
methotrimeprazine Nozinan, generics	75 mg	Low			CPZ and methotrimeprazine are useful if sedative effect desirable.	$
loxapine Loxapac	10–15 mg	Intermediate	Orthostatic hypotension notable with chlorpromazine.			$$–$$$
perphenazine Trilafon, generics	10 mg	Intermediate	Retinal damage with thioridazine > 800 mg/d.	Cardiac effects: pheno-thiazines, pimozide prolong QT interval; interaction with other	Haloperidol has high potency and low cardiac toxicity; is available PO/IM/depot/IV form.	$
trifluoperazine Stelazine, generics	3–5 mg	High	EPS, including parkinsonism, akinesia, akathisia (↑ with HPN).	drugs (e.g., astemizole, terfenadine, antiarrhyth-mics) may promote this.	Pimozide is effective in delusional disorder, tics.	$
fluphenazine HCl π Moditen HCl, generics	2 mg	High			Loxapine is useful if sedation required and in elderly. Has low cardiac toxicity.	$
haloperidol π Haldol, generics	2 mg	High	Cardiac conduction effects with pimozide > 8 mg.	Effects of levodopa may be inhibited.		$
pimozide Orap	1 mg	High				$
flupenthixol π Fluanxol	1 mg	High				$

Atypical Antipsychotics

clozapine Clozaril	50 mg	Low	Agranulocytosis (1–2%). Seizures (5%). Excessive salivation. Weight gain.	Fluvoxamine and erythromycin ↑ clozapine levels. BDZs: ↑ respiratory depression.	Useful in treatment-resistant patients and for negative symptoms. Has very low EPS. Prescribed only by psychiatrist.	\$\$\$\$\$
olanzapine Zyprexa	3 mg	Intermediate	Dizziness. Sedation. Weight gain.		Very low EPS	\$\$\$\$
risperidone Risperdal	1.5 mg	High	Hyperprolactinemia, pronounced hypotension, weight gain, restlessness.		Has low EPS.	\$\$\$

*CPZ equivalence is the equipotent dosage of any antipsychotic compared to 100 mg of chlorpromazine.

† Potency refers to the affinity for dopamine D_2 receptors. High-potency neuroleptics (HPN) are more likely to cause neuromuscular effects (e.g., EPS); low-potency neuroleptics (LPN) are more likely to cause non-neuromuscular effects.

π Depot form available. See Table 2.

‡ Cost of 30-day supply of 300 mg/d CPZ equivalence – includes drug cost only.
Legend: $ < \$50$ \$\$ \$50–100   \$\$\$ \$100–150   \$\$\$\$ \$150–200
         \$\$\$\$\$ \$200–250   \$\$\$\$\$\$ > \$250

olanzapine as first-line treatment in schizophrenia, weighing costs against the favorable side effect profile and impact on negative symptoms.[1,2]

Dosing

Adequate doses should be used to control hallucinations and to reduce delusional thinking gradually over a period of weeks; doses exceeding 600 mg chlorpromazine (CPZ) or equivalent, or 15 mg of haloperidol per day, are associated with poorer patient acceptance and overall function. If there is no response after 4 weeks at a dose of at least 400 mg CPZ or equivalent per day, the dose should be increased to 600 mg per day. If no response after an additional 2 weeks (a total of 6 weeks), another neuroleptic should be tried. For treatment-resistant psychosis, refer to a psychiatrist.

Once therapy is stabilized the regimen should be simplified to once daily dosing, or depot agents should be used to maximize compliance (Table 2).

Maintenance Treatment

Continuous treatment reduces relapse rate in chronic schizo-phrenia from 70 to 20% in a year. The lowest effective daily dose (about 300 mg CPZ or equivalent) of oral or depot medication should be used to prevent relapse. Following a single psychotic episode, after a year of symptom remission, systematic tapering by 20% per month until 50% of the acute dose is reached, may be considered. With repeated episodes, tapering should be attempted after at least 2 months during which residual symptoms have returned to baseline. At the first sign of relapsing symptoms, the patient should be immediately restabilized on higher dose. Patients should be monitored closely for early prodromal symptoms and signs of relapse.

Special Considerations

In the **elderly** lower doses should be used. Loxapine should be considered due to lower cardiac toxicity.

In **pregnancy** no teratogenic effects have been documented, but the risk/benefit of the neuroleptics should be considered, and the drugs should be avoided in the first trimester.

In **neonates** hypertonia has been noted following prepartum antipsychotics.

In **children** most long-term experience has been with thioridazine in psychosis, but pimozide and haloperidol are well tolerated in tic disorders.

---

[1] *Can J Psychiatry 1993;38:S70–S74.*
[2] *J Clin Psychiatry 1996;57(suppl 11):68–71.*

Table 2: **Depot Neuroleptics**

Drug	Usual Dose IM*	Frequency	Cost†
fluphenazine decanoate Modecate	12.5–37.5 mg	Q3 wk	$
haloperidol decanoate Haldol LA	100–200 mg	Q4 wk	$–$$
flupenthixol Fluanxol	20–40 mg	Q2 wk	$–$$
fluspirilene Imap (depot only)	2–10 mg	Weekly	$–$$$
pipotiazine (Piportil)	150–300 mg	Q4 wk	$$$–$$$$$

* A small dose (10% of usual daily dose) should be given to test for allergies.
† Cost of 4-week supply – includes drug cost only.
Legend: $ < $25 $$ $25–50 $$$ $50–75 $$$$ $75–100 $$$$$ $100–125

Side Effects

Tardive dyskinesia (TD) occurs after chronic exposure to dopamine-blocking agents and is characterized by involuntary movements of mouth, face, trunk or extremities. The incidence increases with total neuroleptic exposure; it is about 5% per year of neuroleptic exposure and 20 to 25% in chronically treated schizophrenic patients. The rates are higher with intermittent therapy, drug holidays or affective disorders. The risk is higher in the elderly and females and in the presence of neurological disorders.

TD may be masked by neuroleptics and may emerge with dose reduction or withdrawal. Withdrawal-emergent TD often improves significantly with time.

Treatment is generally unsatisfactory but can include continued suppression with neuroleptics, benzodiazepines, adrenergic agents such as propranolol and clonidine, and experimental use of buspirone. Use of atypical neuroleptics such as clozapine, olanzapine and risperidone may reduce risk. Consider switching to an atypical neuroleptic if TD arises.[3]

Neuroleptic malignant syndrome, a serious side effect of neuroleptic therapy, occurs with an incidence of 1 to 4%. It is characterized by muscle rigidity, fever, autonomic instability, labile blood pressure, clouded consciousness, elevated WBC and elevated creatine kinase. Risk factors include use of high-potency neuroleptics and dehydration. Treatment is primarily supportive (hydration and cooling) but may include amantadine, dantrolene sodium or bromocriptine.

[3] *J Clin Psychiatry 1996;57(suppl 12B):51–58.*

Other serious side effects include **cardiac conduction distur-bances**, which occur with all antipsychotics in higher doses (e.g., pimozide in doses over 8 mg/day). **Seizures** occur at a rate of 1% with all neuroleptics. **Liver damage** may occur with phenothiazine derivatives. **NB:** Neuroleptic-induced hyper-prolactinemia stimulates growth of breast cancer in animals.

Laboratory Monitoring

Laboratory investigations are indicated when adverse effects are suspected and may include liver enzymes, bilirubin and CBC. Clozapine requires continuous weekly monitoring of WBC. (A low incidence of agranulocytosis occurs with phenothiazine derivatives.)

Because there is no consistent relationship between plasma levels and clinical response, monitoring of plasma levels is reserved for nonresponsive patients and for identification of drug interactions that may raise neuroleptic levels excessively.

Adjunctive Medications (Table 3)

Antiparkinson agents are used with high-potency neuroleptics, either prophylactically or PRN to control extrapyramidal motor effects, especially in patients at high risk (young, male, previous history).

Benzodiazepines are used in acute psychosis for sedation and to achieve a reduction in required neuroleptic dose. They may be helpful in controlling akathisia (intense restlessness with resultant pacing and agitation) and reducing incidence of acute dystonias during initiation of emergency antipsychotic treatment.

Propranolol or **amantadine** have some efficacy in akathisia. Antidepressants such as **imipramine** or **fluoxetine** may be considered for secondary depression.

Therapeutic Tips

- A higher dose of antipsychotic agent does not speed resolution of acute psychosis.
- Compliance is key to successful resolution of psychosis and prevention of relapse.
- Successful relapse prevention requires combined psychoeducation and pharmacotherapy.
- It is important to distinguish negative symptoms of schizo-phrenia from extrapyramidal side effects of medication (e.g., akinesia) and secondary depression.
- Adjunctive mood stabilizers should be considered for bipolar or schizoaffective symptoms.
- Informed consent, regarding risks and benefits, must be documented once the patient's mental state renders him/her competent to provide it.

Table 3: **Adjunctive Medications Used in Psychosis**

Drug	Dose (Titrate PRN)	Comments	Cost*
Drugs for Management of Parkinsonism			
benztropine Cogentin, generics	1–2 mg TID PO/IM	IM benztropine or diphenhydramine can be used for acute dystonia. PO benztropine or procyclidine for tremor and rigidity.	$[†]
procyclidine Kemadrin, generics	2.5–5 mg TID PO		$
trihexyphenidyl Artane, generics	2–5 mg TID PO		$
diphenhydramine Benadryl, generics	25–50 mg QID PO/IM	Side effects include dry mouth, blurred vision, constipation, confusion. Toxic in overdose. Amantadine may be helpful for akathisia.	$-$$[†]
amantadine 🐝 Symmetrel, generics	100 mg up to BID		$$
Drugs for Management of Akathisia			
propranolol Inderal, generics	10–40 mg/d	Monitor for hypotension. Contraindicated in asthma. Caution in diabetes.	$
Benzodiazepines			
lorazepam Ativan, generics	0.5–2 mg Q4H PO/IM	Side effects include excessive sedation, impaired memory and poor concentration.	$[†]
clonazepam Rivotril, generics	0.25–2 mg Q6–8H PO		$-$$
alprazolam Xanax, generics	0.25–1 mg Q4H PO		$-$$

🐝 *Dosage adjustment may be required in renal impairment – see Appendix I.*
[†] *Cost for oral tablets; IM formulations may be higher.*
* *Cost of 30-day supply – includes drug cost only.*
Legend: $ < $20 $$ $20–40

Suggested Reading List

Anon. Expert consensus treatment guidelines for schizophrenia. *J Clin Psychiatry* 1996;57(suppl 12B):51–58.

Burnett PL, Galletly CA, Moyle RJ, et al. Low dose depot medication in schizophrenia. *Schizophrenia Bull* 1993;19:155–164, 270.

Cohen S, Kahn A. Adjunctive benzodiazepines in acute schizophrenia. *Neuropsychobiology* 1987;18:9–12.

Jeffries JJ. Ethical issues in drug selection for schizophrenia. *Can J Psychiatry* 1993;38(suppl):S70–S74.

Kane JM. Newer antipsychotic drugs. *Drugs* 1993;46:585–593.

Kane JM, Marder SR. Psychopharmacological treatment of schizophrenia. *Schizophrenia Bull* 1993;19:287–302.

CHAPTER 9

Drug Withdrawal Syndromes

Claudio A. Naranjo, MD

Alcohol, cocaine, opioid and benzodiazepine withdrawal are discussed in this chapter.

Definition

- The development of a substance-specific syndrome due to the cessation of (or reduction in) substance use that has been heavy and prolonged
- The substance-specific syndrome causes clinically significant distress or impairment in social, occupational or other important areas of functioning
- The symptoms are not due to a general medical condition and are not better accounted for by another mental disorder

Withdrawal symptoms develop within hours or days (depending on rate of drug elimination) after cessation or reduction in heavy or prolonged use of alcohol, amphetamines, cocaine, nicotine, opioids, and sedatives, hypnotics or anxiolytics.[1]

Goals of Therapy

- To relieve acute symptoms
- To prevent complications
- To smooth transition into a rehabilitation program
- To prevent relapse

Investigations

- Interview
- Specialized assessment instruments or scales (self-administered or interviewer-administered) [e.g., Clinical Institute Withdrawal Assessment for Alcohol (CIWA-Ar),[2] CIWA-Benzo[3]]
- Physical examination
- Laboratory tests for presence of all suspected psychoactive substances in urine, blood and/or breath
- Rule out organic complications (e.g., infection)

---

[1] *Diagnostic and Statistical Manual of Mental Disorders, 4th Ed, 1994.*
[2] *Br J Addict 1989;84:1353–57.*
[3] *J Clin Psychopharmacology 1989;9:412–416.*

Therapeutic Choices (Figure 1)

Nonpharmacologic Choices

- Monitoring signs and symptoms.
- Reassurance, supportive nursing care.
- Reality orientation.
- Psychosocial treatment program.

Pharmacologic Choices

- Treat specific symptoms of withdrawal and associated complications.
- Substitute abused drug with one of same or similar class (an agonist) that is not likely to be abused.
- Substitute abused drug with one which blocks its reinforcing effects (an antagonist).

Alcohol Withdrawal Syndrome (AWS)

Diagnostic Criteria (Table 1)

Assessment: The symptoms and severity of the AWS vary with the intensity and duration of the preceding alcohol exposure. Severity can be assessed with the CIWA-Ar. Symptoms of a mild reaction are tremor, insomnia and irritability lasting 48 hours or less. In a severe AWS, these are followed by hallucinations, seizures and delusions.

Management: Nonpharmacologic interventions are generally effective for mild AWS (CIWA-Ar score ≤ 20). Patients in moderate to severe withdrawal (CIWA-Ar score > 20) should receive medication (Table 2).

Long-term Rehabilitation: Following successful withdrawal from alcohol, the treatment goal may be abstinence or moderation (defined as drinking < 12 drinks per week, and ≤ 4 drinks per day for males or ≤ 3 drinks per day for females). Medications should be administered only within the context of a relapse prevention (cognitive-behavioral or psychosocial) program in intellectually intact individuals who are motivated (or required, as in judicial programs) to reduce their alcohol consumption. The alcohol-sensitizing drugs, **disulfiram** and **calcium carbimide**, inhibit hepatic aldehyde dehydrogenase, causing increased blood acetaldehyde levels after alcohol ingestion. The result is a very unpleasant episode of flushing, tachycardia, weakness and nausea. Despite several contraindications for use (e.g., pregnancy, liver disease), toxic effects, drug interactions, and little scientific evidence for their efficacy, these drugs may have a limited role when the treatment goal is abstinence.

Naltrexone, a long-acting opioid antagonist, is indicated for alcohol dependence. Although efficacy beyond 12 weeks of

Figure 1: **Management of Drug Withdrawal Syndromes**

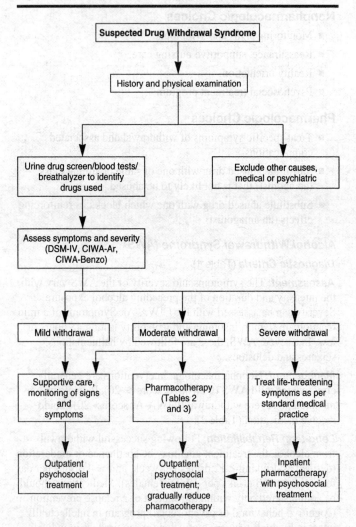

treatment has not been established, it may be advisable to administer it for at least 6 months due to the high risk of relapse within this time period.

Medications should be used within the context of psychosocial treatment.

Patients with comorbid depression or anxiety may benefit from **antidepressants** and **anxiolytics**, particularly if the alcohol dependence was secondary to depression or anxiety.

Generally, follow-up "booster" sessions are required after completion of a cognitive-behavioral or psychosocial relapse

Table 1: **Diagnostic Criteria for Substance-specific Withdrawal Syndromes**

Alcohol	Cocaine	Opioids	Benzodiazepines
• autonomic hyperactivity (e.g., sweating, pulse > 100 bpm)	• fatigue	• dysphoric mood	• autonomic hyperactivity (e.g., sweating, pulse > 100 bpm)
• increased hand tremor	• vivid, unpleasant dreams	• nausea/vomiting	• increased hand tremor
• insomnia	• insomnia or hypersomnia	• lacrimation, rhinorrhea	• insomnia
• nausea/vomiting	• increased appetite	• pupillary dilation, piloerection, sweating	• nausea/vomiting
• transient visual, tactile or auditory hallucinations	• psychomotor retardation or agitation	• diarrhea	• transient visual, tactile or auditory hallucinations
• psychomotor agitation	• craving for cocaine	• yawning	• psychomotor agitation
• anxiety		• fever	• anxiety
• grand mal seizures		• insomnia	• grand mal seizures (only after abrupt cessation of high doses)

Table 2: Pharmacologic Management of Alcohol Withdrawal

Symptom/Severity of Withdrawal	Drug	Dose and Route	Interval	Comments	Cost*
Neurological symptoms	Thiamine	25–50 mg IV	Daily for 3 days	To treat/prevent neurological complications, e.g., Wernicke's encephalopathy. Can administer PO after first dose.	$$
Mild to moderate	Lorazepam	2 mg SL	Q2H	Administer 3 doses, with supportive care.	$
Moderate to severe	Diazepam	20 mg PO	Q1–2H	The initial dose can be repeated every 1–2H until patient shows signs of improvement or mild sedation; median dose is usually 60 mg of diazepam or 300 mg of chlordiazepoxide.	$
	Chlordiazepoxide	100 mg PO			$
Extreme	Diazepam	2.5 mg/min IV	Slow infusion	Rarely needed; most patients respond to adequate dosing with oral diazepam. In those rare cases when needed, should be administered until patient is calm (subsequent dosages must be individualized on the basis of the clinical picture).	$$
Hallucinations	Haloperidol	0.5–5.0 mg IM	Q2H	Until controlled or to a maximum of 5 doses; appropriate doses of diazepam should be used concurrently.	$$

Seizure					
History of seizure disorder or previous withdrawal seizures	Phenytoin	Maintenance: 100 mg PO, Loading dose: 200–300 mg PO	Q8H	Phenytoin detected in blood, maintenance dose: 100 mg; not detected in blood: loading dose: 100 mg, maintenance dose: 100 mg.	$
Repeated seizures requiring acute therapy	Phenytoin	Loading dose: 1 g IV	Infuse at 50 mg/min	Loading dose is 10 mg/kg. Do not dilute in saline or dextrose solution.	$$$$
	Phenytoin	Maintenance: 100 mg PO	Q8H		$
Status epilepticus	Diazepam	5 mg/min IV	Infuse	Until seizures cease or 25–30 mg total has been given.	$$
Long-term reduction in alcohol intake	Naltrexone	50 mg/day	12–24 weeks	Use as part of a comprehensive treatment program. Should not be used in acute hepatitis or liver failure. Hepatotoxicity may occur with very high doses (> 300 mg/day)	$159 for 30 days

*Cost for a single administration – drug cost only.
Legend: $ < $1 $$ $1–10 $$$ $10–20 $$$$ $20–30

prevention program for the long-term maintenance of abstinence or moderation of alcohol use. Self-help groups, e.g., Alcoholics Anonymous (AA), are available in many communities.

Cocaine Withdrawal Syndrome

Diagnostic Criteria (Table 1)

Assessment: Symptoms of cocaine withdrawal are subjective, generally psychological and frequently subtle. Most will decrease steadily over several weeks. Craving for cocaine is the most long-lasting symptom, and can lead to cocaine-seeking behavior and subsequent relapse for up to 1 year after withdrawal.

Management: Medications should be used within the context of psychosocial treatment. Comorbidity, polydrug use (particularly heroin) may influence efficacy of treatment. Currently, there is no standard accepted pharmacologic treatment for cocaine withdrawal. Dopamine agonists (**bromocriptine**, **amantadine**) and tricyclic antidepressants (**desipramine**, **imipramine**) have been shown to reduce craving for cocaine and some symptoms of withdrawal (Table 3).

Long-term Rehabilitation: Psychosocial treatment is the usual initial therapeutic choice. Intensive ($\geq$ 2 times/week) outpatient abstinence-oriented cognitive behavioral treatment is better than once-weekly, as effective as inpatient and probably better than psychotherapy. Legal, financial or medical problems (e.g., HIV infection, pregnancy) must be addressed if present. Adjunctive pharmacotherapy is indicated for patients who do not respond to an adequate trial of psychosocial treatment. No medication has been shown to be consistently efficacious in the long-term maintenance of cocaine abstinence. **Desipramine** may relieve comorbid or subsequent depression and **bromocriptine** has been shown to relieve craving in some studies. **Buprenorphine**, a mixed opioid agonist–antagonist, is under investigation in methadone-maintained cocaine-dependent patients following positive results in preliminary studies.

Opioid Withdrawal Syndrome

Diagnostic Criteria (Table 1)

Assessment: The symptoms of opioid withdrawal are not life-threatening and generally last about 2 weeks if the craving for the abused drug can be overcome.

Management: The best way to avoid craving and subsequent relapse is to make the abused drug completely unavailable. Many opioid abusers can undergo withdrawal in a supportive environment without medications. However, there are effective pharmacologic strategies to reduce the acute symptoms of opioid withdrawal and facilitate long-term abstinence (Table 3). The treatment of choice has been oral administration of **methadone**, a long-acting pure opioid agonist. Many patients begin to experience renewed, but milder, withdrawal symptoms when the dose of methadone drops to below 20 or 30 mg/day. **Clonidine**, a nonopioid antihypertensive medication, can assist in methadone substitution by suppressing nausea, vomiting, cramps and sweating. However, it does little for the muscle aches, insomnia and drug craving symptoms of withdrawal, and its hypotensive effect makes it more suitable for inpatient use, where blood pressure can be monitored.

Buprenorphine is an alternative to methadone but is not available in Canada.

Another protocol involves sequential treatment with **clonidine** and **naltrexone** (an opioid antagonist). Pretreatment with clonidine prevents naltrexone-precipitated withdrawal while the administration of naltrexone ensures a smooth transition into long-term opioid antagonist treatment (see below).

Long-term Rehabilitation: Oral administration of **methadone** for up to 180 days, with gradual decreases of the dose from 60 mg/day to discontinuation, is the current treatment of choice. Patient retention in treatment is high, illicit drug use and needle use are low, and there is time for the patient to achieve improved medical status and psychosocial functioning. Buprenorphine appears to be as effective as methadone in relapse prevention.

Naltrexone, an opioid antagonist, acts by blocking the psychological and physiological effects of the abused opioid such that no euphoric effects will be experienced if the drug is used. Therefore, drug use is unlikely to occur again. An opioid-free interval of 5 to 10 days or pretreatment with clonidine (see above) is necessary to avoid precipitated withdrawal. Naltrexone has a long duration of action, allowing infrequent dosing. It does not prevent drug craving, but is well accepted by motivated patients of higher socioeconomic status.

The nonpharmacologic components of treatment may be continued long-term. Self-help groups, e.g., Narcotics Anonymous (NA), are available in many communities.

Benzodiazepine (BDZ) Withdrawal Syndrome

Diagnostic Criteria (Table 1)

Assessment: A withdrawal syndrome is more likely with higher doses, use more than 1 year, and with short to intermediate half-life BDZs (e.g., lorazepam). The diagnosis of a true withdrawal syndrome must be well established before initiating therapy. Withdrawal symptoms, which appear as behavioral and psychological changes opposite to those observed during acute dosing, must be distinguished from "recurrence" or "rebound" of anxiety, panic disorder or insomnia. Recurrence usually develops slowly after drug discontinuation and remains at a steady level

Table 3: Pharmacologic Management of Cocaine and/or Opioid Withdrawal

Drug	Administration	Comments	Cost*
Cocaine			
Dopamine agonists:			
bromocriptine	0.625–2.5 mg PO QID for 30 days	Reduced symptoms of withdrawal and craving.	$–$$
amantadine	100 mg PO TID for 30 days		$$
pergolide mesylate	.05–1.5 mg PO TID for 7 days†		$$–$$$$
desipramine	200–300 mg/d PO for 12 wks†	Improved depressive withdrawal symptoms in some studies.	$$
Opioids			
methadone	10 mg PO Q2–4H to stabilization (usually 10–40 mg), then taper by 5 mg/d	For acute withdrawal symptoms.	$
	60 mg/d PO for 180 days or longer	For long-term maintenance.	$
clonidine	0.5–1.5 mg/d PO for 8 days, then taper over 3 days	Suppresses nausea, vomiting, cramps, sweating.	$$
buprenorphine	4–8 mg/d sublingual for 4–12 wks	Abruptly discontinue.	‡
clonidine/naltrexone	Clonidine 1 mg/d PO on day 1, taper over 6 days; naltrexone 25 mg/d PO on day 1, increase to 100–150 mg/d over 6 days	Needs careful monitoring for hypotension and precipitated withdrawal. Leads into naltrexone relapse prevention.	$$$$/ $$$$$
Cocaine and Opioid Abusers			
buprenorphine	4–8 mg/d PO suppresses opioid withdrawal symptoms; 12–16 mg/d may be needed for cocaine withdrawal	Promising results treating cocaine withdrawal in methadone-maintained cocaine abusers; still under study.	‡

*Cost for 7 days' treatment — drug cost only.
Legend: $ <$5 $$ $5–25 $$$ $25–50 $$$$ $50–75 $$$$$ $75–100

† Duration of study, not necessarily the recommended clinical treatment regimen.
‡ Not available in Canada.

until drug therapy is reinitiated; rebound is more intense and of short duration; the withdrawal syndrome begins soon after drug discontinuation, particularly if the drug had a short half-life, but eventually resolves.

Management: The withdrawal syndrome usually resolves spontaneously and without complications, depending upon the dose and half-life of the drug and duration of use. Patients who have used a BDZ for > 12 weeks should have the dose gradually reduced and replaced by a medication with a long half-life and cross-tolerance to BDZs, e.g., diazepam or phenobarbital. Patients in withdrawal are usually administered a loading dose of approximately 50% of the reported daily dose of BDZ in diazepam equivalents (Table 4), which is reduced by 10 to 20% per day to discontinuation. Patients who were using low doses (< 60 mg diazepam equivalents) can usually be managed ambulatory. Patients who have used high doses of BDZ or are in acute withdrawal should be hospitalized to facilitate assessment and prevent complications such as seizures, particularly if there is a history of serious withdrawal reactions. After loading with **diazepam** 20 mg Q1H PO, a slower tapering schedule of 5 to 10% each day is recommended. Response to treatment can be monitored with sensitive instruments such as the CIWA-Benzo scale.

Long-term Rehabilitation: The few available data on relapse to BDZ use indicate that approximately 50% of patients remain abstinent after at least 1 year. However, some patients may replace the BDZ with other medications such as chloral hydrate, neuroleptics (e.g., chlorpromazine) or antidepressants (e.g., fluoxetine). The non-BDZ anxiolytic, **buspirone**, has less abuse and dependence potential and produces fewer withdrawal symptoms upon discontinuation than BDZs.

Table 4: **Dose Equivalents of Benzodiazepines**

Benzodiazepine	Elimination half-life	Dose equivalent (mg)
Alprazolam	Intermediate	0.25
Bromazepam	Intermediate	3.0
Chlordiazepoxide	Long	25.0
Clorazepate	Long	3.75
Diazepam	Long	5.0
Flurazepam	Long	15.0
Lorazepam	Intermediate	1.0
Nitrazepam	Long	5.0
Oxazepam	Intermediate	30.0
Temazepam	Intermediate	15.0
Triazolam	Short	0.25

Suggested Reading List

American Psychiatric Association. Practice guidelines for the treatment of patients with substance use disorders: alcohol, cocaine, opioids. *Am J Psychiatry* 1995; 152(11, supplement):1–59.

Ball JC, Ross A. *The effectiveness of methadone maintenance treatment. Patients, programs, services, and outcome.* New York: Springer-Verlag, 1991.

Naranjo CA, Bremner KE. Pharmacotherapy of substance use disorders. *Can J Clin Pharmacol* 1994;1(2):55–71.

Özdemir V, Bremner KE, Naranjo CA. Treatment of alcohol withdrawal syndrome. *Ann Med* 1993;26:101–105.

Sellers EM. Alcohol, barbiturate and benzodiazepine withdrawal syndromes: clinical management. *Can Med Assoc J* 1988;139:113–118.

CHAPTER 10

Chronic Spasticity and Muscle Cramps

John P. Hooge, MD, FRCPC

Chronic Spasticity

Chronic spasticity is the result of disorders of motor pathways in the brain (commonly stroke, head injury or cerebral palsy) or the spinal cord (commonly spinal cord injury or multiple sclerosis). It is one part of the upper motor neuron syndrome in which the patient is disabled by a complex combination of positive and negative symptoms. It can be harmful (reducing functional use of limbs, causing painful spasms and leading to contractures) or helpful (the patient with weakness or paralyzed legs may rely on spasticity of extensor muscles to transfer or stand).

Goals of Therapy

- To improve active function or passive movement of limbs
- To improve comfort
- To reduce extensor or flexor spasms
- To prevent contractures

Therapeutic Choices (Figure 1)

Nonpharmacologic Choices

Rehabilitation assessment: Since spasticity does not occur in isolation, but as one part of the upper motor neuron syndrome, treatment should be tailored to each patient's needs. The rehabilitation team can assist in determining treatment goals. Interventions that help reduce spasticity may include positioning, stretching, casting, seating modifications and other treatments.

Surgery: Various orthopedic and neurosurgical procedures may help severe persistent spasticity that is unresponsive to other treatments.

Pharmacologic Choices

All medications should be started at a low dose and increased gradually with monitoring for effects and side effects (Table 1).

Baclofen

Baclofen is the drug of choice for spasticity of spinal cord origin and in multiple sclerosis. It may be less effective for spasticity of cerebral origin. Its use may be limited by sedation. Baclofen

Figure 1: **Management of Chronic Spasticity**

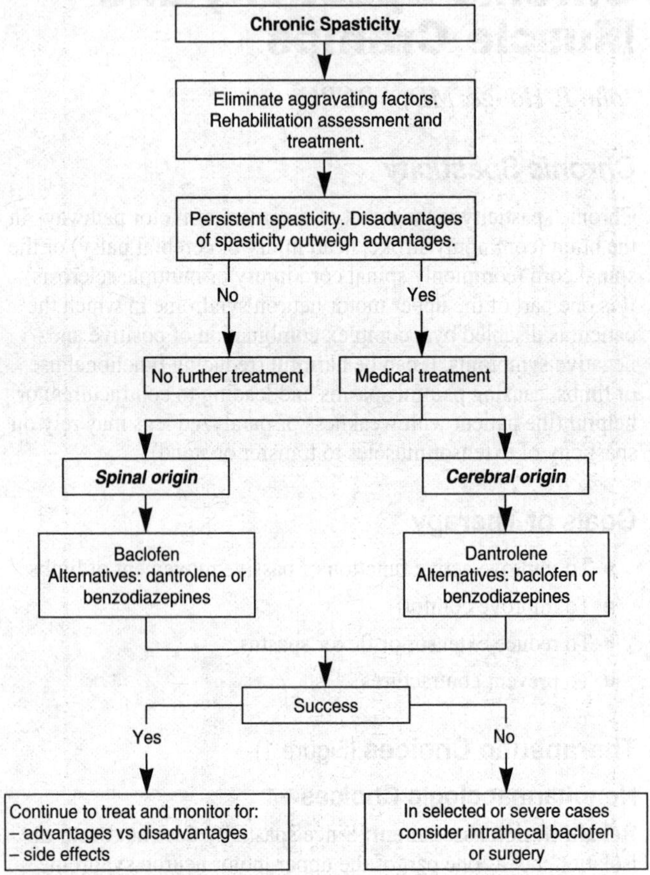

should not be stopped suddenly because abrupt withdrawal can cause hallucinations, confusion or convulsions.

In some patients with very severe spasticity, oral baclofen may have little or no effect. **Intrathecal baclofen** via catheter from a programmable pump to the lumbar subarachnoid space can be very effective,[1] but is expensive.

Dantrolene

Dantrolene is the only antispasticity drug to act peripherally on the muscle fiber. It commonly produces muscle weakness, which limits its usefulness unless the patient has good strength but is restricted by spasticity, or is completely paralyzed. Dantrolene

[1] J Neurosurg 1993;78:226–232.

CHAPTER 10

Chronic Spasticity and Muscle Cramps

John P. Hooge, MD, FRCPC

Chronic Spasticity

Chronic spasticity is the result of disorders of motor pathways in the brain (commonly stroke, head injury or cerebral palsy) or the spinal cord (commonly spinal cord injury or multiple sclerosis). It is one part of the upper motor neuron syndrome in which the patient is disabled by a complex combination of positive and negative symptoms. It can be harmful (reducing functional use of limbs, causing painful spasms and leading to contractures) or helpful (the patient with weakness or paralyzed legs may rely on spasticity of extensor muscles to transfer or stand).

Goals of Therapy

- To improve active function or passive movement of limbs
- To improve comfort
- To reduce extensor or flexor spasms
- To prevent contractures

Therapeutic Choices (Figure 1)

Nonpharmacologic Choices

Rehabilitation assessment: Since spasticity does not occur in isolation, but as one part of the upper motor neuron syndrome, treatment should be tailored to each patient's needs. The rehabilitation team can assist in determining treatment goals. Interventions that help reduce spasticity may include positioning, stretching, casting, seating modifications and other treatments.

Surgery: Various orthopedic and neurosurgical procedures may help severe persistent spasticity that is unresponsive to other treatments.

Pharmacologic Choices

All medications should be started at a low dose and increased gradually with monitoring for effects and side effects (Table 1).

Baclofen

Baclofen is the drug of choice for spasticity of spinal cord origin and in multiple sclerosis. It may be less effective for spasticity of cerebral origin. Its use may be limited by sedation. Baclofen

Figure 1: **Management of Chronic Spasticity**

Figure 1: Management of Chronic Spasticity

```
Chronic Spasticity
        ↓
Eliminate aggravating factors.
Rehabilitation assessment and
treatment.
        ↓
Persistent spasticity. Disadvantages
of spasticity outweigh advantages.
    No          Yes
     ↓            ↓
No further    Medical treatment
treatment
```

Spinal origin	Cerebral origin
Baclofen Alternatives: dantrolene or benzodiazepines	Dantrolene Alternatives: baclofen or benzodiazepines

```
              Success
    Yes                    No
     ↓                      ↓
Continue to treat and    In selected or severe cases
monitor for:             consider intrathecal baclofen
– advantages vs          or surgery
  disadvantages
– side effects
```

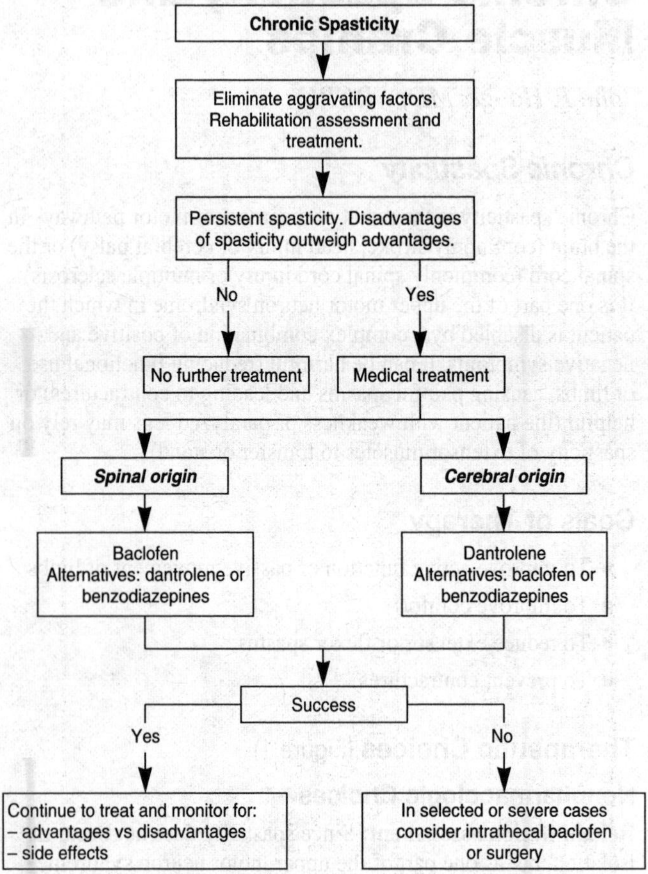

should not be stopped suddenly because abrupt withdrawal can cause hallucinations, confusion or convulsions.

In some patients with very severe spasticity, oral baclofen may have little or no effect. **Intrathecal baclofen** via catheter from a programmable pump to the lumbar subarachnoid space can be very effective,[1] but is expensive.

Dantrolene

Dantrolene is the only antispasticity drug to act peripherally on the muscle fiber. It commonly produces muscle weakness, which limits its usefulness unless the patient has good strength but is restricted by spasticity, or is completely paralyzed. Dantrolene

---

[1] *J Neurosurg* 1993;78:226–232.

Table 1: Drugs Used in Chronic Spasticity

Drug	Adult Dosage	Pediatric Dosage	Adverse Effects	Drug Interactions	Cost*
baclofen ● Lioresal, generics	Starting: 5 mg BID or TID ↑ 5–15 mg Q 3–7 d up to 80 mg/d divided TID (**NB**: some patients can tolerate and benefit from doses up to 120 mg/d)	Starting: same as adults Maximum: 2–7 yrs – 40 mg/d > 8 yrs – 60 mg/d	Sedation, muscle weakness, nausea, dizziness, decreased seizure threshold.	Tricyclic antidepressants may potentiate the effect of baclofen. Baclofen may ↑ the effect of antihypertensives.	$$$$
dantrolene Dantrium	Starting: 25 mg daily or BID; then ↑ by 25 mg Q 3–7 d up to 400 mg/d divided TID–QID	Starting: 0.5 mg/kg/dose BID; then ↑ to TID, QID; then ↑ by 0.5 mg/kg Q 3–7 d to a max 3 mg/kg/dose TID–QID (max. 400 mg/d)	Muscle weakness (frequent), sedation, dizziness, nausea, diarrhea, hepatic injury (especially in women, those > 35 yrs, high dose or long duration of therapy).		$$$$$
Benzodiazepines *diazepam* Valium, Vivol, generics *clonazepam* Rivotril, generics	Diazepam: Starting: 2–5 mg/d; then ↑ by 2–5 mg Q 3–7 d up to 60 mg/d divided BID–TID For nocturnal spasms: Diazepam: 5–10 mg HS Clonazepam: 0.5–2 mg HS	Diazepam: 0.1–0.8 mg/kg/d divided BID–TID Begin low and ↑	Sedation, muscle weakness, confusion, drug dependence.	Drug effects are potentiated by alcohol and CNS depressant drugs, clarithromycin and erythromycin.	$ ● $ ●

* Cost of 30-day supply – includes drug cost only.
Legend: $ < $20 $$ $20–40 $$$ $40–60 $$$$ $60–80 $$$$$ > $80   ● Dosage adjustment may be required in renal impairment – see Appendix I.

may be more effective in spasticity of cerebral origin than
baclofen. Its potential for hepatotoxicity is significant, especially
in women, those > 35 years and those receiving high doses for
prolonged periods; AST and ALT should be monitored during
treatment. If there is no clear benefit after 45 days of treatment,
the drug should be discontinued.

Benzodiazepines

Diazepam and **clonazepam**, the most commonly used benzodiazepines for spasticity, effectively reduce spasticity of cerebral
and spinal origin. Their usefulness is limited by sedation.

Therapeutic Tips

- Spasticity frequently increases in response to any noxious
  stimulus in the body (e.g., urinary tract infections or calculi,
  pressure sores, ingrown toenails and other skin irritations).
  Before treating spasticity with medication, these conditions
  should be ruled out or treated if present.
- The advantages and disadvantages of spasticity to the
  patient should be considered before deciding to treat with
  medication.
- Drugs for spasticity may reduce muscle tone, deep tendon
  reflexes, clonus and muscle spasms but often do little or
  nothing to aid function, ambulation or activities of daily
  living.
- Muscle spasms occurring during the night can interrupt
  sleep. Diazepam or clonazepam can be very helpful in
  reducing these nocturnal spasms.

Muscle Cramps

Ordinary muscle cramps are usually painful, asymmetric, occur at
rest, frequently at night and most often affect the gastrocnemius
muscle and small muscles of the foot. They occur when a muscle
already in its most shortened position involuntarily contracts.

Goals of Therapy

- To prevent or relieve the cramp and associated pain

Investigations

- History and physical examination with attention to:
  – contributing factors, i.e., prolonged or excessive muscle
    use, high heat, salt depletion, hemodialysis or use of drugs
    (nifedipine, clofibrate, salbutamol, penicillamine, excessive
    alcohol)

- muscle weakness, sensory symptoms or fasciculations suggesting an underlying neurological disorder
- symptoms of tetany – paresthesias of the mouth, hands, legs and carpopedal spasm
- Laboratory investigations:
  - sodium if salt depletion is suspected
  - calcium, magnesium, potassium if tetany is suspected

Therapeutic Choices

Nonpharmacologic Choices

- To relieve cramps – passive stretching of the involved muscle.
- To prevent cramps – conditioning exercises and stretching exercises of the involved muscles.

Pharmacologic Choices

Quinine Sulfate

Quinine sulfate is the drug of choice for ordinary muscle cramps. Side effects are rare at the usual dose of 200 to 300 mg HS, but higher doses can cause cinchonism (nausea, vomiting, tinnitus and deafness), visual toxicity or cardiac arrhythmias. Quinine-associated thrombocytopenia occurs rarely, is potentially life threatening, unpredictable and not dose related. A therapeutic trial of 3 to 6 weeks should be tried. If successful, re-evaluate the need for treatment in 3 to 6 months.

Suggested Reading List

Alonso RJ, Mancall EL. The clinical management of spasticity. *Semin Neurol* 1991;11:215–219.

Glenn MB, Whyte J. *The practical management of spasticity in children and adults.* Philadelphia: Lea and Febiger, 1990:1–7, 201–226.

McGee SR. Muscle cramps. *Arch Intern Med* 1990;150:511–518.

Parziale JR, Akelman E, Herz DA. Spasticity: pathophysiology and management. *Orthopedics* 1993;16:801–811.

CHAPTER 11

Headache in Adults

R. Allan Purdy, MD, FRCPC

Goals of Therapy

- To relieve or abolish pain and associated symptoms (e.g., nausea/vomiting)
- To prevent recurrent symptoms in primary headache disorders (e.g., migraine, tension-type and cluster)
- To diagnose and manage serious causes of headache (e.g., tumor, arteritis, infection, hemorrhage)
- To prevent complications of medication usage

Investigations

- A thorough history and physical are most important for a correct diagnosis. Note characteristics of the headache:
  - onset: sudden, gradual, recurrent or chronic
  - quality: severe or mild to moderate intensity
  - temporal profile: progressive or self-limited
  - associated symptoms: nausea, vomiting, sensitivity to light, noise or odors, systemic or other neurologic signs or symptoms
  - interference with activities of daily life (e.g., migraine)
- The physical examination should be normal; if any abnormalities are found (especially visual, motor, reflex, sensory, speech or cognitive), then investigation is warranted
- CT/MRI scans are not routine but must be done if any organic etiology is suspected (see box below)

Red Flags for Serious Headache

- **Age of Onset** – middle aged to elderly patient
- **Type of Onset** – severe and abrupt
- **Temporal Sequence** – progressive severity or increased frequency
- **Significant change in headache pattern**
- **Neurologic Signs** – stiff neck, focal signs, reduced consciousness
- **Systemic Signs** – fever, appears sick, abnormal examination
- **CAUTION:** If headache does not fit typical pattern, a serious diagnosis can be missed

Figure 1: **Diagnosis and Initial Assessment of Headache**

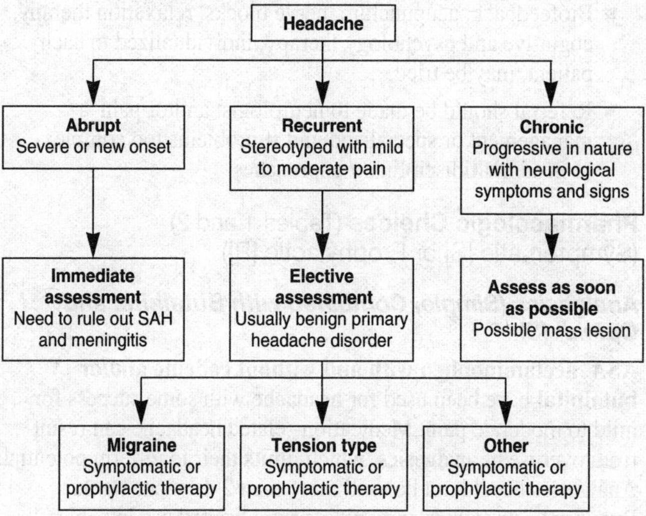

Note: Any headache not recognized as migraine, tension headache or known cause is in the "other" group. Investigate if no response to usual treatments.

Abbreviations: SAH = Subarachnoid hemorrhage.

- Lumbar puncture if subarachnoid hemorrhage, encephalitis, high- or low-pressure headache syndromes or meningitis is suspected
- Laboratory tests (on an individual basis)
  – ESR for suspected temporal arteritis
  – endocrine, biochemical, infection work-up
  – search for malignancy if indicated
- Facial pain may need a thorough assessment by a dental specialist familiar with headaches and facial pain and/or an ENT specialist if sinus or other ENT disorders are suspected

Therapeutic Choices (Figure 1)

If serious structural CNS causes for headache and facial pain have been ruled out, the primary headache disorders and some forms of facial pain can be managed as follows.

Nonpharmacologic Choices

- Explanation and reassurance are most important.
- Triggers, especially in migraine, should be avoided.
- Rest in a dark, noise-free room, application of ice and sleep can help.

- Informal psychotherapy from family doctor, and if psychiatric co-morbidity present, referral to psychiatrist.
- Biofeedback, acupuncture, nerve blocks, relaxation therapy, cognitive and psychology therapy, individualized to each patient, may be tried.
- Referral should be made to neurologist and/or pain management or specialized unit if problems too complex or need multidisciplinary approaches.

Pharmacologic Choices (Tables 1 and 2) (Symptomatic [S] or Prophylactic [P])

Analgesics (Simple, Combined with Butalbital and Opioid) (S)

ASA, acetaminophen with and without codeine and/or butalbital have been used for headache with some success for mild to moderate pain. Medication-related headache can result from overuse of analgesics, which limits their long-term potential. Analgesics should not be used more than 2 days per week. Butalbital compounds and opioids have limited use in benign headache disorders because of potential for dependency.

Ergotamine (S)

Ergotamine acts on 5-HT receptors and is classically used for migraine and cluster but is limited by side effects. It is available in many formulations and routes of administration. Ergotamine may produce rebound headaches if used more than 2 days per week.

Sumatriptan Succinate (S)

Sumatriptan is used to abort migraine but is not yet approved for cluster headaches. It acts on serotonin (5-HT) subclass 1B and 1D receptors on neurons and extracerebral blood vessels. The supposed mechanism of action is to prevent a sterile inflammatory response around such vessels and cause vasoconstriction which reduces pain stimuli. It is safe and effective in most patients, although use in patients with cardiac disorders and sustained hypertension is contraindicated.

Dihydroergotamine (DHE) (S)

DHE has similar actions to sumatriptan but also interacts centrally with dopamine and adrenergic receptors, accounting for some of its side effects. It can be used to treat acute intractable headache or withdrawal from analgesics. It produces no dependence.

Butorphanol Tartrate (S)

Butorphanol is available as a nasal spray to treat acute migraine. It is an opioid receptor agonist-antagonist with potent analgesic effects and rapid onset. It has some risk of abuse and may be of use in infrequent attacks of severe migraine when other treatments are not beneficial. Butorphanol can precipitate withdrawal in individuals addicted to opioids. Its major side effects are dysphoria, drowsiness, nausea and dizziness.

Beta-blockers (P)

Beta-blockers are commonly used and efficacious in migraine prophylaxis; their mechanism of action is uncertain. Effective drugs lack partial agonist activity, but CNS penetration, membrane stabilization and cardioselectivity do not influence efficacy. **Propranolol** is the most widely used, but others, especially **nadolol**, which does not appreciably cross the blood-brain barrier, can be used.

Calcium Channel Blockers (P)

These drugs may work by modulating neurotransmitter function rather than producing vasodilation or protecting against hypoxia. **Diltiazem, verapamil** and **nifedipine** are useful in migraine prophylaxis. Verapamil is useful in cluster prophylaxis. **Flunarizine** is nonselective for cardiac receptors and has good efficacy.

Tricyclic Analgesics (P)

Amitriptyline, nortriptyline and **doxepin** are effective for migraine and tension-type headache. They act as analgesics at doses lower than those required for affective disorders. They do not produce dependence and are relatively safe medications. Amitriptyline is useful in facial pain and other pain disorders.

Valproate/Divalproex Sodium (P)

These agents are effective in migraine prophylaxis. Guidelines for use have been published.[1] They may work by modulating GABA receptors in the peripheral trigeminovascular system. Teratogenicity (neural tube defects) occur. ASA should be avoided with valproic acid because of effects on hemostasis and coagulation.

Serotonin Antagonists (P)

Methysergide is a potent prophylactic medication for migraine and cluster headaches but has potentially serious long-term side effects which can be avoided by limiting duration of treatment. Although less potent than methysergide, **pizotyline** (pizotifen) is helpful in migraine if tolerated at maximal dosage. Although the mechanism of action is questionable, these drugs may work by antagonizing $5\text{-}HT_2$ receptors of the smooth muscle of blood vessels, causing vasoconstriction.

---

[1] *Headache 1996;36:547–555.*

Table 1: **Medications for Symptomatic Treatment of Headache**

Drug	Dosage per Attack	Selected Adverse Effects	Comments	Cost*/Dose
Analgesics				
ASA/acetaminophen with codeine and/or butalbital 282, 292; Tylenol w/Codeine (#2, 3, 4); Fiorinal plain, C1/4, C1/2; generics	ASA, acetaminophen 650–1 300 mg Q4H × 2 Codeine varies with formulations Butalbital as per formulation	GI with ASA/NSAIDs. Dependence and tolerance to barbiturates and narcotics. Potential liver and kidney dysfunction for acetaminophen with chronic use of high doses or in acute overdose.	Analgesics may be simple or compounds with or without narcotics or barbiturates. Symptomatic treatment only.	$
ibuprofen Motrin, Advil, Actiprofen, generics	Ibuprofen 400–800 mg Q6H × 2		Use only 2 d/wk. Great risk of rebound headache (less for naproxen). Naproxen sodium useful in perimenstrual attacks. Repeat dosages must be individualized.	$
naproxen Naprosyn, Anaprox (sodium), generics	Naproxen sodium 275–550 mg Q2–6H			$
opioids (many formulations)	Opioids require individual consideration			$
Ergot Derivatives				
ergotamine Ergomar	**Ergotamine and caffeine tablets:** 2 × 1 mg tablets at onset and 1 mg Q1H × 3	Nausea, vomiting, paresthesias, cramps, vasoconstriction for ergots. Ergot dependence producing ergotism.	Use only 2 d/wk. Contraindicated in pregnancy, cardiac disorders, hypertension, sepsis, peripheral vascular disease, peptic ulcer disease, renal or liver disease. Caution in elderly.	$
compounds Cafergot, Cafergot-PB, Megral, Wigraine (many formulations, routes: PO, SL, inhaled and rectal suppositories)	**Ergotamine and caffeine suppositories:** 1/2 of a 2 mg supp at onset (maximum 3 mg within 24 h)			$

Drug	Dosing	Adverse Effects	Comments	Cost*
dihydroergotamine (DHE) parenteral and nasal (Migranal) formulations	DHE: 0.5–1 mg SC, IM or IV. May repeat at 1 h; maximum 4 doses/24 h. Preceded by 10 mg metoclopramide IV or 5 mg prochlorperazine IV (watch for hypotension, rare) **Deliver IV meds SLOWLY** See Raskin Protocol for use in intractable headache (*Neurology* 1986;36:995–997)	Same as for ergotamine but less frequent and less prolonged.	Not as potent a vasoconstrictor as ergotamine, mainly venoconstrictor. Same contraindications as ergotamines; no dependence. Good for attacks beginning in ER and in treating medication-associated headaches.	$ plus cost of administration and parenteral antiemetics if given IV
	Nasal: 1 spray 0.5 mg in each nostril, repeat in 15 min if no effect. Maximum 2 mg/d	Rhinitis, nausea, taste disturbance.	Convenient. Bypasses GI tract.	$
Sumatriptan Imitrex tablets, SC autoinjector, nasal spray	PO: 50–100 mg at start or during attack, not to exceed 300 mg/24 h SC: 6 mg at start or during attack, not to exceed 2 injections/24 h with at least 1 h interval. **Patients not responding to 1st dose of PO or SC sumatriptan should not take 2nd dose for same attack. May be used for a subsequent attack**	Chest discomfort, paresthesias, drowsiness, nausea, throat symptoms.	Do not use if **any** cardiac-like symptoms. Contraindicated in ischemic heart disease, sustained hypertension, pregnancy, basilar or hemiplegic migraine, or with selective serotonin reuptake inhibitors, MAO inhibitors, ergotamine-containing products.	Injection $$$$$ Tablets $$$ Nasal $$$
	Nasal: Minimum effective dose: 5 mg. Maximum recommended: 20 mg. Maximum daily dose: 40 mg. Administer in one nostril only	Taste disturbance, nausea.	Faster onset than oral. Bypasses GI tract.	

* Cost per dose – includes drug cost only.
Legend: $ < $5 $$ $5–10 $$$ $10–20 $$$$ $20–30 $$$$$ > $30

Table 2: **Medications for Prophylactic Treatment of Headache**

Drug	Daily Dosage Range	Selected Adverse Effects	Comments	Cost*
Beta-blockers				
propranolol Inderal, generics	Propranolol 40–240 mg	Fatigue, impotence, bradycardia and hypotension, GI symptoms, bronchospasm, CHF, depression.	Contraindicated in asthma, insulin-dependent diabetes, heart block or pregnancy. Avoid abrupt withdrawal. Consider long-acting formulations. Nadolol has fewer CNS side effects and is excreted by kidneys.	$
nadolol 🔵 Corgard, generics	Nadolol 20–160 mg			$
atenolol 🔵 Tenormin, generics	Atenolol 50–150 mg			$–$$
metoprolol Lopresor, Betaloc, generics	Metoprolol 100–200 mg			$
Calcium Channel Blockers				
flunarizine Sibelium	Flunarizine 5–10 mg (QHS)	Bradycardia, hypotension, constipation (verapamil), weight gain, extrapyramidal effects, drowsiness, depression with flunarizine.	Long latency to onset. Many patients have side effects. Contraindicated in hypotension, heart failure and arrhythmia. Avoid if severe constipation, especially verapamil. Do not use flunarizine in depressed patients or with extrapyramidal disorders.	$$–$$$$
verapamil 🔵 Isoptin, generics	Verapamil 240–320 mg			$$

Tricyclic Analgesics

Drug	Dosage	Adverse Effects	Comments	Cost
amitriptyline Elavil, generics	Amitriptyline 10–150 mg (QHS)	Weight gain, drowsiness, anticholinergic symptoms (e.g., dry mouth, constipation), lower seizure threshold, confusion.	Dose can be cumulative, adjustments needed. Contraindicated if significant cardiac disease, glaucoma, prostate disease or hypotension. Start low dosage in elderly or in patients sensitive to these agents.	$
doxepin Sinequan, Triadapin, generics	Doxepin 25–100 mg (QHS)			$
nortriptyline Aventyl, generics	Nortriptyline 10–150 mg (QHS)			$–$$$

Serotonin Antagonists

Drug	Dosage	Adverse Effects	Comments	Cost
pizotyline Sandomigran	Pizotyline: Start with 0.5 mg QHS, gradually ↑ to TID; if necessary ↑ to 3 or 6 mg/d (usual dose: 1–6 mg)	Weight gain, retroperitoneal cardiac and pulmonary fibrosis with methysergide; drowsiness, weight gain with pizotyline.	Consider QHS dosing of pizotyline at increasingly higher doses. NEVER use methysergide for more than 6 mos without a 1 mo drug holiday. ↓ dosage gradually before discontinuation. Methysergide not a first-line medication, many contraindications to use; review every time medication prescribed.	$–$$$$
methysergide Sansert	Methysergide: Start with 2 mg QHS, gradually ↑ to TID; if necessary ↑ to 8 mg/d (usual dose: 4–8 mg)			$$–$$$$

Antiepileptics

Drug	Dosage	Adverse Effects	Comments	Cost
valproate Depakene	500–1 500 mg/d	Nausea, alopecia, tremor, weight gain, ↑ hepatic enzymes.	Neural tube defects can occur. Start low dosage 250–500 mg/d. Do CBC, liver function tests initially; if ↑, ↓ dosage; if 2–3 × normal, stop medication.	$–$$$
divalproex sodium Epival				$$–$$$$

● *Dosage adjustment may be required in renal impairment – see Appendix I.*
* *Cost of 30-day supply – includes drug cost only.*
Legend: $ < $20 $$ $20–40 $$$ $40–60 $$$$ > $60

Others (S, P)

Carbamazepine and **phenytoin** have been used to treat facial pain. These antiepileptic medications have potentially significant side effects and drug interactions but can benefit some patients. Teratogenic effects (neural tube defects) have been reported with carbamazepine.

Corticosteroids, including dexamethasone, can be useful in many headache disorders, including status migraine, cluster headache and cerebral neoplasms with edema (especially metastatic lesions). Steroids in temporal arteritis relieve headache and prevent blindness.

Lithium is useful in the treatment of chronic cluster headache. Phenothiazines (e.g., **prochlorperazine** or **chlorpromazine**) have been used in the emergency room for treatment of migraine and other intractable headaches. **Indomethacin** has been found useful in chronic paroxysmal hemicrania and coital cephalgia.

Antinauseants (e.g., **dimenhydrinate** 50 to 100 mg PO PRN) and antiemetic/prokinetic agents (e.g., **metoclopramide** 10 mg PO or IV and **domperidone** 10 to 20 mg PO) are useful as adjunctive or primary therapy in headache disorders associated with nausea and vomiting.

Headaches Associated with Medication Use

Many medications (e.g., nitrates) can produce headaches as a side effect and should be discontinued or changed if possible. Some drugs used for headache treatment (e.g., ergotamine) can result in more headache.

Analgesics, especially opioids, can produce **rebound headaches** if used for more than 2 days per week. In some patients inter-mittent migraine changes to a continuous headache. The headache occurs daily or almost daily and has characteristics of tension-type with superimposed migraine. If the analgesics can be stopped, the headache may return to the former migraine pattern, which is treatable. Analgesics not only perpetuate this chronic headache but also preclude efficacy of other migraine medications.

Management includes recognizing the problem, stopping the offending agent, starting a prophylactic medication such as amitriptyline, and using an abortive agent such as DHE or sumatriptan for migraine headache if it emerges. The Raskin protocol for inpatient management of medication-induced headaches (using DHE) is very useful.[2,3]

[2] *Neurology 1986;36:995.*
[3] *Neurol Clin 1990;8:850–865.*

Therapeutic Tips

The management of headache is as much an art as science; the science is improving, but the art remains important. Communicating with patients to let them know their headache is real, and that they have a specific diagnosis, is of paramount importance. Patients' expectations should be determined and management options explained to them. After serious causes are excluded, the interaction with the patient is the first and most important therapeutic choice.

- Abortive treatment without exceeding recommended dosages should be given as soon as possible.
- Use of analgesics more than 2 days per week should be avoided.
- Calendar or diary of headaches is very useful in follow-up assessment.
- A record of medications, their usefulness, dosage and side effects should be kept.
- If migraine occurs more than 2 or 3 times per month, prophylactic medications should be tried for several months and then discontinued.
- Different medications may need to be tried.
- Follow-up is most important in managing chronic headache.
- Reassurance and explanation are most important in the long term.
- Always offer hope to patients with chronic headache even if no cure is available; most primary headaches can be controlled.

Pharmacoeconomic Considerations

Jeffrey A. Johnson, PhD

Given the considerable morbidity and health care resource utilization by patients with migraine headache, this condition has been considered most often in terms of the pharmacoeconomic impact. Effective migraine treatment is clearly the most cost-effective in terms of both direct and indirect costs. For the prophylaxis of migraines there are many older low-cost medications (e.g., amitriptyline and imipramine, or propranolol and atenolol) that have equal or better effectiveness than newer, more expensive agents. However, there is little published evidence for the relative cost-effectiveness of these agents. Similarly, there are many useful medications options for acute migraine treatment, with a wide cost range among these drugs. Effective migraine abortive therapy will decrease the cost of repeated dosing and disability. Considerable cost savings can be achieved through self-treatment, thus avoiding expensive ER visits. Initial evidence regarding the use of sumatriptan suggests that patients tend to seek medical attention less often and incur fewer costs following initiation of this drug. The pharmacoeconomic impact of sumatriptan is currently being evaluated by CCOHTA.

Suggested Reading

Adelman JU, Von Seggern R. *Cost considerations in headache treatment. Part 1: prophylactic migraine treatment. Headache 1995;35:479–487.*

Von Seggern R, Adelman JU. *Cost considerations in headache treatment. Part 2: acute migraine treatment. Headache 1996;36:493–502.*

Litaker DG, Solomon GD, Genzen JR. *Impact of sumatriptan on clinic utilization and costs of care in migraineurs. Headache 1996;36:538–541.*

To T, Wu K. *Health care utilization and disability of migraine: the Ontario Health Survey. Can J Public Health 1995;86:196–199.*

Suggested Reading List

Mathew NT, ed. Advances in Headache. *Neurology Clinics* 1997;15(1).

Pryse-Phillips WEM, Dodick DW, Edmeads JG, et al. Guidelines for the diagnosis and management of migraine in clinical practice. *Can Med Assoc J* 1997; 156:1273–1287.

CHAPTER 12

Headache in Children

Sharon Whiting, MBBS, FRCPC

Headaches occur commonly in children and adolescents. They may occur as a primary disorder such as migraine or accompany systemic disorders or infectious diseases. It is estimated that 25% of children will have experienced a significant headache by age 10.

Goals of Therapy

- To make an accurate diagnosis of headache
- To relieve or abort pain and associated symptoms
- To prevent further headaches

Investigations (Figure 1)

- The history is the key to the diagnosis of headache and should be obtained from both parent and child
  - specific questions — where pain began, progress, duration, frequency, relieving and aggravating factors (especially sleep loss, excitement and certain foods, relief with activity) and associated symptoms such as vomiting and photophobia
  - specific neurological symptoms — seizures, visual disturbance, difficulty with balance, personality change, weakness
  - interference with school and social life
  - general — pregnancy, labor, delivery, growth and development, behavior, academic function

NB: During the interview, observe interaction between parent and child.

- Physical examination:
  - blood pressure, vital signs, palpation of sinuses, neck stiffness, examination of optic fundi
  - height, weight, head circumference
  - a thorough neurological examination including cranial nerves, muscle tone, power and reflexes, and tests of coordination
- Investigations:
  - sinus x-rays if sinusitis
  - CT followed by lumbar puncture with measurement of opening pressure if pseudotumor cerebri suspected
  - lumbar puncture if infectious process suspected

– CT and/or MRI if abnormal neurological examination, decreased visual acuity, recent behavior change, increasing severity and frequency of headaches, headache does not fit a known pattern

Figure 1: Identifying the Temporal Profile of the Headache

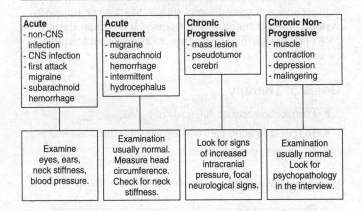

Acute	Acute Recurrent	Chronic Progressive	Chronic Non-Progressive
- non-CNS infection - CNS infection - first attack migraine - subarachnoid hemorrhage	- migraine - subarachnoid hemorrhage - intermittent hydrocephalus	- mass lesion - pseudotumor cerebri	- muscle contraction - depression - malingering
Examine eyes, ears, neck stiffness, blood pressure.	Examination usually normal. Measure head circumference. Check for neck stiffness.	Look for signs of increased intracranial pressure, focal neurological signs.	Examination usually normal. Look for psychopathology in the interview.

Therapeutic Choices

Nonpharmacologic Choices

After exclusion of mass lesion or other causes:

- Reassure and explain.
- Discuss triggers of migraine, e.g., lack of sleep, too much sleep, excitement, foods, stress.
- Encourage sleep at the time of headache and medication early in the course of the headache.
- Biofeedback and relaxation therapy are effective.

Pharmacologic Choices

These can be divided into medication given at the time of the headache (symptomatic) and medication to prevent headache (prophylactic).

Symptomatic Treatments (Table 1)

Analgesic Drugs

Intermittent oral analgesics, given as early in the course of the headache as feasible, are the mainstay of pharmacologic management of childhood migraine. Acetaminophen, ibuprofen and ASA at appropriate doses are effective.

Combination drugs such as ASA with caffeine and butalbital, with or without codeine (Fiorinal), play secondary roles should the initial agents fail. These sedating drugs have abuse potential and should be reserved for adolescents for brief periods only. Care must be taken to avoid unnecessary opioids.

Antiemetics

Nausea and vomiting occur in up to 90% of young migraine sufferers and besides being disabling, inhibit oral administration of analgesics. Antiemetics alone are surprisingly effective in elimination of all symptoms including the headache, e.g., chlorpromazine, prochlorperazine, metoclopramide. Chlorpromazine with chloral hydrate to induce sleep is an effective combination in childhood migraine.

Ergotamine and Dihydroergotamine

Ergotamine compounds have very limited use in pediatrics for the following reasons:

- Auras are uncommon and inconsistent; therefore, warning indicators that trigger the time to treat with ergot are often unreliable
- Ergot can exacerbate gastrointestinal upset
- Ergots are contraindicated in complicated migraine syndromes because of the risk of increasing vasospasm

In severe intractable headache, dihydroergotamine can be used IV in combination with an antiemetic in the emergency department.

Sumatriptan

This 5-HT agonist is an effective agent in adults. While there are some studies of sumatriptan in pediatrics, it is not currently approved for children.

Prophylactic Agents (Table 2)
Serotonin Antagonists

Pizotyline, a less potent prophylactic medication than methysergide, is helpful in migraine. Methysergide is not used in pediatric headache because of potentially serious long-term side effects.

Beta-blockers

The beta-blocker **propranolol** has been commonly used and is effective in some cases. It is contraindicated in reactive airway disease, diabetes mellitus and bradyarrhythmias. Depressive symptoms are an under-reported but common effect in adolescents.

Antihistamines

Cyproheptadine, an antihistamine with antiserotonergic and calcium channel blocking properties, is firmly entrenched as a prophylactic agent, although it has never been subject to controlled study. Its use in older children and adolescents is limited by sedative properties and associated weight gain.

Calcium Channel Blockers

Flunarizine has been shown to significantly reduce headache frequency and severity in children.

Antidepressants

Amitriptyline has shown efficacy of 50 to 55% in adults. No controlled trials in children have been reported.

Nonsteroidal Anti-inflammatory Agents

Several studies in adults show these medications reduce headache frequency and severity when used as prophylaxis, presumably through prostaglandin inhibition. One series in adolescent children showed a 60% reduction in headache frequency and severity using **naproxen sodium.**

Anticonvulsants

Carbamazepine and valproic acid have been studied in adults but not in children. Phenobarbital and phenytoin are no longer used.

Therapeutic Tips

- There are very few controlled trials of pharmacologic management of childhood migraine; hence, anecdotal experience prevails. Most young patients with migraine do not require daily medication but need access to reliable analgesia at home and at school.

- Children are debilitated by nausea and vomiting and benefit greatly from antiemetics. Rest and sleep are usually very helpful.

- Consider prophylactic agents for children who cycle through periods of time when they experience such frequency of headache that their lifestyle is disrupted or when isolated or infrequent events are severe and complex.

- Calendars are helpful in identifying triggers, headache patterns, frequency and severity and are invaluable for management and evaluation of response to therapy.

- Prophylactic medication should be considered, using medications with the least side effects first. Pizotyline or propranolol are the drugs of first choice. Cyproheptadine is usually used in younger children. For adolescents, propranolol, amitriptyline, naproxen sodium and flunarizine are used in that order.

Table 1: Drug Treatment of Headache in Children

Drug	Daily Dosage Range	Adverse Effects	Comments	Cost*
Analgesics				
acetaminophen	10–15 mg/kg/dose Q4H	All: Gastrointestinal upset.	Medication most often used at time of headache.	$
ASA	Age ≥ 12 yrs: 500–650 mg PRN		Because of the concern of Reye's syndrome, ASA should not be used in the context of fever or a viral illness.	$
ibuprofen Motrin, Advil, generics	5–10 mg/kg/dose 4 times daily			$
naproxen sodium Anaprox, generics	Age > 2 years: 5–7 mg/kg/dose Q8–12H			$
Combination Therapy				
butalbital, caffeine, ASA Fiorinal, generics	1–2 tablets 4 times daily	Gastrointestinal upset; dependence and tolerance to barbiturates and opioids.	Reserved for adolescents. No more than 2 days/week. Risk of tolerance, addiction and misuse.	$
orphenadrine citrate, ASA, caffeine Norgesic	1–2 tablets 4 times daily			$$
Antiemetics				
chlorpromazine Largactil, generics	1 mg/kg PO/IM to a maximum of 25 mg Q8H	Hypotension.	Can be used with PO chloral hydrate 25–50 mg/kg PO Q8H	$
	0.1 mg/kg IV Q10–15 minutes to a maximum of 30 mg		Can cause hypotension when given IV. Use in the emergency department.	$$
prochlorperazine Stemetil, generics	2.5–5 mg twice daily PO 10 mg IV	Extrapyramidal dysfunction.	Use IV in adolescents in the emergency department.	$ $$
metoclopramide Maxeran, Reglan, generics	1–2 mg/kg (<10 mg) PO 10 mg IV	Extrapyramidal dysfunction.	Use IV in adolescents in the emergency department.	$ $$$

(cont'd)

Table 1: Drug Treatment of Headache in Children *(cont'd)*

Drug	Daily Dosage Range	Adverse Effects	Comments	Cost*
Ergot Derivatives *dihydroergotamine*	0.1–0.25 mg/dose IV. May be repeated Q20 minutes × 3. Give metoclopramide 0.2 mg/kg/dose 30 minutes prior to IV dihydroergotamine (maximum 20 mg).	Flushed feeling. Tingling in extremities. Nausea and vomiting.	Useful in patients with severe and prolonged migraine headache. This protocol to take place in hospital. Contraindicated in complicated migraine, coronary heart disease, abnormal blood pressure, abnormal ECG.	$$$$
sumatriptan			Not currently indicated for children under age 18.	

* Cost per dose (based on 20 kg) – includes drug cost only.
Legend: *$ < $0.50*   *$$ $0.50–1.00*   *$$$ $1.00–1.50*   *$$$$ > $1.50*

Table 2: Prophylactic Treatment of Headache in Children

Drug	Daily Dosage Range	Adverse Effects	Comments	Cost*
Beta-blockers *propranolol* Inderal, generics	0.6–1.5 mg/kg/d PO	Fatigue, bradycardia, hypotension, depression.	Contraindicated in asthma, diabetes, heart block, bradyarrhythmias, pregnancy. Avoid abrupt withdrawal.	$
Serotonin Antagonists *pizotyline* Sandomigran	0.5–1.5 mg/d PO	Sedation and weight gain.	Start medication slowly and increase over 1–3 weeks.	$–$$
Calcium Channel Blockers *flunarizine* Sibelium, generics	5 mg/d PO	Bradycardia, hypotension, depression.	May take several weeks before effective. Do not use in depressed patients or those with extrapyramidal disorders.	$$
Tricyclics *amitriptyline* Elavil, generics	10–150 mg/d	Weight gain, drowsiness. Anticholinergic symptoms such as dry mouth and constipation.	Contraindicated in significant cardiac disease or hypotension.	$

(cont'd)

Table 2: Prophylactic Treatment of Headache in Children *(cont'd)*

Drug	Daily Dosage Range	Adverse Effects	Comments	Cost*
Antihistamines *cyproheptadine* Periactin, generics	Age 2–6 years: 2 mg Q8–12H (maximum 12 mg/d) Age 7–14 years: 4 mg Q8–12H (maximum 16 mg/d)	Drowsiness.		$–$$
Nonsteroidal Anti-inflammatory Agents *naproxen sodium* Anaprox, generics	275–550 mg twice daily	GI upset.	Use in adolescents.	$–$$

* *Cost of 30-day supply – includes drug cost only.*
Legend: $ < $20 $$ $20–40

- The prognosis for children with migraine is favorable with 50% of patients reporting improvement within 6 months after medical intervention, regardless of treatment methods used.
- Most children respond to reassurance, general advice and simple remedies for attacks when they occur.

Suggested Reading List

Smith S. Comprehensive evaluation and treatment of recurrent paediatric headache. *Pediatr Ann* 1995;24:450–457.

Graf W, Riback P. Pharmacologic treatment of recurrent pediatric headache. *Pediatr Ann* 1995;24:477–484.

Singer H. Migraine headaches in children. *Pediatr Rev* 1994;15:94–101.

CHAPTER 13

Acute Pain

Jane E. Gloor, MD, FRCPC

Definition

An unpleasant sensory and emotional experience associated with actual or potential tissue damage or described in terms of such damage.[1]

Goals of Therapy

- To identify the patient experiencing pain
- To relieve the pain to a level acceptable to the patient
- To minimize possible adverse effects

Investigations

The expression of pain will depend on the patient's age, anxiety, developmental level, coping skills, ethnocultural background, previous pain experience and pain severity. Individuals who have difficulty communicating their needs (including infants, young children, patients with psychoses or severe emotional problems, the developmentally challenged, demented patients and patients with language barriers) require particular attention to pain assessment and management.

Asking the patient how much it hurts is a quick **cognitive** measure of pain intensity. Self-reporting is the single most reliable indicator of acute pain severity and location in children and adults.

Physiological signs of acute pain (e.g., tachycardia, hypertension, sweating and pallor) are present for the first few hours after an injury. They can be used in all age groups but are most useful in infants and young children for whom a cognitive assessment cannot be performed.

Behavioral pain indicators are age-dependent and include crying, agitation or paradoxical withdrawal from activity, information seeking, fist clenching and teeth gritting.

Physiological and behavioral measures infer the amount of pain being experienced and are influenced by anxiety and fear. They are most useful for people unable to directly communicate about the pain they are experiencing.

---

[1] *Pain 1979;6:249.*

Analgesia can be administered during the initial assessment. The early aggressive treatment of pain allows for a more complete assessment by ensuring cooperation from the patient.

Therapeutic Choices

A multifaceted approach to pain management, incorporating nonpharmacologic methods in conjunction with medication, will usually be the most efficacious.

Nonpharmacologic Choices

- **Education** – inform the patient about procedures, expected discomfort, and what he or she can do to decrease the expected pain.
- **Relaxation** – instruct the patient to perform deep rhythmic breathing, inhaling through the nose to a count of 3 and exhaling through the mouth to a count of 3, allowing the tension to leave their body.
- **Imagery** – ask the patient to imagine a favorite spot in as much detail as possible; a beach or a forest is often chosen.
- **Distraction** (auditory or visual) – provide music, talk about enjoyable activities, place pleasant pictures on the ceiling.
- **Physical measures** – apply cold or heat, immobilize fractures, and instruct the patient on exercise, stretching and massage.

Pharmacologic Choices
Systemic Analgesics (Table 1)

Acetaminophen is used for mild to moderate pain; it can be given orally or rectally.

NSAIDs are used for mild to moderate pain (Chapter 50). They are usually given orally; ketorolac is available in parenteral form. NSAIDs should be avoided in patients with a history of peptic ulcer disease, renal failure, congestive heart failure or asthma.

Opioids are used for moderate to severe pain. They can be given by oral, rectal and parenteral routes and are often used in combination with acetaminophen, ASA or NSAIDs.

Topical

Eutectic mixture of local anesthetics (EMLA) provides good local anesthesia for superficial skin injuries. Peak effect occurs in 1 to 2 hours after application. A mixture of **tetracaine + epinephrine (Adrenalin) + cocaine** (TAC) is useful for small facial lacerations. A combination of bupivacaine-norepinephrine is as effective as TAC and does not contain cocaine. Viscous lidocaine can provide analgesia for cleaning surface wounds.

Table 1: Selected Analgesic Drugs*

Drug	Dose	Route	Comments	Cost†
acetaminophen 🌢 Tylenol, many others	P: 10–15 mg/kg/dose Q4H A: 650–975 mg Q4H	PO, PR	Equianalgesic to NSAIDs, no anti-inflammatory effect.	$
ASA 🌢 Aspirin, many others	Same as above	PO	Rarely used in children. See Chapter 50 for adverse effects and drug interactions.	$
ibuprofen 🌢 Motrin, Advil, generics	P: 10 mg/kg/dose Q6H A: 400 mg Q4–6H	PO	See Chapter 50 for adverse effects and drug interactions.	$
naproxen 🌢 Naprosyn, generics	P: 5–7.5 mg/kg/d Q12H A: 250 mg Q8H	PO	Available as suspension, 25 mg/mL. See Chapter 50 for adverse effects and drug interactions.	$
ketorolac 🌢 Toradol	Oral: 10 mg Q6–8H IM: 30 mg Q6H	PO, IM	Recommended for short-term use only; IM use not to exceed 5 days. Contraindications, adverse effects and drug interactions are similar to other NSAIDs.	PO: $$ IM: $$$$
codeine generics	P: 1–1.5 mg/kg PO Q4–6H A: 60 mg PO Q4H	PO	Available as 5 mg/mL syrup. Analgesic effect potentiated by combination with NSAIDs, acetaminophen. For adverse effects and drug interactions see Chapter 16.	$
morphine ‡ Statex, MS•IR, M.O.S., generics	IV: P: 0.1–0.2 mg/kg/dose A: 2.5–5 mg/dose PO: P: 0.3 mg/kg/dose Q2–3H A: 30 mg Q3–4H	IV PO	Give repeated small boluses Q10–15 min until patient is comfortable in both pediatric and adult patients. For adverse effects and drug interactions see Chapter 16.	PO: $ IV: $

meperidine ‡ 🐝 Demerol, generics	IV	P: 1–1.5 mg/kg/dose Q2–3H A: 1 mg/kg/dose Q3H	Not recommended for oral administration. Contraindicated in patients with renal impairment and in those using MAOIs.	$
fentanyl ‡ generics	IV	P: 1–3 µg/kg/dose Q1–2H A: 50–100 µg/dose Q1–2H	Titrate to patient comfort.	$$$–$$$$

* This table is not inclusive of all available analgesics nor all available routes.
‡ Use lower doses in debilitated or elderly patients.
🐝 Dosage adjustment may be required in renal impairment – see Appendix I.

Abbreviations: P = pediatric; A = adult; MAOI = monoamine oxidase inhibitor.
† Cost per adult dose (assuming 50-kg patient) – includes drug cost only.
Legend: $ < $0.50 $$ $0.50–1.00 $$$ $1.00–3.00 $$$$ > $3.00

Inhalation

Inhaled **nitrous oxide** is an alternative in some situations involving moderate to severe pain such as childbirth, procedural pain and pre-hospital care of trauma patients. Contraindications to use include impaired level of consciousness (whether from injury or intoxication), hypotension, decompression sickness, pulmonary injury or disease (COPD) and bowel obstruction.

Regional Analgesia

Regional analgesia may reduce the amount of parenteral analgesia necessary for pain control in certain situations (e.g., hematoma block for fracture reduction, nerve block for rib fractures). It has few systemic side effects, excellent pain relief and decreases the need for systemic analgesia. NB: The administration of regional analgesia requires special skills and should be performed by specially trained personnel.

Patient Controlled Analgesia (PCA)

Optimal acute pain management occurs when a steady state concentration of analgesic is maintained. This is best achieved by a continuous infusion of medication with additional boluses given as needed. Opioids are used most commonly in PCA infusion pumps for postoperative pain control. Local anesthetics, either alone or in combination with opioids, can be infused into the epidural space for analgesia. Local anesthetics are used alone to maintain a regional block of peripheral nerves.

PCA requires a special infusion pump that is programmed to deliver a preset amount of drug either by continuous infusion or repeated small boluses. A lockout interval is preset to prevent overadministration. PCA pumps cannot be used in severely ill patients with a decreased level of consciousness. They can be used by children as young as 6 years of age.

Treatment Based on Pain Severity

Mild pain (e.g., otitis media, pharyngitis, simple lacerations, scrapes, minor sprains and strains, musculoskeletal pain) is usually treated with oral analgesics such as acetaminophen, ASA or NSAIDs.

Moderate pain (e.g., mild pain not responding to usual therapy, sprains and strains, fractures, burns, minor surgical conditions) may be treated orally with codeine or morphine alone or in combination with acetaminophen, ASA or NSAIDs. IV analgesia with an opioid may be required acutely; IM analgesia is painful, and absorption can be variable. Treatment with combination agents in children is limited by the amount of acetaminophen or NSAID in the preparation.

If **procedural** pain (e.g., fracture reduction) is anticipated, regional anesthesia should be used with IV analgesia and sedation

meperidine ‡ 🍂 Demerol, generics	P: 1–1.5 mg/kg/dose Q2–3H A: 1 mg/kg/dose Q3H	IV	Not recommended for oral administration. Contraindicated in patients with renal impairment and in those using MAOIs.	$
fentanyl ‡ generics	P: 1–3 µg/kg/dose Q1–2H A: 50–100 µg/dose Q1–2H	IV	Titrate to patient comfort.	$$$–$$$$

This table is not inclusive of all available analgesics nor all available routes.
‡ *Use lower doses in debilitated or elderly patients.*
🍂 *Dosage adjustment may be required in renal impairment – see Appendix I.*

Abbreviations: P = pediatric; A = adult; MAOI = monoamine oxidase inhibitor.
† *Cost per adult dose (assuming 50-kg patient) – includes drug cost only.*
Legend: $ < $0.50 $$ $0.50–1.00 $$$ $1.00–3.00 $$$$ > $3.00

Inhalation

Inhaled **nitrous oxide** is an alternative in some situations involving moderate to severe pain such as childbirth, procedural pain and pre-hospital care of trauma patients. Contraindications to use include impaired level of consciousness (whether from injury or intoxication), hypotension, decompression sickness, pulmonary injury or disease (COPD) and bowel obstruction.

Regional Analgesia

Regional analgesia may reduce the amount of parenteral analgesia necessary for pain control in certain situations (e.g., hematoma block for fracture reduction, nerve block for rib fractures). It has few systemic side effects, excellent pain relief and decreases the need for systemic analgesia. NB: The administration of regional analgesia requires special skills and should be performed by specially trained personnel.

Patient Controlled Analgesia (PCA)

Optimal acute pain management occurs when a steady state concentration of analgesic is maintained. This is best achieved by a continuous infusion of medication with additional boluses given as needed. Opioids are used most commonly in PCA infusion pumps for postoperative pain control. Local anesthetics, either alone or in combination with opioids, can be infused into the epidural space for analgesia. Local anesthetics are used alone to maintain a regional block of peripheral nerves.

PCA requires a special infusion pump that is programmed to deliver a preset amount of drug either by continuous infusion or repeated small boluses. A lockout interval is preset to prevent overadministration. PCA pumps cannot be used in severely ill patients with a decreased level of consciousness. They can be used by children as young as 6 years of age.

Treatment Based on Pain Severity

Mild pain (e.g., otitis media, pharyngitis, simple lacerations, scrapes, minor sprains and strains, musculoskeletal pain) is usually treated with oral analgesics such as acetaminophen, ASA or NSAIDs.

Moderate pain (e.g., mild pain not responding to usual therapy, sprains and strains, fractures, burns, minor surgical conditions) may be treated orally with codeine or morphine alone or in combination with acetaminophen, ASA or NSAIDs. IV analgesia with an opioid may be required acutely; IM analgesia is painful, and absorption can be variable. Treatment with combination agents in children is limited by the amount of acetaminophen or NSAID in the preparation.

If **procedural** pain (e.g., fracture reduction) is anticipated, regional anesthesia should be used with IV analgesia and sedation with a benzodiazepine as necessary. The IV route is preferred because it allows titration of dose until the desired effect is achieved and provides venous access should reversal of either the narcotic or benzodiazepine be necessary. Inhaled nitrous oxide is an alternative to IV analgesia for moderate to severe pain associated with procedures and can be safely used for patients of a sufficient age to cooperate with its use.

Severe pain (e.g., moderate pain not responding to usual therapy, renal colic, trauma, burns, fractures, postoperative) requires aggressive management with IV opioids as the simplest way to achieve patient comfort. The opioids can be given in small boluses until the patient is comfortable. Hemodynamic and respiratory status should be watched closely during adminis- tration. Inhaled nitrous oxide is an alternative in some situations including childbirth, procedural pain and pre-hospital care of trauma patients.

The analgesic effects of opioids are potentiated by combination with other pain management techniques.

Therapeutic Tips

- Measure pain severity and treat the pain experienced, not the pain expected.
- Specific agents (e.g., glyceryl trinitrate for cardiac ischemic pain) are preferable to analgesics.
- A **pain-free** route with predictable absorption for analgesia administration should always be chosen; oral or IV routes are preferred over SC or IM injections.
- Whichever route is chosen, an **appropriate amount of time** for the drug to be effective must be allowed; even IV administration requires 5 to 10 minutes for peak effect.

Suggested Reading List

Acute Pain Management Guideline Panel. *Acute pain management: operative or medical procedures and trauma.* Clinical Practice Guideline. AHCPR Publ. No. 92-0032. Rockville, MD: Agency for Health Care Policy and Research, Public Health Service, U.S. Department of Health and Human Services, February 1992.

Schechter NL, ed. Acute pain in children. *Pediatr Clin North Am* 1989;36:781–794.

Stewart RD. Nitrous oxide sedation/analgesia in emergency medicine. *Ann Emerg Med* 1985;14:139–148.

Yaster M, Tobin JR, Fisher QA, et al. Local anesthetics in the management of acute pain in children. *J Pediatr* 1994;124:165–176.

CHAPTER 14

Chronic Nonmalignant Pain

Eldon Tunks, MD, FRCPC

Goals of Therapy

- To define and treat medical and psychological factors associated with chronic pain according to evidence-based principles
- To promote or restore healthy behavior, fitness, and appropriate role functions
- To prevent or minimize work absence

Investigations

- History for:
  - current pain and function, pre-existing pain, disability, headache, analgesic intake, psychological distress (especially anxiety, depression), adversarial factors (e.g., compensation, family problems)
  - particularly with headache, self-monitoring may be useful to determine headache patterns and associated factors
- Physical examination:
  - to determine if other treatable causes are present
- Laboratory tests:
  - where indicated by physical examination to rule out underlying disease
- Psychological testing may be helpful in some cases

Therapeutic Choices

Nonpharmacologic Choices

Treatment should include simultaneous use of appropriate nonpharmacologic and pharmacologic treatments and detoxification if needed. Multidisciplinary chronic pain programs combine withdrawal of excessive analgesics and sedatives, treatment of depression, nonpharmacologic treatments (e.g., exercise, pacing, improving body mechanics) and psychological treatments (e.g., patient education, family intervention, relaxation therapies, coping skills training and goal setting). In some areas, "Early Intervention Units" have been established for workers whose return to the workplace is delayed unduly by persistent pain or coping problems.

Figure 1: **Management of Chronic Nonmalignant Pain**

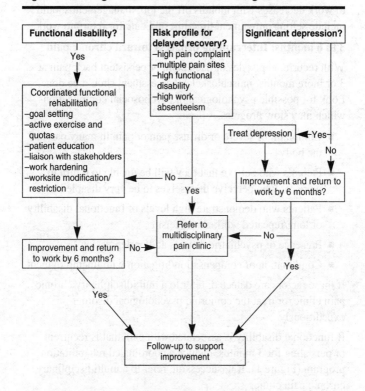

Pharmacologic Choices

Chronic pain syndromes differ in response to various analgesic agents, depending on pain mechanisms. Nonmalignant chronic pain may be treated effectively with analgesics with or without opioids when the physician knows the patient and any history of substance abuse, addiction, drug escalation or a compliance problem (Table 2, Chapter 15). The analgesic should be effective for the pain condition in a low to moderate dosage, improve function and quality of life; otherwise, it should be discontinued. For chronic pain, longer-acting drugs are preferred.

Chronic Back Pain (Figure 1)

0 to 30 days: Promoting early recovery (Chapter 48)

30 to 90 days: Restoring function

Providing information about the usually benign history of low back pain and treatment options, generally improves patient adherence in the recovery process. Active exercise is more beneficial than passive treatment or bed rest. Probability of return to work decreases with months off the job; management should include setting a treatment time-line and date for return to work.

3 to 6 months: Interrupting progress toward chronic pain

With recurrent episodes of back pain, or persistent back pain at 3 or more months, musculoskeletal assessment should be done. Look for possible psychological or psychosocial complications which may slow progress.

- Complaint of severe or diffuse pain or pain in many parts of the body
- Patients who believe that they will be unable to return to work, or who perceive themselves to be very disabled
- Patients who demonstrate high levels of functional disability or long/repeated work absenteeism
- Presence of psychiatric distress and/or depression
- Combination of compensation/litigation with unemployment

If these factors are detected, refer to a multidisciplinary chronic pain clinic, or treat the comorbid psychological disorder expeditiously.

If functional disability is associated with pain that is recurrent or persisting for 3 months, include a coordinated rehabilitation program (Figure 1). If unsuccessful, refer to a multidisciplinary chronic pain clinic.

Persistent pain after 6 months or more

Multidisciplinary chronic pain clinics which include active exercise, functional restoration, patient goal-setting, patient education, and training in coping skills are more efficacious by this point than passive physiotherapy, injections, biofeedback, prescription medications, back school or patient education, unless an active exercise component is included.

Engaging the patient to actively collaborate in setting treatment goals and quotas and in monitoring progress is a key ingredient.

Recurrent or persistent problems after multidisciplinary chronic pain clinic programs

Patients who have "failed" treatment in a comprehensive chronic pain program will not usually benefit from further attempts at the same thing unless barriers to progress are identified and corrected. Barriers include: an Axis I disorder (especially major depression, dysthymia, or anxiety disorder); a significant attitude problem (such as unwillingness to set goals for change "despite pain"); underlying medical/surgical problem.

Therapeutic Tips

About 30% of chronic pain sufferers have comorbid depression, anxiety, or dysthymia, often "masked" by the pain presentation. To reveal the underlying mood disorder, inquire about insomnia, nightmares, panic spells, persistent fearfulness, poor concentration, lack of enjoyment, irritability, passive suicidal thoughts. Comorbid depression often responds to treatment using antidepressants, with improvement in coping with pain. Antidepressants may have an analgesic or coanalgesic effect, even when depression is not a diagnosis (Table 1).

Chronic Headache (Figure 1)

The foregoing also applies to treatment of chronic headache, with some additional considerations.

Chronic headache occurs continuously for 3 days or more per week, for 6 months or more. Although most patients have a previous history of migraine which has gradually "transformed" into a chronic daily headache, some began with tension or post-traumatic headaches. In the majority of cases, chronic overuse of abortive medication (ergotamine, ASA or acetaminophen with caffeine, barbiturate, opioid, or even excessive prolonged use of nonprescription preparations of acetaminophen) is an important cause. In patients dependent on mixed analgesics, the majority will improve significantly within a few days or weeks of ceasing the abuse. Many will require the addition of prophylactic medications as analgesics are withdrawn. These may be introduced singly or in combination (Chapter 11). **Beta-blockers** (e.g., propranolol, metoprolol), tricyclic **antidepressants** and other antidepressants, **calcium channel blockers** (e.g., verapamil, flunarizine), and sometimes **NSAIDs** (e.g., naproxen) are effective in chronic headache prophylaxis.

Because patients often present initially in a great deal of distress, it may be necessary to taper and stop the analgesic while introducing prophylactic medication, or to use **dihydroergotamine** (IV, IM, or inhaled) or **corticosteroids** (IV or oral) in order to break the headache cycle. It is sometimes necessary to arrange a short-term admission to hospital to ensure that oral intake of abortive medication has stopped, there is compliance with the prophylactic regime and emotional support is available to the patient.

The majority of chronic headache can be managed in the primary care setting. If psychosocial risk factors are present or the patient fails to respond to appropriate management after 3 to 6 months, consider referral to a multidisciplinary chronic pain clinic. Depression should be treated.

Table 1: Antidepressants Used in Chronic Pain*

Drug	Applications in Pain	Dosage	Main Adverse Effects†	Drug Interactions	Cost‡
Tricyclics *amitriptyline* Elavil, generics *doxepin* Sinequan, generics *clomipramine* Anafranil, generics *desipramine* Pertofrane, Norpramin, generics *imipramine* Tofranil, generics	Chronic headache Diabetic neuropathy Postherpetic neuralgia Atypical facial pain Chronic fibromyalgia Pain with depression	**Amitriptyline, clomipramine, doxepin or imipramine** Begin 10–25 mg QHS, ↑ by 10–25 mg QHS weekly until effect. For chronic pain 25–75 mg QHS may be effective; for depression higher doses may be needed. **Desipramine** Begin 10 mg – QAM may be preferable. Eventual dosage 25–75 mg.	Hypotension, dry mouth, blurred vision, drowsiness, confusion, weight gain, agitation, nightmares, lowered seizure threshold, constipation, urinary retention, ECG changes. Pregnancy/lactation – safety not established.	Guanethidine: inhibition of antihypertensive effect. Cimetidine: ↑ serum levels of tricyclics. Alcohol: excess sedation. MAOIs: contraindicated. Anticholinergics, sympathomimetics: additive effects. SSRIs: ↑ serum levels of TCA.	$ $ $ $ $
Monoamine Oxidase Inhibitors *phenelzine* Nardil	Atypical facial pain^π Headache with depression^π	Begin 15 mg/d, ↑ by 15 mg weekly; 60–75 mg/d may be needed in some cases. QAM dosage usually preferable – dose may be split to ↓ side effects.	Dizziness, hypotension, drowsiness, insomnia, elevated liver transaminase, precipitation of mania.	Contraindicated with reserpine, meperidine, SSRIs, TCAs, levodopa. Can cause hypertensive crisis with sympathomimetics. Restrict vasopressor-containing foods (e.g., dopamine, tyramine, caffeine); follow MAOI diet.	$$–$$$

	Use	Dosing	Side Effects	Interactions/Contraindications	Cost[‡]
Selective Serotonin Reuptake Inhibitors *fluoxetine* Prozac, generic *fluvoxamine* Luvox, generic *paroxetine* Paxil *sertraline* Zoloft	Chronic headache[π] Pain with depression[π]	Morning or evening may be appropriate, depending on drowsiness or insomnia. Take with food. **Fluoxetine or paroxetine** 20–60 mg/d. **Fluvoxamine or sertraline** 50–200 mg/d.	Headache, gastric pain, diarrhea, nervousness, insomnia, nausea, drowsiness (side effects ↑ with dose). Pregnancy/lactation – safety not established.	MAOIs: contraindicated. Other antidepressants: blood levels may greatly ↑. May interfere with protein-bound drugs. Astemizole and terfenadine: contraindicated.	$$–$$$$ $–$$$$ $$$–$$$$$ $$$–$$$$$
Heterocyclics *maprotiline* Ludiomil, generic	Neuralgia[π]	Evening or morning dose. Begin 10 mg/d, ↑ by 25 mg weekly. Eventual dosage range 25–200 mg.	Dry mouth, drowsiness, blurred vision, constipation, headache, nervousness, lowered seizure threshold. Pregnancy/lactation – safety not established.	MAOIs: contraindicated. May block effect of antihypertensive drugs (e.g., clonidine, methyldopa). Additive effects with sympathomimetics, anticholinergics.	$–$$$
Others *trazodone* Desyrel, generics	Pain with insomnia and depression[π]	Start 50 mg/d, ↑ by 50–100 mg weekly. May be used QHS or daytime in divided doses.	Drowsiness, nausea, dry mouth, headache, nasal stuffiness, priapism. Pregnancy/lactation – safety not established.	May ↑ digoxin and phenytoin levels.	$–$$

*Drugs were chosen on the basis of an established literature of controlled trials. However, other antidepressants may also be effective; this is not intended to restrict use of other drugs.
π Literature is limited.

† See Gillis MC, ed. Compendium of Pharmaceuticals and Specialties (CPS). Ottawa: Canadian Pharmacists Association, 1998, for complete list of adverse effects.
‡ Cost of 30-day supply – includes drug cost only.
Legend: $ < $20 $$ $20–40 $$$ $40–60 $$$$ $60–80 $$$$$ > $80

Therapeutic Tips

Patients often declare that all prophylactic drugs have failed.

- First, determine whether adequate doses were used consistently for a sufficient time, and whether the patient continued to use OTC or abortive medications during the trial.

- Alcohol abuse may be an important factor, and in resistant headache, should be considered a possibility.

- It may be worthwhile to try some of the prophylactic regimes again if previous trials were insufficient, or contaminated with concurrent OTC use or alcohol abuse.

Note that Neuralgias are discussed in Chapter 15.

Suggested Reading List

Basmajian JV, Banerjee SN, eds. *Clinical Decision Making in Rehabilitation*. New York: Churchill Press, 1996.

Bigos SJ, Bowyer O, Braen G, et al. *Acute low back problems in adults*. Clinical Practice Guide Number 14. AHCPR Publication No. 95–0642. Rockville, MD: Agency for Health Care Policy and Research, Public Service, U.S. Dept. of Health and Human Services. December 1994.

Lane NE, Wolfe F, eds. Musculoskeletal Medicine. *Rheum Dis Clin North Am* 1996;22(3).

Saper JR, et al. *Handbook of headache management: A practical guide to diagnosis and treatment of head, neck, and facial pain*. Baltimore: Williams and Wilkins, 1993.

Sternbach RA. *Mastering pain. A twelve step program for coping with chronic pain*. New York: Ballantyne Books, 1987.

Tunks E, Bellissimo A. *Behavioral medicine: concepts and procedures*. New York: Pergamon Press, 1991.

CHAPTER 15

Neuralgia

C. Peter N. Watson MD, FRCPC
Eldon Tunks MD, FRCPC

Neuralgia implies pain in the distribution of a nerve or group of nerves. Common usage suggests a paroxysmal, brief, lancinating quality. Only specific, more common types of peripheral neuropathic (nerve injury) pain are dealt with here.

Goals of Therapy

- To diagnose lesions causing neuropathy that may require surgery (herniated discs and tumors) by appropriate imaging (CT and MR)
- To reduce pain from severe or moderate to mild and tolerable. It is important that both patient and physician understand that total pain relief is not realistic for most of these difficult problems.
- To balance pain relief against acceptable side effects
- To plan gradual drug withdrawal after initial control of pain (which may resolve spontaneously, e.g., postherpetic neuralgia)

Investigations

- History for:
  - the temporal profile and characteristics of the pain
  - depression, insomnia, disability and previous treatments
  - history of chemical dependency, especially if opioids are considered
- Physical examination:
  - to determine areas of sensory loss (hypoesthesia) and skin sensitivity characteristic of neuralgia, i.e., causalgia, allodynia, hyperpathia, hyperalgesia[1]
  - to determine other neurological findings which might indicate a progressive lesion requiring imaging and surgery
  - to determine concurrent conditions that contribute to the pain problem, e.g., metabolic, vascular, myofascial, psychogenic

---

[1]*Causalgia – a burning pain due to injury of a peripheral nerve.*
Allodynia – pain resulting from a non-noxious stimulus to normal skin.
Hyperpathia – abnormally exaggerated subjective response to painful stimuli.
Hyperalgesia – abnormally increased pain sense.

Figure 1: **Pharmacologic Management of Neuralgia**

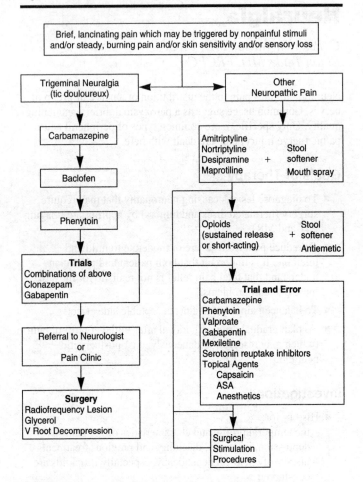

- Other investigations:
  - imaging with CT or MR scanning if a space-occupying lesion is suspected
  - diagnostic sympathetic blockade if reflex sympathetic dystrophy (complex regional pain syndrome) is suspected
  - during pharmacotherapy, blood levels help to assess compliance and guide dosage

Therapeutic Choices

Acute Neuralgia – Herpes Zoster (HZ)

The varicella-zoster virus, dormant in dorsal root ganglia, is reactivated by such factors as trauma, decreased immunological competence and lymphoma. HZ occurs more commonly in persons over age 50. Severe pain, stabbing and dysesthesia are soon followed by vesicular eruption in the affected dermatomes (thoracic dermatomes in about 50% of cases, and cranial in about 15%). Motor deficits occur in more severe cases. When it affects the forehead, observation for eye complications is essential.

The risk of chronic postherpetic neuralgia increases with age and with severity of the eruption. Early treatment of HZ may reduce the incidence of postherpetic neuralgia. Antivirals (**acyclovir**, **valacyclovir** and **famciclovir**) are most effective if started within 72 hours of the onset of the pain. Even if the rash has not appeared, the sudden appearance of severe, acute neuropathic pain unilaterally in the forehead or thoracic area in an individual over age 60 is a reasonable basis to initiate an antiviral drug since these agents are safe and well tolerated. Valacyclovir or famciclovir may be preferred for reasons of efficacy, compliance and cost.

Concurrently with instituting an antiviral agent, it is important to relieve the acute pain. This may be accomplished with **opioids** if necessary, nerve blocks, and early treatment with **amitriptyline**.

Recurrent Neuralgia – Trigeminal Neuralgia (TN)
(Figure 1)

TN is confined to the face and shows a predilection for the 2nd or 3rd trigeminal divisions. Always unilateral, it generally afflicts persons over the age of 50, and often follows a remitting course. It may occur with other craniofacial neuralgias. TN usually responds very well to therapy with **carbamazepine** (CBZ) (Table 1), which should be slowly increased to 400 to 800 mg/day in divided doses, until good control is obtained, unless there are intolerable side effects. The sustained-release form may improve compliance, lessen untoward effects and provide a more sustained effect. Blood levels are a useful guide to compliance and dose increments.

Other pharmacologic approaches are far inferior to CBZ. Therefore if some relief is achieved with CBZ but side effects are unacceptable, a good strategy is to reduce the dosage to toler-ability and add **baclofen**, beginning at 10 mg/day, and slowly increase. Should this fail, add **phenytoin** or replace baclofen with phenytoin. **Clonazepam**, **valproate** and **gabapentin** may be tried if other strategies fail.

Should medical therapy fail, neurosurgical options, e.g., decom-pression of the gasserian ganglion, or ablative procedures to the gasserian ganglion have a high success rate in experienced hands.

Chronic Neuralgia

The following conditions are grouped together because the pharmacologic approaches are similar.

Nerve Root Compression: Cervical and Lumbar Radiculopathy

Although the great majority of low back pains and sciatic pains are not attributable to herniated disc and compromised nerve roots, occasionally disc material is extruded through the ligamentum flavum, and this sequestrum, or less likely the bulging disc itself, causes nerve root compression (cervical and lumbar radiculopathies). In the acute phase, anti-inflammatories (**NSAIDs**) are effective. Where necessary, additional pain relief is achieved with strong **opioids** (Table 1), an appropriate regimen of rest and avoidance of further aggravation. This pain often settles with conservative management. Consider surgical treatment: if medical treatment fails over 6 to 12 weeks and if neuroimaging with CT or MR shows a surgically treatable lesion; if acute pain is excruciating and intractable; if a neurological deficit and a correctable lesion are present. Signs of a progressive neurological deficit should prompt surgical consultation as early as possible. Investigation is needed if pain does not resolve within a reasonable time frame, or if this is the first episode in an elderly person (because of possible malignancy or other serious illnesses).

Complex Regional Pain Syndrome (CRPS)

CRPS is the new term for reflex sympathetic dystrophy (RSD) or sympathetically-maintained pain. CRPS is described by causalgia, neurovascular and dystrophic changes and may result from penetrating or crush injuries to nerve but sometimes from other causes such as stroke or myocardial infarction. Charac-teristics include aching, burning, causalgic pain, hyperalgesia, hyperpathia and allodynia, sweating, rubor, and coldness of the limb.

If symptoms persist, after a few months one may see widening of the painful area, cool cyanotic skin, a glossy appearance to the skin with the odor of sweat, decreased hair growth, and progressive loss of function.

Some will go on to dystrophic changes, osteoporosis, nail changes, subcutaneous thinning with pointed digits, and further loss of function with contractures or frozen shoulder, with continued severe pain. A larger proportion of chronic cases lose the neurovascular picture and end up with more of a chronic diffuse myofascial pain with poor function.

While RSD was thought to be due to sympathetic overactivity, evidence now points to a disorder of upregulation of adrenergic

Table 1: **Drugs Used in Neuropathic Pain**

Drug	Dosage	Adverse Effects	Cost*
Antidepressants	Begin 10–25 mg QHS. Increase by same dose weekly to relief or side effects. Give with mouth spray and stool softener. Caution re: weight gain.	dry mouth constipation drowsiness blurred vision urine retention (in elderly male) weight gain confusion	
amitriptyline Elavil, generics			$
desipramine Norpramin, generics			$
nortriptyline Aventyl, generics			$
maprotiline Ludiomil, generics			$
Anticonvulsants			
carbamazepine Tegretol, generics Tegretol CR	Start with 100 mg 2–3 × day. Increase by 100 mg every few days to side effects or relief. Blood levels may be guide to compliance and dosage increases. Consider controlled-release preparations.	drowsiness ataxia dizziness nausea hyponatremia	$ $$
phenytoin Dilantin	100–300 mg QHS. Depending on age. Blood levels may guide therapy and assess compliance (therapeutic range 40–80 μmol/L).	ataxia drowsiness nausea	$
Baclofen Lioresal, generics	Start 10 mg BID. Maximum 20 mg TID.	drowsiness	$$–$$$
Opioids	Start low and go slow (starting dose and increments)		
oxycodone Percocet, Percodan, OxyContin, generics	5–10 mg Q6H	nausea (antiemetic) constipation (stool softener) drowsiness (reduce dose)	$
morphine MS Contin, M-Eslon	10–15 mg Q12H		$$–$$$
hydromorphone Dilaudid, Hydromorph Contin	1–2 mg Q6H		$ $$$
fentanyl patch Duragesic	25 μg/h Q 3 days		$8.50 per patch

* *Legend: Cost of 1-day supply – includes drug cost only*
$ < $0.50 $$ $0.50–1.00 $$$ $1.00–1.50.

receptors. Although sympathetic blocks often provide temporary relief, sympathectomy does not necessarily result in permanent resolution. Bier blocks using guanethidine are ineffective. Physical therapy, corticosteroids, sympathectomies and repeated sympathetic blocks have limited success. At follow-up, two-thirds are likely to have continued pain, and only about one-quarter return to fully normal activity. Some of these patients may require chronic opioid therapy.

Postherpetic Neuralgia (PHN) and Other Chronic Peripheral Neuropathic Pain Such as Diabetic Neuropathy and Phantom Limb Pain

Tricyclic antidepressants (Table 1) are the only proven therapy for PHN. The standard therapy is **amitriptyline**. If this fails, then **nortriptyline**, **desipramine** and **maprotiline** may be tried in sequence as some patients may respond better to one of these agents. A stool softener and mouth spray of artificial saliva will pre-empt the common side effects of constipation and dry mouth. If pain is severe, **opioid** therapy (Table 1) may be prescribed. Extensive evidence shows that psychological dependence, tolerance and physical dependence are not major problems when opioids are used for chronic, severe, nonmalignant pain. Guidelines are suggested in Table 2.

All other treatments, such as topical **capsaicin** or **SSRI anti-depressants**, are scientifically unproven or of modest efficacy. However, a trial and error approach may be helpful in refractory patients for a possible analgesic response, placebo benefit,

Table 2: Guidelines for Opioid Therapy of Nonmalignant Pain

1. Consider after other reasonable therapies have failed.

2. Perform a complete pain and psychosocial history and physical examination. A history of substance abuse, tension-type headaches and pain that appears largely determined by psychologic factors is a relative contraindication to the use of opioid therapy.

3. A single physician who sets up a contract with the patient should be responsible for opioid prescriptions. The agreement should specify the drug regimen, possible side effects, the functional restoration program and that violations will result in the abrupt termination of opioid therapy.

4. The opioid analgesic of choice should be administered around the clock without a provision of "rescue doses" for breakthrough pain. Drug administration should include a titration phase to minimize side effects. If a graded analgesic response to incremental doses is not observed, the patient may not be opioid-responsive and opioid treatment should probably be terminated.

5. The patient should be seen monthly for the first few months and every two months thereafter. At each visit the patient should be assessed for analgesia, opioid-related side effects, compliance with functional goals and presence of aberrant drug-related behavior.

6. The goal of opioid therapy is to make the pain tolerable. For some patients with nonmalignant pain (i.e., postherpetic neuralgia), the administration of an opioid analgesic can make the difference between bearable and unbearable pain.

general antidepressant effect, while waiting for the possibility of spontaneous pain resolution and for psychological support.

Surgical treatment has no role in PHN in the majority of patients.

Therapeutic Tips

- While patients frequently say they have used amitriptyline or carbamazepine or other agents, these drugs have often been used in too high or too low a dose and for too short a period of time. It is useful to re-institute these drugs according to the guidelines (start low, go slow, increase to side effects or relief, treat side effects if possible).

- Be sure the patient understands the goals of therapy: reduction in pain from moderate or severe, to mild at the price of some side effects, which may be tolerable or treatable.

- A rating scale, such as a scale of 0 to 10 where 0 is no pain and 10 the worst pain imaginable, may be used to evaluate pain relief.

- After a period of relief of 1 to 3 months it may be possible to reduce or stop the drugs. Gradual reduction is preferable.

- If opioids are used, guidelines are important and should be worked through with the patient (Table 2).

- A trial and error approach of scientifically unproven treatments is reasonable if standard therapy fails.

- Repeated visits can provide important psychological support and hope for desperate patients as trial and error approaches are also utilized.

- If chronic neuralgia is being managed in general practice, semi-annual or annual visits with a pain specialist help to provide support to the family practitioner for contentious approaches such as opioids, as well as the chance of a novel therapy for the patient.

Suggested Reading List

Merskey H, Bogduk N. *Classification of Chronic Pain.* 2nd ed. Seattle: IASP Press, 1994.

Fromm GH, Sessle BJ, eds. *Trigeminal neuralgia.* Stoneham: Butterworth-Heinmann, 1991.

Watson CPN, ed. Herpes zoster and postherpetic neuralgia. New York: Elsevier, 1994.

Moulin DE. Opioid analgesics for chronic nonmalignant pain. The Canadian Journal of CME, February 1996.

CHAPTER 16

Pain Control in Palliative Care

Elizabeth J. Latimer, MD, CCFP, FCFP

Palliative care is the active and compassionate care of the patient when the goals of cure and prolongation of life are no longer paramount.

Goals of Therapy

- To relieve pain and other symptoms while maintaining as alert a sensorium as possible
- To support patient and family
- To enhance the quality of life remaining

Investigations

- A careful **pain history** and **physical examination** to determine the nature, etiology and severity of the pain (Figure 1)
  - *neuropathic pain* is often described as burning or hot (dysesthetic) or shooting and electric shock-like (lancinating)
  - *bone pain* is aching and may increase on movement
  - *liver capsular stretch* is a deep aching that may be referred to the shoulder and have a pleuritic component
  - if able, the patient should **quantify** the pain on a 0–5 scale (5 being the worst pain imaginable and 1 being minimal)
  - the level of pain at the time of analgesic dosing, the level of pain relief achieved at maximum effect and the duration of the best relief achieved should be noted
- A detailed **medication history**
- **Laboratory tests:** minimum required for diagnosis

Therapeutic Choices (Figure 1)

Nonpharmacologic Choices

- **Team approach** to total patient care (physical, emotional, spiritual).
- **Relaxation and imagery** to enhance well-being.
- **Physical and occupational therapy** to maximize function and reduce strain.

Figure 1: **Approach to Pain Management**

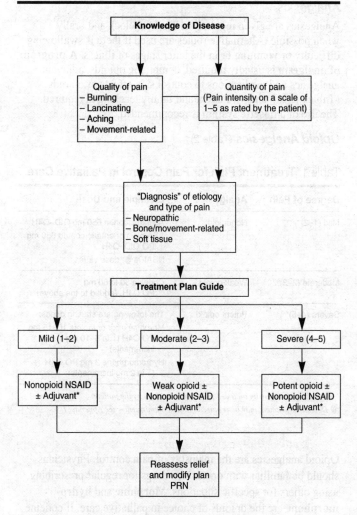

* Depending on etiology and quality of pain, appropriate adjuvant (tricyclic antidepressant, anticonvulsant, corticosteroid) is added (Table 4).

- **Disease-directed treatment** to enhance symptom control e.g., radiotherapy (bone pain, tumor pressure), chemotherapy (generalized bone pain), antibiotics (infection) anticholinergics (troublesome secretions), antianginals (ischemic cardiovascular pain).

- **Transcutaneous nerve stimulation** for pain relief.

- **Acupuncture and hypnosis** for pain and other symptoms and general distress.

Pharmacologic Choices (Table 1)
Analgesics

Analgesics are given regularly around the clock and orally when possible. Alternative routes are used if there is swallowing difficulty or vomiting or in the latter stages of illness. A **program of analgesia** is usually required, combining opioids, adjuvant analgesics and medications to control side effects of opioids (Tables 1, 2, 3 and 4). Patient and family teaching is required. The use of a **dosette system** is recommended.

Opioid Analgesics (Table 2)

Table 1: Treatment Plan for Pain Control in Palliative Care

Degree of Pain	Analgesic	Example and Dose
Mild (1–2)*	Nonopioid	Acetaminophen 650 mg QID–Q4H
		ASA plain or enteric-coated 650 mg PO QID–Q4H
		NSAIDs🌑: dose varies
Moderate (2–3)*	Weak opioid	Codeine 30 to 60 mg PO Q4H (added to the above)
Severe (4–5)*	Potent opioid	The following are starting doses:
		Morphine elixir or tablets 10–15 mg PO Q4H (↑ in 5–10 mg increments)
		Hydromorphone 2 mg PO Q4H (↑ in 2 mg increments)

* Refers to pain intensity on a 0–5 point scale as rated by the patient.
🌑 *Dosage adjustment may be required in renal impairment – see Appendix I.*

Opioid analgesics are the mainstay of pain control. Physicians should be familiar with one or two drugs for regular prescribing, using others for specific situations. **Morphine** and **hydromorphone** are the opioids of choice in palliative care. If codeine phosphate 60 mg PO Q4H does not relieve pain, morphine 10 to 15 mg or hydromorphone 2 to 4 mg PO Q4H should be started. Because the medication is new to the patient, dosing may be on a Q4H PRN basis for the first 24 hours, then Q4H regularly thereafter.

There is no ceiling dose of opioid analgesics. Dose requirements are highly individual, ranging from a few to several hundred milligrams Q4H; escalation should be titrated against pain relief achieved and level of side effects, particularly sedation. Dramatic or continued increases in analgesic requirements indicate the need to reassess the patient to rule out new complications (e.g., pathological fracture, epidural cord compression). **Initial doses of opioids should be lowered** in patients with impaired renal or hepatic metabolism or those who have not recently been taking potent opioids and who have not developed tolerance to the side effects.

Breakthrough pain should be treated with half the regular dose of analgesic. For example, a regular dose of hydromorphone 16 mg would require a standard order for 8 mg Q2H PRN for breakthrough pain.

Short-acting (4 hour half-life and Q4H dosing) preparations of **morphine** and **hydromorphone** are used to achieve analgesia. Sustained-release formulations (oral, transdermal, or rectal) can follow for ease of dosing. **Transdermal fentanyl** patches are effective for patients who are unable to use oral analgesics. Hydromorphone may cause less confusion in the **elderly** than morphine, and is viewed by some as the drug of choice in this group.[1]

Fortunately, true **morphine allergy** (anaphylaxis) is rare but does occur. Anileridine or fentanyl may be used in this situation. Meperidine can be used but is a poor alternative.

Meperidine is not recommended for regular use in chronic pain because of its short duration of action, poor oral absorption and potential accumulation of the metabolite normeperidine, which can cause CNS excitation and seizures. **Heroin** has no proven superiority over morphine in equianalgesic doses.

Alternative Routes for Opioid Analgesia

Opioids can be given by oral, parenteral, transdermal or rectal routes; match route to individual patient need. **Equivalent doses** are noted in Table 2. Subcutaneous doses are usually given intermittently by butterfly needles inserted subcutaneously. Continuous infusion pumps are required in about 5% of cases (high doses, severe pain problem, need for bolus extra dosing).

If suppositories are not available, individual **rectal doses** can be created by placing oral tablets inside gelatin capsules and inserting rectally.

Use of Adjuvant Analgesics (Table 4)

Particular pain syndromes require special analgesic modalities.

Careful reassessment of relief achieved with appropriate adjustments in therapy is necessary for effective management.

---

[1] *Mayo Clin Proc 1994;69:384–390.*

Table 2: Narcotic Analgesics

Opioid	Equianalgesic Dose	Interval	Dosage Forms	Comments	Cost*
Weak				**For all Opioids**	
codeine various	180–240 mg PO 120 mg SC†	4 h	Oral elixir: 3 mg/mL Tablets: 30, 60 mg Injection: 30, 60 mg/mL Oral combinations with acetaminophen or ASA	**Adverse Effects‡** Nausea and vomiting, constipation, sedation or drowsiness, confusion, psychotomimetic effects, respiratory depression, myoclonus, urinary retention, dry mouth.	$$$
Potent					Soln $$ Tab $ Inj $$ Supp $$$$
morphine M.O.S., MS•IR, Morphitec, Statex, Morphine HP, generics	20–30 mg PO 10–15 mg SC†	4 h	Oral solution: 1, 5, 10, 20, 50 mg/mL Tablets: 5, 10, 15, 20, 25, 30, 40, 50, 60 mg Injection: 2, 10, 15, 50 mg/mL Suppository*: 5, 10, 20, 30 mg	**Drug Interactions** CNS depressants including narcotics, sedatives, tranquilizers, alcohol may ↑ CNS depression. For fentanyl and meperidine: MAO inhibitors.	
morphine (sustained-release) M.O.S.-SR, MS Contin, Oramorph SR, M-Eslon	60–90 mg PO	12 h	SR tablets: 15, 30, 60, 100, 200 mg SR capsules: 10, 30, 60, 100 mg		$$
hydromorphone Dilaudid, Dilaudid-HP, generics	4–6 mg PO 2–3 mg SC†	4 h	Oral solution: 1 mg/mL Tablets: 1, 2, 4, 8 mg Injection: 2, 10, 20, 50 mg/mL Suppository*: 3 mg		$$

fentanyl Duragesic	Based on total daily morphine dose (or equianalgesic dose of other opioid) 100 µg/h patch is approximately equivalent to a total daily morphine dose of 360 mg PO or 180 mg SC† Patch is usually worn for 72 h		Transdermal patch: 25, 50, 75, 100 µg/h		$$$
anileridine Leritine	75 mg PO 25 mg SC†	3–4 h	Tablets: 25 mg Injection: 25 mg/mL	Anileridine and meperidine should not be used routinely because of short duration of action and potential for side effects in higher doses. Main indication use is in case of true morphine allergy.	$$
meperidine Demerol	300 mg PO 75 mg IM, SC†	3–4 h	Tablets: 50 mg Injection: 50, 75, 100 mg/mL		$

† *The SC route is almost always preferred. The IM route is more painful and unnecessary.*
π *Suppository dose is equal to oral dose.*
‡ *See Table 3 for management of adverse effects.*

* *Cost per day of doses equianalgesic to 360 mg/d of oral morphine – includes drug cost only.*
Legend: $ *< $4* $$ *$4–8* $$$ *$8–12* $$$$ *> $12*

Table 3: **Management of Opioid Adverse Effects**

Nausea and vomiting	**Haloperidol** 1–2 mg PO/SC BID–TID (may be given as a single daily dose)
	If persistent, add **metoclopramide** ❥ 10–20 mg PO/SC/IV TID–QID
	If there is a clear vestibular component (motion-type sickness) **dimenhydrinate** 50–100 mg PO/PR Q8H–Q6H or **scopolamine** 0.4 mg SC Q4H
Constipation	Regular doses of stool softener + stimulant laxative (e.g., **docusate** 100–200 mg + **sennosides** 2–3 tablets or **bisacodyl** 10–15 mg PO BID–TID)
	The softener may be replaced with **lactulose** 30 mL BID–TID
	Bisacodyl suppositories, phosphate enemas or oil retention enemas may be required at intervals
	Magnesium hydroxide/mineral oil mixture 30 mL + **cascara** 5 mL daily–BID may be used at intervals in addition to regular regimens
Confusion and/or agitation	**Haloperidol** 1–2 mg PO/SC BID–TID (may be given as a single daily dose)
Multifocal myoclonus	May occur when opioid doses ↑ or clearance ↓ or in presence of other metabolic disturbances. Opioid dose should be ↓ slightly; consider rehydration if appropriate in the clinical context. **Lorazepam** 1–2 mg SL, **midazolam** 0.5–1.0 mg SC Q3–4H PRN (or regularly) or **diazepam** 5 mg PO/PR Q8H–Q6H PRN (or regularly) for myoclonus

❥ *Dosage adjustment may be required in renal impairment – see Appendix I.*

Table 4: **Adjuvant Analgesics**

Type of Pain	Adjuvant
Neuropathic pain *Dysesthetic/ burning pain*	Add tricyclic antidepressant* (**imipramine** or **amitriptyline**) 25 mg PO BID–TID; may ↑ gradually up to 150 mg/d (may be given as a single bedtime dose if tolerated)
Lancinating/ shock-like pain	Add **carbamazepine*** 100–200 mg PO TID–QID
If severe	**Dexamethasone** 4 mg PO/SC/IV TID–QID (may need as much as 24–32 mg/d in some cases)
Bone pain	Add NSAID with cytoprotective agent (e.g., **naproxen** 500 mg PO/PR BID with **misoprostol** 200 µg PO BID)
If severe	**Dexamethasone** 4 mg PO/SC/IV TID–QID (may need as much as 24–32 mg/d in some cases)
Closed space pain	**Dexamethasone** as described above
Pleuritic pain	NSAID as described above

NB: Doses of tricyclics and carbamazepine* **should be lowered by 50% *in frail or elderly patients or in hepatic or renal impairment; dose increments should be made cautiously.*

Suggested Reading List

Doyle D, Hanks GWC, MacDonald N. *Oxford textbook of palliative medicine.* 2nd ed. New York: Oxford University Press, 1998.

Librach SL, Squires BP. *The pain manual: principles and issues in cancer pain management.* Toronto: Pegasus Health Care International, 1997.

CHAPTER 17

Parkinson's Disease

Donald B. Calne, DM, FRCPC

Goals of Therapy

- To start treatment only when symptoms interfere with a patient's social or economic life
- To reduce symptoms to a level that allows the patient to perform usual activities
- To balance benefit against side effects as disease advances
- To manage side effects with nonpharmacologic intervention if possible or, with pharmacologic agents if necessary

Investigations

- History with attention to dopamine-blocking drugs that may cause parkinsonism (e.g., neuroleptics, metoclopramide)
- Neurologic examination with attention to extrapyramidal deficits, disturbances of conjugate ocular gaze, cerebellar signs, pyramidal signs, autonomic deficits and intellectual impairment
- Salient clinical features of idiopathic parkinsonism are tremor, rigidity, bradykinesia, impaired postural reflexes
- Assessment for depressive illness (increased prevalence in patients with Parkinson's disease)
- In atypical young patients, a slit-lamp examination of the eye to exclude Kayser-Fleischer rings (Wilson's disease)
- In atypical patients of any age, a magnetic resonance imaging (MRI) scan of the head or a CT scan if MRI unavailable

Therapeutic Choices

Nonpharmacologic Choices

- The patient should be counseled on maintaining independence and dealing with emotional stress, since anxiety exacerbates symptoms that increase the level of agitation. If the patient has difficulty adjusting, psychiatric help should be sought.
- Rehabilitation services should be consulted for information and advice on safety, posture, energy conservation, speech, swallowing and adaptive devices.
- Moderate exercise is recommended. A physical therapist can suggest suitable activities and community programs.

- Patients should be made aware of local Parkinson's support groups.

Pharmacologic Choices (Table 1)

Levodopa Plus a Decarboxylase Inhibitor

Levodopa combined with a peripheral decarboxylase inhibitor (carbidopa or benserazide) is the cornerstone of treatment. A longer-acting form of levodopa/carbidopa (Sinemet CR) is helpful in patients encountering "wearing-off" reactions. Theoretically, starting therapy with controlled release (CR) levodopa/carbidopa, which provides a more even delivery of levodopa to the brain, may reduce long-term side effects such as dyskinesias and troublesome fluctuations. CR levodopa/carbidopa also tends to cause less nausea and hypotension than standard preparations when starting treatment. Because CR levodopa/carbidopa may be slow to achieve its beneficial effects at the start of the day, it is often helpful to combine the first dose with the more rapidly acting standard preparation.

Dopamine Agonists

Dopamine agonists are added as the disease advances. **Bromo-criptine** stimulates the D_2 receptor, whereas **pergolide** stimulates both the D_1 and the D_2 receptors. There is no convincing evidence that either agonist is better, although patients may have a preference.

Ropinirole and **pramipexole** are new artificial dopamine agonists which activate D_2 and D_3 receptors but have negligible D_1 activity. Neither drug is an ergot derivative, unlike bromo-criptine, pergolide and **cabergoline** (another dopamine agonist not yet available). Therefore, they should be useful in patients who develop pulmonary reactions or erythromelalgia while on ergot congeners.

Selegiline

Selegiline alleviates symptoms in some patients and may delay the need for levodopa. Unfortunately, there is no proof of a neuroprotective action.[1]

COMT Inhibitors

Tolcapone inhibits catechol-O-methyl-transferase (COMT), thereby increasing the plasma half-life of levodopa. It is an adjunct to levodopa and should be useful in patients who have a deterioration in mobility at the end of the interval between doses of levodopa (wearing-off reactions). **Entacapone** is another COMT inhibitor that is in development.

---

[1] *Ann Neurol 1992;32:795–798.*

Table 1: Drugs Used in the Treatment of Parkinson's Disease

Drug	Dosage	Adverse Effects	Drug Interactions	Cost*
Levodopa *levodopa/carbidopa* Sinemet, generics Sinemet CR	**Levodopa/carbidopa (regular) –** **levodopa/benserazide** initial: 50/12.5 mg BID usual: 100/25 mg QID max dose: single 200/50 mg, daily 1 600/400 mg	Nausea, vomiting, orthostatic hypotension, dyskinesias, hallucinations, delusions.	Neuroleptics ↓ effect of levodopa. Antihypertensives, diuretics, tricyclic antidepressants may ↑ hypotensive action.	Sinemet, Prolopa $–$$ Sinemet CR $$$
levodopa/benserazide Prolopa	**Levodopa/carbidopa** **(controlled release)** initial: 100/25 mg BID usual: 200/50 mg QID max dose: single 400/100 mg, daily 2 000/500 mg			
Dopamine Agonists *bromocriptine* Parlodel, generics	initial: 1.25 mg BID usual: 10 mg TID max dose: single 15 mg, daily 60 mg	Nausea, vomiting, orthostatic hypotension, hallucinations, erythromelalgia, pleural effusions (do a baseline chest x-ray before initiating therapy).	Antihypertensives, diuretics, tricyclic antidepressants may ↑ hypotensive action of dopamine agonists.	$$$$
pergolide Permax	initial: 0.05 mg daily usual: 1 mg TID max dose: single 1.5 mg, daily 6 mg			$$$$
pramipexole Mirapex	initial: 0.125 mg TID usual: not yet established max: 4.5 mg/d	Orthostatic hypotension, somnolence, insomnia, hallucinations, dyskinesia, nausea.	↑ Levodopa levels.	$$$$†
ropinirole Requip	initial: 0.25 mg TID usual: not yet established max: 24 mg/d	Orthostatic hypotension, hallucinations, nausea, headache, somnolence.		$$$–$$$$‡

Drug	Dose	Adverse Effects	Drug Interactions	Cost
selegiline (deprenyl) Eldepryl, generics	initial: 2.5 mg BID usual: 5 mg BID Give before 1 p.m.	Insomnia.	Avoid use with meperidine, dextromethorphan, SSRIs and dextroamphetamine.	$$
tolcapone Tasmar	initial: 100 mg TID max: 200 mg TID (100 mg TID in cirrhosis)	Dyskinesia, nausea, sleep disorder, anorexia, dystonia, diarrhea, ↑ LFTs.		$$$$–$$$$$
Anticholinergic Agents	usual doses:	Dry mouth, blurred vision, constipation, urinary retention, aggravation of glaucoma, confusion.	Amantadine may ↑ anticholinergic effects.	
trihexyphenidyl Artane, generics	2 mg QID			$
orphenadrine Disipal	50 mg TID			$
benztropine Cogentin, generics	2 mg BID			$
procyclidine Kemadrin, generics	5 mg QID			$
amantadine ● Symmetrel, generics	usual: 100 mg BID	Same as anticholinergics. Also livedo reticularis, ankle edema.	Anticholinergic agents may ↑ effects.	$

● *Dosage adjustment is required in renal impairment – see Appendix I.*
* *Cost of 30-day supply of usual dose – includes drug cost only.*
† *Price based on 0.5 mg TID.*
‡ *Price based on 4–5 mg TID.*
Legend: $ < $50 $$ $50–100 $$$ $100–150 $$$$ $150–200 $$$$$ > $200

Anticholinergic Agents

Trihexyphenidyl, orphenadrine, benztropine or **procyclidine** can be helpful in treating parkinsonian tremor, and sometimes improve rigidity. Unfortunately, they do not alleviate brady-kinesia or akinesia, which become the major problems as Parkinson's disease advances.

Amantadine

Although similar to anticholinergics, it often has a mild but useful effect on tremor, rigidity, bradykinesia and akinesia.

Long-term Management

It has been usual to start treatment with standard levodopa plus carbidopa or benserazide, but increasingly there is a trend to begin therapy with CR levodopa/carbidopa. As deficits increase, most neurologists prefer to add a dopamine agonist since long-term results appear to be more satisfactory with these two categories of drug combined in relatively low dose, rather than one category of drug in high dose. A dopamine agonist is generally indicated when the daily dose of levodopa is in the range of 750 to 1 000 mg for the standard preparations of levodopa plus carbidopa or benserazide, or 1 000 to 1 200 mg for CR carbidopa/levodopa (which has a lower bioavailability).

Surgery

Pallidotomy is now being employed for patients whose parkinsonism cannot be controlled with medications. The procedure is very effective for patients who are encountering substantial dyskinesia as a side effect of levodopa preparations. At present, experience suggests that unilateral pallidotomy has a good risk–benefit trade off but bilateral pallidotomy often leads to serious complications. Current studies suggest that deep brain stimulation may be helpful and relatively safe if surgical treat-ment is necessary on the side opposite a unilateral pallidotomy.

Management of Adverse Effects

Nausea

When starting levodopa or a dopamine agonist the most common adverse effect is nausea, especially when the drug is taken on an empty stomach. Nausea is reduced, and benefit is generally longer if these medications are taken after a snack or a meal. Prophylactic **domperidone** (10 to 20 mg given 30 to 60 minutes before each dose of levodopa or dopamine agonist) is a valuable adjunct against nausea.

The protein content of meals should be spread evenly through the day since a single high-protein intake may interfere with the entry of levodopa into the brain because of competition for transport systems between large neutral amino acids.

Orthostatic Hypotension

Orthostatic hypotension, also a common early management problem, can often be corrected by increasing salt and water intake. Fluids should be restricted after 4:00 p.m. to prevent nocturia. The salt can be well tolerated in small amounts of tomato juice. If necessary, **fludrocortisone** (0.1 to 0.2 mg daily) or occasionally **midodrine** (5 to 30 mg daily) may be given.

Dyskinesias

Dyskinesia is a common late side effect of dopaminomimetic drugs. It is more likely to be precipitated by levodopa than by a dopamine agonist. Reducing the dose of levodopa and increasing the dose of the dopamine agonist is helpful.

Psychiatric Side Effects

Hallucinations and **delusions** are more likely to be caused by dopamine agonists; thus, it is generally helpful to reduce their dosage and increase levodopa. Dopaminomimetics taken late in the day can cause nightmares and vivid dreams. Specialist advice should be sought when psychotic symptoms cannot be managed by reduced medication. Low doses of **clozapine** or **olanzapine** may be helpful.

Confusion caused by antiparkinson drugs should be treated by reducing, and if necessary stopping, in order of priority, selegiline, anticholinergics, amantadine, dopamine agonists and levodopa. Neuroleptics should be avoided.

Fluctuations in Response

CR levodopa/carbidopa is the most helpful preparation in patients who are encountering wearing-off effects. Dopamine agonists are also useful because their duration of action is longer than standard levodopa plus carbidopa or benserazide.

Therapeutic Tips

- Ensure patient understands the drug rationale and plan.
- The doses of antiparkinson drugs should be increased gradually. Sudden changes should be avoided unless there are prominent side effects.
- The patient should be taught to distinguish dyskinesia from tremor, because the history is helpful in guiding the physician's decision on dose adjustments.
- Antihypertensive agents, diuretics or tricyclic antidepressants can exacerbate the hypotensive action of dopaminomimetics.

134 Neurologic Disorders

Suggested Reading List

Calne DB, ed. *Neurodegenerative diseases*. Philadelphia: WB Saunders, 1994.

Calne DB. Treatment of Parkinson's disease. *N Engl J Med* 1993;329:1021–1027.

Fahn S, suppl. ed. Therapy of Parkinson's disease: Four critical issues. *Neurology* 1994;44(suppl 1).

Koller WC, Paulson G, eds. *Therapy of Parkinson's disease*. 2nd ed. New York: Marcel Dekker, Inc., 1995.

CHAPTER 18

Seizures

Adrian R.M. Upton, MB, BChir, LRCP, MRCS, FRCPC

Goals of Therapy

- To control seizure disorder and prevent recurrence (occurs in 20–80% of untreated patients after a single seizure)
- To minimize side effects/teratogenic effects of medications
- To achieve good compliance over a long period
- To return patient to a normal lifestyle (e.g., work, driving, social interaction)
- To withdraw medication eventually with continuing control

Investigations

- Obtain a thorough history with information from witnesses or relatives about the seizure:
  - type of seizure, description and frequency
  - duration/age of onset/change with time
  - precipitating causes, e.g., alcohol, drugs (antidepressants, neuroleptics, etc.), cardiac arrhythmia, flickering lights, poor compliance
  - postictal state, e.g., drowsiness, confusion, behavioral change
  - previous problems, e.g., stroke, head injury, hypoxia, encephalitis, toxic exposure, developmental problems
  - family history
- Physical examination:
  - localizing neurologic signs
  - evidence of trauma
  - skin lesions, e.g., tuberous sclerosis, port wine stain, hyperpigmented or hypopigmented patches
  - retinal changes, e.g., pigment, cherry red spots, atrophy
  - dysmorphic features
  - organomegaly
  - systemic illness, e.g., diabetes, thyroid, cardiac, renal, hepatic dysfunction
  - neurologic changes, e.g., head circumference, cognitive assessment, muscle tone, reflexes, sensory changes, cerebellar findings
  - exclude noncranial factors and nonseizures (Figure 1)

Figure 1: **Management of Seizure Disorders**

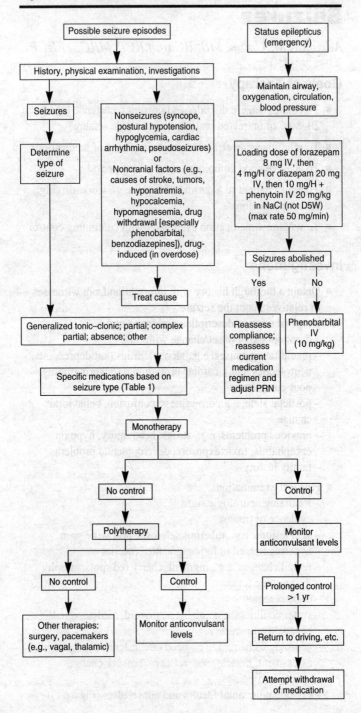

- Laboratory tests:
  - EEG (including in some cases 24-hour portable)
  - CT or MRI scan of head
  - serum albumin

Therapeutic Choices (Figure 1)

Nonpharmacologic Choices

- Avoidance of precipitating factors (see Investigations).
- Regulation of eating and sleeping.
- Reduction of stress or fatigue.
- Biofeedback, relaxation therapy, cognitive therapy.
- In emergency situations support of airway, circulation, blood glucose.

Pharmacologic Choices

Anticonvulsants should be tailored to the seizure disorder (Table 1). For characteristics of drugs used in seizure disorders, see Table 2.

The newer antiepileptics (i.e., gabapentin, lamotrigine, vigabatrin, clobazam) are indicated as adjunctive therapy in patients with refractory seizures. There is increasing evidence that lamotrigine, gabapentin and topiramate may be alternatives to first choice drugs, even for monotherapy.

Table 1: **Drugs for Specific Seizure Types**

Seizure Type	Drug(s)
Generalized tonic–clonic (primary and secondary), focal	Phenytoin, carbamazepine, phenobarbital, valproic acid, lamotrigine
Secondarily generalized seizures	Gabapentin, vigabatrin
Absence (petit mal)	Valproic acid, ethosuximide, phenobarbital
	Adjuncts: vigabatrin, lamotrigine, clobazam, clonazepam
Complex partial, partial	Carbamazepine, phenytoin, phenobarbital, valproic acid, topiramate
	Adjuncts: lamotrigine, gabapentin
Myoclonic	Valproic acid, clonazepam
Status epilepticus	IV diazepam or lorazepam, IV phenytoin, IV phenobarbital
Infantile spasm	ACTH*, corticosteroids (may help)
Unclassified seizures (e.g., neonatal cry, eye movement, jerks, chewing, swimming)	Complex drug regimen

Supplementary drugs: acetazolamide (may be useful in menstrual epilepsy; tolerance develops in weeks), clorazepate (no advantage over other benzodiazepines). Although not available in Canada, felbamate is used in the US; however, the benefits of therapy must be weighed against the risks of aplastic anemia and acute hepatic failure.

* 20–40 units/d or 80 units Q2D IM × 3 mos or until 1 mo after seizures stop.

Available through the Special Access Program (formerly the Emergency Drug Release Program), Therapeutic Products Directorate, Health Canada.

Table 2: Characteristics of Antiepileptic Drugs

Drug/ Usual Adult Dose	Therapeutic Range (μmol/L)	Half-life (hours)	Time to Steady State	Mechanism of Action/ Comments	Side Effects*/ Drug Interactions†	Cost‡
Benzodiazepines						
clobazam Frisium 5–80 mg/d	Not established	10–30 h Metabolite: 36–46 h	2–6 d Metabolite: 7–9 d	Suppresses action potentials. Not for monotherapy. May produce good initial control, followed by recurrence after 6 mos; withdrawal of BDZ associated with ↑ risk of seizure recurrence.	Personality change/aggression, ataxia, tolerance. ↑ side effects when used with other medications, e.g., valproic acid. Alcohol may ↑ levels significantly.	$–$$
clonazepam Rivotril 0.05 mg/kg/d (1.5–10 mg/d)	Not established	22–33 h	14 d			$
carbamazepine Tegretol, generics 20–80 mg/kg/d (800–1 400 mg/d)	Monotherapy: 17–42 Polytherapy: 17–34	8–20 h	3–5 d	Inhibits burst firing. May induce its own metabolism. Up to 40% of patients may experience toxicity if start drug at full dosage; slow titration (↑ by 100 mg/wk) reduces this problem.	Neutropenia (leukocyte count <3.0 × 10⁹/L requires careful monitoring and possible cessation). Weight gain. SIADH.	$
ethosuximide Zarontin 20 mg/kg/d (750–2 000 mg/d)	280–700	20–60 h	5–8 d	Inhibits calcium currents.	Nausea, headache, hiccups. ↓ levels with carbamazepine. ↑ levels with valproic acid.	$–$$

gabapentin ● Neurontin 900–4 800 mg/d	Not established	6–7	1–2 d	Enhances GABA inhibition. Renal excretion; not metabolized.	Drowsiness, dizziness, fatigue, ataxia. Rash (0.54%). Antacids ↓ absorption 20%. No interaction with other anticonvulsants, oral contraceptives. Not significantly bound to plasma proteins.	$–$$$$$
lamotrigine Lamictal 100–500 mg/d	Not established	22–36 h (longer in elderly and Gilbert's syndrome)	5–7 d	Inhibits burst firing.	Headache, nausea, vomiting, dizziness, ataxia, tremor, diplopia. Rash (3–5%). May require cessation of therapy. No interaction with oral contraceptives and warfarin. Shorter $t_{1/2}$ (15–29 h) with carbamazepine, phenobarbital and phenytoin. Prolonged $t_{1/2}$ with valproic acid. Neurotoxicity with high dose carbamazepine (↓ carbamazepine dose if symptoms—headache, nausea, dizziness, ataxia, diplopia).	$–$$

(cont'd)

Table 2: **Characteristics of Antiepileptic Drugs** (cont'd)

Drug/ Usual Adult Dose	Therapeutic Range (μmol/L)	Half-life (hours)	Time to Steady State	Mechanism of Action/ Comments	Side Effects*/ Drug Interactions†	Cost‡
phenobarbital generics 2 mg/kg/d (30–240 mg/d)	80–200	50–150 h	2–3 wks	Enhances GABA inhibition. Withdraw carefully to ↓ risk of recurrent seizures.	Enzyme induction may ↓ blood levels of phenytoin, other drugs. Concurrent BDZ use may cause severe somnolence.	$
primidone Mysoline, generics 10–15 mg/kg/d (500–1 000 mg/d)	23–69	6–18 h phenobarbital: 50–150 h phenylethyl–malonamide: 16–24 h	2 d metabolites: 2–3 wks	Similar effects to pheno-barbital. Low initial dosage (125–250 mg/d) ↓ risk of toxicity (sedation).	Valproate may ↑ phenobarbital levels. May displace other medications from protein binding sites. Conversion of primidone to phenobarbital may be ↑ by phenytoin and ↓ by valproate.	$
phenytoin Dilantin, generics 4–6 mg/kg/d (300–400 mg/d)	40–80	10–40 h (average 24 h)	5–7 d	Inhibits burst firing. Therapeutic drug monitoring difficult due to zero-order kinetics. Dosage increments should be small, e.g., 50 mg. IM administration not recommended. Poor oral absorption in children < 3 yrs.	Gum hypertrophy (↓ by regular brushing of teeth), acne, lymphadenopathy, lupus-like syndrome, hirsutism, vitamin D/ folate deficiency, nystagmus and ataxia with ↑ serum levels. ↓ levels with antacids, carbamazepine, primidone. Enzyme induction may ↓ plasma concentration of other drugs.	$

topiramate Topamax 200–600 mg/d	Not established	20–30 h	4–6 d	Enhances GABA inhibition, suppresses action potentials and attenuates activation of some glutamate receptors. 15% plasma protein bound. Excreted unchanged in urine (80%).	Nervousness, fatigue, dizziness, language problems. Phenobarbital, phenytoin, carbamazepine ↓ $t_{1/2}$; May ↑ phenytoin levels. May ↓ efficacy of oral contraceptives.	$$$–$$$$$
valproic acid (valproate, sodium valproate) Depakene, generics Epival 15–70 mg/kg/d 750–3 000 mg/d	280–700	8–12 h	3–4 d	Enhances GABA inhibition.	Alopecia (usually reversible), hepatitis in children <2 yrs, weight gain. ↑ phenobarbital levels. May inhibit conversion of carbamazepine to inactive metabolites and of primidone to phenobarbital.	$–$$$ $–$$$$
vigabatrin Sabril 1 000–4 000 mg/d	Not established	7 h	2–3 d	Enhances GABA inhibition.	Weight gain, behavioral disturbances. May ↓ phenytoin levels.	$–$$$$

All anticonvulsants can cause rash, drowsiness, cognitive effects, memory reduction and balance problems.

†*Anticonvulsants interact with many medications (e.g., warfarin, narcotics, antidepressants, tranquilizers, neuroleptics); they may ↓ the effectiveness of birth control medication with breakthrough bleeding and possible pregnancy (↑ dosage of oral contraceptive may be required for effective contraception).*

‡*Cost of 30-day supply – includes drug cost only:*
Legend: $ < $50 $$ $50–100 $$$ $100–150 $$$$ $150–200 $$$$$ > $200

Control of Seizures (Table 3)

General factors determining control of seizures include compliance, stress and shift work.

Duration of Treatment

Some seizures (e.g., pyrexial seizures in children < 5 years old, absence) will resolve over time. Others (e.g., complex partial) are more resistant to treatment.

After 5 years of complete seizure control with anticonvulsants, there is a 20 to 34% chance of recurrence if the medication is withdrawn (usually within 6 months to 2 years). Risk factors are similar to the predictors of seizure control (Table 3).

Special Problems

Allergic reactions to one anticonvulsant increase the risk of allergic responses to other medications, even if they are from different chemical groups.[1] This risk is increased if drugs are used in quick succession, which may be necessary for seizure control.

Behavioral change and aggression can occur with some medications (e.g., clobazam, barbiturates, vigabatrin).

Zero-order kinetic drugs (e.g., phenytoin) tend to have a **narrower therapeutic range** than first-order kinetic drugs (e.g., barbiturates).

Seizure control may be lost at higher blood levels (especially phenytoin and carbamazepine).[2] The wide range of recommended therapeutic levels reflects lack of consensus among experts.

Table 3: **Predictors of Control and Recurrence of Seizures**

Good Risk	Bad Risk
Onset age 1–14 yrs	Onset before age 1 yr
Few seizures in total	Many seizures
Generalized tonic–clonic seizures	Mixed seizures (e.g., tonic–clonic and complex partial)
Absence seizures	Prolonged seizures
Early control	Poor early control
Response to monotherapy	Need for multiple medications
Patient does not drive or use machinery	Focal onset of seizures
	Focal neurologic signs
	Injury during seizures
	Structural brain abnormality, EEG abnormality
	Psychological or psychiatric problems
	Use of alcohol, barbiturates or benzodiazepines

---

[1] *J Clin Invest 1988;82:1826–1832.*

[2] *Chadwick D. Drug-induced convulsions. In: Rose FC, ed. Research progress in epilepsy. London: Pitman Press, 1983:151–160.*

Although **monotherapy** is favored over polytherapy, 10 to 15% of patients require 2 or more medications. It is often necessary to use a combination of anticonvulsants for patients with complex partial seizures or intractable epilepsy. Two medications at low therapeutic levels may be better tolerated than one medication near toxic levels.[3]

Poor compliance with anticonvulsant therapy is the major cause of seizure recurrence and the most common cause (40%) of status epilepticus in a known epileptic patient. About 60% of patients take their medications correctly. Compliance (including avoidance of aggravating agents such as alcohol and street drugs) can be maintained or improved by:

- recognition of high-risk groups (e.g., teenagers)
- monitoring of blood levels (failure to take the medication can be a reason to withdraw a driving licence)
- use of the return of a driving licence as an inducement
- follow-up clinic visits
- counseling on importance of maintaining blood levels
- using long-acting preparations and once-daily or BID dosing
- use of drug distribution boxes and dosage boxes

For problems related to **anticonvulsant use in pregnancy,** see Table 4.

Monitoring Therapy

Measurement of blood levels is of proven value in managing anticonvulsant therapy. The therapeutic range of antiepileptic medication reflects both antiseizure effects and toxic effects (e.g., increasing phenobarbital levels improves seizure control, but patients become less and less responsive until they are comatose). For patients in good control, blood levels should be measured every 6 to 12 months. When poor compliance is suspected, even weekly levels may be necessary.

Status Epilepticus

The management of status epilepticus is described in Figure 1.

---

3 Antiepileptic drugs: Optimal use and future prospects. Epilepsia: 2nd International Merrit-Putnam Symposium 1994;35(suppl 4):S1–S60.

Table 4: **Antiepileptic Drugs in Pregnancy**

Problem	Treatment
Anticonvulsants decrease efficacy of birth control pill.	Warn patient of risk of pregnancy. Use higher-dose birth control pill if there is break-through bleeding.
Teratogenic effects of first trimester use of anticonvulsants including cleft palate, atrial septal defect of heart, epicanthic folds, spina bifida, minor dysmorphic features.	Advise patient of potential risks. Withdraw anticonvulsants weeks before conception if possible. If unable to withdraw, inform patient of potential risk to offspring. There may be problems with driving licences, use of machinery and work that limit withdrawal. Withdrawal carries risks of seizures. Folic acid supplements ↓ risk of spina bifida (Chapter 99).
Alteration (↑) of unbound fractions of anticonvulsants during pregnancy (particularly phenytoin).	Measure blood levels, correct for low albumin; it is usually not necessary to alter dosage.
↑ risk of seizures in last trimester.	Monitor blood levels during last trimester; encourage good compliance.
Vomiting in early pregnancy.	Give medications later in the day. Use slow-release carbamazepine. Change from valproic acid or sodium valproate to carbamazepine, phenytoin.
Transfer of anticonvulsants to fetus.	No specific therapy.
Much longer half-life of anti-convulsants in infant.	No specific therapy; withdrawal effects may be ↓ by breast-feeding.
Withdrawal effects in infant after birth (prolonged because of longer half-lives).	Recognize irritability in infant.
Transfer of anticonvulsants in breast milk (except valproic acid).	Should not prevent breast-feeding.

Suggested Reading List

Antiepileptic drugs: Optimal use and future prospects. *Epilepsia: 2nd International Merrit-Putnam Symposium* 1994;35 (suppl 4):S1–S60.

Chadwick D, Brodie MJ, Bruni J, Guberman A, Wilder BJ. New generation antiepileptic drugs. Recent developments in the treatment of epilepsy. *Can J Neurol Sci* 1996;23: (suppl 2):S1–S23.

CHAPTER 19

Cataract Surgery Postoperative Care

Raymond P. LeBlanc, MD, FRCSC

Goals of Therapy

- To control inflammation
- To prevent infection
- To maintain eye comfort
- To promote early visual rehabilitation

Investigations

- Pain: the postoperative eye should be comfortable
  - at worst patient may have a mild foreign-body sensation; more intensive pain suggests increased IOP, increased inflammation and/or infection
- History of recent trauma:
  - any trauma to the eye in the early postoperative phase requires thorough reassessment
- Change in vision: darkened, loss of detail
  - any significant change could indicate a hemorrhage, retinal detachment or other acute intraocular pathology requiring immediate attention
- Visual phenomena: flashing lights or dark shadows
  - requires thorough reassessment
- Itchy, red eye:
  - suggests allergy to medications
- Examination of eye for:
  - swelling of lids and/or conjunctiva suggests drug allergy or infection
  - red reflex (should be confirmed with ophthalmoscope)
  - hyphema/corneal opacity
- Review of ocular medications:
  - reinforce use
  - clarify any confusion
  - discuss with family member
- Verify follow-up visits with surgeon

Figure 1: **Management of Postop Cataract Patient**

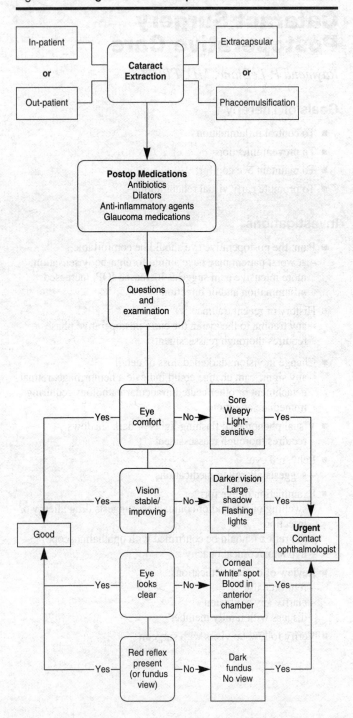

Therapeutic Choices (Figure 1)

Postoperative medications may include:

- Antibiotics: used for 7 to 14 days to prevent endophthalmitis; usually a broad-spectrum antibiotic.
  – either **Polysporin, tobramycin** or **sulfacetamide** drops.

- Dilators: used to keep iris away from implant during early healing period; also help for comfort.
  – either **cyclopentolate, phenylephrine** or **tropicamide** drops.

- Anti-inflammatory agents: used for 5 to 15 days to reduce postoperative inflammation.
  – **corticosteroids** include **prednisolone, dexamethasone, fluorometholone** or **rimexolone** drops.
  – **nonsteroidal anti-inflammatory drugs** include **flurbiprofen, indomethacin, ketorolac** or **diclofenac** drops.

- Glaucoma medications: often pre-existing regimen that may be modified in postoperative period to protect against early postoperative intraocular pressure rise.
  – includes any or all beta-blockers, miotics, alpha-adrenergics, prostaglandins, and/or carbonic anhydrase inhibitors, either topical or oral.

- No changes to medications should be made without discussion with treating ophthalmologist.

- Mild analgesic may be required: acetaminophen 500 mg Q4–6H.

- Sedation is rarely needed.

- Other systemic medications should be continued.

Suggested Reading List

American Academy of Ophthalmology. *Basic ophthalmology for medical students and primary care residents*. 6th ed. San Francisco: American Academy of Ophthalmology, 1993.

American Academy of Ophthalmology. *Preferred practice pattern: cataract in the otherwise healthy adult eye*. San Francisco: American Academy of Ophthalmology, 1989.

Coles W. *Ophthalmology: a diagnostic text*. Baltimore: Williams & Wilkins, 1989.

Reinecke R, Tarrell T. *Fundamentals of ophthalmology: a programmed text*. 2nd ed. San Francisco: American Academy of Ophthalmology, 1987.

Stein H, Slatt B, Stein R. *A primer in ophthalmology*. St. Louis: Mosby-Year Book, 1992.

CHAPTER 20

Glaucoma

Paul Rafuse, MD, PhD, FRCSC

Definition

A group of ocular diseases that have in common an optic neuropathy that causes visual loss. Characteristically, the optic disc is cupped and peripheral field loss precedes deterioration of visual acuity. Elevated intraocular pressure (IOP) is the most important, and only modifiable risk factor for glaucoma. A full understanding of the pathogenesis remains obscure as some people can have high IOPs without glaucoma and others glaucoma without elevated IOPs.

Goals of Therapy

- To prevent, halt or slow progressive visual loss
- To preserve the structure and function of the optic nerve
- To eliminate pain and improve vision in acute forms

NB: The therapeutic goals are achieved (with medications, laser and/or surgery) by decreasing the IOP.

Investigations

- Thorough history with special attention to:
  - nature of any ocular disturbances (e.g., loss of peripheral vision, halos around lights, decreased visual acuity)
  - quality of any pain (e.g., deep orbital, brow or headache)
  - associated systemic symptoms (e.g., abdominal pain, nausea and vomiting)

NB: The most common varieties are chronic. Generally, only the acute types are accompanied by symptoms.

- Careful assessment of risk factors (Table 1)
- History of drug use that can cause or worsen glaucoma
  - corticosteroids (common)
  - drugs with antimuscarinic activity (e.g., antihistamines, decongestants, antidepressants, antispasmodics, etc.; rare)
- Physical examination (i.e., assessment of visual acuity, visual field, IOP and optic disc)
- Comprehensive eye examination by an ophthalmologist
- Laboratory tests:
  - automated perimetry
  - optic disc photography

Table 1: **Risk Factors for the Development of Glaucoma**

Acquired (Primary)	Open-Angle	Closed-Angle
	Elevated IOP	Female[1]
	Advanced age	Advanced age[1,2]
	Black	Black[2]
	Positive family history	Positive family history[1,2]
	Myopia	Hyperopia[1,2]
	Diabetes mellitus	White[1]
	Systemic hypertension	
Acquired (Secondary)	Blunt and penetrating trauma	
	Previous intraocular surgery	
	Previous intraocular inflammation	
	Corticosteroid use	
Congenital	Positive family history	

Closed-angle glaucoma can be either acute[1] or chronic.[2]

Therapeutic Choices (Figure 1)

Nonpharmacologic Choices

- There are no lifestyle modifications proven to be of benefit before, or subsequent to, the use of drug therapy.
- Surgical or laser procedures are options if drug therapy is unsuccessful (Figure 1).

Pharmacologic Choices (Table 2)

- Reversible causes of **secondary** and **angle-closure** glaucoma should be treated.
- Excessive IOP, the only modifiable risk factor in chronic primary **open-angle** glaucoma (the most prevalent form), should be treated; all treatment measures in Figure 1 are believed to exert their therapeutic effect by lowering IOP.

Beta-blockers

Topical **timolol maleate, levobunolol hydrochloride** and **betaxolol hydrochloride** are efficacious ocular hypotensive agents that lack significant ocular side effects. They decrease IOP by inhibiting the formation of aqueous humor. The principal deterrents to their use are coincident pulmonary and cardiac diseases (Table 2). Betaxolol hydrochloride is relatively specific for beta$_1$-receptor blockade and may be used with caution in selected patients with mild obstructive pulmonary disease.

NB: Systemic absorption of eye drops occurs through the nasal mucosa. This can be reduced by digital occlusion of the nasolacrimal drainage system for several minutes following instillation of the drops.

Figure 1: **Management of Open-angle Glaucoma**

Treatment is stepped up if optic disc cupping progresses, the visual field
deteriorates or IOP control is inadequate.

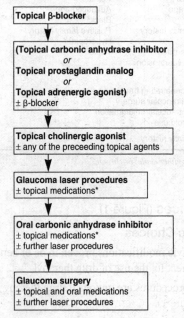

* *β-blockers, cholinergic agonists, adrenergic agonists and prostaglandin analogs.*

Topical Carbonic Anhydrase Inhibitors

Dorzolamide hydrochloride is the first available agent in this
new class. Like oral carbonic anhydrase inhibitors, it decreases
IOP by inhibiting an enzyme involved in the formation of
aqueous humor. It has limited systemic effects when compared
to the oral products and has more favorable ocular tolerability
than the cholinergic agonists. Dorzolamide may be the drug of
choice in patients with cardiopulmonary contraindications to
beta-blockers.

Prostaglandin Analogs

Latanoprost, a prostaglandin $F_{2\alpha}$ analog with a novel mechanism
of action, lowers IOP by increasing uveoscleral outflow. It is
highly efficacious and is administered using a single daily dosage
schedule. Early clinical experience shows this agent to have no
measureable cardiopulmonary effects. It may also be considered
as a first-line agent in patients with systemic contraindications
to beta-blockers. Ocular tolerability is generally good; however,
some brown colored irides may be darkened irreversibly with
long-term use.

Table 2: **Drugs Used in Glaucoma**

Drug	Dosage	Adverse Effects	Comments	Cost*
Beta-blockers (topical)				
levobunolol hydrochloride – Betagan, generics	Q12H	Local adverse effects usually minimal – stinging, dry eyes, rarely conjunctivitis.		$
betaxolol hydrochloride – Betoptic, Betoptic S	Q12H	Bronchospasm, exacerbation of CHF, bradycardia, syncope, depression, impotence, altered response to hypoglycemia, reduction of high-density lipoproteins.		$$
timolol maleate – Timoptic, generics	Q12H			$
timolol maleate gelan – Timoptic-XE	once daily			$$
timolol maleate + pilocarpine – Timpilo-2, -4	Q12H			$$
Carbonic Anhydrase Inhibitors (topical)				
dorzolamide hydrochloride – Trusopt	Q8H	Metallic taste, local allergic reaction.	Cross reactivity in patients allergic to sulfonamides.	$$
Prostaglandin Analogs (topical)				
latanoprost – Xalatan	once daily	Foreign body sensation, burning, stinging, itching, increased iris pigmentation.	Once daily dosing should not be exceeded. More frequent administration may ↓ IOP lowering effect of the medication.	$$$
Cholinergic Agonists (topical)				
pilocarpine hydrochloride – Isopto Carpine, generics, Minims, Pilopine HS gel	QID (drops) QHS (gel)	Reduced vision in patients with cataracts, blurred vision due to refractive shift, headache, GI upset.	Inhibition of plasma cholinesterase by echothiophate can markedly prolong action of succinylcholine.	$ drops $$ gel
carbachol – Isopto Carbachol, Miostat	Q8H			$
echothiophate (irreversible cholinesterase inhibitor) – Phospholine Iodide	Q12H	Iris cysts, cataracts (echothiophate).		$$$

(cont'd)

Table 2: **Drugs Used in Glaucoma** *(cont'd)*

Drug	Dosage	Adverse Effects	Comments	Cost*
Adrenergic Agonists (topical)				
dipivefrin hydrochloride – Propine, DPE	Q12H	Local allergic reaction, tachycardia, hypertension, headache, tremor.	Dipivefrin has fewer systemic adverse effects than epinephrine.	$
epinephrine bitartrate + pilocarpine – E-Pilo	QID			$
apraclonidine hydrochloride – Iopidine	1% once daily 0.5% Q8H			$$$
brimonidine tartrate – Alphagan	0.2% Q12H		Brimonidine: early clinical experience suggests lower frequency of allergy than other drugs in this class. Shows promise as a 1st or 2nd-line agent.	$$
Carbonic Anhydrase Inhibitors (oral)				
acetazolamide ✿ – Diamox, Diamox Sequels, generics	250 mg QID (acetazolamide) 500 mg Q12H (Sequels)	Paresthesias of extremities, metabolic acidosis, hypokalemia, GI upset, urolithiasis, lethargy and depression, aplastic anemia (rare), Stevens-Johnson syndrome (rare).	Cross reactivity in patients allergic to sulfonamides.	$4/mo Sequels $45/mo
methazolamide ✿ – Neptazane	25–50 mg Q8H			$24–35/mo

Dosage adjustment may be required in renal impairment – see Appendix I.
* *Cost per mL or g – includes drug cost only.*
Legend: $ < $2 $$ $2–4 $$$ $4   > $4

Cholinergic Agonists

Topical cholinergic agonists may act either directly on the muscarinic receptors activating the ciliary muscle or indirectly through inhibition of ciliary cholinesterase. Both lower IOP by causing an increase in trabecular outflow. Rarely is enough drug absorbed systemically to cause abdominal cramping or diarrhea. **Pilocarpine hydrochloride** and **carbachol** are direct-acting agents. **Echothiophate** is also an irreversible inhibitor of plasma cholinesterase. Because it can markedly prolong the action of succinylcholine, topical echothiophate should be discontinued 2 weeks before elective surgery requiring general anesthesia.

Adrenergic Agonists

Topical **epinephrine**, the prototype in this class, is no longer widely used as a single agent in Canada. A prodrug, **dipivefrin hydrochloride**, is used to enhance aqueous humor outflow and lower IOP. **Apraclonidine hydrochloride** is an $alpha_2$-specific agonist used for acute IOP elevations following anterior segment laser procedures. Long-term use has been associated with a high rate of local allergic responses. **Brimonidine tartrate** is a newer $alpha_2$ agonist with similar efficacy to apraclonidine. It may be better tolerated and shows promise as an adjuvant agent or as a first-line drug for patients unable to use beta-blockers.

Carbonic Anhydrase Inhibitors

Acetazolamide and **methazolamide** lower IOP by decreasing the production of aqueous humor. Their use is normally reserved for advanced chronic cases or acute emergencies because of serious side effects. Approximately 50% of patients are unable to use these drugs. Both these agents and topical dorzolamide can show cross reactivity in patients allergic to sulfonamides.

Therapeutic Tips

- OTC antihistamine products (which carry a caution against use in glaucoma patients due to anticholinergic side effects) will rarely cause a problem in open-angle glaucoma. The caution is made to advise those people without glaucoma but who are at risk for acute angle closure.

Suggested Reading List

LeBlanc RP. A current approach to medical management in glaucoma with a topical carbonic anhydrase inhibitor. *Ophthalmic Pract* 1996;14:190–193.

Quigley HA. Medical progress: open-angle glaucoma. *N Engl J Med* 1993;328:1097–1106.

Shields MB. *Textbook of glaucoma*. 3rd ed. Baltimore: Williams and Wilkins, 1992.

CHAPTER 21

Red Eye

Sueda Akkor, MD, FRCSC

Definition

Red eye is common in a wide variety of ocular conditions, some with serious consequences that require immediate referral to an ophthalmologist.

Goals of Therapy

- To preserve eyesight
- To control infection
- To control inflammation
- To provide symptomatic relief

Etiology

- Infections – conjunctivitis/keratitis: bacterial, viral (herpetic, non-herpetic), other
- Allergy
- Dry eyes: keratoconjunctivitis sicca
- Blepharitis and secondary conjunctivitis/keratitis
- Toxic/chemical/other irritants: topical drugs, contact lens solutions, acids/alkalis, smoke, wind, UV light
- Traumatic injury: corneal abrasions, foreign bodies, hyphema, other
- Ocular inflammation: iritis, episcleritis, scleritis
- Glaucoma: acute angle-closure glaucoma
- Others: lacrimal system infections, pterygium, subconjunctival hemorrhage

Investigations

The first step is to differentiate the major/serious causes from the minor causes. The following warning signs require referral to an ophthalmologist:

- Limbal/ciliary injection (redness dominant at the corneo-scleral junction)
- Pain **not** relieved by test dose of topical anesthetic drop (proparacaine, tetracaine)
- Pupil abnormalities: miotic or mid-dilated and fixed

Figure 1: **Management of Red Eye**

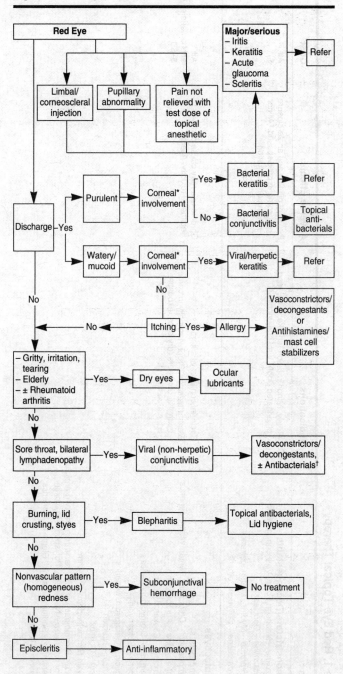

* Corneal staining with fluorescein strip indicates corneal involvement.
† Rarely used to prevent secondary bacterial infection.

Table 1: Red Eye Topical Therapy

Drugs	Indications	Adverse Effects	Cost*
Vasoconstrictors/Decongestants *naphazoline* – Naphcon Forte, Vasocon, generics *oxymetazoline* – Ocuclear *phenylephrine* – Mydfrin, Prefrin, generics *tetrahydrozoline* – Collyrium, others	Allergy. Minor irritation (smoke, dust, wind, chlorinated pool). Viral conjunctivitis.	Pupillary dilation and angle-closure glaucoma in predisposed.† Minor stinging on instillation.	All $
Anti-infectives **Antibacterials** *chloramphenicol* – Chloroptic, Pentamycetin, generics *chlortetracycline* – Aureomycin *ciprofloxacin* – Ciloxan *erythromycin* – Diomycin, generics *framycetin* – Soframycin *gentamicin* – Garamycin, generics *norfloxacin* – Noroxin *ofloxacin* – Ocuflox *polymyxin B/trimethoprim* – Polytrim *polymyxin B combinations with bacitracin and/or gramicidin and/or neomycin* – Neosporin, Polysporin, Polycidin *sulfacetamide* – Sodium Sulamyd, Bleph-10, generics *tobramycin* – Tobrex	Bacterial conjunctivitis/keratitis. Blepharitis/styes. Prophylactically in corneal epithelial disorders (dry eyes, exposure, lid malpositions).	Chronic use may cause corneal epithelial toxicity. Allergy.	All antibacterials $–$$

Antivirals
idoxuridine – Herplex
trifluridine – Viroptic
acyclovir 🔴 – Zovirax ‡

Herpes simplex, Herpes zoster (acyclovir is the only effective antiviral).

Chronic use may cause corneal epithelial toxicity.

All antivirals $ – $$$

Antihistamines/Mast Cell Stabilizers
sodium cromoglycate – Opticrom
lodoxamide tromethamine – Alomide
levocabastine – Livostin
nedocromil – Mireze
antazoline/naphazoline – Albalon-A Liquifilm, Vasocon-A
antazoline/xylometazoline – Ophtrivin-A
pheniramine maleate/naphazoline – Naphcon-A, Opcon-A

Allergies. Sodium cromoglycate in contact lens wear-related giant papillary conjunctivitis.π

Minor stinging on instillation.

$
$$
$$
$$
$
$

Ocular Lubricants
carboxymethylcellulose – Cellufresh, Celluvisc
dextran/polyethylene glycol – Aquasite
hydroxypropyl methylcellulose – Isopto Tears, Moisture Drops, Tears Naturale, Tears Naturale II, others
methylcellulose – Murocel
polysorbate – Tears Encore
polyvinyl alcohol – Hypotears, Liquifilm Tears, Liquifilm Forte, Refresh, Tears Plus, generics
mineral oil/petrolatum – Duolube, Hypotears, Lacri-Lube S.O.P., Oculube, generics
sodium hyaluronate – Eyestil
sorbitol/carbomer – Tear-Gel

Dry eyes, exposure, lid malpositions, blepharitis, minor irritations.

Preservative toxicity, filmy vision.

All $ – $$ (preservative-free unit dose products are more expensive)

(cont'd)

Table 1: Red Eye Topical Therapy *(cont'd)*

Drugs	Indications	Adverse Effects	Cost*
Anti-inflammatory Agents	Episcleritis, iritis, scleritis, some keratitis, ocular allergy.		
Steroids		Minor stinging on instillation.	
dexamethasone – Decadron, Maxidex, generics		Steroids may worsen herpetic/fungal keratitis.	$
fluorometholone – FML, FML Forte, Flarex		Long-term steroids may cause glaucoma, cataracts.	$$
prednisolone – Inflamase Mild/Forte, Pred Mild/Forte, generics			$
prednisolone/sulfacetamide – Metimyd, generics			$$
rimexolone – Vexol			$$
Nonsteroidals			
diclofenac – Voltaren Ophtha			$$
flurbiprofen – Ocufen			$$$
indomethacin – Indocid			$$$
ketorolac – Acular			$$

* Cost of smallest unit – includes drug cost only. (For OTC products, add retail mark-up.)
  Legend: $ < $10 $$ $10–20 $$$ > $20–30
† See Glaucoma, Chapter 20.
● Dosage adjustment may be required in renal impairment – see Appendix I.
‡ Not available as a topical ophthalmic agent. Systemic acyclovir is used 800 mg 5 × day for 6 days in H. zoster; 200 mg QID for 2 weeks in H. simplex.

π Giant papillary conjunctivitis is a hypersensitivity disorder seen in patients with contact lenses or artificial eyes. The family practitioner may suspect it in patients complaining of itching and ropy whitish discharge, but diagnosis is made with slit lamp exam by an ophthalmologist.

- Raised intraocular pressure
- History of iritis/angle-closure glaucoma
- Recent history of trauma

Therapeutic Choices (Figure 1)

Nonpharmacologic Choices

- Contact lens wear should be stopped.
- Make-up, smoke, wind, other irritants should be avoided.
- Cold wet compresses should be applied in allergic or viral conjunctivitis.
- Hot wet compresses should be applied in blepharitis/styes.
- Lid hygiene should be used in blepharitis.

Pharmacologic Choices (Table 1)

Choice depends on underlying cause.

Therapeutic Tips

- Once the major/serious conditions are ruled out, treatment can be initiated.
- If no improvement is seen after one week, refer.
- Most topically administered eyedrops used in therapy are themselves capable of causing irritation/toxicity.
- Antibiotic–steroid combinations and steroids may worsen herpetic/fungal keratitis and should not be used indiscriminately.
- Long-term use of topical steroids may cause glaucoma and/or cataracts.
- Topical decongestants/vasoconstrictors may provoke angle-closure glaucoma in those predisposed.

Suggested Reading List

Berson FG, ed. *Basic ophthalmology for medical students and primary care residents*. 5th ed. San Francisco: American Academy of Ophthalmology, 1987:58–77.

Chawla HB. *Ophthalmology*. 2nd ed. New York: Churchill Livingstone, 1993:89–97.

Vaughan DG, Asbury T, Riordan-Eva P. *General ophthalmology*. 13th ed. Los Altos, CA: Lange, 1992:63–77, 96–124.

CHAPTER 22

Acute and Postmyocardial Infarction

Ernest L. Fallen, MD, FRCPC

Acute Myocardial Infarction

Goals of Therapy

- To decrease mortality
- To reduce or contain infarct size
- To salvage functioning myocardium/prevent remodeling
- To quickly re-establish patency of infarct related vessel
- To prevent complications

NB: There is undeniable evidence that IV thrombolytic therapy administered **early** in the course of an evolving acute myocardial infarction (MI) substantially reduces mortality and morbidity.

Investigations

- 12-lead ECG STAT and once daily × 3 days
- Creatine kinase (CK) STAT and Q8H × 3 for the first 24 hours and then once daily × 3
- If indicated, an echocardiogram or a resting radionuclide angiocardiogram within the first 72 hours may identify:
  – the site and severity of wall motion abnormalities
  – infarct site in cases of left bundle branch block
  – endocardial thrombus
  – candidates for ACE inhibitor therapy by assessing left ventricular function
- Total and LDL cholesterol during the first 24 hours of infarct. The complete lipid profile should be obtained 6 to 8 weeks post-MI. However, it is useful to know the early cholesterol level to initiate dietary advice when the patient is most receptive to risk factor modification

Therapeutic Choices (Figure 1, Table 1)

Therapeutic Tips

- **Time is of the essence!** It is far more important to begin thrombolytic treatment as rapidly as possible than to debate which thrombolytic agent to use.

Figure 1: **Treatment of Acute Myocardial Infarction**

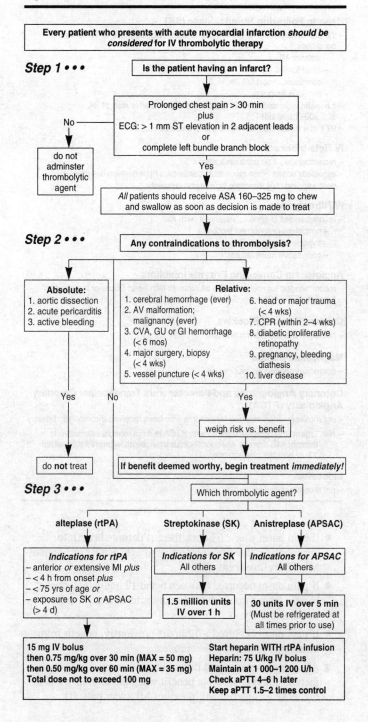

Every patient who presents with acute myocardial infarction *should be considered* for IV thrombolytic therapy

Step 1 • • •   **Is the patient having an infarct?**

Prolonged chest pain > 30 min
plus
ECG: > 1 mm ST elevation in 2 adjacent leads
or
complete left bundle branch block

No — do not adminster thrombolytic agent

Yes

All patients should receive ASA 160–325 mg to chew and swallow as soon as decision is made to treat

Step 2 • • •   **Any contraindications to thrombolysis?**

Absolute:
1. aortic dissection
2. acute pericarditis
3. active bleeding

Relative:
1. cerebral hemorrhage (ever)
2. AV malformation; malignancy (ever)
3. CVA, GU or GI hemorrhage (< 6 mos)
4. major surgery, biopsy (< 4 wks)
5. vessel puncture (< 4 wks)
6. head or major trauma (< 4 wks)
7. CPR (within 2–4 wks)
8. diabetic proliferative retinopathy
9. pregnancy, bleeding diathesis
10. liver disease

Yes — do **not** treat

No

Yes — weigh risk vs. benefit

If benefit deemed worthy, begin treatment *immediately!*

Step 3 • • •   Which thrombolytic agent?

alteplase (rtPA)

Indications for rtPA
– anterior *or* extensive MI *plus*
– < 4 h from onset *plus*
– < 75 yrs of age *or*
– exposure to SK *or* APSAC (> 4 d)

Streptokinase (SK)

Indications for SK
All others

1.5 million units IV over 1 h

Anistreplase (APSAC)

Indications for APSAC
All others

30 units IV over 5 min
(Must be refrigerated at all times prior to use)

15 mg IV bolus
then 0.75 mg/kg over 30 min (MAX = 50 mg)
then 0.50 mg/kg over 60 min (MAX = 35 mg)
Total dose not to exceed 100 mg

Start heparin WITH rtPA infusion
Heparin: 75 U/kg IV bolus
Maintain at 1 000–1 200 U/h
Check aPTT 4–6 h later
Keep aPTT 1.5–2 times control

Table 1: **Adjuvant Therapy for Acute MI**

Heparin Following Streptokinase (SK)
– the use of heparin after SK remains unclear. Consider use in the following conditions:
  – anterior MI
  – atrial fibrillation
  – congestive heart failure
  – previous embolus
– if heparin indicated, start IV heparin infusion 4 h after start of SK at 1 000–1 200 U/h
– PTT at 4 h and maintain aPTT 1.5–2 times control

IV Beta-blockers
– recommended if no contraindications
– especially useful when sinus tachycardia plus hypertension are present
– best withheld until thrombolytic infusion complete

IV Nitroglycerin
– recommended in specific instances such as:
  – persistent or recurrent ischemia
  – hypertension
  – congestive heart failure

Angiotensin Converting Enzyme Inhibitors
– recommended for routine use in all patients with heart failure or impaired LV function (EF < 40%)

Calcium Channel Blockers
– not recommended for *routine* use

Magnesium Sulfate
– not recommended for *routine* use

Coronary Angiography and Percutaneous Transluminal Coronary Angioplasty (PTCA)
– not routinely recommended for patients who have received thrombolytic therapy

– **NB:** urgent angiography together with PTCA is a reasonable alternative to thrombolytic therapy when local circumstances allow intervention within 1 h of hospital presentation

Lidocaine
– not recommended for *routine* use

- If pain onset was < 6 hours, there is definite benefit to thrombolytic therapy irrespective of age, gender or previous MI. **Therefore treat all!**

- If pain onset occurred between 6 and 12 hours, potential benefit from thrombolytic therapy is less clear. Therefore treat selectively.

- If pain onset occurred > 12 hours previously, benefit from thrombolytic therapy is unproven.

- All groups benefit from thrombolytic therapy. However, there is a higher absolute benefit when the mortality risk is higher (e.g., anterior MI, previous MI, older patient).

Management of Early Complications

Post-MI Angina

Nitrates (oral, IV or topical) and/or beta-blockers are treatments of choice if there are no contraindications. A calcium channel blocker may also be used to control persistent post-MI angina unresponsive to above agents. Although controversial, concern about the safety of short-acting calcium channel blockers in the post-MI patient has been raised. If rest angina persists despite treatment, coronary angiography should be considered.

Dysrhythmias

- Treatment of asymptomatic ventricular ectopy or brief episodes of nonsustained ventricular tachycardia is not warranted.

- With symptomatic ventricular ectopy, beta-blockers are sometimes useful. Caution is urged in the use of any Class IA agents (e.g., quinidine, disopyramide, procainamide). Class IC agents (flecainide and propafenone) are contraindicated.

- In the post acute phase of an MI, patients with sustained ventricular tachycardia requiring electric shock or post cardiac arrest should undergo coronary angiography with or without electrophysiologic studies (Chapter 26).

- Patients with frequent PVCs, complex ventricular ectopy or nonsustained VT plus LV dysfunction may be considered for amiodarone therapy.

- With atrial fibrillation, the ventricular rate can be brought under control with digoxin at a dose that maintains the ventricular rate < 90 beats/minute. A beta-blocker or calcium channel blocker (verapamil or diltiazem) should be considered if rate remains high and patient is not in heart failure (Chapter 25).

- With symptomatic bradycardia, the dose of beta-blocker, calcium channel blocker or digoxin should be reduced or another drug should be substituted. If patient is on no medication and symptomatic bradyarrhythmia persists longer than 2 weeks, consider pacemaker implantation.

Heart Failure (See also Chapter 24)

- ACE inhibitor, especially if low output syndrome (fatigue, weakness, dyspnea).
- Salt restriction.
- Diuretic, especially for cases with dyspnea and pulmonary rales (important to monitor potassium levels).

- Beta-blockers, calcium channel blockers and other cardiac depressants should be avoided.
- Digoxin should be considered if:
  – rapid atrial fibrillation
  – dilated left ventricle and S3 gallop rhythm.

Hypertension

Systemic hypertension causes an increased demand for myocardial oxygen and may extend the infarct. It is necessary to restore the BP toward the normal range. An ACE inhibitor is the treatment of choice. The addition of a beta-blocker or calcium channel blocker should be considered if systolic BP remains > 160 mm Hg or diastolic BP > 95 mm Hg.

Pericarditis

Pericarditis is common within 72 hours after an acute transmural MI. If symptomatic, ASA should be increased to 650 mg QID for 1 to 2 weeks. If pain persists, an NSAID or corticosteroid should be considered. Peri-infarction pericarditis usually resolves spontaneously by the 3rd or 4th day.

Discontinuation of anticoagulants is unnecessary if pericarditis presents as part of acute phase MI.

Postmyocardial Infarction

The post-MI phase is defined as the time from transfer to the ward (day 3 to 5) up to 1 year from hospital discharge.

Goals of Therapy

- To develop a risk stratification profile
- To prevent recurrent ischemic events
- To reduce mortality and morbidity
- To return the patient to an optimum quality of life
- To reduce or reverse modifiable risk factors
- To educate the patient and his/her family

Investigations

- Symptom-limited exercise test (or submaximal exercise test depending on the risk stratification profile)
- A predischarge 24-hour Holter recording for patients with suspected ventricular arrhythmias or symptomatic bradyarrhythmias

- A follow-up echocardiogram (2 to 3 weeks post-MI) in patients with a suspected or previously documented endocardial thrombus
- A lipid profile (total cholesterol, LDL, HDL, triglycerides) no sooner than 6 to 8 weeks postdischarge

Risk Stratification Profile (Figure 2)

The first step in the rehabilitation of the post-MI patient is to assign a risk assessment.

NB: It is just as important to identify the very-low-risk patient, thus sparing him/her unnecessary aggressive investigation and therapy, as it is to identify the high-risk patient for whom aggressive therapy may be life saving.

A risk stratification profile (Figure 2) should be done at three strategic stages: on first arriving on the ward from the acute coronary unit; at the time of discharge (a time when patient education ought to be reinforced); following a symptom-limited exercise test at around 2 to 4 weeks postdischarge. At each stage, the patient may stay within the risk group or be reassigned up or down. Further preventive strategies and treatment decisions rest on the respective risk group, as illustrated in Figure 2.

The intermediate-risk group has the potential for further episodes of ischemia.

Post-MI Prophylaxis at Time of Hospital Discharge

Routine Prophylaxis

All patients, regardless of risk category or age, should receive **ASA** (160 to 325 mg/d) indefinitely.

All patients should be prescribed a **beta-blocker** to be continued indefinitely unless contraindicated as below:

Absolute	Relative
1. 2nd or 3rd degree heart block, sick sinus syndrome	1. Insulin-dependent diabetes with history of hypoglycemic attacks
2. *Overt* CHF	2. Persistent hypotension (systolic BP < 100 mm Hg)
3. Chronic obstructive lung disease	3. Heart rate persistently < 60 beats/min

Special Circumstances

Warfarin is recommended following acute MI complicated by severe LV dysfunction, CHF, previous emboli, atrial fibrillation

Figure 2: **Three Phase Post-MI Risk Stratification**

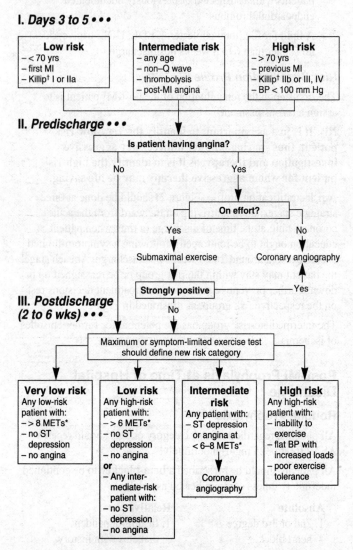

I. *Days 3 to 5* •••

Low risk
– < 70 yrs
– first MI
– Killip† I or IIa

Intermediate risk
– any age
– non–Q wave
– thrombolysis
– post-MI angina

High risk
– > 70 yrs
– previous MI
– Killip† IIb or III, IV
– BP < 100 mm Hg

II. *Predischarge* •••

Is patient having angina?

No — Yes

On effort?

Yes — No

Submaximal exercise — Coronary angiography

Strongly positive — Yes

III. *Postdischarge* (2 to 6 wks) •••

No

Maximum or symptom-limited exercise test
should define new risk category

Very low risk
Any low-risk
patient with:
– > 8 METs*
– no ST
 depression
– no angina

Low risk
Any high-risk
patient with:
– > 6 METs*
– no ST
 depression
– no angina
or
– Any inter-
 mediate-risk
 patient with:
– no ST
 depression
– no angina

**Intermediate
risk**
Any patient with:
– ST depression
 or angina at
 < 6–8 METs*

Coronary
angiography

High risk
Any high-risk
patient with:
– inability to
 exercise
– flat BP with
 increased loads
– poor exercise
 tolerance

* 1 MET is the amount of energy expended by a person at rest. It is equivalent to
 3.5 mL O₂/kg/min (e.g., walking 4 km/h = 3 METs).

*Reprinted with permission from Fallen EL, et al. Management of the postmyocardial
infarction patient: A consensus report – Revision of 1991 CCS Guidelines. Can J Cardiol
1995;11:478.*

† The Killip classification is a scoring system for heart failure:

Class	Clinical Findings
I	No rales, no S3
IIa	Rales < 50% of lungs; no S3
IIb	Rales < 50% of lungs; S3 present
III	Rales > 50%, pulmonary edema
IV	Shock

or 2D echocardiographic evidence of mural thrombosis. After 1 to 3 months, warfarin should be switched to ASA.

An **ACE inhibitor** is recommended for patients with > Killip Class IIa (see Figure 2 footnote) or reduced LV function (LV ejection fraction < 40%).

Verapamil or **diltiazem** may be considered in patients **with non–Q wave MI who are free of CHF** if beta-blockers are contraindicated.

No substantive evidence to date warrants **routine** prophylaxis with the following agents: organic nitrates, antiarrhythmic agents, antiplatelet agents other than ASA, calcium channel blockers.

For prescribing information see Table 2.

Figure 3: **Activities Prescription**

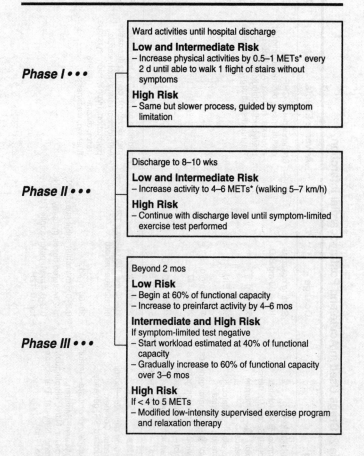

Phase I • • •

Ward activities until hospital discharge

Low and Intermediate Risk
– Increase physical activities by 0.5–1 METs* every 2 d until able to walk 1 flight of stairs without symptoms

High Risk
– Same but slower process, guided by symptom limitation

Phase II • • •

Discharge to 8–10 wks

Low and Intermediate Risk
– Increase activity to 4–6 METs* (walking 5–7 km/h)

High Risk
– Continue with discharge level until symptom-limited exercise test performed

Phase III • • •

Beyond 2 mos

Low Risk
– Begin at 60% of functional capacity
– Increase to preinfarct activity by 4–6 mos

Intermediate and High Risk
If symptom-limited test negative
– Start workload estimated at 40% of functional capacity
– Gradually increase to 60% of functional capacity over 3–6 mos

High Risk
If < 4 to 5 METs
– Modified low-intensity supervised exercise program and relaxation therapy

* 1 MET is the amount of energy expended by a person at rest. It is equivalent to 3.5 mL 0_2/kg/min (e.g., walking 4 km/h = 3 METs).

Table 2: Drugs Used in Acute and Postmyocardial Infarction

Drug	Dosage	Adverse Effects	Drug Interactions	Cost*
Beta-blockers	*Starting dosages*	Bronchospasm, CHF, sleep disturbances, dizziness, fatigue, anorexia, nausea, A-V block, bradycardia, claudication, Raynaud's, lethargy, drowsiness.	Enhanced cardiodepressant effect with: calcium channel blockers, antiarrhythmics, anesthetics.	
acebutolol ◑ – Monitan, Rhotral, Sectral, generics	100–200 mg BID			$
atenolol † ◑ – Tenormin, generics	50 mg/d		Increased bradycardia with digoxin.	$
metoprolol ◑ – Betaloc, Lopresor, generics	50 mg BID		Hypertension with alpha-agonists.	$
nadolol ◑ – Corgard, generics	40–80 mg/d		Reduced effect with cimetidine.	$
oxprenolol – Trasicor, generics	20 mg TID			$
pindolol – Visken, generics	5 mg BID			$
propranolol † – Inderal, generics	40 mg BID/TID			$
timolol † – Blocadren, generics	5–10 mg BID			$
Nitrates	*Starting dosages*	Headache (up to 50%; tolerance may develop), contact dermatitis with topical forms, tachycardia, palpitation, hypotension, syncope (rare), dizziness, nausea, flushing, weakness.	Potential hypotensive effect with vasodilators.	
isosorbide dinitrate – Isordil, Coradur, Coronex, Cedocard SR, generics	10–30 mg TID (allow a 12H nitrate-free period)			$
isosorbide mononitrate – Imdur	30–60 mg/d			$
nitroglycerin – Minitran, Nitro-Dur, Nitrol, Nitrolingual, Nitrong, Nitrostat, Transderm-Nitro, Tridil	0.3–0.6 mg tablet sublingual PRN; 1–2 metered doses by spray PRN; 0.2–0.4 mg/h patch applied daily for 10–12H			SL tablets, spray $; Transdermal $$

	Starting dosages		Cost
ACE Inhibitors			
captopril ♥ – Capoten, generics	test dose 6.25 mg then 6.25–50 mg TID	↑ risk of neutropenia with antiarrhythmics, allopurinol, corticosteroids.	$$
enalapril ♥ – Vasotec, generics	start with 2.5 mg/d then up to 10–20 mg/d	Hyperkalemia with spironolactone, triamterene, amiloride. Hypotension with diuretics.	$$
lisinopril ♥ – Zestril, Prinivil, generics	5–10 mg/d (single dose)	Proteinuria (1%), neutropenia, rash, hypotension, alterations in taste, nausea, anorexia, dizziness, dry cough. Caution in patients with renovascular hypertension.	$
Anticoagulants			
heparin sodium – Hepalean, Heparin Leo warfarin – Coumadin, Warfilone	These drugs must be individualized according to aPTT for heparin and prothrombin time or INR for warfarin at 1.5–2 × control	Hemorrhage, hypersensitivity reactions, alopecia, thrombocytopenia. / Many drugs may affect prothrombin time. (Check PT or INR with introduction of any new drug.)	Varies
Antiplatelets			
ASA – Entrophen, Aspirin, generics	ASA 160–325 mg/d	Nausea, vomiting, GI hemorrhage, tinnitus, vertigo, hypersensitivity.	$
Thrombolytics			
streptokinase – Streptase	(Figure 1)	Bleeding, allergy to streptokinase, hypotension, nausea, fever, reperfusion arrhythmias. / ↑ risk of hemorrhage with oral anticoagulants, heparin and NSAIDs.	SK $275/dose
anistreplase – Eminase		Cross allergenicity is seen with streptokinase.	APSAC $1 700/dose
alteplase – Activase rtPA		↑ risk of bleeding as for SK.	rtPA $1 350/dose

♥ Dosage adjustment may be required in renal impairment – see Appendix I.
† Proven efficacy for prophylaxis in post-MI patients.

* Cost of 30-day supply – includes drug cost only.
Legend: $ <$25 $$ $25–50 $$$ $50–75

Rehabilitation

Rehabilitation is the sum of activities required to ensure the best possible physical, psychologic and social conditions so the patient may, by his/her own efforts, regain as normal as possible a place in the community and lead an active, productive life. It includes exercise, risk factor and lifestyle modification, attention to psychosocial factors and management of dyslipidemias (Chapter 27).

Exercise

Guidelines for graduated physical activities post-MI are provided by established cardiac rehabilitation programs in many communities. For general guidelines refer to Figure 3.

Risk Factor and Lifestyle Modification

Compelling evidence shows that modifying risk factors such as hyperlipidemia, smoking and hypertension improves outcome, delays progression of atherosclerosis, reduces mortality and improves functional capacity. For instance, ex-smokers can look forward to a 35 to 50% reduction in mortality whereas the relative risk of sudden cardiac death is 1.6 to 2.2 times in those who continue to smoke. For those willing to comply, psychosocial support, education, exercise programs, relaxation therapy and special teaching programs are helpful as adjunctive measures.

Pharmacoeconomic Considerations

Jeffrey A. Johnson, PhD

Among proven therapies in acute MI, ASA would appear to have a large benefit to cost ratio, given the number of deaths and nonfatal MI that would be prevented in both the short and long term, at a very low cost for the drug itself. Similarly, use of IV beta-blockers in acute MI prevents a significant number of subsequent events at a relatively small cost, as does its continued oral use as post-MI prophylaxis.

Thrombolytic therapy is also cost-effective when compared to other cardiovascular interventions in terms of dollars per years of life saved. Cost-effectiveness studies clearly show that shortening the time to treatment has a critical impact on the cost-effectiveness of thrombolytic therapy, as does the age of the patient. Initiating treatment within 6 hours of AMI is associated with better outcomes, and is therefore more cost-effective. The relative cost-effectiveness of the thrombolytic agents (i.e., SK and alteplase [rtPA]) remains somewhat controversial. The most effective strategy may be one of selective use of the two drugs based on time of presentation, age of the patient and location of the infarction. For the vast majority of patients presenting with AMI with either ST segment elevation or bundle branch block, streptokinase is more cost-effective. The exception would be in younger individuals with a large anteroseptal infarction, who may receive greater benefit from alteplase.

As noted above, continued use of ASA and beta-blockers is economically justified in terms of post-MI prophylaxis. Use of an ACE inhibitor to prevent development of CHF and reduce mortality in MI survivors with low ejection fraction is also associated with a favorable cost-effectiveness ratio when compared to other interventions. Furthermore, participation in cardiac rehabilitation initiated soon after acute MI has shown to be an efficient use of health care resources in terms of the cost per quality-adjusted life years gained.

Suggested Reading

Castillo PA, Palmer CS, Halpern MT, et al. Cost-effectiveness of thrombolytic therapy for acute myocardial infarction. Ann Pharmacother 1997;31:596–603.

Collins R, Sleight P, Baigent C, Peto R. Aspirin, heparin, and fibrinolytic therapy in suspected acute myocardial infarction. N Engl J Med 1997;336:847–860.

Tsevat J, Duke D, Goldman L, et al. Cost-effectiveness of captopril therapy after myocardial infarction. J Am Coll Cardiol 1995;26:914–919.

Oldridge N, Furlong W, Feeny D, et al. Economic evaluation of cardiac rehabilitation soon after acute myocardial infarction. Am J Cardiol 1993;72:154–161.

Suggested Reading List

Cairns J, Armstrong P, Belenkie I, et al. Canadian consensus conference on coronary thrombolysis – 1994 update. *Can J Cardiol* 1994;10:517–529.

Fallen EL, Cairns J, Dafoe W, et al. Management of the post-myocardial infarction patient: a consensus report – revision of the 1991 CCS guidelines. *Can J Cardiol* 1995;11:477–486.

The GUSTO Investigators. An international randomized trial comparing four thrombolytic strategies for acute myocardial infarction. *N Engl J Med* 1993;329:673–682.

ISIS-2 Study Group. Randomized trial of intravenous streptokinase, oral aspirin, both or neither among 17,187 cases of suspected acute myocardial infarction. *Lancet* 1988;2:349–360.

ISIS–4 Collaborative Group. A randomised factorial trial assessing early oral captopril, oral mononitrate and intravenous magnesium sulphate in 58 050 patients with suspected acute myocardial infarction. *Lancet* 1995;345: 669–685.

Yusuf S, Peto R, Lewis JA, et al. Beta-blockade during and after myocardial infarction: a review of the randomized trials. *Prog Cardiovasc Dis* 1985;27:335–371.

CHAPTER 23

Angina Pectoris

John O. Parker, MD, MSc(Med), FACP, FRCPC and
John D. Parker, MD, FRCPC

Stable Angina Pectoris

Goals of Therapy

- To decrease or abolish symptoms
- To improve exercise tolerance
- To retard disease progression
- To prevent complications

Investigations

- Thorough history with special attention to:
  - pain: quality, severity, location, radiation, precipitating and relieving factors
  - effect of nitroglycerin
- Physical examination:
  - presence of hypertension, valvular disease, cardiomegaly, heart failure
- Laboratory tests:
  - CBC, blood glucose, creatinine, cholesterol
- Exercise test:
  - not universally required; helps to confirm diagnosis and assess functional status and provides prognostic information

Therapeutic Choices (Figure 1)

Nonpharmacologic Choices

- The patient should be educated to understand the pathophysiology of myocardial ischemia.
- Lifestyle changes should include, when appropriate: dietary modifications to reduce cholesterol, weight reduction, smoking cessation (Chapter 40), avoidance of strenuous exercise (particularly isometric), increased activities (e.g., walking).
- Strenuous activity after meals or in cold weather should be avoided.

Figure 1: **Management of Stable Angina Pectoris**

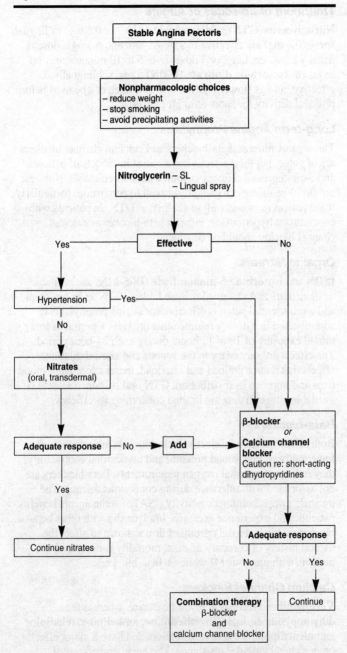

Abbreviations: SL = sublingual.

Pharmacologic Choices (Table 1)
Treatment of Episodes of Angina

Nitroglycerin (GTN) sublingual tablets (0.3 or 0.6 mg) or lingual spray (0.4 mg) are effective in 95% of patients. A single dose is usually adequate, but 2 or 3 doses over 5 to 10 minutes may be required. **Isosorbide dinitrate (ISDN)** 5 mg, sublingually, is effective but has slower onset than GTN. Each can be used before physical activity for short-term prophylaxis.

Long-term Angina Prophylaxis

The organic nitrates, beta-blockers and calcium channel blockers are of value, but their effectiveness varies in subsets of patients and their degree of efficacy is somewhat unpredictable. Nitrates are first-line therapy in patients without hypertension, particularly if the patient responds well to sublingual GTN. In patients with concomitant hypertension, either a beta-blocker or calcium channel blocker should be considered.

Organic Nitrates

ISDN and **isosorbide-5-mononitrate (IS-5-MN)** are available as immediate and sustained-release tablets. GTN as an ointment and a transdermal patch is effective for angina prophylaxis if administered in a dosing regimen that provides a period of low nitrate exposure of 10 to 12 hours during each 24-hour period. The effects are secondary to the venous and arterial dilating effects that reduce preload and afterload, increase coronary blood flow and improve its distribution. GTN oral sustained release is available although data are limited concerning its efficacy.

Beta-blockers

Both selective and nonselective beta-blockers are effective. By lowering heart rate, blood pressure and myocardial contractility, they reduce myocardial oxygen requirements. Beta-blockers are not associated with tolerance during continuous therapy. The intrinsic sympathomimetic activity (ISA) of some agents benefits patients who experience excessive bradycardia with other beta-blockers. This is the only group of drugs shown to affect the natural history of coronary disease; mortality is decreased in patients with previous MI while on beta-blockers.

Calcium Channel Blockers

Verapamil and **diltiazem** lower heart rate, whereas the dihydropyridines, including **nifedipine, amlodipine, felodipine** and **nicardipine,** are arteriolar dilators and have a major effect on peripheral vascular resistance. The beneficial effects of the calcium channel blockers are secondary to their effect on lowering arterial blood pressure and the reduced heart rate seen with verapamil and diltiazem. They also increase coronary blood

Table 1: Drug Therapy for Stable Angina

Drug	Dosage	Drug Interactions	Comments	Cost*
Nitrates		For all nitrates: Potential hypotensive effect with vasodilators.	For all nitrates: Headache, hypotension, tachycardia, flushing, edema, contact dermatitis with topical forms.	
nitroglycerin – Nitrolingual Spray, Nitrong SR, Nitrostat ointment: Nitrol transdermal: Nitro-Dur, Transderm-Nitro, Minitran	SL: 0.3–0.6 mg PRN Spray: 0.4 mg PRN Nitrong SR: 2.6 mg BID (7 h apart) Patch: 0.2–0.8 mg/h for 12 h per 24 h period Ointment: 1.25–5 cm BID–TID; remove for 12 h per 24 h period			$ Patches $$
isosorbide dinitrate – Isordil, Cedocard SR, generics	SL: 5 mg PRN Regular: 10–30 mg TID on QID schedule (allow 12 h nitrate-free period) SR: 20–40 mg BID (7 h apart)			$
isosorbide-5-mononitrate – Imdur, ISMO	Regular: 20 mg BID (7 h apart) SR: 30–120 mg once daily			$$
Beta-blockers		For all β-blockers: With digoxin ↑ bradycardia. Calcium channel blockers and amiodarone may ↑ cardiodepressant effect.	For all β-blockers: Bradycardia (less common with pindolol), hypotension, fatigue, depression, sleep disorders, dyspnea. Monitor HR, caution in patients with CHF, COPD, diabetes mellitus.	
propranolol – Inderal, generics	20–80 mg QID			$
metoprolol – Betaloc, Lopresor, generics	25–200 mg BID			$–$$
atenolol 🌂 – Tenormin, generics	50–400 mg daily			$–$$$
nadolol 🌂 – Corgard, generics	20–160 mg daily			$
pindolol – Visken, generics	5–20 mg BID			$–$$
acebutolol 🌂 – Monitan, Rhotral, Sectral	50–400 mg BID			$–$$

(cont'd)

Table 1: Drug Therapy for Stable Angina (cont'd)

Drug	Dosage	Drug Interactions	Comments	Cost*
Calcium Channel Blockers†		Additive myocardial depressant effects with β-blockers, digoxin, amiodarone. Monitor for excessive bradycardia.		
amlodipine – Norvasc	5–10 mg once daily		Hypotension, flushing, headache, edema.	$$-$$$
diltiazem – Cardizem, Cardizem CD, Cardizem SR, generics	Regular: 30–120 mg TID–QID CD: 120–480 mg once daily SR: 60–240 mg BID		Caution in patients with CHF or bradycardia.	Regular $-$$$$ CD $$-$$$$ SR $-$$$
nifedipine – Adalat PA, Adalat XL, generics	PA: 10–40 mg BID XL: 30–120 mg once daily		Hypotension, tachycardia, flushing, edema.	PA $$-$$$$ XL $$-$$$$
verapamil – Isoptin, Isoptin SR, generics	Regular: 80–240 mg BID SR: 180–480 mg daily		Bradycardia, heart block, hypotension, constipation, flushing, edema.	Regular $-$$ SR $$-$$$$

Cost of 30-day supply – includes drug cost only.
Legend: $ < $25 $$ $25–50 $$$ $50–75 $$$$ > $75

Dosage adjustment may be required in renal impairment – see Appendix I.
Abbreviations: SL = sublingual; SR = sustained release; CD = controlled delivery;
XL = extended release.
† The short-acting dihydropyridine calcium channel blockers should be avoided; long-acting/sustained-release preparations are preferred.

flow by dilating conductive arteries. The dihydropyridines also have an effect on coronary resistance vessels, which may lead to deleterious effects in some patients by inducing coronary steal with redistribution of flow away from ischemic zones. There is mounting evidence that the use of short-acting calcium channel blockers may be associated with adverse cardiac events. Although no clear data are available concerning the patient with stable angina, it would seem prudent to **avoid the use of short-acting dihydropyridines** in patients with coronary artery disease. The rationale for using a short-acting agent when long-acting agents are available must be questioned.

Combination Therapy

Nitrates and either beta-blockers or calcium channel blockers are usually very effective. The increased heart rate seen during nitrate therapy may be blunted by the beta-blocker or rate-limiting calcium channel blocker. Adding a beta-blocker to a rate-limiting calcium channel blocker can be undesirable because excessive bradycardia may occur. Combination therapy allows for titration of doses of individual agents to maximize benefits and to minimize side effects. There are little data to support the use of combination therapy despite the fact that this approach is widely used.

Coronary Artery Revascularization

Coronary artery bypass surgery or percutaneous transluminal coronary artery angioplasty may be indicated for the patient who is significantly limited by recurrent symptoms despite maximal medical therapy.

Unstable Angina Pectoris

Definition

Patients with unstable angina are a heterogeneous group: those on no medication with new onset exertional angina and those already on maximal antianginal therapy presenting with rest pain and electrocardiographic changes.

Goals of Therapy

- To reduce episodes of chest pain or other symptoms of myocardial ischemia
- To prevent the onset of MI
- To treat or reverse secondary causes of unstable angina

Investigations

- Thorough history with special attention to:
  - pain: quality, severity, location, radiation, precipitating and relieving factors
  - effect of nitroglycerin
  - duration of anginal symptoms, previous cardiac events, risk factors
- Physical examination:
  - presence of hypertension, valvular heart disease, heart failure, cardiomegaly
- Laboratory tests:
  - ECG, CBC, electrolytes, creatinine, CPK (MB), blood glucose and cholesterol
- Treadmill exercise test:
  - in patients with atypical pain or no ECG changes to clarify if symptoms are cardiac in origin
  - for predischarge risk stratification
  - to determine severity of underlying coronary artery disease and relative risk of future events

Treadmill exercise testing can be carried out safely in patients with unstable angina who respond well to medical therapy. It is useful in determining whether further invasive diagnostic procedures are required.

Therapeutic Choices (Figure 2)

Nonpharmacologic Choices

- Patients generally should be admitted to hospital for bed rest. The presence of a quiet atmosphere, reassurance, explanation of the nature of the problem, analgesia and mild sedation are helpful initial measures.
- Attention to potential secondary causes (i.e., anemia, fever, concurrent infection, congestive heart failure, tachy- or bradyarrhythmias) is mandatory since their management may control the symptoms of unstable angina.

Pharmacologic Choices (Table 2)
Anticoagulant and Antiplatelet Therapy

Many patients have evidence of thrombus formation involving one or more atherosclerotic plaques within their coronary circulation. ASA and full-dose heparin are effective in reducing the number of episodes of ischemia and the incidence of progression to infarction. During the hospital phase, heparin and ASA appear superior to ASA alone in preventing refractory symptoms and the progression to MI. Following discharge from

Figure 2: **Management of Unstable Angina Pectoris**

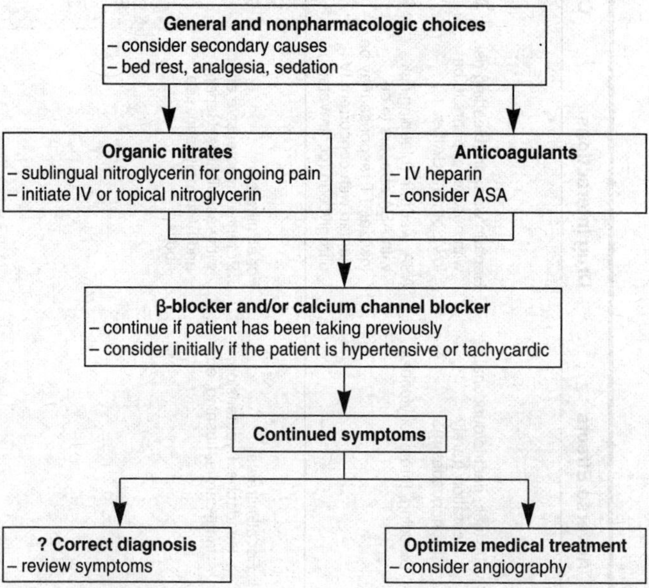

hospital, long-term prophylactic therapy with ASA reduces the incidence of reinfarction and has beneficial effects on mortality.

Antianginal Therapy
Nitrates

Organic nitrates have potent preload reducing effects and lower myocardial oxygen demand. Their effects on epicardial diameter may increase coronary blood supply and myocardial oxygen supply in some patients with severe, epicardial stenoses. There is growing evidence that the nitrates, particularly nitroglycerin, have primary antiplatelet effects. The latter 2 effects may be of particular importance in unstable angina with pain occurring at rest, since these transient episodes of ischemia are probably caused by reductions in coronary blood flow rather than increased cardiac demand.

Although IV nitroglycerin is widely employed, nitroglycerin ointment or an oral formulation may be appropriate. IV nitroglycerin is easily titrated to the patient's symptoms and its effect on systemic arterial blood pressure. Nitrates are usually well tolerated although headache is a prominent side effect. Intermittent topical nitrate regimens should not be used in patients with unstable angina. **Caution should be used when changing from continuous nitrates to an intermittent regimen in patients recovering from unstable angina.**

Table 2: Drug Therapy for Unstable Angina

Drug	Dosage	Dosage Adjustment	Adverse Effects	Drug Interactions	Cost*
Anticoagulants and Antiplatelets					
ASA Aspirin, Entrophen, generics	325 mg/d	None.	Gastritis, gastric/duodenal ulceration (rarely bronchospasm).	Heparin/warfarin (bleeding risk with heparin appears to be low); other NSAIDs.	$
heparin Hepalean, Heparin Leo, generics	5 000 unit bolus IV, then 1 000 units/h; adjust dosage based on aPTT	Follow aPTT (should be maintained at 2–2.5 × control). Draw first aPTT 4 h after initial bolus.	Bleeding, thrombocytopenia.	ASA, warfarin (bleeding risk with ASA appears to be low); aPTT response may be blunted with concurrent IV nitroglycerin (controversial).	$†
Organic Nitrates					
IV nitroglycerin Tridil, generics	10–150 mg/min IV (titrate dose to symptoms and blood pressure)	If symptoms recur ↑ infusion rate by 15–25%. No maximum dosage, although high infusion rates associated with significant ethanol dose in diluent.	For all nitrates: Headache, hypotension, tachycardia, flushing, edema.	For all nitrates: Potential hypotensive effect with vasodilators. Heparin and IV nitroglycerin, see above.	$†
topical nitroglycerin Nitrol	2.5–5 cm Q4–6H				$–$$
isosorbide dinitrate Isordil, generics	10–30 mg PO TID (on QID schedule)	Often started after stabilization on IV nitroglycerin.			$

Drug	Dose	Comments	Cost
Calcium Channel Blockers‡			
Nondihydropyridines			
verapamil 🔔 Isoptin SR, generics	180–480 mg daily	All: Caution in CHF.	$–$$$
diltiazem Cardizem CD & SR, generics	120–360 mg daily	Bradycardia, heart block, hypotension, constipation, flushing, edema.	$$–$$$
		Bradycardia, hypotension.	
Dihydropyridines			
amlodipine Norvasc	5–10 mg daily	Hypotension, flushing, marked peripheral edema.	$$–$$$
nifedipine Adalat PA, Adalat XL, generics	30–120 mg once daily	Hypotension, tachycardia, flushing, edema.	$$–$$$$
		All: additive effect with β-blockers, digoxin, amiodarone. Monitor for excessive bradycardia.	$–$$$
Beta-blockersπ			
metoprolol Betaloc, Lopresor, generics	25 mg PO BID; max. 200 mg BID	For all β-blockers: Caution in patients with CHF, reactive airway disease. Monitor carefully in diabetics.	$–$$
atenolol 🔔 Tenormin, generics	25 mg PO daily; max. 200 mg BID	For all β-blockers: Bradycardia, hypotension, dyspnea, fatigue, depression.	$–$$$
		For all β-blockers: With digoxin: ↑ bradycardia. Ca++ channel blockers, amiodarone, antiarrhythmics may ↑ cardiodepressant effect.	

π β-blockers suggested are examples only. Both metoprolol and atenolol are β₁-selective; however, any β-blockers may be used. Probably best to avoid those β-blockers with intrinsic sympathomimetic activity (e.g., pindolol) in the acute setting.
Abbreviations: SR = sustained release; CD = controlled delivery; XL = extended release.

* Cost of 30-day supply – includes drug cost only.
† Cost of average 1-day supply because duration of therapy varies.
Legend: $ < $25 $$ $25–50 $$$ $50–75 $$$$ > $75
🔔 Dosage adjustment may be required in renal impairment – see Appendix I.
‡ The short-acting calcium channel blockers should be avoided in unstable angina.

Beta-blockers

The role of beta-blockers in the treatment of unstable angina is being re-examined because many ischemic episodes are not preceded by increases in heart rate or blood pressure and appear secondary to a primary decrease in myocardial oxygen supply. When used alone, they may not be effective in preventing ischemic episodes. Patients already on a beta-blocker should continue and their antianginal therapy intensified with another agent. For those not on a beta-blocker, one in combination with nitrates may be appropriate. This is particularly true if the patient is anxious and/or has underlying tachycardia and hypertension. In the patient with refractory symptoms despite treatment with nitrates and heparin, a beta-blocker is appropriate.

Calcium Channel Blockers

Calcium channel blockers can be effective if the patient continues to have symptoms despite therapy. Diltiazem may be beneficial in the occasional patient with clinical evidence of coronary vasospasm with intermittent episodes of pain accompanied by electrocardiographic evidence of ST segment elevation. The short-acting calcium channel blockers should be avoided in light of clinical trials suggesting that these agents, particularly the short-acting form of nifedipine, are potentially dangerous in the setting of unstable angina.

Coronary Artery Revascularization

Coronary artery bypass surgery or percutaneous transluminal coronary artery angioplasty may be indicated in patients with continued symptoms of myocardial ischemia on medical therapy.

Pharmacoeconomic Considerations

Jeffrey A. Johnson, PhD

Available cost-effectiveness data suggest that medical therapy or coronary angioplasty are the preferred initial strategies for low-risk coronary disease; whereas, CABG is recommended for many high-risk patients, particularly those with triple-vessel disease and impaired LV function. For patients with milder symptoms and milder coronary disease, revascularization therapy is likely to be less cost-effective. Any assessment of cost of treatment must take into account the cost of investigation, treatment, the morbidity associated with procedures or side effects of drugs, together with that of recurrent hospitalization, prolonged life, and premature death. Taking these factors into account, medical therapy is the least expensive short- and long-term treatment for angina pectoris (Cleland 1996).

Suggested Reading

O'Rourke RA. Cost-effective management of chronic stable angina. Clin Cardiol 1996;19:497–501.

Cleland JG. Can improved quality of care reduce the costs of managing angina pectoris? Eur Heart J 1996;17(Suppl A):29–40.

Suggested Reading List

Cairns J, Theroux P, Armstrong P, et al. Unstable angina—report from a Canadian expert roundtable. *Can J Cardiol* 1996; 12:1279–1292.

Maseri A. Aspects of the medical therapy of angina pectoris. *Drugs* 1991;42 Suppl 1:28–30.

Opie LH. Calcium channel antagonists in the management of anginal syndromes: changing concepts in relation to the role of coronary vasospasm. *Prog Cardiovasc Dis* 1996;38: 291–314.

Packer M. Drug therapy. Combined beta-adrenergic and calcium-entry blockade in angina pectoris. *N Engl J Med* 1989; 320:709–718.

Ribeiro PA, Shah PM. Unstable angina: new insights into pathophysiologic characteristics, prognosis, and management strategies. *Curr Probl Cardiol* 1996;21: 669–731.

CHAPTER 24

Congestive Heart Failure

Jean L. Rouleau, MD, FRCPC

Goals of Therapy

- To limit factors that precipitate or aggravate heart failure
- To control symptoms and signs
- To improve quality of life
- To prevent progression of the disease
- To improve survival

Classification

Of the two broad categories, the most common is **systolic heart failure**, which is due to the impaired pumping ability of the heart. This usually occurs in patients with a left ventricular ejection fraction $\leq 35\%$. Those with systolic dysfunction but no overt heart failure have been identified as a subgroup.

In **diastolic heart failure**, the systolic function is preserved but filling of the heart is impaired. The left ventricular ejection fraction is $\geq 45\%$. Two broad subgroups are patients with hypertrophic cardiomyopathy and those without.

Investigations (Figure 1)

The history and physical are used to assess the severity of congestive heart failure (CHF), to identify precipitating or aggravating causes, and to exclude other causes of symptoms and signs of heart failure.

- Routine laboratory tests (Figure 1) should be done in all patients and, if possible, should include assessment of cardiac function by echocardiography.
- Special laboratory tests are reserved for those patients whose precipitating causes or complications are being sought or re-evaluated.

Therapeutic Choices (Figures 2 and 3)

Nonpharmacologic Choices

The treatment of precipitating or aggravating causes is essential in either systolic or diastolic heart failure.

- The treatment of myocardial ischemia is a top priority since these patients are the most likely to benefit from coronary revascularization. Percutaneous transluminal coronary

Figure 1: **Investigation of Congestive Heart Failure**

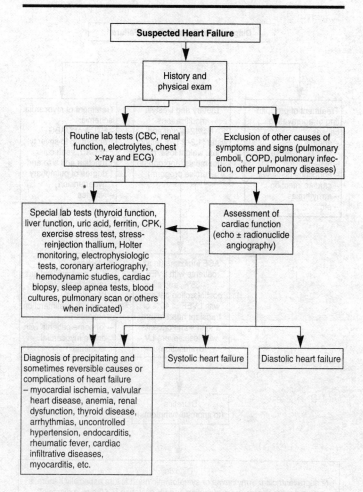

angioplasty (PTCA) has expanded the indications for coronary revascularization. However, little information exists on the effects of PTCA on survival in patients with severe heart failure. Although there are no prospective randomized studies evaluating the effects of coronary artery bypass surgery on the survival of patients with severe heart failure, current evidence suggests that survival is improved in patients with angina and/or extensive myocardial ischemia. In patients with less severe heart failure, it has been conclusively demonstrated that bypass surgery improves the prognosis of patients with more extensive coronary artery disease. Nevertheless, in patients with severe left ventricular dysfunction and marked left ventricular dilatation or pulmonary hypertension, any invasive investigation or therapy is risky

Figure 2: **Management of Systolic Heart Failure**

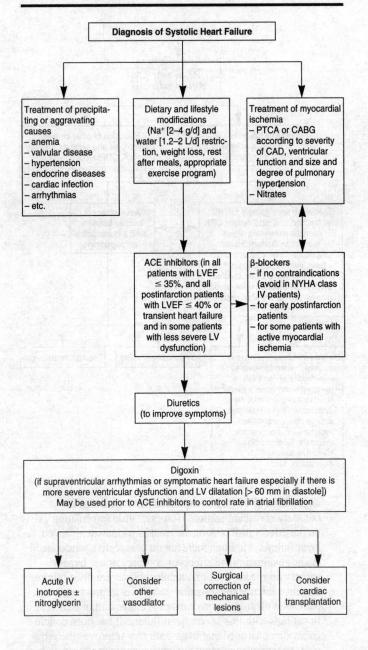

Abbreviations: LV = left ventricle; LVEF = left ventricular ejection fraction; PTCA = percutaneous transluminal coronary angioplasty; CAD = coronary artery disease; CABG = coronary artery bypass graft; NYHA = New York Heart Association.

Figure 3: **Management of Diastolic Heart Failure**

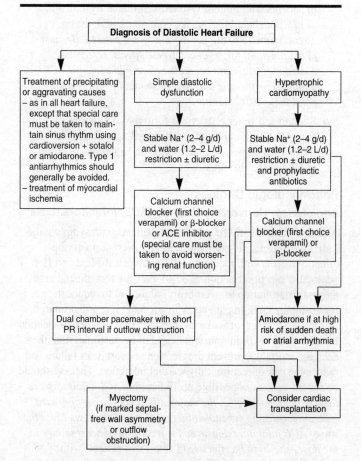

and should be reserved for cases where no other therapeutic options exist or reversible mechanical factors are present.

- The maintenance of sinus rhythm is extremely important, particularly in patients with diastolic dysfunction. Once adequate systemic anticoagulation therapy is sustained for 3 to 4 weeks, cardioversion should be attempted in all patients with atrial fibrillation of less than 6 months duration. In atrial fibrillation of longer duration, where maintenance of sinus rhythm is thought to be particularly important, cardioversion can be attempted in selected cases once loading with an antiarrhythmic drug has been completed (Chapter 25). The maintenance of sinus rhythm in patients with CHF and dilated atria is surprisingly successful when adjunctive therapy is used. In patients with less severe ventricular dysfunction or idiopathic cardiomyopathy, the use of **sotalol** (160 to 320 mg per day) is recommended; in patients with more severe left ventricular dysfunction or in whom beta-blockers are contraindicated, the use of **amiodarone** (200 mg per day) is recommended. *Because of the potential for serious adverse effects, referral to a cardiologist should be made before initiation of amiodarone therapy and sotalol should be initiated under continuous ECG monitoring.*

■ Sodium and water restrictions form the cornerstone of therapy and should be adjusted according to the severity of CHF. Weight loss, rest after meals and appropriate exercise programs are also important.

Pharmacologic Choices
Angiotensin Converting Enzyme (ACE) Inhibitors (Table 1)

ACE inhibitors should be given to all patients with symptomatic CHF unless a specific contraindication is present. In asymptomatic patients with moderate left ventricular dysfunction (left ventricular ejection fraction ≤ 35%), they are recommended to prevent deterioration to overt heart failure and to reduce the need for hospitalization. In patients with a recent myocardial infarction and moderate left ventricular dysfunction (left ventricular ejection fraction ≤ 40 %) or in transient heart failure postinfarction, they decrease mortality, prevent progression to overt heart failure and reduce the risk of recurrent myocardial infarction. Therapy should be started as soon as possible postinfarction. *ACE inhibitors are largely interchangeable, the major differences being approved indications, dosing schedule and cost. Nevertheless, we favor the use of ACE inhibitors approved for treatment of heart failure in the doses shown to be effective* (Table 1). In patients with diastolic heart failure, ACE inhibitors are not first-line drugs but can be used to control arterial hypertension and to help induce regression of left ventricular hypertrophy where this is thought to be a precipitating factor.

Nitrates

Either topical or oral nitrates are recommended to improve symptoms and exercise tolerance in patients intolerant of ACE inhibitors or who remain symptomatic despite optimal therapy with ACE inhibitors, diuretics and digoxin or in whom myocardial ischemia is thought to be a factor. Doses of isosorbide dinitrate 30 mg PO TID before meals, or topical preparations 0.4 to 0.6 mg from 8 a.m. to 8 p.m. are recommended. Newer mononitrate preparations are also effective. A nitrate-free period of at least 10 and preferably 12 hours each day is necessary to prevent loss of nitrate effect.

Table 1: ACE Inhibitors

Drug	Equivalent Dose	Dosage ❦	Adverse Effects (common to all ACEIs)	Drug Interactions (common to all ACEIs)	Cost*
benazepril Lotensin	10–20 mg	10–60 mg/d given daily to BID	Hypotension, hyperkalemia, dry cough, renal insufficiency, angioedema (rare), skin rashes, taste disturbance, proteinuria, neutropenia (rare), headache, dizziness.	Diuretics → hypotension (monitor BP).	$$–$$$$
captopril † Capoten, generics	50 mg	75–150 mg/d divided BID–TID		Potassium-sparing diuretics → hyperkalemia (monitor K⁺).	$$–$$$
cilazapril † Inhibace	2.5 mg	2.5–5 mg/d given daily		Potassium → hyperkalemia (monitor K⁺).	$$
enalapril † Vasotec	5–10 mg	10–40 mg/d given daily to BID		NSAIDs → decreased hypotensive effect (monitor BP).	$$–$$$$
fosinopril † Monopril	10 mg	10–40 mg/d given daily		Lithium → lithium toxicity (monitor lithium levels).	$$–$$$
lisinopril † Prinivil, Zestril, generics	5–10 mg	10–40 mg/d given daily			$$–$$$
perindopril Coversyl	4 mg	2–8 mg/d given daily			$–$$$
quinapril † Accupril	10 mg	10–40 mg/d given daily to BID			$$
ramipril † Altace	2.5 mg	2.5–20 mg/d given daily			$$–$$$
trandolapril † Mavik	1 mg	1–4 mg daily			$$–$$$

❦ All ACE inhibitors are excreted primarily by the renal route except fosinopril, which is excreted by the renal/hepatic routes. Dosage adjustments may be required in renal impairment for ACEIs excreted primarily by the renal route – see Appendix 1; fosinopril does not require dosage adjustment.

* Cost of 30-day supply – includes drug cost only.
Legend: $ < $20 $$ $20–40 $$$ $40–60 $$$$ > $60

† All ACE inhibitors are indicated for hypertension. Captopril, cilazapril, enalapril, fosinopril, lisinopril, quinapril and ramipril are also indicated for heart failure. Only captopril, enalapril, lisinopril and ramipril have been shown to reduce morbidity and prolong survival in heart failure.

Hydralazine

Hydralazine combined with nitrates is indicated in patients with symptomatic systolic heart failure who are intolerant of ACE inhibitors and angiotensin II receptor blockers or have refractory CHF despite use of ACE inhibitors, diuretics and digoxin. Doses of 75 to 100 mg PO TID are recommended. Some patients may require lower doses, but these higher doses were used in studies where hydralazine in combination with nitrates prolonged survival.

Diuretics (Table 2)

Diuretics should be used as required to control signs and symptoms of CHF. In patients with diastolic dysfunction, they can be a first-line drug; in patients with systolic dysfunction, they are generally reserved for those who are symptomatic despite the use of ACE inhibitors.

Digoxin

Digoxin should be used to control ventricular response in patients with atrial fibrillation and in patients with symptomatic systolic dysfunction to improve symptoms and exercise tolerance. It appears to be particularly effective in those with more severe ventricular dysfunction and ventricular dilatation (diastolic diameter $\geq$ 60 mm). Maintenance doses should be 0.125 to 0.25 mg PO daily depending on the patient's size and renal function.

Beta-blockers (Table 3)

Beta-blockers can be used in patients with chronic heart failure to preserve or improve ventricular function. Started in extremely low doses (i.e., **carvedilol** 3.125 mg PO BID or **metoprolol** 6.25 mg PO BID), these *beta-blockers are increased slowly over a period of weeks to months* to maintain doses that average carvedilol 25 mg PO BID or metoprolol 50 mg PO BID. In patients with left ventricular dysfunction postinfarction, they should be started before hospital discharge and continued indefinitely. Beta-blockers should be avoided in all patients with very low cardiac output. They can be used to control symptoms of myocardial ischemia in patients with CHF and angina. Although not first-line drugs for diastolic dysfunction, they are beneficial in some patients, controlling heart rate at rest and during exercise and permitting better filling of the ventricle. Beta-blockers can be particularly useful in patients in whom myocardial ischemia is an associated problem.

Table 2: Diuretics

Drug	Dosage	Comments	Adverse Effects	Drug Interactions	Cost*
Thiazides and Related Diuretics			**(Common to thiazide and loop diuretics)**	**(Common to thiazide and loop diuretics)**	
chlorthalidone Hygroton, generics	50–200 mg/d given daily	Mild diuretic; acts on distal tubule. Use: mild heart failure or with loop diuretic.	Dehydration, hypokalemia, nausea, anorexia, hyperglycemia (more with thiazides), hyperuricemia, weakness, fatigue, rash, increased total cholesterol, ototoxicity (with high doses of loop diuretics).	Lithium → lithium toxicity (monitor lithium levels). Digoxin → digoxin toxicity if K^+ depleted (monitor K^+). Antidiabetic agents → increased blood glucose (monitor glucose). Corticosteroids → hypokalemia (monitor K^+). NSAIDs → decreased diuretic effect; increased renal toxicity (monitor).	$
hydrochlorothiazide HydroDiuril, generics	25–200 mg/d given daily to BID	Mild diuretic; acts on distal tubule (+ proximal tubule). Use: mild heart failure or with loop diuretic.			$
metolazone Zaroxolyn	2.5–10 mg/d given daily to BID	Strong diuretic; acts on dilutional distal + proximal tubules. Use: refractory heart failure.			$
Loop Diuretics					
bumetanide Burinex	1–4 mg/d	Strong diuretic; acts on ascending loop of Henle. Use: alternative to furosemide particularly when renal blood flow is reduced.	See above.	See above.	$–$$
ethacrynic acid Edecrin	50–400 mg/d given daily to BID	Strong diuretic; acts on ascending loop of Henle (+ other portions of nephron). Use: alternative to furosemide.			$–$$$$

(cont'd)

Table 2: **Diuretics** (cont'd)

Drug	Dosage	Comments	Adverse Effects	Drug Interactions	Cost*
furosemide Lasix, generics	20–500 mg/d given daily to BID	Strong diuretic; acts on ascending loop of Henle (+ proximal + distal tubules). Use: moderate to severe heart failure.			$–$$$$
Potassium-sparing Diuretics			**(Common to potassium-sparing diuretics)**	**(Common to potassium-sparing diuretics)**	
amiloride Midamor	2.5–10 mg/d given daily to BID	Moderate diuretic; acts on distal tubule. Use: with K+ wasting diuretic.	Hyperkalemia, gynecomastia (with spironolactone).	ACE inhibitors → hyperkalemia (monitor K+).	$
spironolactone Aldactone, generics	12.5–200 mg/d daily to BID	Mild diuretic; acts on distal tubule. Use: with K+ wasting diuretic.		Potassium supplements → hyperkalemia (avoid).	$
triamterene Dyrenium	50–200 mg/d given daily to BID	Mild diuretic; acts on distal tubule. Use: with K+ wasting diuretic.			$–$$

* Cost of 30-day supply – includes drug cost only.
Legend:　$ < $20　$$ $20–40　$$$ $40–60　$$$$ $60–80

Table 3: Beta-blockers

Drug	Dosage	Comments	Adverse Effects	Drug Interactions	Cost*
carvedilol Coreg	3.125–25 mg PO BID	Nonselective, also alpha-blocker resulting in some vasodilating effects.	Orthostatic hypotension, fluid retention.	↑ cardiodepressant effect with calcium channel blockers, antiarrhythmics.	$$$$
metoprolol Betaloc, Lopressor, generics	6.25–50 mg PO BID	Selective β-blocker. 6.25 mg strength not commercially available.	All: bronchospasm, dyspnea, bradycardia, malaise, fatigue, asthenia, may mask hypoglycemia.		$

* Cost of 30-day supply – includes drug cost only.
Legend: $ < $20 $$ $20–40 $$$ $40–60 $$$$ $60–80

Antiarrhythmic Drugs, Pacemakers and Devices

These should generally be reserved for symptomatic or sustained ventricular arrhythmias or to help maintain sinus rhythm in atrial fibrillation. Class IC agents (flecainide, propafenone) and Class IA agents (quinidine, procainamide) should be avoided. The Class III drug (**sotalol** 160 to 320 mg per day according to severity of heart failure) may be used with caution. **Amiodarone** (200 to 300 mg per day) is effective and usually considered the drug of choice in patients with severe CHF. Serum potassium should be kept ≥ 4 mmol/L in all patients. Antiarrhythmic drug therapy, when indicated, should be started in the hospital setting. Implantable cardiac defibrillators should be used when pharmacologic therapy has failed. A dual chamber (DDD) pacemaker with a short PR interval (0.08 s) may improve symptoms and exercise tolerance in patients with hypertrophic cardiomyopathy and outflow obstruction.

Anticoagulation

The guidelines for systemic anticoagulation therapy in patients with or without CHF are similar. Anticoagulation is strongly recommended in all patients with heart failure and associated atrial fibrillation, demonstrated intraventricular thrombi, acute myocarditis and for the first 3 to 6 months postacute anterior myocardial infarction. It is not recommended for routine use in sinus rhythm with no other risk factors for emboli. The INR to be achieved is 1.8 to 2.5. In patients at risk from **warfarin** therapy or where warfarin therapy is not indicated, **ASA** 325 mg daily is recommended (Chapter 32).

Calcium Channel Blockers

In systolic heart failure and in postinfarction patients with left ventricular dysfunction, the use of calcium channel blockers is generally contraindicated. In systolic left ventricular dysfunction, the calcium channel blocker, **amlodipine**, may be used in specific cases: hypertension not controlled with ACE inhibitors or with associated angina or where ACE inhibitors are contraindicated and the combination of hydralazine and nitrate is inadequate or not tolerated. In patients with diastolic dysfunction, calcium channel blockers may be used to control arterial hypertension and to help induce regression of myocardial hypertrophy. They also provide symptomatic relief in up to 60% of patients with hypertrophic cardiomyopathy. In diastolic dysfunction, the calcium channel blocker most commonly used is **verapamil** (240 mg per day). **Diltiazem** (180 to 240 mg per day) has also shown benefit. In hypertrophic cardiomyopathy, calcium channel blockers should in some patients be started in hospital as they may cause significant deterioration.

Angiotensin II Receptor Blockers

These medications block the effects of angiotensin II better than ACE inhibitors but do not have the beneficial effects on vasodilator systems that ACE inhibitors have. Short-term studies suggest that **losartan** 50 mg daily for 48 weeks is beneficial in elderly patients in heart failure.[1] Long-term data are also emerging but more data is necessary before they can be recommended in heart failure.

IV Inotrope or Vasodilator Therapy

Dobutamine (5 to 10 μg/kg/min), **milrinone** (0.375 to 0.75 μg/kg/min) or IV **nitroglycerin** (1 to 2 μg/kg/min) $\pm$ **dopamine** (5 to 10 μg/kg/min) infusions for 48 to 72 hours can be used to treat patients with acute decompensation of severe systolic heart failure. Special care must be taken to avoid ventricular arrhythmias and hypokalemia.

Surgical Correction of Mechanical Lesions

Although a number of cardiac reduction and cardiomyoplasty procedures are being offered today, at this time only aneurysm resection and valvular repair are recommended in patients where this is deemed responsible for the progression of heart failure.

Continuous Positive Airways Pressure (CPAP)

There is mounting evidence that sleep apnea contributes to the progression of heart failure in some patients. CPAP should be considered in these patients.

Therapeutic Tips

- ACE inhibitors should be used with care in patients with renal dysfunction, particularly those with a history of hypertension, and are contraindicated in bilateral renal artery stenosis. Although the risks of hyperkalemia and deterioration of renal function are higher in patients with diabetes, the long-term use of ACE inhibitors (when tolerated) has been useful in preserving renal function.

- When ACE inhibitors cause hypotensive symptoms or deterioration of renal function, a reduction in the dosage of diuretics frequently reduces hypotensive symptoms and recuperates lost renal function.

- Cough is unrelated to the use of ACE inhibitors in the majority of patients with CHF. Whenever possible the ACE inhibitor should be continued despite the cough. When the cough is intolerable, changing ACE inhibitor type may reduce the cough.

[1] *Lancet 1997;349:747–752.*

■ Diastolic heart failure, although due to impaired filling of the left ventricle, is generally associated with hypertension and renal dysfunction and is much more common in older patients. These are all complicating factors that must be considered when choosing one form of therapy over another.

■ Patients in periods of acute decompensation of otherwise chronic heart failure should receive furosemide IV to assure rapid and complete delivery of the dose as edematous and sluggish bowels may lead to erratic absorption of oral doses.

Suggested Reading List

Johnstone DE, Abdulla A, Arnold JMO, et al. Diagnosis and management of heart failure. *Can J Cardiol* 1994;10: 613–631.

Louie EK, Edwards LC III. Hypertrophic cardiomyopathy. *Prog Cardiovasc Dis* 1994;36:275–308.

Maron BS. Hypertrophic cardiomyopathy. *Curr Probl Cardiol* 1993;18:637–704.

Report of the American College of Cardiology/American Heart Association Task Force on Practice Guidelines (Committee on Evaluation and Management of Heart Failure). Guidelines for the evaluation and management of heart failure. *J Am Coll Cardiol* 1995;26:1376–1398.

Stauffer JC, Gaasch WH. Recognition and treatment of left ventricular diastolic dysfunction. *Prog Cardiovasc Dis* 1990;32:319–332.

Tardif J-C, Rouleau J-L. Diastolic dysfunction. *Can J Cardiol* 1996;12:389–398.

CHAPTER 25

Supraventricular Tachycardia

Anne M. Gillis, MD, FRCPC and
D. George Wyse, MD, PhD, FRCPC

The most common causes of supraventricular tachycardia (SVT) are atrial fibrillation, atrial flutter, atrioventricular node reentrant tachycardia or reciprocating tachycardia utilizing the atrioventricular node and an extra-nodal accessory electrical connection between atria and ventricles (e.g., Wolff-Parkinson-White syndrome). In general, it is safest to assume that patients presenting only with atrial flutter have both atrial flutter and fibrillation, although the atrial fibrillation may not be documented.

Goals of Therapy

- To convert to sinus rhythm
- To control ventricular rate (chronic atrial fibrillation/flutter)
- To relieve associated symptoms: palpitations, fatigue, dyspnea, presyncope, syncope, angina, heart failure
- To prevent recurrence
- To prevent complications: life-threatening arrhythmia (e.g., Wolff-Parkinson-White syndrome), stroke, other systemic thromboembolism, tachycardia-induced heart failure, myocardial infarction

Investigations

- Thorough history and physical examination with special attention to detecting underlying structural heart disease
- 12-lead ECG, during SVT and sinus rhythm
- Thorough attempt to document SVT with ECG, including 24-hour ambulatory monitoring and/or event recorders
- Chest x-ray
- 2-D echocardiogram, transesophageal echocardiogram in special circumstances (see Therapeutic Tips)
- TSH, CBC, INR, PTT (for patients with atrial fibrillation/flutter)

Table 1: Acute Therapy of Persistent Paroxysmal Atrial Fibrillation/Flutter

Patient Unstable	Patient Stable*
Electrical cardioversion 100–400 J (repeat if necessary) →	**Achieve heart rate control:** propranolol 2–10 mg by IV infusion in 1 mg boluses Q1 min
	or
	metoprolol 5–15 mg by IV infusion in 5 mg boluses Q5 min
	or
	verapamil 5–20 mg IV push in 5 mg boluses Q5 min
	or
	diltiazem 0.25 mg/kg IV infusion then 0.35 mg/kg IV 15 min later if necessary
	or
	procainamide 10–15 mg/kg given as 25 mg/min IV infusion if blood pressure stable, then maintenance dose 2–4 mg/min IV (Wolff-Parkinson-White syndrome), depending on assessment of need for antithrombotic therapy†
	or
	digoxin 0.5–0.75 mg by IV infusion over 30 min, followed by an additional 0.75 mg in divided doses over next 12–24 h

*Procainamide is the drug of choice for Wolff-Parkinson-White-Syndrome. See Therapeutic Tips.
†See Therapeutic Tips concerning antithrombotic therapy.

Figure 1: Approach to Management of Atrial Fibrillation

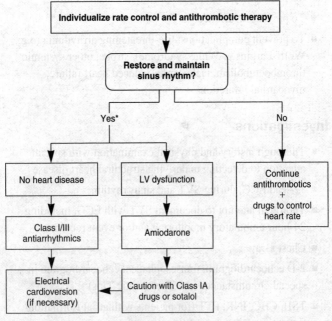

*See Therapeutic Tips concerning antithrombotic therapy.

Paroxysmal Atrial Fibrillation/Flutter
(Table 1, Figure 1)
Pharmacologic Choices

Drugs that slow conduction in the AV node are administered to achieve heart rate control (Tables 1 and 2). Beta-blockers and calcium channel blockers are more effective than digoxin but must be used cautiously in patients with heart failure.

Heart Rate Control
Digoxin

Digoxin is effective at rest, has relatively few side effects, can be administered once daily and is inexpensive. It is frequently ineffective for heart rate control during exercise.

Beta-blockers

Beta-blockers effectively control heart rate at rest and during exercise but must be prescribed cautiously in patients with heart failure or bronchospastic lung disease.

Calcium Channel Blockers

Verapamil effectively controls heart rate at rest and during exercise. Diltiazem is less effective, but synergistic effects are observed with digoxin. Nifedipine and other dihydropyridine calcium channel blockers are ineffective as they have no effects on AV node conduction.

Restoration and Maintenance of Sinus Rhythm

Drugs that alter the electrophysiology of atrial muscle (atrial conduction velocity and/or action potential duration) are effective in converting atrial fibrillation/flutter to sinus rhythm and maintaining it (Table 3). The initial drug of choice remains empiric. Consideration must be given to a strategy for anti-thrombotic therapy prior to restoration of sinus rhythm when paroxysmal atrial fibrillation is persistent (i.e., does not stop spontaneously). Atrial fibrillation which is continuous for ≥ 48 hours requires specific antithrombotic therapy prior to restoration of sinus rhythm (see Therapeutic Tips). Intermittent, self-administered therapy at the onset of atrial fibrillation to achieve pharmacologic cardioversion can be used in selected patients.

Class IA Drugs

These cause mild to moderate prolongation of conduction velocity that may manifest in some QRS interval prolongation and moderate prolongation of the action potential duration that manifests as QT interval prolongation. Torsades de pointes ventricular tachycardia is the most serious side effect in the setting of marked QT interval prolongation.

Table 2: Heart Rate Control of Fibrillation/Flutter or Termination/Prevention of PAT

Drug	Dosage	Dosage Adjustment	Adverse Effects	Drug Interactions	Cost*
digoxin 🔹 Lanoxin	PO or IV: loading: 1–1.5 mg IV or PO: maintenance 0.125–0.375 mg/d	↓ maintenance dose in renal insufficiency.	Bradycardia, nausea, vomiting, visual disturbances, proarrhythmia.	With β-blockers, Ca⁺⁺ channel blockers, amiodarone, propafenone, quinidine, in hypokalemia: ↓ digoxin dose by 25–50%.	$
Beta-blockers *propranolol* Inderal, Inderal-LA, generics	IV: 4–8 mg PO: 80–240 mg/d	Monitor carefully in diabetic patients; caution in patients with CHF or bronchospastic lung disease.	Bradycardia, hypotension, dyspnea, fatigue, depression.	With digoxin, Ca⁺⁺ channel blockers, amiodarone: ↓ dose 25–50%. Hypoglycemic agents.	$ LA $–$$
atenolol 🔹 Tenormin, generics	PO: 50–150 mg/d	As per propranolol and ↓ dose in moderate to severe renal insufficiency.	As per propranolol.	As per propranolol.	$
metoprolol Betaloc, Lopresor, generics	IV: 5–15 mg PO: 100–300 mg/d	As per propranolol.	As per propranolol.	As per propranolol.	$
nadolol 🔹 Corgard, generics	PO: 20–160 mg/d	As per propranolol and ↓ dose in moderate to severe renal insufficiency.	As per propranolol.	As per propranolol.	$

Calcium Channel Blockers			
verapamil Isoptin, Isoptin SR, generics	IV: 5–15 mg 80 mg PO TID; max. dose 120 mg QID – 240 mg BID	Caution in patients with CHF.	Bradycardia, hypotension, constipation, flushing.	β-blockers, digoxin, amiodarone.	$–$$ SR $$–$$$
diltiazem Cardizem, Cardizem CD, Cardizem SR, generics	IV: 0.25–0.35 mg/kg PO: 180–540 mg/d	Caution in patients with CHF.	Bradycardia, hypotension.	As per verapamil.	$$–$$$$ SR/CD $$–$$$$$

NB: *The β-blockers suggested are examples only. Atenolol and metoprolol have β₁ selectivity; both atenolol and nadolol are hydrophilic agents and less likely to cause CNS side effects. Acebutolol, labetolol and timolol would also be effective. Sustained-release preparations for some agents are available.*

* *Cost of 30-day supply of oral doses – includes drug cost only.*
Legend: $ < $30 $$ $30–60 $$$ $60–100 $$$$ $100–140 $$$$$ > $140

Table 3: Drug Therapy for Long-term Prophylaxis of Atrial Fibrillation/PAT

Drug	Dosage	Dosage Adjustment	Adverse Effects	Drug Interactions	Cost*
Class IA *quinidine* ♥ Biquin Durules, generics	200–250 mg PO Q8H ↑ by 200–250 mg doses if QTc < 460 msec. ↓ dose if QTc ≥ 500 msec. Max. dose 1 g PO Q8H	↓ initial dose 50% + ↑ dosing interval Q12H in renal failure. Active metabolites accumulate in renal failure but therapeutic blood monitoring of them is not readily available. Careful monitoring of the ECG intervals should guide dosing decisions.	Diarrhea, stomach cramps, tinnitus, fever, rash, thrombocytopenia, torsades de pointes VT.	↓ digoxin dose by 50%.	$ Biquin Durules $$–$$$$$
procainamide SR ♥ Procan SR, Pronestyl SR	250 mg PO Q6H ↑ by 250 mg increments if QTc < 460 msec. ↓ dose if QTc ≥ 500 msec. Max. dose 1 g PO Q6H	Metabolism depends on rate of acetylation. The active metabolite NAPA accumulates in fast acetylators and in renal failure. Monitor procainamide + NAPA levels and keep sum < 80 μM; monitor ECG intervals.	SLE syndrome, torsades de pointes VT.		$$
disopyramide ♥ Norpace, Norpace CR, Rythmodan, Rythmodan-LA	100 mg PO Q8H CR and LA: 150–250 mg Q12H ↑ by 100 mg increments if QTc < 460 msec. Max. dose 300 mg PO Q8H	↓ initial dose 50% and ↑ dosing interval Q12H in renal failure.	Urinary retention, constipation, dry mouth, torsades de pointes VT.		$–$$ CR/LA $$–$$$

Class IC			
flecainide ▶ Tambocor	50 mg PO Q12H ↑ by 50 mg increments Max. dose 200 mg PO Q12H. ↓ dose if ↑ QRS > 20% from baseline	↓ initial dose 50% in renal failure; titrate dose based on QRS intervals.	VT proarrhythmia, tremor, blurred vision, CHF.	$–$$$$
propafenone ▶ Rythmol	150 mg PO Q8H Max. dose 300 mg PO Q8H. ↓ dose if QRS prolonged > 20% from baseline	↓ initial dose 50% in renal and hepatic failure and ↑ dosing interval to Q12H. Active metabolites accumulate in rapid metabolizers. Monitor QRS duration carefully.	Constipation, headache, metallic taste, VT proarrhythmia.	$$$–$$$$
Class II			
sotalol ▶ Sotacor, generics	80 mg PO Q12H ↑ by 80 mg increments if QTc < 460 msec Max. dose 240 mg PO Q12H. ↓ dose if QTc ≥ 500 msec	↓ initial dose in renal failure. ↓ initial dose to 40 mg PO Q12H in the elderly.	Torsades de pointes VT, hypotension, bradycardia, wheezing.	Digoxin/verapamil/other β-blockers may cause AV block, bradycardia.	$–$$
amiodarone ▶ Cordarone	200 mg PO TID × 2 wk then 200 mg daily or accelerated loading dose in hospital	Avoid high loading dose in setting of sinus bradycardia (HR < 50 beats/min).	Pulmonary toxicity, CNS effects, hyper-/hypo-thyroidism, photosensi-tivity, corneal deposits, hepatic toxicity.	→ quinidine/procainamide dose by 50%. → digoxin dose by 50%. → β-blockers dose by 50%. → warfarin dose by 50%.	$$–$$$$

* Cost of 30-day supply – includes drug cost only.
Legend: $ < $30 $$ $30–60 $$$ $60–100 $$$$ $100–140 $$$$$ > $140

Class IC Drugs

These cause marked prolongation of conduction velocity that manifests as significant QRS interval prolongation.

Class III Drugs

These cause significant prolongation of action potential duration and QT interval prolongation. Torsades de pointes ventricular tachycardia can occur with marked QT interval prolongation.

Nonpharmacologic Choices

- Direct-current cardioversion is the most rapid method for restoring sinus rhythm in a patient with significant hemodynamic compromise, angina or heart failure. It is also effective when used electively, particularly after initiation of antiarrhythmic therapy.

- When heart rate control cannot be achieved or medications are not well tolerated, catheter ablation of the AV node and implantation of a permanent pacemaker should be considered.

- Catheter ablation techniques may prevent recurrent atrial flutter without inducing complete heart block.

- Antitachycardia pacemakers are effective in terminating some episodes of atrial flutter.

- Some surgical techniques may prevent atrial fibrillation and preserve sinus rhythm; the role of atrial-based pacing is being investigated. The implantable automatic atrial defibrillator is at an early stage of investigation.

Chronic Atrial Fibrillation

Pharmacologic Choices

- When sinus rhythm cannot be maintained, therapy is aimed at achieving heart rate control (Table 2).

- Chronic anticoagulation is indicated to reduce the risk of systemic thromboembolism (Table 4).

Nonpharmacologic Choices

- When heart rate control cannot be achieved with drug therapy, catheter ablation of the AV node and implantation of a permanent pacemaker should be considered.

Table 4: **Anticoagulation for Paroxysmal and Chronic Atrial Fibrillation***

Condition	Drug
Patient with no risk factors and Age < 65 yrs	ASA 325 mg/d

Patient with any one of the following risk factors:
  Age < 75 yrs and
    congestive heart failure
    left ventricular dysfunction
    mitral valve disease
    hypertension
    diabetes mellitus
    previous stroke or embolism
    left atrial enlargement
	Warfarin (INR 2.0–3.0)

Age ≥ 75 yrs	Individualize therapy: warfarin (INR 1.8–2.5)

See Therapeutic Tips for anticoagulation prior to restoration of sinus rhythm.

Therapeutic Tips (Atrial Fibrillation/Flutter)

- If atrial fibrillation has been present for ≥ 48 hours, anti-coagulation with heparin should be initiated followed by oral anticoagulation. Attempts to convert atrial fibrillation should be delayed for at least 3 weeks if present for more than 48 hours before initiation of anticoagulation. An increasingly acceptable alternative is immediate anticoagulation with heparin followed by transesophageal echocardiography and then immediate restoration of sinus rhythm if no intra-cardiac clot is noted on the echo. **Warfarin must be started and continued for 4 weeks after restoration of sinus rhythm (regardless of whether it is done immediately or delayed ≥ 3 weeks).**

- Antithrombotic therapy should be considered for all patients with paroxysmal atrial fibrillation or chronic atrial fibrillation based on risk for systemic thromboembolism (Table 4).

- **Digoxin, beta-blockers and calcium channel blockers are contraindicated for atrial fibrillation in Wolff-Parkinson-White syndrome; these drugs favor conduction down the accessory pathway and/or hypotension, which may precipitate ventricular fibrillation.** IV procainamide is the drug of choice (Table 1).

- Prophylactic therapy with Class I/III antiarrhythmic drugs is indicated in high-risk patients and in patients with frequent symptomatic episodes of atrial fibrillation. **These drugs must be used with caution in patients with severe left ventricular dysfunction.**

- **The use of Class IC drugs (flecainide and propafenone) for maintenance of sinus rhythm is contraindicated in patients with coronary artery disease and cannot be recommended for patients with significant ventricular dysfunction.**

- Bradycardia, hypokalemia and hypomagnesemia predispose patients to ventricular proarrhythmia on Class I/III drugs. If patients are taking diuretics, K^+ and Mg^{++} levels should be measured before initiation of therapy; regular monitoring during therapy is also required. Twelve-lead ECGs should be performed at each steady-state dose to assess QTc.

- Since antiarrhythmic agents may precipitate bradyarrhythmia, permanent pacemaker implantation may be required in some patients. Twenty-four hour ambulatory ECG monitoring should be performed at each steady-state dose in high-risk patients.

- Because of the toxicity profile, referral to a cardiologist should be made before initiation of amiodarone therapy.

Supraventricular Tachycardia

The approach to therapy for an acute episode of supraventricular tachycardia is illustrated in Table 5.

The chronic therapy for prevention of paroxysmal supraventricular tachycardia is illustrated in Table 6.

Table 5: Acute Therapy for Paroxysmal SVT

Termination of Acute Episode

A. QRS is ≤ 0.1 s or Patient Known to Have Bundle Branch Block
1. maneuvers to activate the vagus nerve: Valsalva maneuver, carotid sinus massage, pressure on orbit, diving reflex

2. adenosine 6–12 mg by IV push (max. dose 24 mg)
   or
3. verapamil 5–20 mg by IV push in 5 mg boluses Q5 min

4. metoprolol 5–15 mg by IV infusion in 5 mg increments Q5 min
   or
5. diltiazem 0.25 mg/kg IV infusion; then 0.35 mg/kg 15 min later
   or
6. digoxin 0.5–0.75 mg by IV infusion over 15–30 min, followed by additional 0.75 mg in divided doses over 12–24 h

B. QRS is > 0.1 s and No Previous ECG or Patient Known to Have QRS ≤ 0.1 s
1. (Suspect Wolff-Parkinson-White syndrome) procainamide 15 mg/kg given as 25 mg/min infusion if blood pressure stable, then maintenance dose 2–4 mg/min IV

2. electrical cardioversion under anesthesia

Table 6: **Chronic Therapy for Paroxysmal SVT**

A. Recurrences Rare and/or Brief and Hemodynamically Stable; QRS ≤ 0.1 s during PAT or Patient Known to Have Bundle Branch Block

1. vagal maneuvers

or

2. verapamil PO at onset 80 mg Q2H for up to 3 doses

or

3. metoprolol PO at onset 50–100 mg Q2H for up to 3 doses

or

4. propranolol PO at onset 40–80 mg Q2H for up to 3 doses

B. Recurrences Frequent and/or Prolonged and Hemodynamically Stable; QRS ≤ 0.1 s during PAT or Patient Known to Have Bundle Branch Block

1. catheter ablation

or

2. continuous prophylaxis with verapamil 160–480 mg/d

or

3. continuous prophylaxis with diltiazem 180–540 mg/d

or

4. continuous prophylaxis with propranolol 80–240 mg/d

or

5. continuous prophylaxis with metoprolol 100–400 mg/d

or

6. continuous prophylaxis with atenolol 50–200 mg/d

or

7. continuous prophylaxis with equivalent doses of alternative beta-blocker

or

8. continuous prophylaxis with digoxin 0.25–0.5 mg/d

or

9. surgical therapy

C. Recurrences Frequent and/or Prolonged and Hemodynamically Stable; QRS > 0.1 s during PAT in Patient with Known Wolff-Parkinson-White Syndrome

1. catheter ablation

or

2. continuous prophylaxis with sotalol 160–480 mg/d

▼

3. continuous prophylaxis with propafenone 450–900 mg/d plus calcium channel blocker or beta-blocker listed above in B

▼

4. continuous prophylaxis with flecainide 100–400 mg/d plus calcium channel blocker or beta-blocker listed above in B

▼

5. continuous prophylaxis with amiodarone 200–300 mg/d

D. Recurrence Hemodynamically Unstable Regardless of Frequency, Duration or QRS Width

1. catheter ablation or surgical therapy

Pharmacologic Choices

- Drugs that slow conduction in the AV node (e.g., adenosine, beta-blockers, calcium channel blockers, digoxin) are effective in terminating and preventing recurrence of SVT. Maintenance doses are shown in Table 2.

- Drugs that prolong conduction and action potential duration in atrial muscle effectively terminate and prevent recurrence of SVT in the Wolff-Parkinson-White syndrome (Table 3).

Nonpharmacologic Choices

- **Catheter ablation is the treatment of choice in patients with Wolff-Parkinson-White syndrome who do not respond to therapy or do not tolerate drug therapy.** AV node ablation of the slow or fast pathway is an effective therapy for AV node reentrant tachycardia. Catheter ablative therapy as a primary alternative to pharmacologic therapy is becoming increasingly popular. There are some data to suggest that catheter ablation is the most cost-effective approach to the management of SVT.

- Antitachycardia pacing is occasionally effective.

- Surgical ablation of the AV node or accessory pathway may be considered when catheter ablation has been unsuccessful.

Therapeutic Tips (Supraventricular Tachycardia)

- Beta-blockers and calcium channel blockers should be used with caution in patients with congestive heart failure.

- Digoxin and verapamil **as monotherapy** are relatively contraindicated in patients with Wolff-Parkinson-White syndrome.

- Combination calcium channel blockers or beta-blockers with Class I/III antiarrhythmic drugs may be required to prevent recurrence of SVT in patients with Wolff-Parkinson-White syndrome.

Suggested Reading List

Gilligan DM, Ellenbogen KA, Epstein AE. The management of atrial fibrillation. *Am J Med* 1996;101:413–421.

Kalbfleisch SJ, Calkins H, Langberg JJ, et al. Comparison of the cost of radiofrequency catheter modification of the atrioventricular node and medical therapy for drug-refractory atrioventricular node reentrant tachycardia. *J Am Coll Cardiol* 1992;19:1583–1587.

CHAPTER 26

Ventricular Tachyarrhythmias

Paul Dorian, MD, FRCPC

Definitions

Ventricular tachycardia (VT) is defined as ≥ 3 consecutive ventricular complexes at a rate > 100 beats/minute on an ECG recording. By itself, VT is only an electrical phenomenon – its clinical and prognostic importance and management depend on its specific features and the presence, if any, of associated structural heart disease.

Ventricular fibrillation (VF) is defined as a rapid, disorganized rhythm without recognizable QRS complexes on the ECG and is invariably associated with cardiovascular collapse. VF frequently results from VT. If VF occurs in the absence of reversible causes, recurrence rates are high.

Goals of Therapy

- To relieve symptoms, including restoring sinus rhythm as quickly as possible in sustained VT or cardiac arrest
- To prevent the potentially fatal occurrence or recurrence of sustained VT or cardiac arrest

Classification of VT

- **Asymptomatic:** usually discovered during routine screening ECG or other electrocardiographic monitoring
- **Symptomatic:** may cause palpitations, dyspnea, chest discomfort, presyncope, loss of consciousness, cardiac arrest
- **Sustained:** lasting ≥ 30 seconds or requiring immediate medical intervention; for management decisions, > 15 beats is a reasonable working definition
- **Nonsustained:** < 30 seconds but usually lasting only a few seconds; most commonly < 10 consecutive ventricular complexes
- **In the presence of structural heart disease:** usually coronary, valvular or hypertensive heart disease; left ventricular dysfunction is the most important distinguishing characteristic
- **Unaccompanied by structural heart disease** (in a normal heart)

- **Monomorphic:** all the ventricular (QRS) complexes appear the same
- **Polymorphic:** beat-to-beat variability in the QRS complex morphology

Investigations

- Careful history with special reference to:
  – syncope or severe presyncope
  – angina, heart failure
  – history suggesting structural heart disease
  – symptom correlation with exercise or stress
- Physical examination:
  – signs of structural heart disease
- 12-lead ECG:
  – signs of MI
  – repolarization abnormalities (prolonged QT interval)

NB: A 12-lead ECG documenting ventricular tachycardia is very important. If available, ECG at tachycardia onset (or offset) is very useful.

- Echocardiogram with special reference to:
  – left ventricular size and function
  – right ventricular size
- Holter monitoring with special reference to:
  – presence and morphology of ventricular ectopy and symptom–rhythm correlation
- Treadmill exercise test with special reference to:
  – exercise-induced VT
  – ECG signs and symptoms of myocardial ischemia (or scintigraphic evidence of ischemia if necessary)

All wide-complex (QRS duration ≥ 0.12 seconds) tachycardias in patients over 50 should be considered VT until proven otherwise.

Wide-complex tachycardia in an older patient with a history of heart disease *is almost always* VT, regardless of the morphology of ECG complexes.

Most wide-complex tachycardias in any patient of any age group are due to VT.

Significance of VT/VF

Asymptomatic tachycardia is rarely serious in itself. In the presence of structural heart disease, especially left ventricular dysfunction, asymptomatic VT (usually nonsustained) may indicate a risk of serious, symptomatic, sustained VT or VF.

Symptomatic: The prognostic importance of VT and its management are determined by the underlying cardiac status and the type of VT rather than the severity of symptoms (e.g., even severe symptoms in a patient with nonsustained VT and no structural heart disease are prognostically benign and the patient requires reassurance but not necessarily specific antiarrhythmic therapy).

Sustained VT is most often associated with structural heart disease, typically coronary disease with previous MI. It requires investigation and therapy: antiarrhythmic drugs, implanted cardioverter defibrillators or antitachycardia surgery.

Nonsustained VT usually has minimal or no symptoms and requires treatment only if likelihood of subsequent sustained VT or cardiac arrest is high.

VT associated with structural heart disease is usually symptomatic and associated with a high risk of sudden death or recurrence (if sustained) or asymptomatic but associated with at least a moderate risk of sudden death (if nonsustained).

VT associated with a structurally normal heart may be symptomatic but rarely life threatening even if sustained; it requires no therapy if asymptomatic and nonsustained.

Monomorphic VT usually implies an abnormal automatic focus in the ventricle or a fixed reentrant pathway associated with a scar. It does not by itself suggest prognosis or therapy.

Polymorphic VT is usually present as long runs of nonsustained VT. Myocardial ischemia and VT related to prolonged repolarization (torsades de pointes VT with QT prolongation) need to be considered.

Significance of VF

VF may complicate acute MI. However, the prognosis for resuscitated patients is similar to that in patients with equivalent severity infarction uncomplicated by VF.

Most episodes of VF are not caused by acute MI or obvious acute ischemia, although they generally occur in patients with coronary artery disease and prior MI. Most patients with VF are at high risk of recurrence and need to be investigated in a similar fashion to patients with sustained VT as well as treated to prevent recurrences.

Therapeutic Choices (Figures 1 and 2)

Immediate Therapy for Sustained VT or VF

If the patient is unstable (e.g., has hypotension, angina, heart failure or marked symptoms), **cardioversion** is effective and safe. A synchronized shock of 50 to 100 J is usually effective for VT.

If immediate conversion to sinus rhythm is not considered necessary, antiarrhythmic drug therapy can be given. For VF, an immediate nonsynchronized shock of 200 to 300 J is required, repeated as necessary at 300 to 360 J until defibrillation is achieved.

Lidocaine: 1 to 1.5 mg/kg IV followed by a 1 to 3 mg/minute infusion will occasionally be effective and rarely causes hypotension. If conversion does not occur within 10 to 15 minutes lidocaine will probably be ineffective.

Procainamide: 10 to 15 mg/kg IV over 30 to 45 minutes will often slow VT and terminate tachycardia. Hypotension may occur, especially at the more rapid infusion rates, and blood pressure should be carefully monitored.

Bretylium: 5 to 10 mg/kg IV over 5 to 10 minutes may prevent VF. Data on efficacy in monomorphic VT are limited. It frequently causes severe hypotension and should be used with caution.

Magnesium: 2 to 5 g IV over 3 to 5 minutes is the treatment of choice for torsades de pointes VT associated with QT prolongation and a characteristic long–short initiating sequence, and may be useful in the presence of myocardial ischemia. It is of unclear benefit in monoform VT. Magnesium may rarely cause hypotension but is generally safe.

Amiodarone: IV amiodarone appears to be effective in terminating VT and especially in preventing early recurrence. The usual dose is 3 to 5 mg/kg IV over 5 to 10 minutes followed by a 0.5 to 2 mg/minute infusion. Hypotension may occur, especially if the drug is administered very rapidly. It is likely the most effective therapy for electrical storm characterized by frequent recurrences of VT/VF.

Chronic Therapy – Prevention of VT/VF Recurrence

Therapeutic choices for long-term management of sustained VT/VF include both drug therapy (Table 1) and nondrug therapy (implanted cardioverter defibrillators, map guided endocardial resection, catheter ablation).

Sustained monomorphic VT or VF is likely to recur in the absence of treatment. Empiric treatment (i.e., without some objective documentation of drug efficacy) is generally not recommended. Indicators of drug efficacy include the inability to deliberately induce VT in the presence of a drug when VT can be induced in its absence, and the marked reduction of the frequency or elimination of nonsustained VT episodes or PVCs by the given antiarrhythmic agent.

Figure 1: **Management of Nonsustained Ventricular Tachycardia (VT) (< 15 beats)**

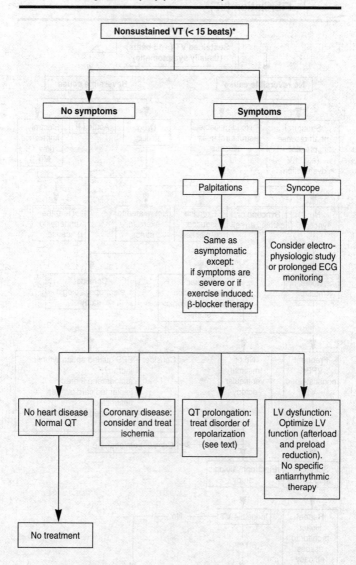

*Evidence from a controlled clinical trial suggests that patients with nonsustained VT and severe LV dysfunction (ejection fraction < 35%) are at high risk of serious arrhythmias and may profit from electrophysiologic evaluation. (Moss AJ et al, N Engl J Med 1996; 335: 1933–40)

Figure 2: **Management of Sustained Ventricular Tachycardia (VT) (> 15 beats) or Ventricular Fibrillation (VF)**

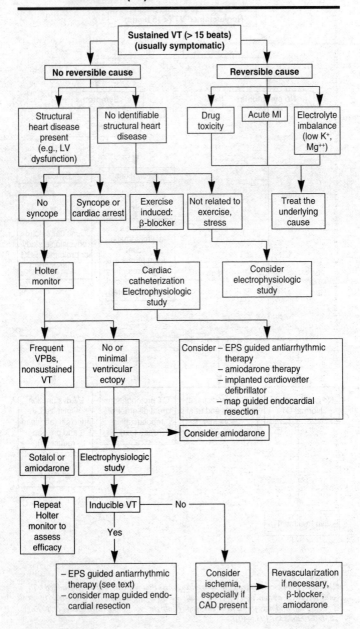

NB: Implanted cardioverter defibrillator therapy may be considered for any patient with sustained VT.

Abbreviations: LV = left ventricle; MI = myocardial infarction; VPB = ventricular premature beat; EPS = electrophysiologic study; CAD = coronary artery disease.

Table 1: Drug Therapy for VT/VF

Drug	Dosage	Dosage Adjustment	Drug Interactions	Comments	Cost*
Drugs that slow conduction and prolong repolarization (Class IA)					
quinidine † 🔾 generics, Biquin Durules	800–1 600 mg/d (sulfate equivalent)	↓ initial dose by 50% + ↑ dosing interval to Q12H in renal failure. Active metabolites accumulate in renal failure, but therapeutic blood monitoring is not readily available. Careful monitoring of the ECG intervals should guide dosing decisions.	↓ digoxin dose by 50%.	Long history of use. Frequent GI intolerance. Rare fever, thrombocytopenia. May cause torsades de pointes; (proarrhythmic) VT.	Generics $ Biquin Durules $$–$$$
procainamide † 🔾 Pronestyl, generics, Pronestyl SR, Procan SR	2–4 g/d	Metabolism depends on rate of acetylation. The active metabolite NAPA accumulates in fast acetylators and in renal failure. Monitor procainamide + NAPA levels; monitor ECG intervals.		Frequent arthralgias after long term use. May cause SLE syndrome. Rare granulocytopenia. Occasional torsades de pointes.	$$–$$$
disopyramide † 🔾 Norpace, Norpace CR, Rythmodan, Rythmodan-LA	400–800 mg/d	↓ initial dose by 50% and ↑ dosing interval to Q12H in renal failure.		Depresses LV function. Should not be used in patients with LV dysfunction. Dry mouth, urinary retention, blurred vision May cause torsades de pointes.	$–$$

(cont'd)

Cardiovascular Disorders

Table 1: **Drug Therapy for VT/VF** *(cont'd)*

Drug	Dosage	Dosage Adjustment	Drug Interactions	Comments	Cost*
Drugs that slow conduction (Class IB & IC)					
mexiletine † 🐾 Mexitil	600–900 mg/d	↓ dose by 50% and ↑ dosing interval to Q12H in renal failure.	Phenytoin and rifampin may ↓ effect. May need to ↑ mexiletine dose.	Frequent CNS side effects.	$$$
flecainide † 🐾 Tambocor	100–200 mg/d	↓ initial dose by 50% in renal failure. Titrate dose based on QRS intervals.		Moderately frequent proarrhythmia. Should not be used in patients with LV dysfunction, especially prior MI. Increases mortality compared to placebo in patients who have frequent PVCs following MI.	$$
propafenone † 🐾 Rythmol	600–900 mg/d	↓ initial dose by 50% in renal and hepatic failure and ↑ dosing interval to Q12H. Active metabolites accumulate in rapid metabolizers. Monitor QRS duration carefully.	↓ digoxin dose by 25–50%.	Weak β-blocking effect. Depresses LV function. Should be used with great reservation, if at all, in patients with LV dysfunction, especially prior MI.	$$$–$$$$
Drugs that primarily prolong repolarization (Class III)					
sotalol 🐾 Sotacor, generics	160–480 mg/d	↓ initial dose in renal failure. ↓ initial dose to 40 mg PO Q12H in the elderly.	Digoxin, verapamil, other β-blockers may cause AV block, bradycardia.	Potent β-blocker and bradycardic agent. Often causes fatigue. May cause torsades de pointes, especially at higher doses or with renal dysfunction. May be especially effective in exercise-related arrhythmias. Likely more effective than other drugs in suppressing inducibility of VT. Contraindicated in bronchial asthma.	$–$$$

Drug	Dosage	Precautions	Drug Interactions	Comments	Cost
amiodarone Cordarone	Loading dose: 800–1 600 mg/d × 7–10 d Maintenance dose: 200–400 mg/d	Avoid high loading dose in setting of sinus bradycardia (HR < 50 beats/min).	↓ quinidine/procainamide dose by 50%. ↓ digoxin dose by 50%. ↓ β-blocker dose by 50%. ↓ warfarin dose by 50%.	Very complex drug; also slows conduction, blocks adrenergic activity, blocks Ca++ channels. Very long half-life. Frequent adverse effects in many organ systems. Requires close monitoring. May be the most effective antiarrhythmic drug. Usually used as empiric therapy.	$$$–$$$$
Other					
beta-blockers	Individualized according to chosen agent	Monitor carefully in diabetic patients. Caution in patients with CHF.	Digoxin. Ca++ channel blockers. Amiodarone. ↓ dose of hypoglycemic agents by 25–50%.	Especially useful in exercise-induced VT, with ischemia, or VT in the absence of structural heart disease. Of probable but unclear benefit in patients with sustained VT and prior MI. May enhance efficacy of other antiarrhythmic drugs in this setting. Very low proarrhythmic risk. Contraindicated in bronchial asthma.	Varies

† Should be used with great caution in any patient with a history of structural heart disease and LV dysfunction. Circumstantial and limited clinical trial evidence suggests these drugs are less effective for VT or VF recurrence in patients with structural heart disease than sotalol or amiodarone.

* Cost of 30-day supply – includes drug cost only.
Legend: $ < $30 $$ $30–60 $$$ $60–100 $$$$ > $100

Patients with a history of VF or cardiac arrest are at risk of recurrence of VF or VT, since their original arrhythmia may have been VT degenerating to VF. Their treatment is similar to that of patients with sustained VT, although markers to judge drug efficacy (inducible VT or VF, PVCs or nonsustained VT on Holter monitoring) are less often present.

Nonpharmacologic Choices for VT

- Map guided endocardial surgery:
  - requires careful patient selection, specialized facilities and complex open heart surgery; may be very effective in certain patient subsets.
- Implanted cardioverter defibrillator (ICD):
  - extremely effective in treating VT or VF but requires complex evaluation and follow-up. The AVID trial reported 39% total mortality reduction in ICD-treated patients compared to antiarrhythmic therapy.
- Catheter ablation using radiofrequency energy:
  - may be especially effective for VT arising from the right ventricle in patients with apparently normal hearts; experimental for VT following myocardial infarction.

Suggested Reading List

The Antiarrhythmics versus Implantable Defibrillators (AVID) Investigators. A comparison of antiarrhythmic-drug therapy with implantable defibrillators in patients resuscitated from near-fatal ventricular arrhythmias. *N Engl J Med* 1997;337:1576–1583.

Kowey PR, Levine JH, Herre JM, et al. Randomized, double-blind comparison of intravenous amiodarone and bretylium in the treatment of patients with recurrent hemodynamically destabilizing ventricular tachycardia or fibrillation. *Circulation* 1995;92:3255–3263.

Nattel S. Antiarrhythmic drug classifications: a critical appraisal of their history, present status, and clinical relevance. *Drugs* 1991;41:672–701.

Teo KK. Evaluation of therapeutic modalities in patients with life threatening arrhythmias. *Can J Cardiol* 1994;10:333–341.

CHAPTER 27

Dyslipidemias

Ghislaine O. Roederer, MD, PhD

Goals of Therapy

- To reduce cardiovascular disease (CVD)
- To prevent pancreatitis (from severe hypertriglyceridemia)

Investigations

- Medical history with attention to CVD (past or present), major negative cardiovascular risk factors (Figure 1) and possible causes of secondary hyperlipidemia (Table 1)
- Family history:
  - premature CVD (before age 45 in males, age 55 in females) in first-degree relatives
  - hyperlipidemia
- Physical examination:
  - weight
  - bilateral brachial blood pressure
  - arcus corneae (especially in the young patient)
  - funduscopy (lipemia retinalis, retinopathies)
  - peripheral pulses
  - cardiac auscultation
  - arterial bruits
  - hepatosplenomegaly
  - lipid deposits (xanthomas)
- Laboratory tests: lipid and lipoprotein levels[1]
  - use the same laboratory for repeated measurements
  - a 12-hour fast is required for triglyceride levels
  - for initial diagnosis of the dyslipidemic phenotype, obtain 2 or 3 measurements at 4- to 6-week intervals to establish a baseline. At least 1 measurement should include a lipoprotein profile (high-density lipoprotein cholesterol [HDL-C], low-density lipoprotein cholesterol [LDL-C])
  - other lab investigations to rule out frequent causes of secondary dyslipidemias (Table 1)

Classification of Dyslipidemias

Primary (genetic) vs secondary dyslipidemias: Possible causes for secondary dyslipidemia must be sought and addressed directly

---

[1] *NB: The Friedwald equation routinely used to calculate LDL-C values (all units mmol/L)* **LDL-C = TOTAL-C − (HDL-C + TRG/2.2)** *cannot be used if triglyceride levels > 4.52 mmol/L or if dealing with type III dysbetalipoproteinemia.*

Figure 1: **Management of Dyslipidemia**

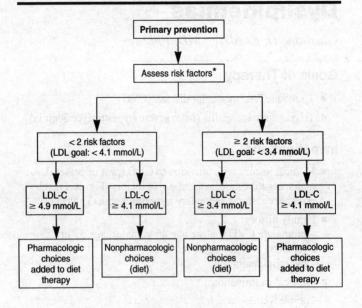

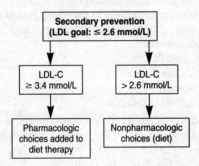

Primary prevention: for patients with no previous CVD.
Secondary prevention: for patients with prior CVD/atherosclerotic disease.

* Positive Risk Factors:
 – *male ≥ 45 yrs, female ≥ 55 yrs*
 – *premature menopause without hormone replacement therapy*
 – *family history of premature CVD*
 – *cigarette smoking*
 – *hypertension*
 – *diabetes mellitus*
 – *low HDL-C (< 0.9 mmol/L)*
NB: *High HDL-C (≥ 1.6 mmol/L) is considered a **negative** (i.e., protective) risk factor for CVD.*

Table 1: **Common Causes of Secondary Hyperlipidemia**

Hypothyroidism	Medication:
Pregnancy	Thiazide diuretics
Excess weight	β-blockers without intrinsic sympathomimetic or alpha blocking activity
Alcohol excess	Oral contraceptives
Obstructive liver disease	Hormone replacement therapy
Nephrotic syndrome	Corticosteroids

if present. If secondary dyslipidemia persists despite proper management of the underlying disease and constitutes an additional risk factor for the condition, then lipid-lowering treatment becomes mandatory (e.g., diabetic dyslipidemia).

- Primary dyslipidemias carrying a risk for **CVD** are (in *decreasing* order of risk):
  - **heterozygous familial hypercholesterolemia** (hzFH) – associated with severe hypercholesterolemia (LDL-C), premature atherosclerosis and characteristic xanthomas. When diagnosed, family screening (including children) is recommended for early prevention and treatment.
  - **familial combined hyperlipidemia** (FCH) – associated with premature atherosclerosis and characterized by elevated cholesterol and/or triglyceride levels; however, in time, affected persons may display various lipoprotein phenotypes.
  - **type III dysbetalipoproteinemia** – associated with coronary and peripheral vascular disease, pathognomonic xanthomas and almost exclusively an E2/E2 phenotype.
- Primary dyslipidemias carrying a risk for **pancreatitis** are (in *decreasing* order of risk):
  - **familial hyperchylomicronemia** – lipid-lowering drugs are not effective; a strict fat-poor diet (< 10% fat) is the cornerstone of treatment.
  - **familial hypertriglyceridemia** (FHTG) – with a type V phenotype.

Phenotypic expression (the description of the lipoprotein anomaly, Table 2) provides no information about the etiology of the disorder. However, proper recognition of the phenotype will provide guidance as to which medication to use.

Criteria for Intervention

Current recommendations from the Expert Panel of the American National Cholesterol Education Program[2] include **clinical status**

---

[2] *JAMA* 1993;269:3015–3023.

Table 2: **Classification of Dyslipidemia Phenotypes***

Phenotype	Lipoproteins				Lipids	
	Chylomicrons	VLDL	IDL	LDL	Cholesterol	TG
I	↑↑					↑↑
IIa				↑	↑	
IIb		↑		↑	↑	↑
III			↑		↑	↑
IV		↑				↑
V	↑	↑				↑↑

* Fredrickson-Levy classification, based on electrophoretic data.
Abbreviations: VLDL = very-low-density lipoproteins; TG = triglycerides;
IDL = intermediate-density lipoproteins; LDL = low-density lipoproteins.

(primary vs secondary prevention), **risk factors** and **HDL-C levels** in the decision tree (Figure 1). Triglycerides may also have an atherogenic role.[3] High triglyceride levels (2.3 to 11.3 mmol/L) are an additional cardiovascular risk factor when associated with atherogenic dyslipidemias (e.g., FCH, insulin resistance, diabetes, renal insufficiency). Individuals with triglycerides in the very high range (> 11.3 mmol/L) are at increased risk for pancreatitis.

Therapeutic Choices (Figure 1)

Nonpharmacologic Choices

Diet, aimed at reducing blood lipid levels and weight (if needed), should *always* be the first approach to treating all dyslipidemias. A 6-month dietary trial (Table 3) is mandatory before considering medication; during this time, 2 (ideally 3) lipid and lipoprotein measurements should be taken.

Increased physical activity may help decrease cholesterol and triglyceride levels while increasing HDL.

Other lifestyle changes that reduce the risk of CVD (e.g., weight loss, smoking cessation) should be encouraged.

Pharmacologic Choices (Table 4)
Resins

The bile-acid-sequestering resins **cholestyramine** and **colestipol** reduce plasma LDL and can slightly increase HDL levels. They have a strong safety record. Resins are the only lipid-lowering agents appropriate for use in children (> 2 years) or in pregnant or lactating women. Some recommend concurrent supplementation with fat soluble vitamins.

---

[3] *Am J Cardiol 1992;70:19H–25H.*

Table 3: **Dietary Interventions**

Step I (Primary Prevention) (patients with no previous CVD)	Step II (Secondary Prevention)* (patients with prior CVD/ atherosclerotic disease)
↓ dietary cholesterol intake to < 300 mg/d	↓ dietary cholesterol intake to < 200 mg/d
Restrict fat intake to 30% of calories	Restrict fat intake to 20% of calories
Distribute fat intake equally between saturated, polyunsaturated and monosaturated fats	7% of daily calories as saturated fat
Favor high-fiber intake	
Limit simple sugars to 8% of total calories	
Limit alcohol consumption to 5% of total calories	

The help of a dietitian is usually required to reach and maintain these goals.

HMG CoA Reductase Inhibitors or "Statins"

HMG CoA reductase inhibitors, the most potent LDL-lowering agents, interfere with the atherosclerotic disease process.[4] Significant reductions in CVD morbidity, CVD mortality and total deaths in both primary[5] and secondary[6] prevention have been associated with their use.

Effect on HDL is modest. Within the range of currently recommended dosages, atorvastatin has the greatest triglyceride-lowering effect (Table 5). Statins differ in their structure, pharmacokinetics, in vitro properties and efficacy; no dose-to-dose equivalence can be drawn between them.[7] Increasing the dose may result in further decrease in LDL.

Nicotinic Acid (Niacin)

Niacin is a B vitamin that, at high doses, lowers triglycerides and LDL and raises HDL. It also reduces hepatic VLDL synthesis and secretion. The unpleasant side effects of niacin make patient compliance difficult, limiting its usefulness. Slow-release formulations appear to be more hepatotoxic than standard-release products.[8]

Fibrates

Clofibrate, gemfibrozil, fenofibrate and **bezafibrate** lower triglyceride levels and raise HDL. They are useful in diabetic dyslipidemia. The effect of fibrates on LDL is variable; third

[4] *NEJM 1997;336:153–162.*
[5] *NEJM 1995;333:1301–1307.*
[6] *Lancet 1994;344:1383–1389.*
[7] *Am J Cardiol 1994;73:3D–11D.*
[8] *JAMA 1994;271:672–677.*

Table 4: Lipid-lowering Agents

Drug	Dosage	Effect on Lipoproteins LDL	HDL	TG	Adverse Effects	Comments	Cost*
Resins							
cholestyramine Questran, Questran Light	Given daily to TID, AC 4–24 g/d	↓↓	↑		Constipation, bloating, abdominal fullness, flatulence, ↑ triglycerides, ↑ transaminases (reversible).	Administer 1 h before or 4 h after concurrent medications due to possible adsorption of anionic molecules in the GI tract.	$–$$$$$
colestipol Colestid	5–30 g/d					Recommend high-fiber diet to ↓ constipation. Monitor liver function and triglycerides.	$$–$$$$$
HMG CoA Reductase Inhibitors							
lovastatin Mevacor, generics	Usually given as a single daily dose: 20–40 mg with evening meal, up to 80 mg/d (40 mg BID)	↓↓↓	↑	↓ ↔	Mild upper GI disturbances, myalgias, sleep disturbances, ↑ CPK, ↑ transaminases (reversible).	Monitor liver function and CK at 3, 6, 12 mos then yearly. Extreme caution if combination therapy with fibrates, erythromycin, cyclosporine or niacin (↑ risk of hepatotoxicity, myopathy/myositis): start with low doses.	$$–$$$$$$
simvastatin Zocor	5–40 mg with evening meal					Excellent safety profile.	$$–$$$$$
pravastatin Pravachol	10–40 mg QHS						$$$–$$$$
fluvastatin Lescol	20–40 mg with evening meal						$$
atorvastatin Lipitor	10–40 mg at any time			(↓↓)†			$$–$$$$$

Drug	Dose				Adverse Effects	Comments	Cost
Niacin (Nicotinic Acid) generics (regular and slow-release formulations)	Regular: 1.5–6 g/d divided TID, PC Slow release (not recommended): 0.5–2 g/d divided BID, PC	↓↓	↑↑	↓↓	Hot flushes and pruritus, (symptoms of vasodilation which abate with time) dry skin, acanthosis nigricans (reversible), reactivation of peptic ulcer, GI disturbances. Severe hepatotoxicity may occur (more frequent with slow-release formulation). ↑ blood glucose, uric acid, transaminases.	Greatest HDL-raising effect. Monitor blood glucose, uric acid, transaminases at 3, 6, 12 mos then yearly. Avoid in diabetic patients. Caution if using in combination with statins (potential hepatotoxicity). Reassure and instruct the patient of the following: ↑ medication stepwise (start with 50 mg TID; double dose Q5d to 1.5–2 g/d. If tolerated, max. dose is 6 g/d) after meals. To reduce flushing: avoid hot drinks, hot showers, spicy food, alcohol for 1–2 h after a dose; low-dose ASA daily in the first few weeks of treatment may be helpful. Avoid missing a dose.	$–$$$
Fibrates ❓ *clofibrate* Atromid-S, generics	1–2 g/d divided BID	↑ ↔ ↓	↑↑	↓↓↓	Upper GI disturbances (nausea, abdominal pain, flatulence), myalgias, ↑ bile lithogenicity, ↑ CPK, occasionally ↑ creatinine.	Monitor CK, CBC, liver and renal function at 3, 6 and 12 mos. May ↑ oral anticoagulant activity. Caution when combining with statins. Very useful in diabetic dyslipidemias.	$
gemfibrozil Lopid, generics	1200 mg/d divided BID						$$$
fenofibrate Lipidil, generics, Lipidil-Micro (micronized)	100 mg BID–QID with meals Micro: 200 mg/d (given once daily with largest meal)						$$–$$$
bezafibrate Bezalip (immediate-release, slow-release [SR] formulations)	200 mg BID–TID SR: 400 mg/d with evening meal						$$$

* Cost of 30-day supply -- includes drug cost only.
Legend: $ < $20 $$ $20–40 $$$ $40–60 $$$$ $60–80 $$$$$ > $80
† At doses ≥ 40 mg, atorvastatin has a greater TG lowering effect than other statins.
❓ Dosage adjustment may be required in renal impairment – see Appendix I.

Table 5: **Dose vs Efficacy of HMG CoA Reductase Inhibitors**

Drug	Efficacy		
	LDL	HDL	TG
Lovastatin			
20 mg	−24%	+7%	−10%
40 mg	−34%	+7%	−14%
80 mg	−40%	+9%	−16%
Simvastatin			
5 mg	−24%	+7%	−10%
10 mg	−28%	+7%	−10%
20 mg	−35%	+10%	−17%
40 mg	−41%	+13%	−19%
Pravastatin			
10 mg	−22%		
20 mg	−32%		
40 mg	−34%	+14%	−25%
Fluvastatin			
20 mg	−20%	+2%	−7%
40 mg	−25%	+7%	−10%
Atorvastatin			
10 mg	−39%	+6%	−19%
20 mg	−43%	+9%	−26%
40 mg	−50%	+6%	−29%
80 mg	−60%	+5%	−37%

Abbreviations: LDL = low-density lipoproteins; HDL = high-density lipoproteins; TG = triglycerides.

generation agents (e.g., bezafibrate, fenofibrate) show a more consistent LDL-lowering effect. The newer fibrates have supplanted clofibrate because of their better safety record and greater potency.

Therapeutic Tips

- Lipid-lowering drugs must **always** be an adjunct, not a substitution, to diet therapy.
- Except for resins, lipid-lowering drugs should be avoided in children and pregnant or lactating women.
- Therapy should be maintained at the lowest dosage required to reach the desired effect.
- Different agents within the same class should be tried in cases of intolerance or lack of efficacy.
- Clinical and laboratory follow-up is essential to monitor lipid-lowering efficacy and adverse effects of therapy.

- Allow 3 months for plasma lipid stabilization after a coronary or other major medical event.
- Because some combination therapies carry an increased risk of drug toxicity, referral should be considered for such patients.

Pharmacoeconomic Considerations

Jeffrey A. Johnson, PhD

Two economic evaluations of simvastatin therapy have been conducted using the results of the 4S study, one of which was specific for the Canadian context. The original cost-effectiveness analysis included both direct and indirect costs (Appendix II), and indicated that in patients with coronary heart disease, simvastatin therapy is cost-effective among both men and women at ages 35 to 70 years and total cholesterol levels prior to treatment of 5.5 to 8.0 mmol/L. Data for secondary prevention of coronary artery disease in Canada also indicate that simvastatin is a cost-effective approach, with cost-effectiveness ratio of $6 108 to $9 876 per year of life gained, depending on the length of time that the clinical benefits were assumed to accumulate.

Suggested Reading

Johannesson M, Jonsson B, Kjekshus J, et al. Cost-effectiveness of simvastatin treatment to lower cholesterol levels in patients with coronary heart disease. N Engl J Med 1997;336:332–336.

Riviere M, Wang S, Leclerc C, et al. Cost-effectiveness of simvastatin in the secondary prevention of coronary artery disease in Canada. Can Med Assoc J 1997;156:991–997.

Suggested Reading List

Expert Panel on Detection, Evaluation, and Treatment of High Blood Cholesterol in Adults. Summary of the Second Report of the National Cholesterol Education Program (NCEP) Expert Panel on Detection, Evaluation, and Treatment of High Blood Cholesterol in Adults (Adult Treatment Panel II). *JAMA* 1993;269:3015–3023.

Jialal I. A practical approach to the laboratory diagnosis of dyslipidemia. *Am J Clin Pathol* 1996;106:128–138.

Grundy SM. Atherogenic dyslipidemia: lipoprotein abnormalities and implications for therapy. *Am J Cardiol* 1995;75: 45B–52B.

Levine GN, Keany JF Jr., Vita JA: Cholesterol reduction in cardiovascular disease. *N Engl J Med* 1995;332:512–521.

Schectman G, Hiatt J: Dose-response characteristics of cholesterol-lowering drug therapies: Implications for treatment. *Ann Intern Med* 1996;125:990–1000.

CHAPTER 28

Hypertension

S. George Carruthers, MD, FRCP, FACP, FRCPC

Goals of Therapy

- To decrease morbidity and mortality attributable to high blood pressure, particularly from stroke, cardiovascular disease, kidney disease
- To provide patients with effective, well-tolerated and convenient treatment that does not diminish quality of life

Investigations

- Office blood pressure (BP) recordings on at least 3 separate occasions[1]
- Thorough history including family history of hypertension, heart disease and stroke; personal history of diabetes, cardiovascular disease
- Physical examination focusing on evidence of arterial or arteriolar disease (e.g., diminished pulses, carotid or abdominal bruits, abdominal aneurysm, retinal vascular tortuosity or narrowing)
- Laboratory tests:
  – CBC, urea, creatinine, electrolytes
  – routine urinalysis (in diabetics check for microalbuminuria)
  – total cholesterol, LDL- and HDL-cholesterol
  – ECG

NB: Routine echocardiography, home BP monitoring or ambulatory BP monitoring is not recommended but may be useful in selected patients.

- Special investigations for secondary hypertension as indicated (e.g., radionuclide renogram, captopril test, digitized renal arteriography for suspected renal artery stenosis; plasma and urinary catecholamines, CT scan, MRI for adrenal medullary and cortical tumors)

---

[1] *Refer to Can Med Assoc J 1993;149:575–584 for detailed description of correct procedure for measuring blood pressure.*

Figure 1: **Pharmacologic Treatment of Hypertension**

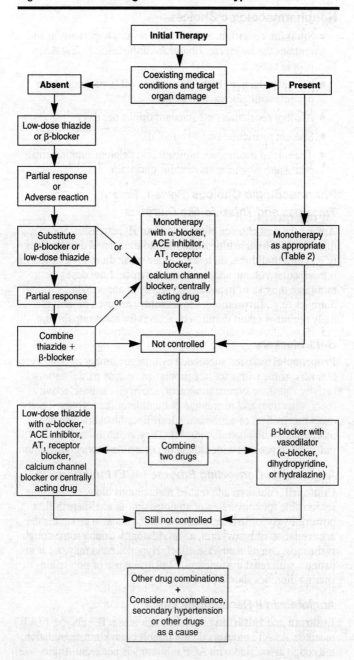

Adapted with permission from Ogilvie RI, et al. Report of the Canadian Hypertension Society Consensus Conference: 3. Pharmacologic treatment of essential hypertension. Can Med Assoc J 1993;149:575–584.

Therapeutic Choices

Nonpharmacologic Choices

- **Smoking cessation.** Smoking aggravates hypertension and remains the major contributor to cardiovascular disease in people under 65.
- Weight reduction (body mass index < 27), particularly in patients with glucose intolerance.
- Alcohol restriction (< 2 standard drinks per day).
- Sodium restriction (< 150 mmol/d).
- The role of meditation, biofeedback, calcium supplements, potassium supplements remains uncertain.

Pharmacologic Choices (Figure 1, Table 1)

Thiazides and Thiazide-like Diuretics

Among the first choices of the Canadian Hypertension Society, thiazides like **hydrochlorothiazide** and the related quinazolines (e.g., **chlorthalidone**, **metolazone**) are weak diuretics that reduce intravascular volume and vascular resistance. Low doses minimize the risk of hypokalemia and lipid abnormalities. Loop diuretics (e.g., **furosemide**, **bumetanide**) are used in multiple daily regimens (short duration of action) for renal impairment.

Beta-blockers

Propranolol has been succeeded by a large number of other beta-blockers, some with ancillary properties such as partial agonist activity (intrinsic sympathomimetic activity), cardioselectivity (beta$_1$ selective) and membrane or quinidine-like activity. Their exact mechanism of action is unclear. Beta-blockers reduce mortality in patients following MI. They are absolutely contra-indicated in patients with asthma or reversible airway obstruction.

Angiotensin Converting Enzyme (ACE) Inhibitors

Captopril, **enalapril** and related medications block the enzyme responsible for conversion of angiotensin I to angiotensin II, a powerful vasoconstrictor. Kininase inhibition also promotes the accumulation of bradykinin, a vasodilator. A troublesome cough is the most common adverse effect. Hyperkalemia may occur in patients with renal dysfunction. Concurrent use of potassium-sparing diuretics should be avoided.

Angiotensin II Receptor Blockers

Losartan and **valsartan** block the angiotensin II, subtype 1 (AT$_1$) receptor. As AT$_1$ blockers do not inhibit bradykinin degradation, the cough associated with ACE inhibitors is not seen. Angio-edema is a possible side effect. These drugs are useful alone or in combination therapy. Long-term effects on morbidity and mortality are unknown.

Table 1: Commonly Used Antihypertensive Drugs

	Daily Dose		
	Starting	Full	Cost*
Thiazide Diuretics			
chlorthalidone (Hygroton, Uridon, generics)	12.5 mg	25 mg	$
hydrochlorothiazide (HydroDiuril, Esidrix, generics)	12.5 mg	50 mg	$
indapamide (Lozide)	2.5 mg	2.5 mg	$
metolazone (Zaroxolyn)	2.5 mg	5 mg	$
β-blockers			
acebutolol (Monitan, Sectral) [ISA]	200 mg	800 mg	$$
atenolol (Tenormin, generics)	25 mg	100 mg	$
labetalol (Trandate)	200 mg	1200 mg	$$$$
metoprolol (Lopresor, Betaloc, generics)	50 mg	200 mg	$
nadolol (Corgard, generics)	20 mg	160 mg	$$
oxprenolol (Trasicor) [ISA]	80 mg	320 mg	$$$$
pindolol (Visken, generics) [ISA]	10 mg	30 mg	$$
propranolol (Inderal, generics)	80 mg	320 mg	$
timolol (Blocadren, generics)	10 mg	40 mg	$$
ACE Inhibitors			
benazepril (Lotensin)	10 mg	40 mg	$$$
captopril (Capoten, generics)	25 mg	100 mg	$$
cilazapril (Inhibace)	2.5 mg	10 mg	$$$
enalapril (Vasotec, generics)	5 mg	20 mg	$$$
fosinopril (Monopril)	10 mg	40 mg	$$$
lisinopril (Prinivil, Zestril, generics)	5 mg	20 mg	$$
perindopril (Coversyl)	4 mg	8 mg	$$$
quinapril (Accupril)	10 mg	40 mg	$$$
ramipril (Altace)	2.5 mg	10 mg	$$
trandolapril (Mavik)	1 mg	4 mg	$$$
Angiotensin II Receptor Blockers			
losartan (Cozaar)	25 mg	50 mg	$$
valsartan (Diovan)	80 mg	160 mg	$$
Calcium Antagonists			
amlodipine (Norvasc) [D][V]	5 mg	10 mg	$$$
diltiazem (Cardizem, generics)	120 mg	360 mg	$$$
felodipine (Plendil, Renedil) [D][V]	5 mg	20 mg	$$$
nicardipine (Cardene) [D][V]	60 mg	120 mg	$$$$
nifedipine (Adalat, generics) [D][V]	20 mg	80 mg	$$$
verapamil (Isoptin, generics)	120 mg	480 mg	$$$
Centrally Acting Drugs			
clonidine (Catapres, generics)	0.2 mg	1.2 mg	$$$
methyldopa (Aldomet, generics)	500 mg	2000 mg	$
reserpine (Serpasil, generics)	0.1 mg	0.25 mg	$
α-blockers			
doxazosin (Cardura)	1 mg	8 mg	$$$
prazosin (Minipress, generics)	0.5 mg	20 mg	$$
terazosin (Hytrin)	1 mg	10 mg	$$$
Vasodilators			
hydralazine (Apresoline, generics)	50 mg	200 mg	$$
minoxidil (Loniten)	5 mg	20 mg	$$$

Combination Products

Although there are many preparations combining thiazide diuretics with other antihypertensive agents, initiating therapy with these fixed-dose combinations is not recommended. Individual agents should be titrated to effective dosages; once doses have been stabilized, the clinician may then prescribe the combination best suited to the needs of the patient.

[D] Dihydropyridine [ISA] intrinsic sympathomimetic activity [V] vasodilator.
Doses in this table are intended only as a guide and may be adjusted according to individual physician and patient requirements.
Adapted with permission from Ogilvie RI, et al. Report of the Canadian Hypertension Society Consensus Conference: 3. Pharmacologic treatment of essential hypertension. Can Med Assoc J 1993;149:575–584.
* Cost of 30-day supply of full dose of antihypertensive – includes drug cost only.
Legend: $ < $20 $$ $20–40 $$$ $40–60 $$$$ > $60

Calcium Channel Blockers

The earliest calcium channel blockers, **verapamil**, **nifedipine** and **diltiazem** are chemically unrelated and exert differing effects on vascular smooth muscle, cardiac myocytes and cardiac conducting tissues. All are effective antihypertensives. Side effects of nifedipine and related dihydropyridines reflect the predominant vasodilation of this group (i.e., flushing, palpitations, pedal edema). Verapamil may impair left ventricular function and cause heart block and should not be used with beta-blockers or negative inotropes (e.g., disopyramide). In larger doses constipation is common. Diltiazem's pharmacological profile is intermediate to that of verapamil and nifedipine.

Centrally Acting Antihypertensives

Methyldopa and **clonidine** exert central alpha$_2$-adrenergic agonist effects that reduce sympathetic drive to the peripheral vasculature. They have a minor role in the treatment of hypertension. Methyldopa is considered safe in pregnancy. The rebound hypertension associated with clonidine withdrawal has limited its use, and it must be avoided in patients with poor compliance.

Peripheral Sympatholytics

Reserpine appears safe and effective at very low doses but is associated with suicidal depression when used at higher doses. **Guanethidine** causes orthostatic hypotension and diarrhea.

Alpha-blockers

Prazosin, doxazosin and **terazosin** lower BP without the tachycardia associated with the earlier nonselective alpha-blockers. To avoid the first-dose effect of hypotension and occasional syncope, starting doses should be small and given at bedtime.

Direct Vasodilators

Hydralazine is out of favor because doses in excess of 200 mg daily were associated with an SLE-like syndrome. Reflex tachycardia and activation of the renin–angiotensin–aldosterone system can be controlled by concurrent beta-blocker or diuretic therapy. **Minoxidil** provokes hirsutism. **Nitroprusside** is useful in the management of accelerated hypertension but must be given IV in a critical care unit.

Hypertension with Concurrent Disorders

(Table 2)

Table 2: Therapeutic Choices for Hypertension with Concurrent Disorders

Condition or Risk Factor	Recommended Drugs	Alternative Drugs	Not Recommended
Ischemic Heart Disease			
Angina	β-blockers	CCB (e.g., diltiazem and verapamil) or dihydropyridines + β-blockers.	Dihydropyridines.
Recent MI	β-blockers	CCB (e.g., verapamil and diltiazem) if LV function not severely impaired.	
Congestive Heart Failure	Diuretics, ACEI	Hydralazine + ISDN. Angiotensin II receptor blocker.[1]	β-blockers, CCB.
Peripheral Vascular Disease			
Severe disease, Raynaud's	Vasodilators		β-blockers.
Mild disease		β-blockers may be used.	
Dyslipidemia	α-blockers, ACEI, β-blockers with ISA, CCB, centrally acting drugs*	Low-dose thiazides.	High-dose thiazides, β-blockers without ISA.
Diabetes Mellitus	ACEI, CCB, α-blockers	β-blockers, thiazides, angiotensin II receptor blockers, centrally acting agents or vasodilators if others contraindicated.	High-dose thiazides, β-blockers without ISA.

(cont'd)

Table 2: Therapeutic Choices for Hypertension with Concurrent Disorders *(cont'd)*

Condition or Risk Factor	Recommended Drugs	Alternative Drugs	Not Recommended
Asthma	K⁺-sparing + thiazide diuretic for patients on salbutamol		β-blockers.
Gout			Thiazides, but asymptomatic hyperuricemia is not a contraindication.
Pregnancy	Methyldopa, clonidine, hydralazine, β-blockers		ACEI, CCB, angiotensin II receptor blockers.
Black Patients	Low-dose thiazides, CCB	β-blockers, ACEI are less effective.	

[1] *Lancet* 1997;349:747–752.
Abbreviations: + = combined with; ISA = intrinsic sympathomimetic activity; CCB = calcium channel blocker; ACEI = ACE inhibitor; ISDN = isosorbide dinitrate.
Adapted with permission from Ogilvie RI, et al. Report of the Canadian Hypertension Society Consensus Conference: 3. *Pharmacologic treatment of essential hypertension. Can Med Assoc J* 1993;149:575–584.

Therapeutic Tips

- Consider the patient's age, gender, race, other medical conditions and concurrent medications.
- Start with a low dose of a diuretic or beta-blocker, unless contraindicated.
- Try to achieve BP control with the lowest possible dose of a single medication.
- Consider medications that are of value for other medical conditions (e.g., beta-blockers after MI, ACE inhibitors in symptomatic heart failure).
- Avoid medications likely to aggravate a coexisting disorder (e.g., thiazides with gout, beta-blockers with asthma).
- Unless there are compelling reasons to reduce BP quickly, pressure should be brought to target values (< 140 mm Hg systolic and < 90 mm Hg diastolic) over 3 to 6 months.
- Consider an AT_1 receptor blocker if ACE inhibitor-induced cough is a problem.
- Combination therapy will be necessary when monotherapy is unsuccessful.
- The patient may assist in BP management by monitoring BP at home and work.
- Consider cost-effectiveness of treatment.
- When treatment is ineffective, consider poor compliance. Consider also excessive salt or alcohol consumption, interfering medications such as NSAIDs and secondary causes of hypertension.
- When BP control is lost in an older patient, consider atherosclerotic renal artery stenosis.
- Consider reducing therapy when BP is controlled and stable for at least 1 year.
- Long-term follow-up is essential, even when therapy is reduced and especially if there is a trial of discontinuation of therapy.

Pharmacoeconomic Considerations

Jeffrey A. Johnson, PhD

Costs of antihypertensive therapy include drug acquisition costs, routine physician visits, care of complications such as stroke and MI and laboratory monitoring. For example, inexpensive diuretics require more expensive laboratory monitoring than other first-line antihypertensives.

Given the wide differential of drug costs from thiazides at pennies per day to newer agents costing $1–2 per day, the evidence that less expensive medications are more cost-effective is not particularly robust. Only diuretics and beta-blockers have been definitively shown in long-term studies to reduce "hard" outcomes such as death, MI and stroke. These drugs, with the lowest acquisition costs, appear to be the most cost-effective. Information on newer drugs tends to be speculative, however good the modeling. Cost-effectiveness of antihypertensive agents varies according to risk as the benefit of treatment is dependent on severity of hypertension, concurrent risk factors, age and gender. The greatest value will be seen in the older patients and those with multiple cardiovascular risk factors.

Suggested Reading

Edelson JT, Weinstein MC, Tosteson ANA, et al. *Long-term cost-effectiveness of various initial monotherapies for mild to moderate hypertension. JAMA 1990;263:408-13.*

Kaplan NM. *Cost-effectiveness of antihypertensive drugs. Fact or fancy? Am J Hypertension 1991;4:478-480.*

Suggested Reading List

Recommendations of 1992 Canadian Hypertension Society Consensus Report. *Can Med Assoc J* 1993;149:289–293, 409–418,575–584,815–820,821–826.

Recommendations of U.S. Joint National Committee on Detection, Evaluation and Treatment of Hypertension. *Arch Intern Med* 1993;153:154–183.

CHAPTER 29

Orthostatic Hypotension

Jake Onrot, MD, FRCPC

Definition

Orthostatic hypotension (OH) is defined as a fall in systolic blood pressure (BP) of at least 20 mm Hg and/or diastolic BP of at least 10 mm Hg within 3 minutes of standing. Orthostatic hypotension is a clinical sign and may be symptomatic (usually from cerebral hypoperfusion), or asymptomatic.

OH is characterized symptomatically by anything from transient lightheadedness to syncope, cognitive impairment, visual disturbances ("brownout" or "blackout"), neck or head discomfort, dyspnea, palpitations, nausea, tremulousness or profound weakness.

Goals of Therapy

- To restore adequate upright perfusion pressure to the brain
- To relieve symptoms of brain hypoperfusion
- To avoid side effects of medications

Investigations

Investigations should be directed at quantifying the BP fall and its attendant symptomatology and identifying any causal factors. Orthostatic hypotension must be differentiated from other causes of transient diminution or loss of consciousness.

- Careful drug history to exclude hypotensive agents
- Look for features of autonomic failure (e.g., impotence, constipation or uncontrollable diarrhea, symptoms of urinary retention, reduced sweating)
- In autonomic failure, look for underlying diabetes mellitus, amyloidosis or other rarer causes, and neurological features (e.g., parkinsonism) that suggest multiple system atrophy (Shy-Drager syndrome)
- Standing BP:
  - measurement of the supine and upright pressures is important
  - assess the length of time the patient can stand without symptoms (the standing time); a reasonable goal of therapy is a standing time of 5 minutes
  - supine pressures are often elevated in autonomic failure and may limit pressor therapy directed at upright pressures

Other investigations:

- Assess hypovolemia by postural vital signs, height of the jugular venous pressure, lab parameters (i.e., urea/creatinine ratio)
- Cardiac assessment for underlying heart disease
- Supine and upright plasma catecholamines can confirm an underlying diagnosis of autonomic failure

Therapeutic Choices (Figure 1)

Nonpharmacologic Choices

- Increase venous return:
  - liberalize salt intake
  - discontinue diuretics and hypotensive agents
  - elevate head of bed on blocks at night to reduce nocturnal diuresis
  - use waist-high gradient elastic support garments
- Avoid hypotensive stresses:
  - get up slowly from recumbent position
  - dangle legs at side of bed before rising (especially in the morning)
  - beware of large meals, strenuous exercise (especially isometric with Valsalva), lifting heavy objects, working with hands over head, stairs, hot weather, fever, hot baths, coughing, etc.

Pharmacologic Choices

Fludrocortisone

This long-acting mineralocorticoid is the drug of choice. It acts to increase blood volume and sensitize vessels to endogenous pressors. The initial dose of 0.1 mg per day may be increased by 0.1 mg per day Q1–2 weeks until desired symptomatic response is achieved. The effective dose range is 0.1 to 1.2 mg daily. Mild edema is well tolerated and desirable as it indicates optimal blood volumes, but watch for heart failure. Beware of high supine pressures, which often limit therapy. Hypokalemia often occurs and should be corrected with oral potassium (Chapter 80).

Pressor Amines (Alpha Agonists)

Ephedrine, phenylephrine, phenylpropanolamine and **midodrine** act to constrict veins (to improve venous return) and arterioles (to increase resistance). The first three are rarely used while midodrine is more widely used. Initial midodrine doses of 2.5 mg BID or TID can be titrated by 2.5 mg per day until a satisfactory response is obtained or 30 mg per day is reached. Small doses, ineffective in healthy patients, may have pronounced effects in

Figure 1: **Strategies in Treatment of Chronic Orthostatic Hypotension**

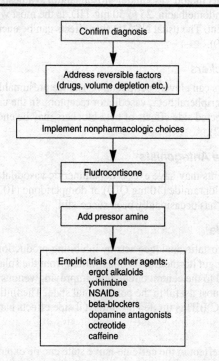

Confirm diagnosis

Address reversible factors
(drugs, volume depletion etc.)

Implement nonpharmacologic choices

Fludrocortisone

Add pressor amine

Empiric trials of other agents:
ergot alkaloids
yohimbine
NSAIDs
beta-blockers
dopamine antagonists
octreotide
caffeine

those with autonomic failure due to denervation supersensitivity. Therapy may be limited by supine hypertension. Side effects include shivering, piloerection and headache.

Yohimbine[1]

This alpha$_2$ antagonist (2.5 to 5 mg BID) stimulates central sympathetic outflow, which may be effective when acting on supersensitive peripheral receptors. In one study, anxiety, tremor and diarrhea limited treatment in 50% of patients.

Ergot Alkaloids[2]

Dihydroergotamine (10 to 40 mg daily) may act more selectively as a venopressor to augment venous return. Bioavailability limits oral therapy, but it has been used successfully SC or via inhalation. Ergotamine can also be used. Side effects are generally due to vasoconstrictor effects (angina, MI, supine hypertension).

---

[1] *Neurology 1987;37:215–220.*
[2] *Ann Intern Med 1986;105:168–173.*

NSAIDs

These agents inhibit vasodilator prostaglandin synthesis to raise pressure. Indomethacin, 25 to 50 mg TID, is the most widely studied agent. The usual NSAID side effects can be encountered (Chapter 50).

Beta-blockers

These drugs can elevate peripheral resistance presumably by blocking peripheral beta$_2$ vasodilator receptors. In the usual doses, expected side effects of beta-blockers may be encountered (Chapter 22).

Dopamine Antagonists

Some patients may have excess dopaminergic vasodilatation; thus metoclopramide (10 mg QID) or domperidone (10 mg TID–QID) has occasionally been successful.

Octreotide[3]

This somatostatin analogue acts by inhibiting production of vasodilator gut hormones; blood is shifted from the splanchnic venous bed to the central circulation, improving venous return. It may be most useful in the postprandial state. The initial dosage of 25 μg SC BID is titrated upwards. GI side effects can occur.

Caffeine[2]

Its pressor effect in the caffeine-naive state can be exploited, especially postprandially, but one rapidly becomes tolerant. Its use should be restricted to 2 cups of coffee once daily with break-fast.

Therapeutic Tips

- Optimize blood volume and avoid vasodepressor drugs and diuretics where possible.
- Supine hypertension often limits therapy; to avoid this, elevate the head of the bed at night, and give shorter-acting pressor agents early in the day. Patients should be instructed not to lie flat during the day; recliner chairs are useful for naps.
- Patients should map out their routes and have prospective rest stops in mind before symptoms can occur; a fold-up tripod chair acts as a cane while walking and can be unfolded to a portable chair for rests.
- Nonpharmacologic adjuncts and patient education are crucial to success of a treatment program.

---

[3] *J Clin Endocrinol Metab* 1989;68:1051–1059.

- The standing time should be assessed; if a patient can stand for 5 minutes, he/she will generally retain good functional capacity for activities of daily living.
- Once symptoms are controlled, the minimum dose of any drug should be sought to maintain control.
- Drug administration should be additive and assessed empirically in each individual.
- Watch for tolerance to drug effects, especially with alpha agonists, once receptors downregulate.

Suggested Reading List

Hoeldtke RD, Boden G, O'Dorisio TM. Treatment of orthostatic hypotension with dihydroergotamine and caffeine. *Ann Intern Med* 1986;105:168–173.

Hoeldtke RD, Israel BC. Treatment of orthostatic hypotension with octreotide. *J Clin Endocrinol Metab* 1989;68: 1051–1059.

Kaufmann H, Brannan T, Krakoff L, et al. Treatment of orthostatic hypotension due to autonomic failure with a peripheral alpha adrenergic agonist (midodrine). *Neurology* 1988;38: 951–956.

Mathias CJ, daCosta DF, Fosbraey P, et al. Cardiovascular, biochemical and hormonal changes during food-induced hypotension in chronic autonomic failure. *J Neurol Sci* 1989;94:255–269.

Onrot J, Goldberg MR, Hollister AS, et al. Management of chronic orthostatic hypotension. *Am J Med* 1986;80: 454–464.

The Consensus Committee of the American Autonomic Society and the American Academy of Neurology. Consensus statement on the definition of orthostatic hypotension, pure autonomic failure, and multiple system atrophy. *Neurology* 1996;46:1470.

CHAPTER 30

Prevention of Cerebral Ischemia

Robert Côté, MD, FRCPC

Goals of Therapy

- To prevent disabling neurologic deficits (stroke) and recurrent transient ischemic attacks (TIA)
- To prevent associated cardiac ischemic events including myocardial infarction (MI)
- To prevent cerebrovascular and cardiovascular-related mortality

Investigations

- Complete history with attention to:
  - nature, frequency, duration and distribution of symptoms (cerebral localization)
  - identification of vascular risk factors
- Physical examination:
  - complete neurologic assessment
  - visual assessment including eye movements, visual fields, acuity and funduscopy
  - complete vascular examination including auscultation (cranium, cervical, cardiac), palpation (temporal artery, peripheral pulses) and blood pressure in both arms
- Laboratory tests – indicated in patients with TIAs or mild strokes (without disabling deficits):
  - CT brain scan (to rule out hemorrhagic process) and cervical and transcranial ultrasonography
  - CBC, coagulation parameters, blood glucose, renal and hepatic profile
  - in selected cases more specialized blood tests (e.g., ESR, immunologic work-up, testing for hypercoagulable states, antiphospholipid antibodies)
  - baseline ECG
  - other cardiac tests (e.g., transthoracic or transesophageal echocardiography, Holter monitoring) may be indicated (usually have a higher yield in patients with established cardiac disease or in young stroke patients)
  - cerebral angiography in selected cases to confirm occlusive cerebrovascular disease and to establish appropriateness of endarterectomy. Magnetic resonance imaging (MRI) and/or

Figure 1: **Prevention of Cerebral Ischemia**

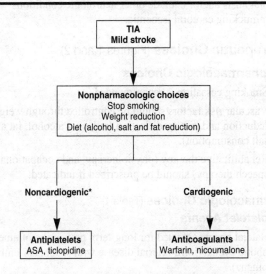

* If carotid symptoms and appropriate severe stenosis, consider surgery.

Figure 2: **Management of Acute Cerebral Ischemia**

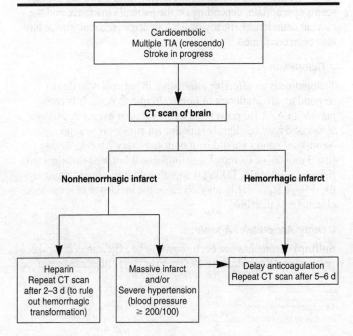

angiography (MRA) may be required to confirm the diagnosis and/or exclude other neurologic conditions mimicking cerebral ischemia.

Therapeutic Choices (Figures 1 and 2)

Nonpharmacologic Choices

- Smoking cessation is recommended.
- Vascular risk factors should be controlled through weight reduction and diet modification (reducing alcohol, fat and salt consumption).
- Rehabilitative therapy (physiotherapy, and occupational and speech therapy) should be prescribed if indicated.

Pharmacologic Choices (Table 1)

Antiplatelet Agents

Antiplatelet agents are used for long-term prevention of athero-thrombotic events (intra-arterial disease with secondary embolic phenomena).

☐ Acetylsalicylic Acid (ASA)

The drug of choice for stroke prevention, ASA has been shown to reduce vascular events (cardiac and cerebral) by about 25%. It is well-tolerated with few (dose-dependent) side effects. Patient acceptability and low cost are advantages. The optimal dosage for stroke prevention remains uncertain; 75 to 1 300 mg per day seems appropriate, depending on the patient's tolerance and the clinical situation.[1] Efficacy of ASA in acute ischemic stroke has also been confirmed.[2]

☐ Ticlopidine

Ticlopidine is an effective alternative in patients who do not respond to, are intolerant of or are allergic to ASA. It is comparable to ASA for prevention of all vascular events in patients at risk and may be slightly superior for stroke prevention. Neutrophil counts should be monitored every 2 weeks during the first 3 months of therapy for an infrequent but well-documented risk of neutropenia. Taking ticlopidine with meals and reducing the dosage temporarily may decrease the incidence of some side effects (e.g., diarrhea).

☐ Other Antiplatelet Agents

Sulfinpyrazone has not been shown to be efficacious in stroke prevention. **Dipyridamole** (400 mg per day) either used alone or

---

[1] *BMJ 1994;308:81–106.*
[2] *Lancet 1997; 349:1641–1649.*

Table 1: Drugs Used in Prevention of Cerebral Ischemia

Drug	Dosage	Adverse Effects	Drug Interactions	Cost*
Anticoagulants				
heparin Hepalean, generics	IV: Initial bolus: 5 000 units (optional) Maintenance: 24 000–32 000 units/24 h continuous infusion (aPTT ratio 1.5–2.5 × control value)	Hemorrhagic complications, usually dose-related. Thrombocytopenia (heparin). Skin necrosis (warfarin and heparin).	With heparin, concomitant use of ASA, NSAIDs or other antiplatelets may ↑ hemorrhagic risk. Effects of oral anticoagulants ↑ by cimetidine, some antibiotics, steroids and ↓ by phenytoin, barbiturates, carbamazepine, alcohol, oral contraceptives.	Varies
warfarin Coumadin, Warfilone	Oral: Dosed to maintain INR between 2.0–3.0 for most cerebrovascular indications; for stroke prevention in patients with **mechanical heart valves**, maintain INR between 2.5–4.5	Oral anticoagulants are contraindicated in pregnancy.		Warfarin 5 mg/d $
nicoumalone Sintrom				Nicoumalone 2 mg/d $
Antiplatelets				
ASA Entrophen, generics (coated); Aspirin, generics	75–1 300 mg/d	Bleeding, usually minor (epistaxis, etc.). ASA: gastric intolerance, GI bleeding (gastric ulcers, erosions), nausea, heartburn, constipation, tinnitus usually dose-related.	Hemorrhagic risk ↑ with concomitant use of anticoagulants. **Ticlopidine:** ↑ half-life of hepatically metabolized drugs ↓ digoxin levels, ↑ theophylline levels.	$
ticlopidine Ticlid	250 mg BID	Ticlopidine: diarrhea, skin rash, neutropenia; contraindicated in severe hepatic impairment.	Absorption ↓ by antacids. When combined with ASA: ↑ antiplatelet effect (not recommended).	$$$$
dipyridamole Persantine, generics	50–100 mg QID	Dipyridamole: headache, dizziness, hypotension.	**Dipyridamole:** effect ↓ by theophylline.	$

* Cost of 30-day supply – includes drug cost only.

Legend: $ < $20 $$ $20–40 $$$ $40–60 $$$$ > $60

in combination with low dose ASA (50 mg per day) was recently found to be of benefit for stroke prevention.[3] As well, dipyridamole (400 mg per day) combined with an oral anticoagulant appears to provide better protection against cardioembolic events in patients with prosthetic heart valves.[4] A new antiplatelet agent, **clopidogrel** (75 mg per day) has been found to be somewhat more efficacious than ASA for the prevention of ischemic events including stroke.[5] This agent is expected to be approved for general use soon.

Anticoagulants

Anticoagulants are used to prevent ischemic attacks from emboli presumed to be of cardiac origin.

❑ Heparin

Although heparin is used to manage acute cerebral ischemic events (e.g., stroke in evolution, multiple recurrent [crescendo] TIAs or cardioembolic infarction), its efficacy has not been proven by evidence from clinical trials. Available data do not support the routine use of heparin in acute partial atherothrombotic stroke. Its only proven efficacy is in the prevention of deep vein thrombosis in acute ischemic stroke. A risk of bleeding complications is always present, and a CT brain scan is mandatory before initiating IV heparin for acute cerebral ischemia.

The dosage is usually 1 000 units per hour via infusion pump, and anticoagulation is monitored using the activated partial thromboplastin time (aPTT) (maintain at 1.5 to 2.5 times control). An initial bolus of 5 000 units is optional to more rapidly attain the desired antithrombotic effect. The optimal duration of treatment is uncertain; 5 to 10 days is suggested.

❑ Warfarin or Nicoumalone

These oral anticoagulants are efficacious in preventing cerebral and systemic emboli in acute MI, in valvular and nonvalvular atrial fibrillation and in patients with prosthetic cardiac valves. The risk of bleeding is influenced by many factors (e.g., the intensity of anticoagulation, and concomitant use of high doses of ASA/other drugs with antiplatelet effects).

❑ Low Molecular Weight Heparins (LMWH)

Dalteparin, enoxaparin, nadroparin and **tinzaparin** are LMWHs approved for thromboprophylaxis after orthopedic surgery and treatment of venous thrombosis. They have an

---

[3] *Journal of Neurological Sciences 1996;143:1–13.*
[4] *Chest 1995;108 (suppl 4):225S–522S.*
[5] *Lancet 1996;348:1329–1339.*

antithrombotic effect equivalent to standard heparin but tend to produce less bleeding. Recently, positive results were reported in acute ischemic stroke with **nadroparin** (Fraxiparine).[6] A larger randomized trial is underway to confirm these preliminary results.

Thrombolytics

At present, the IV use of streptokinase or urokinase in the treatment of acute ischemic stroke cannot be recommended. However, alteplase (rtPA) has been approved in the US for the acute treatment of ischemic stroke and is expected to be approved soon in Canada. Use of this thrombolytic agent should be restricted to a selected group of patients with an acute (< 3 hours) ischemic stroke and subjected to strict guidelines under appropriate neurological supervision.[7]

Others

Several neuronal protective agents (e.g., glutamate antagonists, calcium channel blockers) are presently under investigation in acute ischemic stroke.

Therapeutic Tips

- In most cases antithrombotic treatment should be continued long term, especially in older individuals with atherosclerosis and vascular risk factors.

- If a patient experiences recurrent attacks of cerebral ischemia with a relatively low dose of ASA (i.e., 325 mg per day or less), the dose may be increased up to 1 300 mg per day depending on the patient's tolerance.

- As an alternative to ASA or ticlopidine, consider the combination of low dose ASA (50 mg per day) and dipyridamole (400 mg per day) for stroke prevention.

- Combination therapy (oral anticoagulant plus ASA 100 mg per day) has been shown to be superior to anticoagulant alone in patients with prosthetic heart valves but with an increased risk of minor bleeding episodes. For patients not tolerating ASA, dipyridamole (225 mg per day) plus an oral anticoagulant may be used.

- Patients with carotid symptoms, ipsilateral to a significant (≥ 70%) carotid stenosis documented by angiography, should be considered for carotid endarterectomy in addition to long-term antiplatelet therapy.

---

[6] *N Engl J Med 1995;333:1588–1593.*
[7] *N Engl J Med 1995;333:1581–1587.*

Suggested Reading List

Barnett HJM, Eliasziw M, Meldrum HE. Drugs and surgery in the prevention of ischemic stroke. *N Engl J Med* 1995;332:238–248.

Camarata PJ, Heros RC, Latchaw RE. "Brain Attack": The rationale for treating stroke as a medical emergency. *Neurosurgery* 1994;34:144–158.

Antiplatelet Trialists' Collaboration. Collaborative overview of randomised trials of antiplatelet therapy–I: Prevention of death, myocardial infarction, and stroke by prolonged antiplatelet therapy in various categories of patients. *BMJ* 1994;308:81–106.

CHAPTER 31

Venous Thromboembolism

Alexander G.G. Turpie, MD, FRCP(Lond), FRCP(Glas), FACP, FACC, FRCPC

Prophylaxis

Goals of Therapy

- To prevent deep vein thrombosis (DVT) and pulmonary embolism (PE)
- To reduce mortality
- To prevent the postphlebitic syndrome

Clinical Risk Categories

Venous thromboembolism (VTE) is a common cause of morbidity and mortality in hospitalized patients; the frequency varies according to patients' risk category. Consensus conferences have defined these categories based on clinical criteria and made recommendations for thrombosis prophylaxis according to risk group (Table 1). The risk of VTE is also increased in the presence of the following factors related to venous stasis and coagulopathies:

- age
- varicose veins
- immobility (bed rest > 4 days)
- active cancer
- pregnancy
- puerperium
- high-dose estrogen therapy
- previous DVT or PE
- thrombophilia (tendency to thrombosis)
  - antithrombin III deficiency
  - protein C or protein S deficiency
  - activated protein C resistance
  - antiphospholipid antibody
  - lupus anticoagulant

Nonpharmacologic Choices

Caval interruption by filter is rarely indicated for primary prophylaxis but should be considered in patients in whom anticoagulants have failed or are absolutely contraindicated.

Table 1: Risk Categories and Thrombosis Prophylaxis

Risk Group	Clinical Criteria	Frequency of VTE – Hospitalized Patients (without prophylaxis)			Prophylactic Measures (should be continued for a minimum of 5 to 7 d until the patient is fully ambulant)
		DVT	Proximal vein thrombosis	Fatal PE	
Low	Minor surgery (< 30 min); no risk factors other than age. Major surgery (> 30 min); age < 40 yrs, no other risk factors. Minor trauma or medical illness.	10%	1%	0.01%	Mobilize Graduated compression stockings
Moderate	Major general, urological, gynecological, cardiothoracic, vascular or neurologic surgery; age ≥ 40 yrs or other risk factor. Major medical illness: heart or lung disease, cancer, inflammatory bowel disease. Major trauma or burns. Minor surgery, trauma or illness in patients with previous deep vein thrombosis, pulmonary embolism or thrombophilia.	10–40%	1–10%	0.1–1%	Low-dose heparin (5 000 units SC Q12H or Q8H) Graduated compression stockings External pneumatic compression
High	Fracture or major orthopedic surgery of pelvis, hip or lower limb. Major pelvic or abdominal surgery for cancer. Major surgery, trauma or illness in patients with previous deep vein thrombosis, pulmonary embolism or thrombophilia. Lower limb paralysis (e.g., hemiplegic stroke, paraplegia). Major lower limb amputation.	40–80%	10–30%	1–10%	Low molecular weight heparin* Adjusted-dose heparin (aPTT 1.5 × control) Adjusted-dose warfarin (INR 2.0–3.0) External pneumatic compression Combinations

See individual product monographs for complete information on administration.

Pharmacologic Choices

See Table 1 for prophylactic measures used in different risk categories and Drugs Used in Prophylaxis and Treatment for details on specific drugs.

Treatment

Goals of Therapy

Deep vein thrombosis (DVT)

- To prevent major pulmonary embolism
- To prevent thrombus extension
- To enhance thrombolysis
- To prevent postphlebitic syndrome
- To reduce morbidity of acute event

Pulmonary Embolism (PE)

- To prevent death
- To prevent recurrent thromboembolism
- To prevent chronic thromboembolic pulmonary hypertension

Investigations

Because the clinical diagnosis of DVT and PE is insensitive and nonspecific, objective diagnosis using specific procedures is important for optimal management.

- **DVT:** Ascending venography, impedance plethysmography, B-mode compression ultrasound (most practical and useful clinically)
- **PE:** Pulmonary angiography, perfusion lung scan, ventilation lung scan, DVT tests
- Patients under 40 with recurrent VTE or a family history should be screened for thrombophilia (see Clinical Risk Categories)

Therapeutic Choices

General Measures

Deep Vein Thrombosis

- Immobilize if symptoms warrant (reduces pain, prevents embolization).
- Elevate limb (reduces edema and pain).
- Avoid pressure on the swollen leg.
- Analgesics for pain (including NSAIDs; effective but may ↑ risk of bleeding, especially when used with anticoagulants).

Pulmonary Embolism

- Administer oxygen.
- IV fluids.
- Vasopressor agents.
- Other resuscitory measures (depending on patient's clinical status).

Pharmacologic Choices

Established DVT and/or PE are initially treated with SC **low molecular weight heparin** or IV standard **heparin** for a minimum of 5 days followed by oral anticoagulation with **warfarin** with at least 2 days of overlap with a therapeutic INR. Oral anticoagulation is usually maintained for 3 months in DVT and 3 to 6 months in PE.

Drugs for Prophylaxis and Treatment of Venous Thromboembolism

Low Molecular Weight Heparins (LMWHs)

Enoxaparin (Lovenox) is approved for prophylaxis in high risk orthopedic patients. **Dalteparin** (Fragmin), tinzaparin (Innohep) and **nadroparin** (Fraxiparine) are approved for both prophylaxis in conjunction with surgery and treatment of VTE.

The kinetics of LMWHs are more predictable than those of standard heparin, and their elimination half-life is longer. These properties may make weight-adjusted fixed-dose SC dosing of LMWHs an excellent alternative to adjusted-dose IV heparin in the initial treatment of VTE. LMWHs have become the management of choice for initial treatment of DVT for many outpatients. They are also effective in the treatment of PE.

Heparin

Heparin acts as an anticoagulant by forming a complex with antithrombin III, catalyzing the inhibition of several activated blood coagulation factors. For treatment of VTE, heparin is most commonly given by IV infusion in a dose monitored to prolong the activated partial thromboplastin time (aPTT) to 1.5 to 2.5 times control. It is also effective by SC injection if a sufficiently high dose is given (generally 15 000 to 25 000 units Q12H). An IV bolus (5 000 to 10 000 units) should be given with the SC injection in the initial treatment. Monitoring 4 to 6 hours after the SC dose should aim for an aPTT 2.0 to 2.5 times control. A practical nomogram has been developed for adjusting IV heparin (Table 2).[1]

---

[1] *Arch Intern Med* 1992;152:1589–1595.

Table 2: **Heparin Dosing Nomogram**

Bolus: 5 000 to 10 000 units **Maintenance:** Infusion (20 000 units per 500 mL)

aPTT (s)	Rate Change (mL/h)	Dose Change (units/24h)	Additional Action and Monitoring
< 45	+6	+5760	• Rebolus with 5 000 units Repeat aPTT at 6 h
46–54	+3	+2880	• Repeat aPTT at 6 h
55–85	0	0	• Repeat aPTT next AM
86–110	−3	−2880	• Stop infusion for 1 h Repeat aPTT at 6 h
> 110	−6	−5760	• Stop infusion for 1 h Repeat aPTT at 6 h

Warfarin

Warfarin (Coumadin) inhibits thrombin formation by interfering with vitamin K metabolism, which is essential in the synthesis of coagulation factors II, VII, IX and X. It is given in a dose adjusted to maintain the INR at 2.0 to 3.0.

Monitoring Warfarin Therapy with the INR

A major limitation of the prothrombin time, reported in seconds, is the considerable variability in the results depending on the laboratory technique used. This limitation is largely overcome by the use of the international normalized ratio (INR).

Drug Interactions with Warfarin

The most common cause of poor anticoagulant control is drug interactions (Table 3). ASA and NSAIDs contribute to bleeding by inhibiting platelet function.

Anticoagulation in Pregnancy

- Heparin is the anticoagulant of choice during pregnancy; SC injections twice daily achieve therapeutic levels.
- Heparin should be stopped at the first sign of labor.
- Warfarin or SC heparin may be used for about 6 weeks after delivery for secondary prevention.
- Women can breast-feed while being treated with warfarin.
- The management of pregnant women with a previous DVT or PE is controversial; heparin, 5 000 units SC Q12H throughout pregnancy, is recommended.
- LMWHs do not cross the placental barrier and have been used as alternatives to heparin.

Thrombolytic Agents

Less than 20% of VTE patients are eligible for thrombolytic therapy (i.e., young patients with massive ileofemoral vein thrombosis or patients with major PE). **Streptokinase** (SK), **anistreplase, urokinase** (UK) and **alteplase** are available. The best results are obtained with recent thrombi, but substantial lysis may be obtained in patients with symptoms of up to 14 days' duration.

SK is the least expensive thrombolytic. However, given the prolonged infusions of SK and UK used in VTE, alteplase, with its short infusion, may be more cost effective.

Table 3: **Warfarin Drug Interactions**

Drugs That Increase INR

antimicrobials
Cefamandole
Cefotetan
Chloramphenicol
Ciprofloxacin
Co-trimoxazole
Erythromycin
Metronidazole
Norfloxacin

antifungals
Fluconazole
Itraconazole
Ketoconazole

hormones
Anabolic steroids
Danazol
Thyroid supplements

lipid lowering agents
Bezafibrate
Clofibrate
Fenofibrate
Gemfibrozil
Lovastatin

others
Alcohol (large amounts)
Allopurinol
Amiodarone
Cimetidine
Chloral hydrate
Disulfiram
Paroxetine
Phenylbutazone
Propafenone
Sulfinpyrazone

Drugs That Decrease INR
Antithyroids
Barbiturates
Carbamazepine
Cholestyramine
Griseofulvin
Phenytoin
Primidone
Rifampin
Vitamin K

Drugs That Increase Hypoprothrombinemia
ASA
NSAIDs

Suggested Reading List

Clagett CG, Anderson FA, Heit J, et al. Prevention of venous thromboembolism. *Chest* 1995;108(4):3125–3345.

Hirsh J, Fuster V. Guide to anticoagulant therapy. Part 1: Heparin. *Circulation* 1994;89:1449–1468.

Hirsh J, Fuster V. Guide to anticoagulant therapy. Part 2: Oral anticoagulants. *Circulation* 1994;89:1469–1480.

Hirsh J, Levine MN. Low molecular weight heparin. *Blood* 1992;79:1–17.

Thromboembolic Risk Factors (THRIFT) Consensus Group. Risk of and prophylaxis for venous thromboembolism in hospital patients. *BMJ* 1992;305:567–574.

Turpie AGG. New therapeutic opportunities for heparins: what does low molecular weight heparin offer? *J Thrombosis and Thrombolysis* 1996;3:145–149.

CHAPTER 32

Intermittent Claudication

Richard I. Ogilvie, MD, FRCPC, FACP

Goals of Therapy

- To improve mobility and quality of life
- To increase walking distance and time to claudication
- To increase capacity for regular dynamic leg exercise

Investigations

- History with special attention to cardiovascular disease risk factors and associated conditions:
  - hypertension
  - diabetes mellitus
  - smoking
  - dyslipidemia
  - angina pectoris/MI
  - congestive heart failure
  - TIA/stroke
- Define walking time to claudication (**severe** < 1/2 city block; **moderate** 1/2 to 1 block; **mild** > 1 block)
- Define duration of symptoms (6 to 12 months are required to develop collateral circulation)
- Physical examination:
  - signs of hypertension, dyslipidemia, diabetes mellitus, atherosclerosis (aortic aneurysm, bruits), heart failure
  - signs of peripheral artery obstruction
  - evidence of acute peripheral artery occlusion (acute onset of continuous pain, pale and cool limb or mottled discoloration, thickened swollen stiff muscles plus pain over the muscle)
  - paresthesia and paralysis require immediate surgical revascularization (fibrinolysis may be considered)
  - resting pain, dependent rubor, cyanosis, muscle atrophy, trophic ulcers suggest severe obstruction
- Laboratory tests:
  - fasting blood sugar and lipid profile
  - hemoglobin, hematocrit, platelet count
  - resting Doppler-derived or sphygmomanometric ankle/arm systolic pressure index (Figure 1)

Figure 1: **Treatment of Intermittent Claudication**

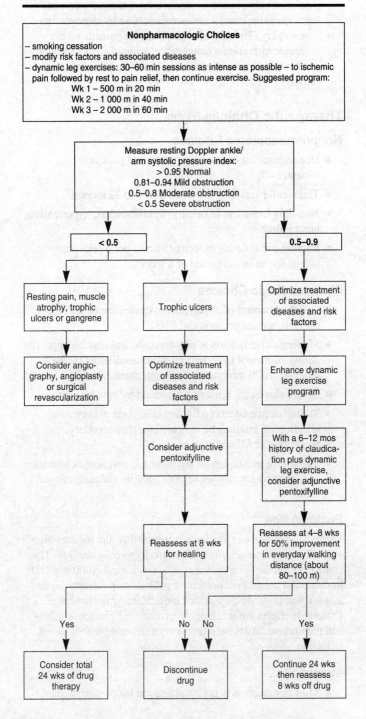

– consider invasive angiography for patients with resting pain, atrophy, cyanosis, nonhealing ischemic ulcers or gangrene for possible revascularization by angioplasty or surgery. The role of angioplasty for patients with chronic intermittent claudication without signs of severe arterial obstruction remains to be defined by clinical trials

Therapeutic Choices (Figure 1)
Nonpharmacologic Choices
- Discontinuation of smoking (active and passive) (Chapter 40).
- Time (collateral flow develops over 6 to 12 months).
- Non-drug treatment of obesity, lipid disorders, hypertension, heart failure.
- Regular dynamic leg exercise (5 times per week continuously for an initial period of 8 weeks).

Pharmacologic Choices
- Optimize control of hypertension, dyslipidemia, diabetes mellitus, angina pectoris and CHF.
- Moderate claudication is not worsened and may be improved during control of hypertension with vasodilators (alpha$_1$-blockers, ACE inhibitors or calcium channel blockers).
- Severe claudication may be worsened by beta-blockers.
- Platelet-active agents (ASA and others) do not improve claudication but may be indicated for the secondary prevention of MI and stroke.
- The role of prostaglandin analogues, L-carnitine or arterial gene therapy has not yet been defined by adequate clinical trials.

Pentoxifylline
Pentoxifylline alters erythrocyte deformability and reduces blood viscosity, platelet reactivity and plasma hypercoagulability. The controlled-release formulation is given with meals (400 mg TID) to reduce GI upset. Five percent of patients stop therapy due to nausea, vomiting, dyspepsia, belching, bloating or flatulence. Other side effects are dizziness, nervousness, agitation, flushing and palpitations. Adverse effects may ameliorate with dose reduction.

Indications
- **Mild** claudication is not an indication for pentoxifylline.

- **Moderate** claudication: cessation of smoking and regular dynamic leg exercise may be more beneficial than pentoxifylline. Dynamic leg exercise for 6 to 12 months after the onset of claudication may allow collaterals to develop. If pentoxifylline is used, a total of 24 weeks of therapy followed by 8 weeks drug-free (as exercise tolerance increases) can decrease or eliminate the need for the drug.

Pentoxifylline may be beneficial adjunctive therapy for trophic ulcers in diabetic and nondiabetic patients; therapy should be assessed at 4-week intervals with a usual maximum duration of 24 weeks (due to cost – approximately $40 per month, drug cost only).

Resting pain, muscle atrophy, trophic ulcers or gangrene should prompt investigation for possible angioplastic or surgical intervention.

Precautions

Pentoxifylline is **contraindicated** in patients with allergy or intolerance to xanthines, during pregnancy or lactation, acute MI, acute hemorrhage or severe hepatic or renal dysfunction. The dose should be reduced in patients with hepatic dysfunction.

Drug Interactions

Pentoxifylline probably reduces the efficacy of adenosine in terminating supraventricular arrhythmias. It may enhance effects of theophylline, warfarin, sympathomimetics, antihypertensives and hypoglycemics.

Suggested Reading List

Gardner AW, Poehlmann ET. Exercise programs for the treatment of claudication pain. A meta-analysis. *JAMA* 1995;274:975–980.

Hood SC, Moher D, Barber GG. Management of intermittent claudication with pentoxifylline: meta-analysis of randomized controlled trials. *Can Med Assoc J* 1996;15: 1053–1059.

Lingarde F, Jelnes R, Bjorkman H, et al. Conservative drug treatment in patients with moderately severe chronic occlusive peripheral arterial disease. *Circulation* 1989;80:1549–1556.

Radack K, Wyderski RJ. Conservative management of intermittent claudication. *Ann Intern Med* 1990;113: 135–146.

Veith FJ, Gupta SK, Wengerter KR, et al. Impact of nonoperative therapy on the clinical management of peripheral arterial disease. *Circulation* 1991;83(suppl 1):I-137–I-142.

CHAPTER 33

Raynaud's Phenomenon

André Roussin, MD, FRCPC

Goals of Therapy

- To decrease symptoms (cold-induced blanching of the fingers) in primary (PRP) or secondary Raynaud's phenomenon (SRP)
- To prevent local and systemic deterioration in SRP
- To heal lesions in SRP

Investigations (Figure 1)

- Thorough history to differentiate between:
  - **PRP** (no associated illness or trauma)
  - **SRP** (secondary to occupational hazards, vascular diseases, connective tissue diseases [CTD], carpal tunnel syndrome, hypothyroidism or other disorders)
  - possible **drug-induced** RP (see Nonpharmacologic Choices)
- Physical examination for:
  - altered pulsations and abnormal Allen's test
  - local signs of CTD (e.g., sclerodactyly) and carpal tunnel syndrome
  - systemic signs of CTD (e.g., telangiectasis, pulmonary fibrosis), vascular diseases and hypothyroidism
- Laboratory tests:
  - nailfold capillary microscopy to detect megacapillaries and other abnormalities suggestive of scleroderma and other CTD
  - ANA (antinuclear antibodies) and ACA (anticentromere antibodies) to detect CTD
  - other tests are less useful as early markers of SRP
  - normal tests suggest PRP

Therapeutic Choices (Figure 1)

Nonpharmacologic Choices

- Minimize cold exposure.
- Avoid prescribing medications with vasoconstrictive potential:
  - ergot derivatives including methysergide
  - beta-blockers (unlikely but controversial)
  - bromocriptine.

Figure 1: **Investigation and Management of Raynaud's Phenomenon**

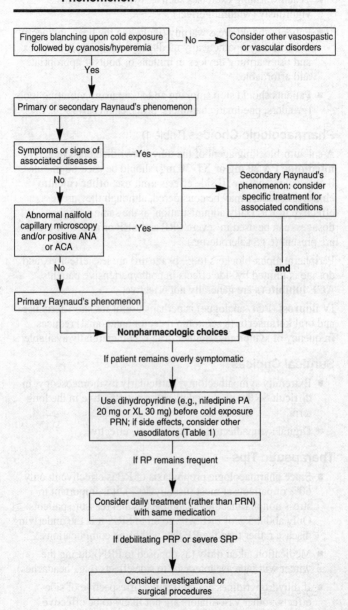

- Reassure patients that no complications arise from PRP.
- Teach warming exercises such as swinging the arms vigorously (windmill effect).
- Patients should dress warmly (including the head and neck) to avoid a sympathetically mediated vasoconstrictive reflex and use warming devices in mittens or boots if appropriate and affordable.
- Patients should stop smoking and avoid using vibrating tools (grinders, pneumatic hammers, drills, chain saws).

Pharmacologic Choices (Table 1)

A calcium-blocking agent of the dihydropyridine class (e.g., **nifedipine PA 20 mg or XL 30 mg**) should be used 60 minutes before cold exposure. If side effects limit use, **other calcium channel blockers** may be considered, although they are less effective in RP. Daily administration, at the same or higher dosages, can be used in severe PRP and SRP or in SRP if ulcers are present (e.g., scleroderma).

Peripheral alpha-blockers (e.g., **prazosin**) are less effective, and dosage is limited by side effects in nonhypertensive patients. **ACE inhibitors** are generally not effective.

IV **iloprost** (PGI_2 analogue) is perhaps useful for short-term use and oral **ketanserin** (a serotonin receptor antagonist) reduces frequency of symptoms. Neither drug is commercially available.

Surgical Choices

- Extremity sympathectomy, particularly by thoracoscopy, in difficult SRP with digital ulcers is not effective in the long term.
- Digital sympathectomy may be more effective.

Therapeutic Tips

- Since pharmacologic prophylaxis of RP is effective in only 60% of patients at most (usually 40%), it is important to stress nonpharmacologic approaches and reassure patients. Only about 5% of PRP will go on to SRP; it is the underlying disease rather than the RP that will bring complications.
- Medication taken **daily** (as opposed to PRN) during the winter will increase tolerance to side effects (e.g., headaches).
- If dihydropyridines are ineffective (irrespective of side effects), other vasodilators are not likely to be effective.
- Laboratory cold-induced tests do not reliably predict a patient's response to any given drug in RP.
- PRP and SRP respond equally well to medications; frequency of attacks, rather than intensity and duration, is most likely reduced.

Table 1: **Dosages of Drugs Used in Raynaud's Phenomenon**

Drug	Dosage	Cost*
Calcium Channel Blockers		
Dihydropyridines		
nifedipine	PA 20 mg or XL 30 mg 30–60 min	$–$$
Adalat PA or XL, generics	before cold exposure	
felodipine	5–10 mg 60 min before cold exposure	$$
Renedil, Plendil		
amlodipine	5 mg 60 min before cold exposure	$$$
Norvasc		
Others		
diltiazem	SR 90 mg or CD 180 mg 60–90 min	$$–$$$
Cardizem SR or CD, generics	before cold exposure	
Alpha₁ Adrenergic Blockers		
prazosin	1–2 mg BID (regular dosage, to avoid	$
Minipress, generics	risk of syncope with irregular use)	

* *Cost per dose – includes drug cost only.*
Legend: $ < 0.50 $$ 0.50–1.00 $$$ 1.00–1.50

Suggested Reading List

Adee AC. Managing Raynaud's phenomenon: a practical approach (review). *Am Fam Physician* 1993;47:823–829.

Coffman JD. Vasospastic diseases. In: Young JR, ed. *Peripheral vascular diseases*. 2nd ed. St. Louis: Mosby, 1996:407–424.

Creager MA, et al. Raynaud's phenomenon and other vascular disorders related to temperature. In: Loscalzo J, ed. *Vascular medicine*. 2nd ed. Boston: Little, Brown and Company, 1996:965–997.

Lowell RC et al. Cervicothoracic sympathectomy for Raynaud's syndrome. *Int Angiol* 1993;12:168–172.

CHAPTER 34

Allergic Rhinitis

D. William Moote, MD, FRCPC

Goals of Therapy

- To prevent the allergic reaction
- To suppress and control symptoms produced by the allergic response

Investigations

- Clinical history and physical examination (Table 1). View nasal mucosa using otoscope
- Skin testing: confirms allergic sensitivity, if present

Table 1: Differential Diagnosis of Rhinitis

Type	Characteristics
Seasonal or perennial allergic rhinitis	Nasal obstruction and rhinorrhea are common.
	Often conjunctival symptoms, sneezing, itching of the nasal mucosa and the oropharynx.
	Seasonal patterns may be recognized, or perennial symptoms may flare up after exposure to allergens like dust mite or animal danders.
	Nasal mucosa is swollen, often pale or bluish, and moist.
Upper respiratory infections	More episodic, often associated with sore throat or fever and not associated with itch.
	Nasal mucosa is often red.
Vasomotor rhinitis	Obstruction and rhinorrhea are prominent and other symptoms infrequent.
	Often triggered by irritant exposures such as smoke, temperature changes, strong odors, etc.
Nasal polyps	Obstruction is the main complaint.
	Anosmia is almost always present.
	Nasal exam will usually detect a polyp.

Therapeutic Choices (Figure 1)

Nonpharmacologic Choices

- Avoidance of allergens allows significant reductions in medication use. Air conditioning reduces pollen exposure. Removing pets from the home will reduce perennial symptoms caused by animal dander.

Figure 1: **Management of Allergic Rhinitis**

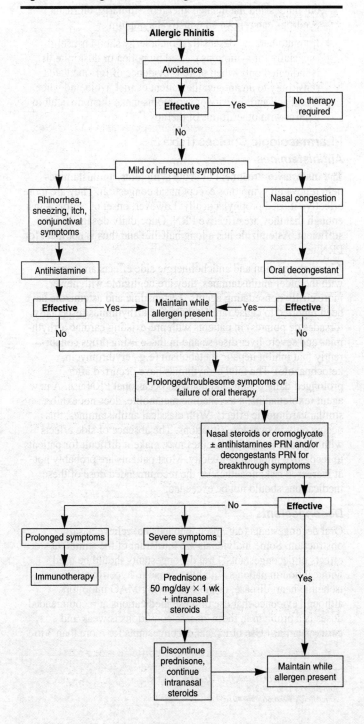

- Saline nose sprays can help relieve symptoms by washing out mucus and the inhaled allergen. Similarly, lubricant eyedrops can relieve conjunctival symptoms.

- Immunotherapy (desensitization, allergy shots) is useful, especially for symptoms caused by pollen or dust mite. It is indicated only when there is evidence of IgE-mediated sensitivity to an antigen the patient cannot avoid and when frequency and severity of symptoms make them difficult to control with other forms of therapy.[1]

Pharmacologic Choices (Table 2)

Antihistamines

The mainstay of treatment of acute symptoms, antihistamines help relieve all symptoms except nasal congestion. They are more effective if used prophylactically; however, onset of action is fast enough that they are effective PRN. Once-daily dosage is often sufficient. Astemizole has a long half-life and thus is not ideal for PRN use.

Although sedation and anticholinergic side effects are common with the older antihistamines, they are negligible with newer, more costly nonsedating agents. Terfenadine and astemizole have been reported to cause rare fatal cardiac arrhythmias (especially torsades de pointes) in patients with pre-existing cardiac arrhythmias and severe liver disease and in those using drugs concurrently that inhibit hepatic metabolism (e.g., erythromycin, ketoconazole). The fatal arrhythmias have occurred after prolonged daily dosing and not with occasional PRN use. A new agent fexofenadine, a terfenadine metabolite, does not exhibit similar cardiotoxic effects. With classical antihistamines, this occurs only in overdose situations. The absence of side effects with nonsedating antihistamines may make it difficult for patients to recognize impending toxicity. Most patients are probably not at increased risk; nonetheless, the recommended dose of these medications should not be exceeded.[2]

Decongestants

Oral decongestants (e.g., pseudoephedrine) relieve nasal obstruction. Some individuals are intolerant of the stimulant side effects of decongestants. Oral decongestants should be used with caution in patients with hypertension, hyperthyroidism or ischemic heart disease, or those receiving MAO inhibitors, although evidence that use of these medications at recommended doses is a problem in these disease conditions is weak and circumstantial.[3] Use of topical decongestants for more than 3 to

---

[1] Can Med Assoc J 1995;152(9):1413–1419.

[2] Ann Allergy 1992;69:276.

[3] Ann Allergy 1986;56:396–401.

7 days results in rhinitis medicamentosa; thus, they should be avoided in allergic rhinitis because long-term therapy is often required.

Antihistamine–Decongestant Combinations

Antihistamines and decongestants have complementary effects. Patients taking both drugs may find combination tablets convenient. Some combinations (e.g., cold preparations) may also contain analgesics and expectorants, which are not helpful in allergic rhinitis and should be avoided.

Topical Therapy

Topical corticosteroids are the mainstay of therapy for chronic rhinitis symptoms. Aqueous preparations of beclomethasone or flunisolide generally have better intranasal deposition than pressurized metered-dose inhalers especially when chronic symptoms have caused significant obstruction or there is ciliary dysfunction, as in smokers. Newer preparations of budesonide or fluticasone have a lower volume spray, which may be preferred by some.

Topical steroids act locally and are quickly metabolized once absorbed. Adrenal suppression has not been seen at therapeutic dosages. Data on inhaled steroids in asthma suggest that systemic effects occur at doses in the range of 1 000 to 2 000 µg – much higher than those recommended for allergic rhinitis. There are anecdotal reports of nasal septal perforation. No reports in controlled studies confirm this; however, patients should be instructed to aim the spray at the turbinates, not at the septum.

Topical cromoglycate sprays have an excellent safety profile but are less effective than the steroids and usually need QID dosing, at least initially.

Levocabastine (antihistamine) nasal spray has a rapid onset but is less potent than topical steroids and is not effective for treatment of congestion.

Pharmacoeconomic Considerations

The therapy of choice based on cost and effectiveness is a topical steroid. Antihistamines are cost effective only for the mildest symptoms.

Quality of life indexes are now being applied in the assessment of allergic rhinitis. They show a significant impairment in day-to-day physical, emotional, occupational, and social functioning.[4] Thirty-nine million persons in the US experienced allergic rhinitis symptoms in 1987, but only 12.3% of those sought medical treatment.[5]

[4] *J Allergy Clin Immunol* 1997;99(2):S742–S749.
[5] *J Allergy Clin Immunol* 1997;99(1):22–27.

Table 2: Drugs Used in Allergic Rhinitis

Drug	Dosage	Adverse Effects	Comments	Cost*
Oral Agents				
Antihistamines: See Chapter 63 (Pruritus).				
Decongestants *pseudoephedrine* Eltor, Sudafed, generics	Adults: 60 mg Q4–6H Sustained release: 120 mg Q12H Children 6–11 yrs: 30 mg Q4–6H (120 mg/d max.) Children 2–5 yrs: 15 mg Q4–6H (60 mg/d max.)	Insomnia, tremor, irritability, headache, nightmares, palpitations.	Rhinitis medicamentosa is not a problem with oral agents but occurs with prolonged use (> 3 days) of topical nasal decongestants.	$†
Antihistamine–Decongestant Combinations – various combinations and products	In accordance with labelled directions	See Chapter 63, Table 1, for antihistamine adverse effects; see above for decongestant adverse effects.	Offer convenience to patient requiring an antihistamine and decongestant.	$†
Topical Agents				
sodium cromoglycate Rynacrom, generics	Adults and children over 5 yrs: 1 spray or cartridge each nostril QID	Nasal stinging, burning, irritation, sneezing.	Slow onset (significant effects may not be seen for 1 wk in seasonal allergic rhinitis and 2–4 wks in chronic allergic rhinitis), low potency, QID dosing, very safe.	$$

Corticosteroids

Drug	Dose	Side effects	Comments	Cost*
beclomethasone Beconase, Vancenase, Beconase AQ	1 spray each nostril QID 2 sprays each nostril BID	Burning or stinging, nosebleeds.	Slow onset (7–14 d for maximal effect), must be used regularly, long duration, very potent, concern about potential steroid side effects, especially in children. Aiming spray up toward turbinates and away from septum helps avoid septal crusting or irritation. Liquid formats may be more effective than metered-dose inhalers.	$–$$$
budesonide Rhinocort Aqua, Rhinocort Turbuhaler	2 sprays each nostril daily			$$
flunisolide Rhinalar, generics	2 sprays each nostril BID			$$
fluticasone Flonase	2 sprays each nostril daily		For once daily dosed medication, administering 1 spray into each nostril BID may be more effective in some situations.	$$$
triamcinolone acetonide Nasacort, Nasacort AQ	2 sprays each nostril daily			$$$

Antihistamines

Drug	Dose	Side effects	Comments	Cost*
levocabastine Livostin	Adults and children over 12 yrs: 2 sprays each nostril BID	Nasal irritation.	Quick onset, short duration, short shelf life. If no improvement in 3 d it should be discontinued. Not effective for congestion.	$$

† Available over the counter – retail mark-up may vary.
* Cost of one unit (spray pump, metered-dose aerosol unit, etc.) or 18 tablets – includes drug cost only.
Legend: $ < $10 $$ $10–20 $$$ $20–30

The cost of illness of allergic rhinitis is also significant. Using data from the National Medical Expenditure Survey, the total cost of illness in the US was $1.23 billion, in 1994 dollars. This represents a significant underestimate of actual medication costs, in that nonprescription medication costs were not captured.

Therapeutic Tips

- If an antihistamine at recommended dosage does not work, little is gained from changing to a different chemical class. Although older studies of long-term dosing with classical antihistamines have demonstrated loss of effectiveness, they are flawed by lack of evidence of compliance. Newer studies show no loss of effectiveness up to 1 year.

- Most antihistamine preparations are available as syrups for children but are not very convenient for portable PRN dosing. Brompheniramine/phenylpropanolamine (Dimetapp Chewtabs) and loratadine (tasteless) tablets can be chewed.

- Medications are usually started at the maximum dose and then tapered to the minimum required for maintenance.

- Patients with predictable seasonal allergic rhinitis can start medications such as intranasal corticosteroids before the allergen exposure period and take them regularly until the end of the season for maximum effectiveness.

- If desired results are not achieved with once-daily dosing of newer topical steroids, a twice-daily regimen may be more effective, even at the same total daily dose.

- Antihistamines can be used in asthmatic patients; many have a slightly beneficial effect on asthma symptoms.

- For conjunctival symptoms, oral antihistamines are useful. Topical ophthalmic levocabastine provides relief in 10 minutes but is short lasting (12 h). Once opened, the bottle should be discarded within a month. Topical cromoglycate or lodoxamide requires several days for onset, but may be more effective.

- In vasomotor rhinitis where rhinorrhea is the major problem, ipratropium bromide spray can be helpful. It is quick in onset.

- Topical steroids will shrink nasal polyps, but long-term treatment is required. Anosmia is not usually improved. If surgery is contemplated, the use of topical steroids after surgery may decrease the recurrence rate.

Suggested Reading List

Anon. Assessing and treating rhinitis: A practical guide for Canadian physicians. Proceedings of the Canadian Rhinitis Symposium. *Can Med Assoc J* 1994;151(4Suppl):1–27.

CHAPTER 35

Viral Rhinitis

William Feldman, MD, FRCPC

Goals of Therapy

- To relieve the embarrassment and discomfort of a drippy nose
- To alleviate the discomfort of breathing through the nose
- To achieve the above with a minimum of adverse effects

Investigations

- No laboratory tests are required for the typical patient with the common cold. Culture for bacterial nasal pathogens has recently been recommended but requires further study before this approach can be accepted

Therapeutic Choices (Figure 1)

Nonpharmacologic Choices

- Although steam inhalation or vaporization is widely recommended to liquefy nasal secretions, there is no evidence that this is effective.
- Vitamin C has not been shown to be of significant therapeutic benefit.
- There is no evidence that bed rest has any effect on severity or duration.
- For infants, removal of nasal mucus with a nasal aspirator may be helpful.
- Zinc gluconate lozenges may reduce rhinitis symptoms and shorten colds, but are associated with unpleasant adverse effects.[1,2]

Pharmacologic Choices

Many patients are able to cope with 4 to 5 days of nasal symptoms without any medication. There is little evidence that preschool children benefit from over-the-counter (OTC) medications other than those used for fever control. Although school-aged and older patients do benefit from OTC medications, the potential for adverse effects must be considered when weighing the benefit/risk ratio.

[1] *Alternative Therapies in Health and Medicine 1996;2(6):63–72.*
[2] *Ann Intern Med 1996;125:81–88.*

Figure 1: **Management of Viral Rhinitis**

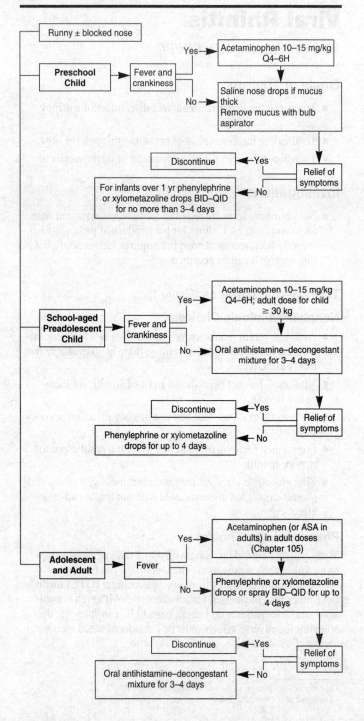

Newer approaches include ipratropium, an anticholinergic nasal spray. Additional comparative clinical trials are needed to determine its place in therapy. Nasal sprays containing antiviral agents, such as pirodavir, are under investigation.

Antibiotics have been recommended for the 20% of adult cold patients who secrete bacterial pathogens from their nose. The number needed to treat, and the benefits in relation to antibiotic side effects and costs need further study before this approach is widely implemented.

Preschool Children

Acetaminophen has been shown to make febrile children with viral infections look and feel better. Oral antihistamines or antihistamine–decongestant combinations are not beneficial. For most, the runny and/or blocked nose can be helped by removing secretions with a nasal aspirator and the use of saline nose drops. This is particularly important in infants before breast- or bottle-feeding, since nasal obstruction will make feeding very difficult. Pharmacologic nose drops or sprays used as decongestants are not recommended for children less than 1 year of age. If used in older children, they should be used for no more than 4 days because of rebound nasal obstruction.

School-aged Children

In the school-aged preadolescent child, oral antihistamine–decongestant combinations are effective. Although one should be mindful of potential side effects (drowsiness, irritability, palpitations, hyperactivity), these agents should be tried before nasal decongestants. If there is no response to the oral medication, or adverse effects occur and symptoms are significant and persistent, a short (4-day) course of nasal decongestants (e.g., phenylephrine 0.125 to 0.25% or xylometazoline 0.05%) can be given.

In preadolescent children, chlorpheniramine has not been shown to cause sedation. However, some children may experience drowsiness or excitation with antihistamines or decongestants.

Adolescents and Adults

Older antihistamines, decongestants (nasal or oral) and antihistamine–decongestant combinations relieve nasal symptoms (congestion, postnasal drip and rhinorrhea). A 4-day course of nasal decongestants should be the initial approach, reserving oral medication for those who do not respond. Side effects due to nasal decongestants include elevated pulse rate, blood pressure, palpitations, fatigue and/or dizziness. Although chlorpheniramine is effective in reducing rhinorrhea in this age group, it causes drowsiness.

Therapeutic Tips

- In **preschool children**
  - OTC preparations are not recommended.
  - nasal aspiration is preferred, if required.

- In **school-aged preadolescent children**
  - oral decongestant–antihistamine combinations are effective in short courses.

- In **adolescents and adults**
  - short courses of nasal medications are preferred initial therapy.

Suggested Reading List

Kaiser L, Lew D, Hirschel B, et al. Effects of antibiotic treatment in the subset of common-cold patients who have bacteria in nasopharyngeal secretions. *Lancet* 1996;347:1507–1510.

Smith MBH, Feldman W. Over-the-counter cold medications: a critical review of clinical trials between 1950 and 1991. *JAMA* 1993;269:2258–2263.

CHAPTER 36

Adult Asthma

David G. McCormack, MD, FRCPC, FCCP

Goals of Therapy

- Maintain normal activity levels
- Prevent symptoms (cough, wheezing, dyspnea)
- Maintain normal (or near normal) spirometry
- Prevent exacerbations
- Avoid side effects of therapy

Investigations

- Thorough history with particular attention to:
  - pattern of symptoms (seasonal, perennial, etc.)
  - precipitating factors (environmental allergens, occupational exposures, irritants such as smoke, drugs such as ASA, beta-blockers, exercise)
  - previous hospitalizations and intensive care admissions
- Physical examination: wheezing, nasal polyps
- Objective measurements needed to confirm diagnosis and assess severity include:
  - spirometry: reduced expiratory flow rates
  - home peak flow monitoring for patients with severe asthma or poor perception of airway obstruction
  - bronchoprovocation challenge test, using methacholine or histamine, if diagnosis in doubt

Therapeutic Choices

Nonpharmacologic Choices

- Known precipitating factors such as environmental allergens and occupational irritants should be avoided.
- Smoking cessation is essential (Chapter 40).
- ASA and other nonsteroidal anti-inflammatory drugs (NSAIDs) should be avoided.
- Hyposensitization therapy to allergens generally is not useful.
- Patient education about asthma symptoms and therapy is essential for optimal management.

Figure 1: **Treatment of Asthma**

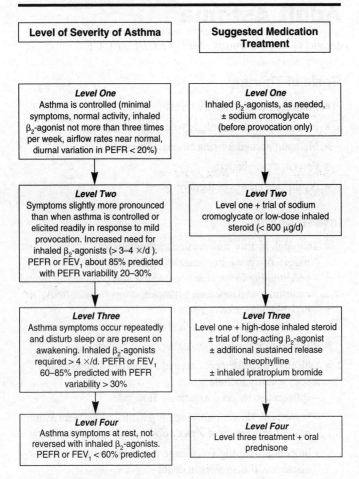

Level of Severity of Asthma	Suggested Medication Treatment
Level One Asthma is controlled (minimal symptoms, normal activity, inhaled β_2-agonist not more than three times per week, airflow rates near normal, diurnal variation in PEFR < 20%)	**Level One** Inhaled β_2-agonists, as needed, ± sodium cromoglycate (before provocation only)
Level Two Symptoms slightly more pronounced than when asthma is controlled or elicited readily in response to mild provocation. Increased need for inhaled β_2-agonists (> 3–4 ×/d). PEFR or FEV_1 about 85% predicted with PEFR variability 20–30%	**Level Two** Level one + trial of sodium cromoglycate or low-dose inhaled steroid (< 800 μg/d)
Level Three Asthma symptoms occur repeatedly and disturb sleep or are present on awakening. Inhaled β_2-agonists required > 4 ×/d. PEFR or FEV_1 60–85% predicted with PEFR variability > 30%	**Level Three** Level one + high-dose inhaled steroid ± trial of long-acting β_2-agonist ± additional sustained release theophylline ± inhaled ipratropium bromide
Level Four Asthma symptoms at rest, not reversed with inhaled β_2-agonists. PEFR or FEV_1 < 60% predicted	**Level Four** Level three treatment + oral prednisone

Note: These are not discrete levels of severity and treatment and are best thought of as a continuum to reflect a dynamic therapeutic approach.

Pharmacologic Choices

The initial level of treatment with medication is chosen after an assessment of asthma severity and previous treatment (Figure 1). Treatment should be reviewed every 3 to 6 months, and if control is achieved a stepwise reduction in treatment should be tried.

Inhaled therapy that maximizes delivery of drugs to the respiratory tract and minimizes systemic side effects is the cornerstone of asthma management. The metered dose inhalers (MDI) or dry powder inhalers deliver drugs as effectively as nebulized therapy. Medications include bronchodilators and anti-inflammatory agents (Table 1).

Bronchodilators

▫ Short-acting Inhaled Beta₂-agonists

Salbutamol, terbutaline, fenoterol, pirbuterol, orciprenaline, isoproterenol and **epinephrine** (the last two are not selective beta₂-agonists) are available in Canada. Selective beta₂-agonists are agents of first choice for treatment of acute exacerbations and for prevention of exercise-induced asthma. They are used best as required rather than on a fixed schedule. Although potent broncho-dilators, they have little effect on the late phase of an exacerbation. If patients use a short-acting beta₂-agonist more than three times per week, initiate therapy with an anti-inflammatory agent.

▫ Long-acting Inhaled Beta₂-agonists

Salmeterol and **formoterol** are long-acting, slow onset beta₂-agonists intended for regular twice daily treatment of asthma and not for immediate symptomatic relief. They should only be used in patients already taking inhaled steroids and may be particularly useful for the prevention of nocturnal symptoms.

▫ Oral Beta₂-agonists

Oral orciprenaline, fenoterol, salbutamol and **terbutaline** offer less bronchodilation, more systemic side effects and a slower onset of action than the inhaled preparations and are therefore not recommended.

▫ Anticholinergic Agents

Ipratropium bromide is a useful alternative for patients who are unusually susceptible to tremor or tachycardia from beta₂-agonists. Although the onset of action is delayed compared to beta₂-agonists, the bronchodilator effect lasts longer.

▫ Theophylline Products

Oral **theophylline, oxtriphylline** and **aminophylline** are third-line therapy, chiefly due to systemic toxicity and mild bronchodilator activity. They should be administered carefully, according to standard regimens with blood levels monitored. In naive patients titrate the dose slowly to minimize side effects. Cimetidine, erythromycin, quinolones and verapamil may increase theophylline levels. Rifampin, cabamazepine and phenytoin may decrease levels.

Anti-inflammatory Agents

▫ Inhaled Corticosteroids

Inhaled **budesonide, beclomethasone dipropionate, fluticasone propionate, flunisolide** and **triamcinolone acetonide** are safe, effective, and cost-effective drugs that block the late phase of asthma. They should be used regularly at the lowest effective dose rather than as needed. They have a higher ratio of topical

Table 1: Drugs Used in the Treatment of Chronic Asthma in Adults

Drugs	Dosage	Adverse Effects	Cost*
Inhaled β₂-agonists, Short-acting		For all:	
salbutamol Ventodisk, Ventolin, generics	100 µg/puff: 1–2 puffs Q4–6H PRN	Nervousness, tremor, tachycardia, palpitations.	Salbutamol: MDI $ Diskhaler/Rotacaps $$
terbutaline Bricanyl	0.5 mg/puff: 1 puff Q4–6H PRN		Terbutaline $
fenoterol Berotec, Berotec Forte	100 µg/puff: 1–2 puffs Q6–8H PRN		Fenoterol $
pirbuterol Maxair	250 µg/puff: 1–2 puffs Q6H PRN		Pirbuterol $
orciprenaline Alupent	0.75 mg/puff: 1–2 puffs Q4H PRN		Orciprenaline $
Inhaled β₂-agonists, Long-acting		See above.	
salmeterol Serevent	25 µg/puff: 2 puffs BID		Salmeterol $$$$
formoterol Foradil	12 µg/puff: 1 puff BID		Formoterol $$$
Anticholinergic Agents			
ipratropium bromide Atrovent	20 µg/puff: 2–4 puffs Q6–8H	Dry mouth, metallic taste; mydriasis and glaucoma (if released into eye).	$$

Theophylline Preparations

theophylline Quibron-T/SR, Slo-Bid, Theo-Dur, Theolair, Uniphyl, generics	For all: serum levels should be monitored 200–300 mg PO Q12H	For all: Nausea, vomiting, abdominal cramps, headache, palpitations.	\$–\$\$
oxtriphylline Choledyl, generics	800–1 200 mg/d PO		\$\$
aminophylline Phyllocontin, generics	225–350 mg PO Q12H		\$–\$\$

Inhaled Corticosteroids

beclomethasone dipropionate Beclovent, Becloforte, Vanceril, generics	200–2 000 μg/d divided BID–QID	For all: Sore mouth, sore throat, dysphonia, oral thrush (can be reduced by rinsing mouth or using spacer).	Beclomethasone: MDI \$ Diskhaler/Rotacaps \$\$ Becloforte \$\$\$\$
budesonide Pulmicort	400–2 400 μg/d divided BID–QID		Budesonide \$\$\$–\$\$\$\$
flunisolide Bronalide	1 000–2 000 μg/d divided BID–QID		Flunisolide \$\$
fluticasone propionate Flovent	100–1 000 μg/d divided BID–QID		Fluticasone \$\$\$–\$\$\$\$
triamcinolone acetonide Azmacort	1 200–3 200 μg/d divided BID–QID		Triamcinolone \$\$
sodium cromoglycate Intal	1 mg/puff: 2 puffs QID	Rare.	\$\$ (112 puffs) \$\$\$ (200 puffs)
nedocromil sodium Tilade	2 mg/puff: 4 mg QID	Rare. Unpleasant taste.	\$\$

Leukotriene Antagonists

zafirlukast Accolate	20 mg PO BID 1 h before or 2 h after meals	Headache, pharyngitis, rhinitis.	\$\$\$

Legend: \$ < \$15   \$\$ \$15–30   \$\$\$ \$30–45   \$\$\$\$ > \$45

* Includes drug cost only. Cost of inhaled agents is per unit; cost of oral medications is per 30-day supply.

to systemic activity than do oral steroids. The incidence of pharyngeal candidiasis from deposition of the inhaled steroid in the pharynx can be reduced by mouth rinsing after use and/or using a spacer device.

❑ Sodium Cromoglycate

This inhaled preparation prevents both the early and late phase of asthma exacerbation. It must be administered regularly to provide significant protection and should not be used to treat exacerbations. It produces few side effects.

❑ Nedocromil Sodium

This medication has comparable indications to sodium cromoglycate.

❑ Systemic Corticosteroids

These are useful in both preventing and treating acute exacerbations. The optimal dosage has not been established. The side effects are significant: glucose intolerance, weight gain, mood alterations and hypertension in the short term and osteoporosis, hypertension, cataracts and myopathy in the long term. These can be reduced by treating patients for short periods (1 to 2 weeks) following an acute exacerbation. Side effects with long-term use may be minimized by using alternate-day dosing regimens.

❑ Leukotriene Antagonists

Zafirlukast is now available and **montelukast** will likely be available in the near future. These agents have anti-inflammatory properties although their exact role in the management of asthma has yet to be established.

Other Therapies

Antihistamines are not useful. The place of **ketotifen** in the treatment of adults has not been established. **Methotrexate** and **gold** have been used in some chronic steroid-dependent asthmatics but should be limited to centers experienced with this therapy.

Asthma in Pregnancy

The best outcome for pregnancy complicated by asthma occurs with optimal management of asthma. In usual therapeutic doses, the drugs used to treat asthma are nonteratogenic.

Emergency Treatment

- Priorities include oxygenation, rehydration, bronchodilation and use of anti-inflammatory medications (Figure 2).

- Bronchodilation with metered dose inhalers is equivalent to nebulized therapy.
- Synergistic effects between ipratropium bromide and the beta$_2$-agonists suggest administering these two medications concomitantly.
- Oral or parenteral steroids should be used early in most patients.

Figure 2: **Emergency Treatment of Asthma**

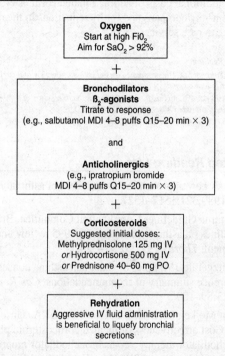

Abbreviations: FiO_2 = fraction of inspired oxygen; SaO_2 = arterial oxygen percent saturation.

Pharmacoeconomic Considerations

Jeffrey A Johnson, PhD

There is considerable evidence that the prevalence and severity of asthma has increased in the past two decades, leading to increased concern about the growing asthma-related morbidity and mortality, and the associated economic burden. Cost-of-illness analyses for asthma have been carried out for several industrialized nations, principally Australia, United Kingdom, New Zealand, and the US. The costs associated with the management of asthma in the US in 1990 were estimated to be $6.2 billion. Direct medical expenditures accounted for $3.6 billion, or approximately 59% of the total estimate. Canadian estimates for the total direct and indirect costs of asthma were between $504 and $648 million in 1990. Hospital and physician services were found to make up approximately one-third of the total costs.

Published cost-effectiveness evaluations of asthma therapy are limited. The few studies that have been conducted indicate that the additional costs of adding inhaled corticosteroids are almost entirely compensated for by reductions in the costs of other health care services.

Suggested Reading

Weiss KB, Sullivan SD. *The economic costs of asthma: a review and conceptual model. PharmacoEconomics 1993;4:14–30.*

Krahn MD, Berka C, Langlois P, et al. *Direct and indirect costs of asthma in Canada, 1990. Can Med Assoc J 1996;154:821–831.*

Suggested Reading List

Barnes PJ. A new approach to the treatment of asthma. *N Engl J Med* 1989;321:1517–1527.

British Asthma Guidelines Coordination Committee. British guidelines on asthma management: 1995 review and position statement. *Thorax* 1997;52:51–524.

Ernst P, Fitzgerald JM, Spier S. Canadian asthma consensus conference summary of recommendations. *Can Respir J* 1996;3:89–100.

Rutten-van Mölken MPMH, Van Doorslaer EKA, Jansen MCC, et al. Cost effectiveness of inhaled corticosteroid plus bronchodilator therapy versus bronchodilator monotherapy in children with asthma. *PharmacoEconomics* 1993;4:257–270.

CHAPTER 37

Asthma in Infants and Children

Mark Montgomery MD, FRCPC

Asthma is defined as airways hyperreactivity (twitchy airways, reactive airways) in the absence of other lung disease. Night cough persisting after a cold, wheeze or shortness of breath limiting activities, all indicate airways hyperreactivity. If there is no evidence of other lung disease such as cystic fibrosis, bronchiolitis or pertussis, the child should be assumed to have asthma and management initiated. If there is little improvement with beta$_2$-agonists or systemic steroids, then the diagnosis of asthma is in doubt, and other respiratory disorders should be considered.

Goals of Therapy

- No cough, wheeze or shortness of breath which interferes with daytime activities, exercise, school attendance or sleep
- No need for regular use of beta$_2$-agonists for symptom relief
- No emergency room visits or hospitalizations
- Normal measures of expiratory airflow, such as peak flows or pulmonary function studies (FEV$_1$)
- No medication side effects

Therapeutic Choices

Nonpharmacologic Choices

Environmental Control

- Avoid exposure to **cigarette smoke.**
- Explore specific allergies to inhalants by history and skin testing.
- For those with **house dust mite allergy**:
  – use vinyl mattress and pillow covers
  – avoid down and feather bedding
  – minimize the number of fluffy toys and upholstered furniture in the bedroom
  – remove bedroom carpeting
  – avoid humidifiers, which raise the relative humidity above 40% and promote growth of house dust mite.
- For those with **allergy to pets**: avoid exposure.

Figure 1: **Maintenance Therapy of Asthma in Children**

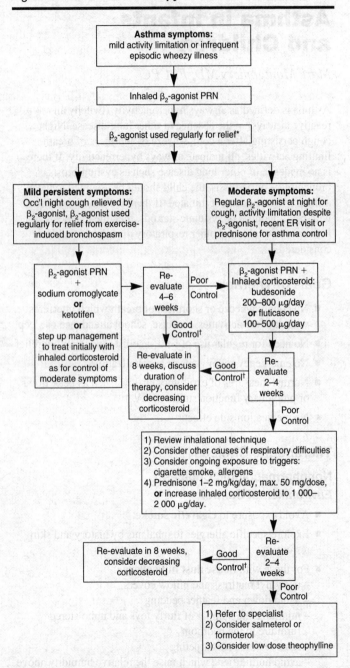

* Regular use β₂-agonist: use ≥ 3 times/week for relief.
† Good asthma control: see Goals of Therapy.

Pharmacologic Choices (Figure 1, Table 1)

Routes of Administration

Inhalation is the preferred route of administration: therapeutic effect is maximized and systemic side effects minimized. Review and advice regarding inhalation technique is required for all individuals on a regular basis. **For infants and young children (age less than 5 years)**, a metered-dose inhaler (MDI) via spacer device with mask attachment is useful. Drug deposition in infants and young children is generally 10 to 20% of the deposition in adults. Therefore, adult doses may be required in children. Wet nebulization is a less attractive alternative due to difficulties with portability and time required for therapy. Furthermore, deposition of drug rapidly decreases as the distance from the mask to the mouth increases. **In older children (age 5 years and over)**, either a dry powder system (Diskhaler, Turbuhaler) or a metered-dose inhaler with spacer device may be used. Incentive spirometers provide visual feedback to children about their inspiratory flows, and can be invaluable teaching devices. Compliance is enhanced when children select the device that works best for them.

Bronchodilator Agents

Inhaled Beta$_2$-agonists

Short-acting beta$_2$-agonists (**salbutamol**, **terbutaline**, **fenoterol**) are effective agents to relieve smooth muscle spasm, but do not reduce airways reactivity or inflammation. Use on an as needed basis provides both rapid relief and valuable information on underlying asthma control. Regular use of beta$_2$-agonists for relief (even once or twice a day) indicates suboptimal control. If the child notes inadequate relief from the beta$_2$-agonist, or relief for less than 2 hours, this suggests ongoing airways inflammation and swelling which requires further assessment, and possibly a course of systemic corticosteroids.

Administration of a short-acting beta$_2$-agonist 5 to 10 minutes before exercise will prevent exercise induced bronchospasm for up to 2 hours.

Long-acting beta$_2$-agonists (**salmeterol**, **formoterol**) provide up to 12 hours protection from exercise-induced bronchospasm. They are useful for control of night cough until an increased dose of inhaled corticosteroids regains asthma control. These agents should not be used as monotherapy in asthma. Moreover, use should be limited to short periods of time (1 to 2 weeks) and then attempts made to discontinue regular use. Long-acting beta$_2$-agonists are presently approved for use only in individuals over 12 years of age.

Anticholinergic Agents

There is little use for **ipratropium bromide** in asthma maintenance therapy in children.

Methylxanthines

Theophylline preparations may have a role in patients receiving optimal anti-inflammatory therapy and requiring more bronchodilation than provided by beta$_2$-agonists. Recent studies suggest a possible anti-inflammatory role for theophylline.

Anti-inflammatory Therapy

Inhaled Corticosteroids

In chronic asthma, inhaled corticosteroids are first-line agents for anti-inflammatory therapy. Regular use improves pulmonary function and controls symptoms. Although long-term studies have demonstrated safety and efficacy, inhaled corticosteroids do not "cure" asthma. Cessation of regular use results in return to the previous status within weeks to months. Regular use reduces the need for oral steroids to treat exacerbations.

Budesonide and **fluticasone** possess better safety and greater potency than **beclomethasone**, **flunisolide** and **triamcinolone**.[1] Both budesonide and fluticasone are only absorbed from the lung and then rapidly cleared from the circulation to an inactive metabolite. Fluticasone has greater potency and risk of systemic side effects (on the hypothalamic-pituitary-adrenocortical [HPA]-axis) than budesonide.[2] Equivalent doses in terms of asthma control and effects on the HPA-axis are fluticasone 500 µg per day and budesonide 800 µg per day. Spacer devices are essential for inhaled corticosteroids. The effect on asthma control begins to plateau above 800–1 000 µg per day. At doses below 800 µg per day the risk of systemic adverse effects such as adrenal suppression, growth suppression and altered bone mineralization is low. The risk of systemic effects of inhaled corticosteroids depends on inherent individual sensitivity, history of systemic corticosteroid use, compliance with therapy, and adequacy of the inhalation technique.

Sodium Cromoglycate

Sodium cromoglycate is a safe anti-inflammatory agent. Mild to moderate asthma is controlled in 60 to 70% of children. It has also proven useful as an adjunct with beta$_2$-agonists to prevent exercise-induced bronchospasm. Regular use 3 to 4 times per day for 4 weeks is required to determine effect.

---

[1] *Allergy 1997;52 (Suppl 39):1–34.*
[2] *Thorax 1997;52:55–58.*

Nedocromil Sodium

Nedocromil sodium is comparable to sodium cromoglycate in anti-inflammatory activity. It prevents antigen-challenge and exercise-induced bronchospasm. Difficulties with taste often limit compliance; a spacer may improve acceptance.

Ketotifen

Ketotifen is an oral prophylactic agent with antihistaminic properties. Side effects include sedation and increased appetite. Its clinical effectiveness is most noted in infants with mild persistent asthma.

Leukotriene Receptor Antagonists

Early trials with leukotriene receptor antagonists (**zafirlukast**, **montelukast**) suggest that these oral agents provide broncho-protection in ASA sensitive asthmatics, and with exercise. Further, these agents may have steroid sparing properties, allowing improved control of asthma at a reduced dose of inhaled corticosteroid. The leukotriene receptor antagonists have not been associated with any significant side effects.

Acute Asthma Management (Figure 2)

An exacerbation of asthma requiring emergency room visit, unscheduled doctor visit or hospitalization is a failure of long-term management. As well as immediate care for respiratory distress, evaluation of the cause of the exacerbation and means of preventing future episodes is essential.

Acute severe asthma should be managed as a pediatric emergency. Initial therapy should be aggressive, and then reduced as the exacerbation settles. Ideally, a child with asthma should not deteriorate once in hospital.

Pulse oximetry or an arterial blood gas should be performed and supplemental oxygen initiated in all asthmatic children with respiratory distress.

The cornerstones of therapy are supplemental oxygen, frequent high dose inhaled beta$_2$-agonist, and systemic corticosteroids. Ipratropium bromide may provide additional bronchodilation. There is no evidence that aminophylline provides additional bronchodilation beyond that produced by frequent high dose beta$_2$-agonist.

Close observation and reassessment of all children with acute severe asthma is mandatory.

Therapeutic Tips

- Where possible, agents or situations which worsen asthma should be avoided.

Table 1: Drugs Used for Maintenance Therapy for Asthma in Children

Drug	Dosage Chronic Therapy	Adverse Effects	Other	Cost*
Bronchodilator Drugs				
Short-acting β₂-agonists		For all agents: Tachycardia, palpitations, nervousness, tremor, hypokalemia.	Prevents exercise-induced bronchospasm for up to 2–4 h. Agents provide relief and provide information on asthma control: regular use indicates poor control, use of ≥ 1 canister per month associated with increased risk of asthma mortality.	$-$$
salbutamol Ventodisk, Ventolin, generics	2 puffs (100 μg/puff) Q4–6H PRN			
terbutaline Bricanyl	1 puff (0.5 mg/puff) Q4–6H PRN			
fenoterol Berotec	1–2 puffs (100 μg/puff) Q4–6H PRN			
Long-acting β₂-agonists		As with β₂-agonists; possibility of tachyphylaxis with regular use.	Not to be used as monotherapy, not for immediate relief, provides protection from exercise-induced bronchospasm for 10 h.	$$$$
salmeterol Serevent	1–2 puffs (25 μg/puff) OD–BID			
formoterol Foradil	1 cap (12 μg) inhaled OD–BID			$$$
Anticholinergic Agents				
ipratropium bromide Atrovent	1–2 puffs (20 μg/puff) TID–QID	Dry mouth, metallic taste, mydriasis and glaucoma (if released into eye).	Also available as nebulizer solution. Not used in maintenance therapy.	$$

Prophylactic Drugs

Inhaled Corticosteroids

Drug	Dose	Adverse effects	Comments	Cost
beclomethasone dipropionate Beclovent, Becloforte, Vanceril, generics	Dose to obtain asthma control 400–1 000 µg/d, divided BID–TID, maintenance dose 200–800 µg/day OD–BID. Regular re-evaluation required to ensure that lowest effective dose of inhaled corticosteroid being used to maintain control.	Oral thrush, dysphonia. Follow linear growth Q3–6 mos with regular asthma reassessments.	Dysphonia and candidiasis can be decreased by use of spacer with MDI and rinsing after use.

Dose response studies show majority of corticosteroid effect on asthma control is achieved with doses under 800 µg/day; children requiring 800 µg/d or more on a regular basis should be assessed by a specialist. | Beclomethasone: MDI $ all others $$$–$$$$ |
budesonide Pulmicort				
fluticasone Flovent				
flunisolide Bronalide				
triamcinolone acetonide Azmacort				
sodium cromoglycate Intal	2 puffs (1 mg/puff) or 1 spincap (20 mg/cap) TID–QID × 4–6 wks, then BID–TID.	Rare.	Used on a regular basis TID–QID Useful for exercise-induced bronchospasm.	$$–$$$
nedocromil sodium Tilade	2 puffs (2 mg/puff) TID–QID	Rare; unpleasant taste.	Useful for exercise-induced bronchospasm.	$$
ketotifen Zaditen, generics	Under 3 yrs: 0.5 mg PO BID Older children: 1 mg PO BID	Sedation, weight gain.	May require 8–12 wks for effect. Clinical effectiveness most noted in infants with mild asthma.	$$–$$$

Leukotriene Antagonists

Drug	Dose	Adverse effects	Comments	Cost
zafirlukast Accolate	20 mg PO BID 1 h before or 2 h after meals.	Headache, pharyngitis, rhinitis.	Indicated for individuals 12 yrs and older.	$$$

* Includes drug cost only. Cost of inhaled agents is per unit; cost of inhalation capsules or oral medications is per 30-day supply.

Legend: $ < $15 $$ $15–30 $$$ $30–45 $$$$ > $45

Figure 2: **Treatment of Acute Asthma in Children**

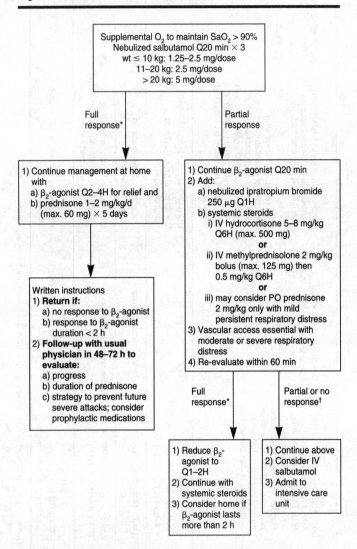

Supplemental O$_2$ to maintain SaO$_2$ > 90%
Nebulized salbutamol Q20 min × 3
wt ≤ 10 kg: 1.25–2.5 mg/dose
11–20 kg: 2.5 mg/dose
> 20 kg: 5 mg/dose

Full response*

Partial response

1) Continue management at home with
   a) β$_2$-agonist Q2–4H for relief and
   b) prednisone 1–2 mg/kg/d (max. 60 mg) × 5 days

Written instructions
1) **Return if:**
   a) no response to β$_2$-agonist
   b) response to β$_2$-agonist duration < 2 h
2) **Follow-up with usual physician in 48–72 h to evaluate:**
   a) progress
   b) duration of prednisone
   c) strategy to prevent future severe attacks; consider prophylactic medications

1) Continue β$_2$-agonist Q20 min
2) Add:
   a) nebulized ipratropium bromide 250 µg Q1H
   b) systemic steroids
      i) IV hydrocortisone 5–8 mg/kg Q6H (max. 500 mg)
      or
      ii) IV methylprednisolone 2 mg/kg bolus (max. 125 mg) then 0.5 mg/kg Q6H
      or
      iii) may consider PO prednisone 2 mg/kg only with mild persistent respiratory distress
3) Vascular access essential with moderate or severe respiratory distress
4) Re-evaluate within 60 min

Full response*

Partial or no response†

1) Reduce β$_2$-agonist to Q1–2H
2) Continue with systemic steroids
3) Consider home if β$_2$-agonist lasts more than 2 h

1) Continue above
2) Consider IV salbutamol
3) Admit to intensive care unit

* *Full response: no indrawing, no wheeze on auscultation, PEFR (if done) > 70% predicted or best, SaO$_2$ > 90% in room air.*
† *May consider IV aminophylline if theophylline used at home. Monitor serum levels to avoid toxicity.*

- When triggers cannot be avoided, use medications at an early stage to improve long-term asthma control.
- Use agents for long-term control (i.e., inhaled corticosteroids) for several weeks after symptoms have resolved to ensure that airways hyperreactivity is controlled.

- Review inhaler techniques regularly and often to ensure optimal use of devices.
- Provide written instructions that relate signs of worsening asthma:
  - cough, wheeze or shortness of breath which interferes with sleep.
  - cough, wheeze or shortness of breath which interferes with activities.
  - regular use of beta$_2$-agonist for relief.
  - drop in peak flow rates.
- Written instructions should also provide the action that the family should initiate when signs of worsening asthma are detected.

Suggested Reading

Ernst P, Fitzgerald M, Spier S. Canadian Asthma Consensus Conference: Summary of Recommendations. *Can Respir J* 1996;3:89–100.

Jackson C, Lipworth B. Optimizing inhaled drug delivery in patients with asthma. *Br J Gen Pract* 1995;45:683–687.

Krahn M, Berka C, Langlois P, Detsky A. Direct and indirect costs of asthma in Canada, 1990. *Can Med Assoc J* 1996;154(6):821–829.

Pederson S. Safety aspects of corticosteroids in children. *Eur Respir Rev* 1994;17:33–43.

Tal A, Golan H, Grauer N, Aviram M, Albin D, Quastel MR. Deposition pattern of radiolabeled salbutamol with mask in young children with airway obstruction. *J Pediatr* 1996;128(4):479–484.

CHAPTER 38

Chronic Obstructive Pulmonary Disease

Tony R. Bai, MD, FRACP, FRCPC

Goals of Therapy

- To decrease or abolish dyspnea
- To decrease sputum production
- To maintain exercise capacity
- To prevent disease progression
- To decrease the frequency of exacerbations
- To maintain arterial blood oxygen saturation above 90%

Investigations

- A thorough history with special attention to:
  - avoidable environmental factors (e.g., cigarette smoking or occupational exposures)
  - the rate of progression of symptoms
  - the degree of disability
- Physical examination: signs of hyperinflation, airflow obstruction, chronic hypoxemia, pulmonary hypertension
- Laboratory tests:
  - CBC
  - chest radiograph
  - spirometry before and after bronchodilator
  - arterial blood gases if $FEV_1 < 30\%$ predicted
  - α_1 antiprotease level if clinical suspicion of genetic predisposition to emphysema

Therapeutic Choices (Figure 1)

Nonpharmacologic Choices

- **Education of patients and their families** through individual and group sessions is essential. Physicians must be aware of patients' expectations and work with them to set realistic goals.
- **Smoking** should be discontinued (Chapter 40).
- **Annual vaccination** against influenza should be given.

Figure 1: **Pharmacologic Management of COPD**

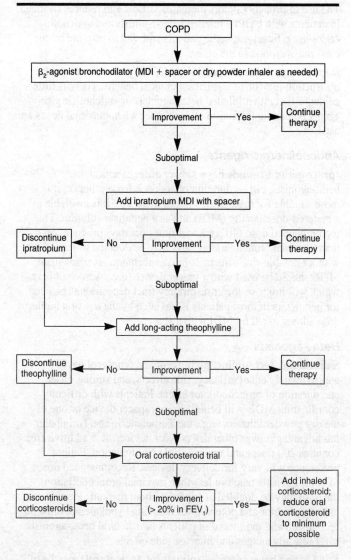

Abbreviations: MDI = metered-dose inhaler; FEV$_1$ = forced expiratory volume in one second.

- **Rehabilitation programs** providing respiratory, physical and occupational therapy, exercise conditioning, nutritional assistance, and psychosocial and vocational rehabilitation benefit patients regardless of the extent of their disease by reducing symptoms and improving exercise performance and quality of life.

Pharmacologic Choices (Table 1)

The use of bronchodilators increases airflow and reduces dyspnea in patients with COPD. Inhaled beta$_2$-agonists and anticholinergics are efficacious; some patients who fail to respond to one class may respond to the other.

A small improvement in airflow in COPD patients with severe obstruction may be of significant clinical benefit. There is little evidence that either inhaled beta$_2$-agonists or anticholinergic agents potentiate the action of each other when maximal doses are used.

Anticholinergic Agents

Ipratropium bromide has a slower onset of action than beta$_2$-agonists, but its duration of action is longer; hence, it is more suitable for regular than intermittent use. It is available as a metered-dose inhaler (MDI) and as a nebulizer solution. The recommended dose (40 µg 3 to 4 times per day) produces less than maximal bronchodilation and may be doubled or tripled without notable side effects. If inhaler technique is inadequate, MDIs should be used with a spacer device (e.g., Aerochamber), which will improve lower respiratory tract deposition. The need for nebulizers in most patients is obviated by the use of a higher dose administered by MDI with a spacer.

Beta$_2$-agonists

Salbutamol, terbutaline, pirbuterol and **fenoterol** have approximately equal efficacy, side effects, and similar onset and duration of bronchodilator effect. Patients with difficulty coordinating MDIs will benefit from a spacer device or one of the dry powder inhalers (e.g., the Turbuhaler). The Turbuhaler has advantages over other dry powder devices: it is additive-free, contains 200 doses and requires little manipulation. Patient preference will vary for delivery devices. Recommended doses of beta$_2$-agonists result in less than maximal bronchodilation; the dose may be doubled or tripled without marked side effects, although tremor and potential for inducing hypokalemia must be recognized and monitored in patients at risk. Oral beta$_2$-agonists offer few advantages and increase side effects.

Long-acting beta$_2$-agonists (**salmeterol, formoterol**) may be of use in COPD, but cost-benefit studies have not been completed.

Theophylline

The role of theophylline in the treatment of COPD is controversial; it may have little bronchodilator effect beyond that of inhaled agents. The use of long-acting theophylline preparations in the evening has been shown to reduce overnight declines in FEV$_1$ and morning respiratory symptoms. Theophylline may offer added nonbronchodilatory effects such as improved respiratory muscle endurance and ventilatory stimulation. Half of patients with severe COPD can show clinically significant improvements in functional capacity (walking distance, dyspnea) following use of slow-release theophylline despite use of inhaled beta$_2$-agonists and anticholinergics. Theophylline is a third-line drug in the treatment of COPD; if it is used, blood levels in the low therapeutic range (55 to 85 µmol/L) should be the goal to minimize adverse effects. Long-acting preparations (12- or 24-hour) provide stable serum levels and reduce side effects. Although combining theophylline with an inhaled anticholinergic or adrenergic agent may be more effective than monotherapy, this will vary among patients. The value of adding theophylline is best judged with a 2- to 4-week trial. The outcome should be measured by improvement in expiratory flow rates, 6- or 12-minute walking distance or objectively observed reduction in dyspnea, medication use or nocturnal symptoms.

Corticosteroids

In acute exacerbations of COPD, a 2-week course of corticosteroids is beneficial in hastening recovery and returning lung function to baseline. However, only 10 to 20% of **stable** COPD patients benefit from either systemic or inhaled corticosteroid therapy. In the assessment of a new patient, if airflow obstruction and symptoms persist following smoking cessation and optimal bronchodilator therapy, the patient's corticosteroid response should be assessed by administering **prednisone** (0.6 mg/kg per day) as a single morning dose for 14 days. Objective end points (e.g., spirometry or 6- or 12-minute walking distance) should be evaluated. An improvement in FEV$_1$ of at least 20% and 0.2 L is evidence of significant corticosteroid responsiveness. In these patients, high-dose inhaled corticosteroids (e.g., 1 500 µg per day of **beclomethasone** or **budesonide** in 2 or 3 divided doses) should be initiated, and the prednisone dose should be tapered to the minimum needed to maintain major benefits. A few severely disabled patients may require maintenance with prednisone 10 mg daily in addition to inhaled steroids. Treatment should be reviewed every 3 to 6 months. If control is achieved, a stepwise reduction in treatment may be possible. For example, inhaled corticosteroid dosage may be reduced to 400 to 800 µg per day.

Antibiotics

The most common infectious agents in exacerbations of COPD are viral. When exacerbations of COPD are accompanied by purulent secretions, broad-spectrum antibiotics directed against typical colonizing bacteria are beneficial. Inexpensive and equally efficacious therapy includes **amoxicillin, co-trimoxazole, erythromycin** or **tetracycline**. The more expensive **quinolones** or newer macrolides may be useful when a resistant gram-negative

Table 1: Medications Used in COPD

Drug	Dosage	Adverse Effects	Comments	Cost*
Inhaled Agents				Cost per unit
β₂-agonists *salbutamol* Ventolin, generics	1–2 puffs Q2–6H PRN not to exceed 8–12 puffs per 24 h	Tremor, nervousness, hypokalemia.	Usual doses are suboptimal for COPD.	Salbutamol: MDI $ Diskhaler/ Rotacaps $$
fenoterol Berotec	Same as above			Fenoterol $
pirbuterol Maxair	Same as above			Pirbuterol $
terbutaline Bricanyl	Same as above			Terbutaline $
Anticholinergics *ipratropium bromide* Atrovent	2–4 puffs TID–QID up to 6–8 puffs TID–QID, if tolerated	Dry mouth, metallic taste.	Usual doses are suboptimal for COPD.	$$
β₂-agonist/Anticholinergic Combinations *salbutamol/ipratropium bromide* Combivent	2 puffs QID	Same as β₂-agonists and anticholinergics above.	May be used as initial therapy in patients with daily symptoms. Fixed dosage leads to some inflexibility.	$$

Corticosteroids

beclomethasone Becloforte, Beclovent, Vanceril, Beclodisk, generics	400–1 500 µg/d in 2–3 divided doses	Oropharyngeal candidiasis, hoarseness (both can be ↓ by using a spacer and rinsing mouth or by using dry powder inhaler).	Poorly absorbed; must be used regularly, not PRN.	Beclomethasone: MDI $ Diskhaler/ Rotacaps $$ (forte) $$$
budesonide Pulmicort	Same as above			Budesonide $$$–$$$$
flunisolide Bronalide	Same as above			Flunisolide $$
fluticasone Flovent	200–1 000 µg/day in 2 divided doses			Fluticasone $$$
triamcinolone Azmacort	Same as beclomethasone			Triamcinolone $$

Oral Agents

			Cost for 30-day supply

Slow-release Theophyllines

Quibron-T/SR, Slo-Bid, Theo-Dur, Theolair-SR, Uniphyl, generics	300–900 mg/d	Nausea, vomiting, abdominal cramps, nervousness, tremor, insomnia, tachycardia.	Cimetidine, fluvoxamine, mexiletine, propranolol, quinolones, erythromycin, may ↑ theophylline levels. Rifampin, carbamazepine, phenytoin may ↓ theophylline levels. Lithium levels may be ↓.	$–$$$$

Corticosteroids

prednisone Deltasone, generics	0.6 mg/kg/d[†]	Glucose intolerance, weight gain, mood alteration, hypertension, osteoporosis, adrenal suppression, cataracts, myopathy.	Barbiturates, phenytoin, rifampin ↓ steroid effect.	$

[†] *Dosage to optimize airflow obstruction, use for 14 days only as single morning dose; no need to taper medication.*

Includes drug cost only. Cost of inhaled agents is per unit; cost of oral medications is per 30-day supply.

Legend: $ < $15 $$ $15–30 $$$ $30–45 $$$$ > $45

organism is suspected (e.g., some strains of *Haemophilus influenzae* or *Moraxella catarrhalis*). However, overall, many of the older antibiotics appear as efficacious as the newer, more expensive ones.

Oxygen Therapy

Oxygen therapy reduces the risk of death in selected patients. In COPD patients with significant hypoxemia (PaO_2 < 55 mm Hg or SaO_2 < 90%), long-term oxygen therapy may increase the lifespan by 6 to 7 years. Improved survival has only been seen when oxygen is administered for at least 12 hours per day, including the nocturnal hours. The greatest survival benefit is with continuously administered oxygen. Patients whose PaO_2 is between 55 and 59 mm Hg may also benefit from supplemental oxygen therapy if there is indirect evidence of hypoxemic end organ damage such as cor pulmonale or polycythemia. Oxygen is usually given through nasal prongs at a flow rate sufficient to produce resting PaO_2 between 65 and 80 mm Hg. Flow rates are often increased by 1 or 2 L/min during exercise and sleep. Oxygen therapy may be prescribed with exercise if oxygen desaturation below 88% occurs and there is **objective** evidence of improvement in exercise duration with oxygen administration.

Other Therapies

Mucolytics and ventilatory stimulants have shown little objective benefit in clinical trials and are not recommended in North American consensus guidelines. Noninvasive nasal or face mask ventilatory assistance is useful in acute exacerbations. For patients with emphysema induced by alpha$_1$ antiprotease deficiency, purified alpha$_1$ antitrypsin protein is available for supplemental IV administration. Resection or collapse of large bullae can be helpful, as can lung transplantation.

Therapeutic Tips

- The most common mistakes in medical management include inadequate education about medications and techniques for using inhalers, suboptimal dosing, inadequate monitoring and failure to advise the patient to take medication before engaging in physical activity.

- If the patient is not corticosteroid-responsive, corticosteroids should not be prescribed.

- To minimize side effects, long-acting theophyllines should be introduced at 50% of the final dosage for the first week.

- The patient should be encouraged to remain active despite the fact that exercise induces often distressing dyspnea; otherwise a vicious cycle of decreasing mobility can develop.

Suggested Reading List

American Thoracic Society. Standards for the diagnosis and care of patients with chronic obstructive pulmonary disease. *Am J Respir Crit Care Med* 1995;152(Suppl):S77–S120.

Canadian Thoracic Society Workshop Group. Guidelines for the assessment and management of chronic obstructive pulmonary disease. *Can Med Assoc J* 1992;147:420–428.

Ferguson GT, Cherniack RM. Management of chronic obstructive pulmonary disease. *N Engl J Med* 1993;328:1017–1022.

CHAPTER 39

Croup

Michael B.H. Smith, MB, BCh, FRCPC

Goals of Therapy

- To evaluate and treat the physiological disturbance
- To determine the cause and initiate appropriate therapy
- To provide symptom relief

Investigations

- Assess degree of airway compromise (Figure 1)
  - **Severe obstruction** is likely when there is marked stridor and drooling accompanied by agitation or lethargy. Infants may refuse to feed and children hold their neck extended forward (the sniffing position) in an effort to maximize the diameter of the airway. Cough is often absent or minimal.
  - **Mild obstruction** is likely when the child has only mild stridor (obvious only on crying with little or none at rest), is alert and consolable. Usually able to drink fluids. Mild hoarseness without stridor may not require treatment beyond symptomatic modalities.
- Review history to determine the most likely cause for symptoms
  - **Acute laryngotracheobronchitis (simple croup)** usually occurs in children aged 6 months to 4 years. There is a preceding viral prodrome with runny nose and mild fever (often < 39°C). The syndrome is characterized by a harsh, barking, seal-like cough, stridor and a hoarse voice peaking at 3 to 5 days before resolution. Symptoms are usually most prominent at night. Some authors separate this syndrome from spasmodic croup which is a nonfebrile version of this syndrome and lasts only 2 to 3 days. In practice it is often not possible to make this distinction and treatment for simple croup is recommended.
  - **Acute bacterial tracheitis** occurs at all ages and can be difficult to diagnose because it may resemble croup in the initial stages, then progresses to more severe disease. Often children present with a persistent, progressive (not barking) cough, stridor and progressive toxicity with high fever and increasing respiratory obstruction.
  - **Acute supraglottitis (epiglottitis)** occurs most commonly in school age children. It presents in the early stages as above but is rapidly progressive with high fever, drooling

Figure 1: **Assessment of Airway Compromise**

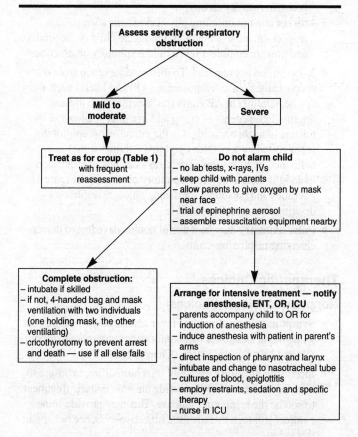

and stridor. Cough is almost always absent. It is now rare since the introduction of the *Haemophilus influenzae* vaccine.

– Other possibilities include **retropharyngeal/peritonsillar abscess** which can cause respiratory obstruction and dysphagia with fever but without stridor, cough and hoarseness. An acute **foreign body obstruction** or **angioneurotic edema** in a child will cause acute respiratory obstruction without fever or other signs of infection.

■ Examination:
  – allow a young child to sit on the parent's lap during examination
  – approach the child gently and observe pattern of breathing at rest
  – fatigue, anxiety, restlessness, altered mental status may indicate impending respiratory obstruction

– hoarse voice, especially on crying, indicates a laryngeal problem (usually croup)
– do not attempt upsetting physical examination (throat inspection, ear examination) unless the child is cooperative and you are confident it is a mild respiratory obstruction

- **X-ray**: often not required. To differentiate croup from other severe causes, an anteroposterior (AP) and lateral neck x-ray can be helpful. On AP views the "steeple" sign indicates the subglottic edema of croup and irregular shadows in the trachea indicate tracheitis. On the lateral view, epiglottitis is suggested by a swollen epiglottis ("thumb sign") and ballooned hypopharynx. The x-ray does *not* alter decision making if there is severe respiratory obstruction (Figure 1). Facilities and personnel for managing acute respiratory deterioration must be available.

- **Pulse oximetry** may be a useful noninvasive test to detect changing respiratory status

Therapeutic Choices

Nonpharmacologic Choices

- **Symptomatic treatment** of fever and associated sore throat with simple analgesics (acetaminophen) will relieve discomfort and help the child sleep (Chapter 105).

- Increasing **humidity** by a cool mist humidifier, exposure to a steamy bathroom or the outside air is an empiric treatment to soothe the respiratory mucosa. This may provide some comfort although there is little objective evidence to support this practice.

- In rare instances, with severe respiratory obstruction, **IV fluids** and **respiratory support** (oxygen and endotracheal intubation) may be required.

Pharmacologic Choices (Table 1)

Therapeutic Tips

- The first priority is assessment of respiratory obstruction, not diagnosis.

- In the majority of patients infectious stridor is simple croup requiring only symptomatic therapy.

- Mild, moderate or severe cases all begin with similar symptoms. While in hospital or the emergency department, frequent reassessment is prudent. On discharge, it is important to inform parents about signs of respiratory compromise and when to return for reassessment.

Table 1: Drugs Used for Treatment of Croup

Drug	Dosage	Adverse Effects	Comments	Cost*
Laryngotracheobronchitis (croup)			Cause: viral, most commonly parainfluenza virus.	
dexamethasone – Decadron, generics	outpatient: 0.15–0.6 mg/kg PO once only inpatient: 0.15 mg/kg/d PO once daily × 3 d	Rare with short-term use.	Use for mild to moderate obstruction. Benefits seen in 1–2 h.	$
budesonide – Pulmicort Nebuamp	By nebulizer: outpatient: 2 mg once inpatient: 2 mg BID × 3 d	Rare with short-term use.	Administering budesonide and dexamethasone together may provide better results but requires further investigation.	$
racemic epinephrine – Vaponefrin	By nebulizer: 0.5 mL/3 mL NS Q1–3H PRN	Pallor, tachycardia, hypertension.	Usually outpatient therapy. Used for moderate or greater obstruction. Requires 3 h period of observation.	$
l-epinephrine 1:1000 – Adrenalin, generics	By nebulizer: < 4 yr: 2.5 mL > 4 yr: 5 mL Q1–3H PRN		Same as above.	$
Bacterial tracheitis		For all: hypersensitivity.	Cause: *S. aureus*, Strep. Group A, *S. pneumoniae*, *H. influenzae*.	
cefuroxime 🐾 – Kefurox, Zinacef **or**	150 mg/kg/d IV divided Q8H (max. 4.5 g/d)	Eosinophilia, phlebitis.	First-line therapy.	$$
cloxacillin – Orbenin, Tegopen **and**	150 mg/kg/d IV divided Q6H	GI disturbance, interstitial nephritis.	Administer together with cefotaxime.	$
cefotaxime 🐾 – Claforan	200 mg/kg/d IV divided Q6–8H	Phlebitis	Use if unimmunized or suspect co-existing meningitis.	$$
Supraglottitis (epiglottitis) same as bacterial tracheitis			Cause: *H. influenzae*.	

Legend: $ < $20 $$ $20–40

* Cost of 1-day supply – includes drug cost only.
🐾 Dosage adjustment may be required in renal impairment – see Appendix I.

Suggested Reading List

Custer JR. Croup and related disorders. *Pediatr Rev* 1993;14: 19–28.

Klassen TP. Recent advances in the treatment of bronchiolitis and laryngitis. *Pediatr Clin North Am* 1997;44:249–261.

Cressman WR, Myer CM. Diagnosis and management of croup and epiglottitis. *Pediatr Clin North Am* 1994;41:265.

CHAPTER 40

Smoking Cessation

Frederic Bass, MD, DSc, SMHyg

Brief clinical tobacco intervention should occur whenever a
smoker receives medical care. Intervention by physicians is
a leading and proven strategy for countering the epidemic
of tobacco addiction. Health reasons are the most common
motivation for stopping to smoke and nicotine replacement
has proven to be one of the most effective aids.

Goals of Clinical Management

- Motivate smokers to stop smoking and youngsters to avoid
  smoking
- Provide key information, skilled counseling, nicotine therapy
  (to those ready to stop), and long-term follow-up
- Educate all patients about environmental tobacco smoke
- Have support staff and a medical record system that ensures
  the above

Investigations

- Initial assessment of all patients aged 9 or older should
  classify smoking status and label the medical record with a
  sticker or computerized prompt (Table 1)

Table 1: **Ask** "Have you ever smoked tobacco regularly?"; if
smoking, "Do you plan to quit smoking in the next
30 days?"; if not smoking, "Are you exposed to other
people's tobacco smoke?"

Label	Description	Definition
	Never smoked*	Has not smoked 100 cigarettes in lifetime; does not smoke now, at risk of starting if < 25 yrs old.
	Smoker	Smokes now (at least some every week) and not quitting in next 30 days.
	Smoker, stopping	Either quitting for good in next 30 days or has stopped and last puff within past 2 weeks.
	Recent ex-smoker*	Last puff 2 weeks to one year ago.
	Long-term ex-smoker*	Last puff more than one year ago.

* If exposed to environmental tobacco smoke, note "ETS" next to sticker.

- History including:
  - pattern of tobacco use: age started, usual and maximum number of cigarettes per day, longest smoke-free period in last 3 years, has patient ever stopped for 1 year
  - nicotine therapy: past use of patch or gum (mg nicotine, manufacturer), duration of use, would patient use it now
  - readiness to stop: rate on a scale of 1 (lowest) to 10 (highest). If < 8, what is required to become a 9. If not planning to stop in next 30 days are they planning to stop within 6 months
  - assessment of nicotine addiction: smokes ≥ 10 cigarettes per day, smokes within 30 minutes of waking, has tobacco withdrawal symptoms if does not smoke

NB: Special attention is required if any of: heavily nicotine-addicted and previous attempts to quit; severe poverty or psychosocial stress; addicted to alcohol or other drugs; history of clinical depression, schizophrenia, or severe anxiety; cessation is medically urgent; or on medication that interacts with nicotine.

- Physical examination: nicotine breath, yellow fingers, signs of early bronchitis, BP, pulse rate
- Biological tests (when available and appropriate):
  - expired carbon monoxide (CO)
  - cotinine, the nicotine metabolite found in saliva, urine and blood
  - $FEF_{0.25-0.75}$ (lung function testing)

Therapeutic Choices

Interventions for smoking cessation are determined by the smoker's readiness to stop (Table 2). Successful treatment must

Table 2: **Behavioral Epidemiology of Smoking**

Smokers (15–30% of population)	Ex-smokers (25–40% of population)	Never smoked (40–60% of population)
40–60% not thinking about stopping (precontemplative)	60% ex-smokers for 5+ yrs (maintenance, long-term)	At risk are children and all adults exposed to environmental tobacco smoke.
25–45% thinking about stopping (contemplative)	20% ex-smokers for 1–5 yrs (maintenance, long-term)	
10–20% smoker stopping (preparation/action)	20% recent ex-smokers for 2 wks to 1 yr	
Among smokers preparing to stop smoking, only 1 in 5 seek any formal stop-smoking help.	Recent ex-smokers are at very high risk of relapse (especially those who have smoked a few cigarettes).	Persons under age 25 are at risk of becoming smokers.

be individualized (Figure 1) and must provide advice, assistance and follow-up (Tables 3 and 4, Figure 2). Light to moderate smokers should be encouraged to try nonpharmacologic approaches on their first attempt.

Table 3: Advise

Individualize advice per patient's medical history and family history:
Recommend stopping smoking now (or staying stopped).
Motivate by:
– asking about the pros and cons of stopping smoking
– listening reflectively to smoker's feelings (anxiety, fear of failure, weight gain)
– expressing confidence in patient's abilities to quit smoking
Offer information: booklets, posters, graphics and videos on:
– health risks of smoking
– how to stop smoking; how to support a friend or spouse to stop smoking
– environmental tobacco smoke and consequences of passive smoking

Table 4: Assist

Offer support	Be ready and willing to help patient stop smoking.
General support	Have available: pamphlets, articles, booklets, videos on how to stop. What have you learned about stopping from earlier attempts? Focus on smoker's positive accomplishments. Repeatedly express your confidence that this person can stop smoking.
Empathy	Listen reflectively to smoker's concerns, feelings: How do you feel now about stopping? What are your greatest concerns?
For smoker ready to stop	When smoker is ready to set a target date (most smokers are not): Write date on a stop-smoking contract or on your prescription pad, sign it and have patient sign it. Suggest patient monitor time/place of each cigarette. Recommend nicotine therapy if patient smokes ≥ 10 cigarettes/day and help patient learn the symptoms of both nicotine withdrawal and toxicity. Refer to available stop-smoking programs when appropriate. Schedule follow-up visit(s).
Describe options to help unready smokers specify plan of action	Patient selects one of the following options: stop in future; patient may set a date to re-decide. Monitor (record) smoking for 2 wks, then decide. Reduce number of cigarettes per day to ≥ 40% of present level (but not to < 8 cigarettes/day). Recommend nicotine Rx to anyone who decides to stop and ≥ 10 cigarettes/day. Cold turkey now; not one more puff! Stop on own; suggest patient set target date. Stop with brief counseling from doctor: suggest patient set target date. Offer nicotine therapy next visit if patient is addicted and ready to stop. Refer to intensive nicotine treatment or to stop-smoking program. If patient has already stopped, remind "not even one puff."

Figure 1: **Stepped–Care Model of Smoking Cessation**

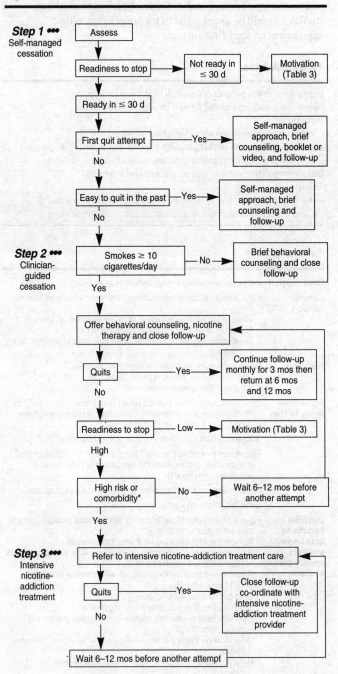

* *See Special Attention under Investigations, History.*

Pharmacologic Choices

Nicotine Replacement Therapy (Table 5)

The purpose of nicotine replacement is to help the motivated patient minimize withdrawal, not to provide the satisfaction of smoking. It is recommended only if $\geq$ 10 cigarettes are smoked per day, the first cigarette is smoked within 30 minutes of waking and tobacco withdrawal symptoms (anxiety, strong cravings, etc.) are experienced. Nicotine replacement should be accompanied by counseling. Patients should be warned not to smoke while using nicotine replacement to avoid adverse effects (hypertensive episodes, stroke, failure to stop smoking).

Nicotine replacement is available as gum (nicotine polacrilex) or patch (transdermal system). Nicotine nasal spray is available in the US. The time to peak venous blood level of nicotine from a single dose varies with the delivery system; smoking a cigarette being the briefest, followed by nasal spray, gum and finally the patch. The briefer the time to peak level, the more addictive the means of delivery. Nicotine gum should be used to anticipate and prevent nicotine withdrawal rather than in response to cravings. It requires proper technique ("chew and park" for 35 to 45 minutes/piece) and avoidance of acidic beverages (e.g., coffee, tea, carbonated beverages, orange and apple juice) because they decrease nicotine absorption. Optimal duration of use of the gum or the patch is unknown. With the patch the usual errors are too short a duration of treatment and too abrupt a reduction in nicotine strength. Symptoms of nicotine withdrawal or toxicity should dictate adjustment in dosage, analogous to adjusting insulin for control of diabetes.

NB: Nicotine 4 mg gum is a simple and very effective aid to treating highly addicted smokers. Nicotine 2 mg gum may be combined with the patches in selected highly addicted patients by experienced nicotine addiction specialists.

The transdermal system provides a continuous release of nicotine which is advantageous in the prevention of withdrawal.

Non-nicotine Agents

Bupropion, an antidepressant likely to become available in Canada, has proven effective for smoking cessation in several well-designed clinical trials.[1]

Clonidine, an antihypertensive agent, has been evaluated in nine randomized, placebo-controlled trials and found to have a pooled odds ratio of 2 compared with placebo. However, it has a high incidence of adverse effects. Clonidine may be a useful second-line agent in patients who have been unsuccessful using closely

---

[1] *N Engl J Med 1997;337:1195–1202.*

Table 5: **Nicotine Replacement Therapy**

Drug	Dosage	Advantages	Disadvantages	Cost*
Nicotine Gum (polacrilex) Nicorette 2 mg, sold without prescription	Usual:10–12 pieces/d initially to a max. of 20 pieces/d for 12 wks; then tapered by 1 piece/d every wk, according to patient's symptoms of nicotine withdrawal.	Fast acting, patient controls delivery rate, can tailor to patient's schedule.	High compliance needed. Often misused (chewed but not parked) with resulting side effects (hiccoughs, stomach ache, burning throat, nausea). Also, sore jaw, air swallowing, denture adhesion. A few become addicted. High relapse rate.	$$
Nicotine Gum (polacrilex) Nicorette Plus 4 mg	Usual:10–12 pieces/d initially to a max. 20 pieces/d for 12 wks; then tapered by 1 piece/d every wk, according to patient's symptoms of nicotine withdrawal.	A very effective nicotine product for highly addicted smokers.	All the above but at greater rate; higher rate of addiction; high relapse rate.	$$$
Nicotine Patch (transdermal) Habitrol, Nicoderm, Nicotrol, Prostep	See Table 6 for dosing.	Ease of use, low compliance requirement, continuous delivery of nicotine, non-addictive.	May not provide sufficient nicotine levels for some patients. Side effects: skin irritation, intense dreams. High relapse rate.	$$$
Combined Nicotine Patch and Gum	Presently under clinical investigation; more closely approximates the nicotine pattern of smoking; might help the more addicted but also might be addicting itself. Must be used under expert supervision.			

Cautions: Patients on nicotine therapy should be closely followed for symptoms of nicotine withdrawal, nicotine toxicity and interaction with other drugs or medical conditions.

Contraindications: Contraindicated in patients in immediate postmyocardial infarction period, or with life-threatening arrhythmias, severe or worsening angina pectoris, recent cerebral vascular accident, generalized skin disorders, hypersensitivity to nicotine, in children and in women who are pregnant or nursing unless women recently failed serious, well-supervised attempts to stop smoking without pharmacological aid and continue to smoke ≥ 15 cigarettes/day.

Comments: Once a patient stops smoking, a decrease in the dose of some concomitant medications may be required, e.g., caffeine, imipramine, insulin, oxazepam, pentazocine, propranolol, propoxyphene, theophylline.

* Cost of 105 pieces of gum or 14 patches – includes drug costs only.
Legend: $ < $20 $$ $20–40 $$$ $40–60

Figure 2: **Follow-up**

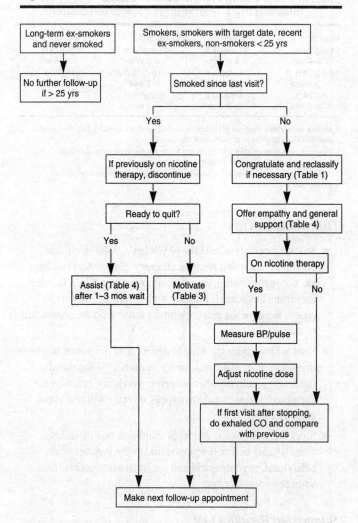

Abbreviation: CO = carbon monoxide.

supervised nicotine replacement therapy. Treatment, using an oral dose of 0.1 mg BID, should begin 3 days prior to smoking cessation and end 3 weeks later.[2]

Other agents such as **naltrexone**, **bromocriptine**, and **mecamylamine** require further evaluation to determine their role in treatment. There is no basis for prescribing **buspirone** or **doxepin**.

---

[2] *Drugs 1995;50(2):197–207.*

Table 6: **Usual Dosage for Nicotine Patches***†
(Manufacturers' recommended dosages and duration)‡

Habitrol:	Nicoderm:	Nicotrol:	Prostep:
21 mg/24 h × 3–4 wks	21 mg/24 h × 6 wks	15 mg/16 h × 8 wks	22 mg/24 h × 6–8 wks
14 mg/24 h × 3–4 wks	14 mg/24 h × 2 wks	10 mg/16 h × 2 wks	11 mg/24 h × 6–8 wks
7 mg/24 h × 3–4 wks	7 mg/24 h × 2 wks	5 mg/16 h × 2 wks	

* *Dosing adjustment required in patients under 45 kg, those smoking less than 10–15 cigarettes/day or those with cardiovascular disease.*
† *If patient smokes more than 2–3 cigarettes while on patch, therapy should be discontinued and reoffered 6–12 mos later.*
‡ *Duration of treatment should be individualized and attention should be paid to recognizing withdrawal.*

Therapeutic Tips

■ Smoking cessation tests the physician's skills in clinical communication and pharmacotherapy. Since most smokers are not ready to stop, the clinician plays two different roles: the strong advocate for health, and the caring, listening coach. Reserve the prescription for those who are committed to stopping!

■ Start asking about smoking at age 9 (after the parent has been invited to leave the room for 30 seconds): "What do you think you would do when someone you know offers you a cigarette? ...You can always speak directly with me about smoking."

■ Stopping to smoke is a chronic condition that often lasts 5 to 10 years before the person makes the biochemical, behavioral, psychological and social transformation from smoker to non-smoker.

Suggested Reading List

Bass F. Mobilizing physicians to conduct clinical intervention in tobacco use through a medical-association program: 5 years' experience in British Columbia. *Can Med Assoc J* 1996;154: 159–164.

Bass F. *Stop smoking: the smoker's approach* (video). (Available through BC Doctors' Stop Smoking Program SSP/BCMA 110–1665 West Broadway, Vancouver BC V6J 5A4).

BC Doctors' Stop Smoking Program (kit – specify GP, specialist). (SSP/BCMA 110–1665 West Broadway, Vancouver, BC V6J 5A4).

Canadian Council on Smoking and Health. *Guide your patients to a smoke free future* (manual). (CCSH, 1000–170 Laurier Ave. W., Ottawa, ON K1P 5V5), 1991.

Fiore MC, Wetter DW, Bailey WC, et al. *Smoking cessation clinical practice guideline*. Rockville, Md: Agency for Health Care Policy and Research, Public Health Service, US Dept of Health and Human Services, 1996. (Summary published in JAMA 1996;275:1270–1280).

Moner SE. Smoking and pregnancy. In: *Canadian task force on the periodic health examination. The Canadian guide to clinical preventive health care*. Ottawa: Minister of Supply and Services Canada, 1994:26–36.

Taylor MC, Dingle JL. Prevention of tobacco-caused disease. In: *Canadian task force on the periodic health examination. The Canadian guide to clinical preventive health care*. Ottawa: Minister of Supply and Services Canada, 1994:500–511.

CHAPTER 41

Chronic Liver Diseases

Mark G. Swain, MD, MSc, FRCPC

This chapter discusses ascites, spontaneous bacterial peritonitis, hepatic encephalopathy, cholestatic disease (including symptom management), autoimmune chronic hepatitis, alcoholic liver disease (including alcoholic hepatitis), hemochromatosis and Wilson's disease. Esophageal varices are discussed in Chapter 44 and viral hepatitis in Chapter 94.

Goals of Therapy

- To manage symptoms associated with chronic liver conditions
- To treat complications of chronic disease (e.g., infection)
- To prevent recurrence
- To delay or prevent disease progression
- To decrease mortality from liver-associated causes

Ascites (Portal Hypertension)

Investigations

- Thorough history with special attention to documented liver disease; other causes of ascites should be ruled out
- Physical examination for features of chronic liver disease (e.g., cutaneous stigmata), hepatosplenomegaly, degree of ascites accumulation (shifting dullness, abdominal protuberance, eversion of umbilicus), signs of portal hypertension (caput medusae, venous hum) or other features of liver failure/complications (GI bleed, asterixis)
- Laboratory tests:
  – ascitic tap (all patients) for neutrophil count, culture, protein/albumin, amylase, lactic dehydrogenase, glucose
  – calculate serum-ascites albumin gradient

Therapeutic Choices (Figure 1, Table 1)

High plasma aldosterone levels in patients with ascites results in sodium/fluid retention; thus, **spironolactone** (a specific aldosterone antagonist) is the diuretic of choice. **Furosemide** can be added at any time to enhance diuresis and/or control serum potassium levels. **Metolazone** (an extremely potent diuretic) can be added to the spironolactone/furosemide combination if ascites is refractory.

Figure 1: **Management of Ascites Secondary to Portal Hypertension**

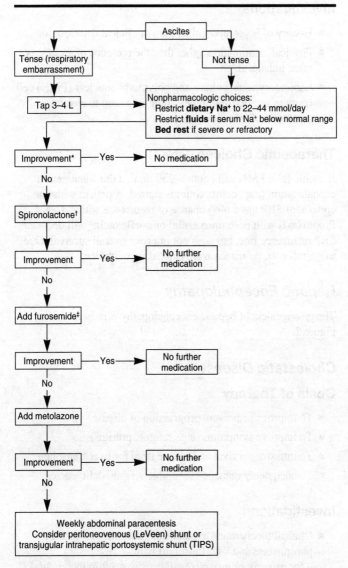

* Aim: 1–1.5 kg/day weight loss if peripheral edema, 0.5–1 kg/day if no edema.

† Patients developing side effects (e.g., painful gynecomastia) can be switched to another potassium-sparing diuretic (e.g., amiloride).

‡ Patients can be started on spironolactone and furosemide simultaneously which often provides a more predictable diuresis with better electrolyte balance.

NB: Diuretics should be given as single doses in the morning. The minimum dose to achieve adequate diuresis should always be used and serum electrolytes, BUN and creatinine monitored before therapy, weekly until stabilized then monthly. Dosage can usually be reduced after diuresis is initiated.

Spontaneous Bacterial Peritonitis (SBP)

Investigations

- History of fever, abdominal pain or clinical deterioration
- Physical examination, other than the presence of ascites, is often unhelpful
- Laboratory tests: culture and polymorphonuclear (PMN) cell count of ascitic fluid; repeat after treatment to ensure resolution of infection

Therapeutic Choices (Table 1)

If ascitic fluid PMN cell count > 250 mm^3, a third-generation cephalosporin (e.g., **cefotaxime**) is started. A patient with one episode of SBP has a 69% chance of recurrence within 1 year. Prophylaxis with **co-trimoxazole**[1] or **norfloxacin**[2] will decrease SBP recurrence rate, but does not improve overall survival. Due to overall cost, co-trimoxazole is the drug of choice.

Hepatic Encephalopathy

The management of hepatic encephalopathy is presented in Figure 2.

Cholestatic Disease

Goals of Therapy

- To improve or prevent progression of disease
- To improve symptoms (e.g., fatigue, pruritus)
- To improve survival and reduce need for liver transplant
- To adequately manage fat-soluble vitamin deficiencies

Investigations

- Clinical/biochemical evidence of cholestasis (↑ alkaline phosphatase and later bilirubin) with:
  - for *primary biliary cirrhosis:* positive antimitochondrial antibody (> 95% of cases); confirmed by liver biopsy
  - for *primary sclerosing cholangitis:* ductular abnormalities (strictures, beading, etc.) on endoscopic retrograde cholangiopancreatography (ERCP)

---

[1] *Ann Intern Med 1995;122:595–598.*
[2] *Hepatology 1990;12:716–724.*

Figure 2: **Management of Hepatic Encephalopathy**

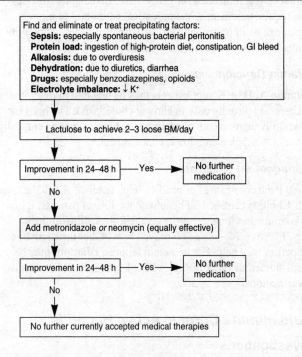

■ Identify vitamin deficiencies by:
  – prothrombin time (↑ if vitamin K deficient)
  – serum calcium, 25(OH)-vitamin D levels
  – serum vitamin A and/or carotene levels

Therapeutic Choices (Figure 3, Table 1)

Primary Biliary Cirrhosis (PBC) and Primary Sclerosing Cholangitis (PSC)

Ursodeoxycholic acid (UDCA) has been shown to improve serum liver biochemical tests in PBC[3–5] and PSC. It appears to have limited effect in preventing disease progression in PSC. In PBC a combined analysis of three trials suggested that UDCA significantly reduced the probability of transplantation and/or death after a median of nearly 4 years. It slows disease progression but is not curative.[6] Its effect on symptoms (i.e., fatigue, pruritus) is controversial but likely minimal.

[3] N Engl J Med 1991;324:1548–1554.

[4] Gastroenterology 1994;106:1284–1290.

[5] Hepatology 1994;19:1149–1156.

[6] Gastroenterology 1995;108:A1082.

Methotrexate is experimental for treating PBC or PSC and cannot be recommended for general use. Cholangitis episodes also require treatment with appropriate antibiotics (e.g., ciprofloxacin in outpatients for early mild episodes; ampicillin/gentamicin/metronidazole for hospitalized patients).

Vitamin Deficiencies

Vitamin A, D or K supplements may be required to treat deficiencies (usually only in chronic cholestasis). The need for **vitamin E** supplements in adults has not been assessed clinically. Vitamin A supplementation is controversial.

Management of Pruritus

Local cutaneous causes of pruritus (e.g., eczema) should be ruled out. **Cholestyramine** will benefit about 90% of patients; it must be continued as long as pruritus is present. **Antihistamines** (e.g., hydroxyzine) are of no proven benefit, but their sedative properties may help. For treatment failures, **rifampin** may be tried. Numerous other therapies have been reported but all are investigational.

Autoimmune Chronic Active Hepatitis

Investigations

- Marked ↑ in serum transaminases and hypergamma-globulinemia; positive antinuclear antibody (ANA) in about 70% of patients

NB: Patient is classically a young woman presenting with either an acute or chronic illness characterized by lethargy, arthralgia, oligomenorrhea, fluctuating jaundice and a cushingoid appearance with striae, hirsutism and acne.

Therapeutic Choices (Table 1)

Immunosuppression with **glucocorticoids,** with or without **azathioprine,** prolongs life, decreases symptoms, improves serum biochemical abnormalities and diminishes hepatic inflammation on liver biopsy. The goal is to induce remission (decreased serum aminotransferase levels to ≤ twice normal and a follow-up liver biopsy that is normal or shows only chronic persistent hepatitis). Most patients will require therapy for at least 2 to 3 years before attempts to stop prednisone can be made; most will require lifelong therapy. If prednisone cannot be lowered below 10 mg per day, azathioprine may be added to the regimen.

Figure 3: **Management of Cholestatic Symptoms**

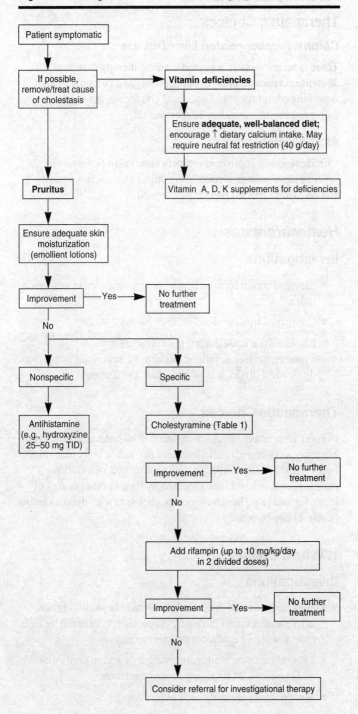

Alcoholic Liver Disease

Therapeutic Choices

Chronic Alcohol-related Liver Disease

There is no universally accepted medical therapy except **abstention from alcohol**. Some trials suggest potential benefit from long-term propylthiouracil and colchicine, but these therapies are still considered experimental.

Alcoholic Hepatitis

Corticosteroids improve short-term survival in patients with severe biopsy-proven alcoholic hepatitis (with encephalopathy and no evidence of GI bleeding or sepsis).

Hemochromatosis

Investigations

- Elevated serum ferritin, fasting percent transferrin saturation index
- Confirmed iron overload on liver biopsy
- Classically, a middle-aged man presents with hyperpigmentation, fatigue, abdominal pain, joint pain, diminished libido, loss of body hair and diabetes

Therapeutic Choices

Dietary iron intake should be reduced. **Phlebotomies** (weekly or biweekly as tolerated) will ultimately normalize body iron stores (with weekly phlebotomies, it may take up to 2 years). If the patient is unable to tolerate phlebotomy (due to other causes of iron overload [e.g., hematological]), chelation with **deferoxamine** (Table 1) can be tried.

Wilson's Disease

Investigations

- Hepatic presentations include fulminant hepatitis, chronic active hepatitis and cirrhosis; diagnosis is confirmed by liver biopsy with ↑ hepatic copper concentrations
- Laboratory tests: ↑ aminotransferase, ↓ serum ceruloplasmin and copper, ↑ 24 h urinary copper excretion
- Most patients are diagnosed before age 30

Table 1: Drugs Used in Chronic Liver Diseases

Drug	Dosage	Adverse Effects	Comments	Cost*
Ascites				
spironolactone ☞ Aldactone, generics	Starting 100–200 mg/d, ↑ to 400 mg/d with dosage adjustments Q5–7 d	Hyperkalemia, gynecomastia, mastalgia.	If intolerable side effects develop, may switch to amiloride (5 mg/d, can be ↑ to 20 mg/d).	$
furosemide ☞ Lasix, generics	Starting 40 mg/d, ↑ daily by 20–40 mg until diuresis achieved (up to 160 mg/d)	Common to thiazides/loop diuretics: hyponatremia, hypokalemia, volume depletion, nausea, anorexia, fatigue, hyperuricemia, hyperglycemia with metolazone, ototoxicity with high-dose furosemide, rash, weakness.		$
metolazone Zaroxolyn	Starting 2.5 mg/d, up to 10 mg/d			$
Spontaneous Bacterial Peritonitis				
Treatment				
cefotaxime ☞ Claforan	2 g IV Q8H × 5 d	Hypersensitivity, GI disturbances, pain at injection site, pseudomembranous colitis.	Alternative: other 3rd-generation cephalosporin.	$$$$
Prophylaxis				
co-trimoxazole ☞ Bactrim, Septra, generics	1 DS tablet 5 ×/week	Hypersensitivities, GI disturbances, blood dyscrasias, skin reactions (rare Stevens-Johnson syndrome).	Prophylaxis to be used only after patient has experienced one confirmed episode of SBP.	$
norfloxacin ☞ Noroxin	400 mg/d	GI disturbances, CNS effects, skin rash.		$$

(cont'd)

Table 1: **Drugs Used in Chronic Liver Diseases** *(cont'd)*

Drug	Dosage	Adverse Effects	Comments	Cost*
Hepatic Encephalopathy				
lactulose Cephulac, generics	30 mL BID–QID	Bloating, flatulence, cramps, diarrhea.	Titrate lactulose to produce 2–3 loose BM/d.	$
metronidazole Flagyl, generics	250–500 mg TID	GI disturbances, headache, metallic taste.	Disulfiram-like reaction with alcohol.	$
neomycin Mycifradin	1 g QID	Malabsorption syndrome, nephrotoxicity, ototoxicity, GI disturbances, rash.	Neomycin and metronidazole are equally effective.	$$
Cholestatic Pruritus				
cholestyramine Questran	4 g before breakfast initially; ↑ in 4 g increments first after break- fast, then at night and then at lunch	Constipation, heartburn, nausea, vomiting.	May bind other drugs given concurrently; separate doses (1 h before or 4–6 h after resin).	$$
Fat-soluble Vitamin Deficiencies				
vitamin K	Vitamin K 10 mg IM monthly			
vitamin A	Vitamin A 5 000–10 000 IU/d† PO (aqueous)		Use of vitamin A is controversial.	$
vitamin D	Vitamin D 1 000 IU Q2 d PO (with 2–3 g elemental calcium/d)		For examples of calcium products, see Chapter 52.	

Drug	Dosage	Adverse Effects	Comments	Cost
Primary Biliary Cirrhosis *ursodeoxycholic acid* Ursofalk	13–15 mg/kg/d	Diarrhea.	A reasonable treatment for PBC; may be of benefit in PSC but is unproven.	$$$‡
Autoimmune Chronic Active Hepatitis *prednisone* Deltasone, generics	Sample dosage regimen (e.g., Mayo Clinic) for *autoimmune chronic active hepatitis:* 60 mg/d × 1 wk, then 40 mg/d × 1 wk, then 30 mg/d × 2 wks, then 20 mg/d *Alcoholic hepatitis:* 40 mg/d for 28 d then taper over 2 wks	Fluid/electrolyte imbalance, suppression of pituitary–adrenal function, hyperglycemia, peptic ulcer, behavioral disturbances, ocular cataracts, glaucoma, cushingoid syndrome, aseptic necrosis of hip.	*Autoimmune chronic active hepatitis:* Gradually taper from 20 mg/d (weeks to months) using serum aminotransferases and clinical status as guides.	$
azathioprine ● Imuran	50–150 mg/d	↓ appetite, leukopenia, thrombocytopenia, infection, biliary stasis, hypersensitivity reactions, rash, rare veno-occlusive disease, nausea, vomiting.	Monitor CBC monthly while on azathioprine.	$–$$
Hemochromatosis *deferoxamine* Desferal	1–4 g by SC minipump over 12 h, adjusted on an individual basis	Allergic reactions, auditory/ocular toxicity, tachycardia, flushing, abdominal discomfort, pain at injection site, hypotension, skin rash, convulsions.	May be beneficial if phlebotomy is not tolerated or contraindicated.	$$$$$

(cont'd)

Table 1: Drugs Used in Chronic Liver Diseases *(cont'd)*

Drug	Dosage	Adverse Effects	Comments	Cost*
Wilson's Disease				
penicillamine Cuprimine, Depen	1–2 g/d in 4 divided doses, on an empty stomach	Proteinuria, hematologic effects, positive ANA, mouth ulcers, diarrhea, ↓ taste sense, ↓ appetite, nausea, vomiting, hypersensitivity.	Use 24 h urinary copper excretion and serum free copper levels to monitor therapy for adequate removal of copper.	$$–$$$$
trientine Syprine π	1–2 g/d in 4 divided doses	Usually well tolerated. Anemia.		π
zinc generics	50 mg (elemental zinc) TID between meals	GI disturbances.	Use in patients intolerant of penicillamine or trientine.	$

† Use minimum effective dose.
‡ Based on 750 mg/day × 30 days.
π Available through the Special Access Program (formerly the Emergency Drug Release Program), Therapeutic Products Directorate, Health Canada.

🔹 *Dosage adjustment may be required in renal impairment – see Appendix I.*
* *Cost of 30-day supply – includes drug cost only.*
Legend: $ < $40 $$ $40–80 $$$ $80–125 $$$$ $125–350 $$$$$ > $350

Therapeutic Choices (Table 1)

Penicillamine is the drug of choice, and treatment is lifelong. Pyridoxine, 25 mg daily, should be given with penicillamine to counteract its antipyridoxine effect. For patients intolerant of penicillamine, **trientine** may be tried. Elemental **zinc** is an option in patients intolerant of penicillamine and trientine. **Foods high in copper** should be avoided (e.g., peanuts, chocolate, liver, shellfish, mushrooms).

Suggested Reading List

Autoimmune Hepatitis. In Rothschild MA, Berk PA, Meyer zum Buschenfelde K-H, eds. *Seminars in liver disease*. Vol 11(3). New York: Thieme Medical Publishers, Inc., 1991.

Mistry P, Seymour CA. Primary biliary cirrhosis – from Thomas Addison to the 1990's. *Q J Med* 1992;82:185–196.

Nichols GM, Bacon BR. Hereditary hemochromatosis: pathogenesis and clinical features of a common disease. *Am J Gastroenterol* 1989;84:851–862.

Runyon BA. Care of patients with ascites. *N Engl J Med* 1994; 330:337–342.

Sternlieb I. Perspectives in Wilson's disease. *Hepatology* 1990;12:1234–1239.

CHAPTER 42

Gastroesophageal Reflux Disease

Eldon A. Shaffer, MD, DABIM, FACP, FRCPC

Gastroesophageal reflux disease (GERD) refers to the symptoms (commonly heartburn) resulting when gastric secretions reflux from the stomach to the esophagus. It may lead to inflammatory histopathologic changes (reflux or peptic esophagitis).

Goals of Therapy

- To relieve symptoms, particularly heartburn
- To promote healing of esophagitis
- To prevent complications (stricture formation, bleeding, progression to Barrett's epithelium)
- To prevent recurrences

Classification of Symptom Severity*

Severity of GERD	Criteria
Mild	Reflux symptoms < 3 times/week Symptoms present for < 6 months Symptoms do not interfere with daily activity Pain (heartburn) severity rated 1–3 out of 10 No major complications
Moderate	As for mild but pain severity rated 4–6 out of 10
Severe	Daily reflux symptoms Symptoms present for > 6 months Symptoms regularly interfere with daily activity and can awaken patient at night Pain severity rated 7–10 out of 10 Complications

* *Classification does not necessarily correspond to histological severity.*

Investigations

- History: identify
  - common symptoms of GERD: heartburn, regurgitation of acid or bile, or dysphagia
  - less common features: chest pain, hypersalivation (water brash), aspiration (cough, asthma, pneumonia), oropharyngeal symptoms (globus sensation, hoarseness), or rarely odynophagia (pain on swallowing)

- predisposing/associated conditions: pregnancy, obesity, scleroderma
- Indications for diagnostic evaluation include:
  - heartburn refractory to 4 to 8 weeks of conservative treatment (lifestyle modification, over-the-counter [OTC] therapy, standard-dose H_2-antagonists)
  - dysphagia
  - atypical chest pain
  - GI bleeding
  - odynophagia
  - extraesophageal symptoms (respiratory, oropharyngeal)
- Types of diagnostic evaluation depend on availability and indication:
  - **esophagogastroscopy,** with biopsy of any suspicious lesion to detect Barrett's epithelium (a premalignant lesion requiring surveillance endoscopy) or carcinoma, is the procedure of choice
  - **barium swallow** to assess peristalsis and detect rings or strictures in dysphagia
  - **Bernstein test** with acid perfusion of the esophagus can sometimes reproduce the symptoms of heartburn and chest pain in questionable cases
  - **esophageal manometry** to document peristalsis is warranted in patients with atypical chest pain and to eliminate a major motility disorder (e.g., scleroderma) before doing antireflux surgery
  - **24-hour pH monitoring** to detect acid reflux into lower esophagus is useful in patients with persistent symptoms but without endoscopic evidence of esophagitis

Therapeutic Choices (Figure 1)

Nonpharmacologic Choices

- Dietary modifications (avoid chocolate, caffeine, acidic citrus juices, large fatty meals).
- Weight loss if 20% greater than ideal body weight.
- No snacks before bedtime.
- No lying down after meals.
- Reduce alcohol intake.
- Legs under the head of the bed should be elevated on 10- to 15-cm blocks.
- Stop smoking (Chapter 40).
- Avoid tight clothing.

Figure 1: **Management of GERD**

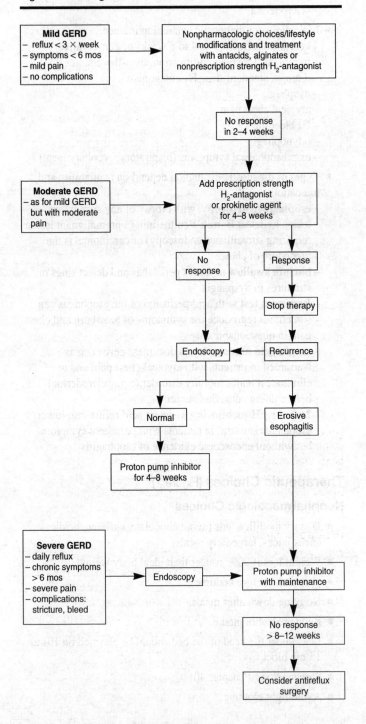

Pharmacologic Choices (Tables 1 and 2; refer also to Chapter 44)

Mild GERD

Drugs that impair esophageal motility and lower esophageal sphincter tone should be eliminated when possible (e.g., calcium channel blockers, theophylline, tricyclic antidepressants, beta-blockers, anticholinergic agents).

Most people with mild symptoms frequently do not seek medical attention and will obtain symptomatic relief with **antacids**, **alginates** or nonprescription strength **H$_2$-antagonists**. The latter are a high-expense commodity for the yield in acid reduction. Additional therapy becomes necessary as GERD severity increases.

Moderate to Severe GERD

Antacids or nonprescription strength H$_2$-receptor antagonists are *not* effective alone.

Histamine (H$_2$) Antagonists

Cimetidine, ranitidine, famotidine and **nizatidine** are equally effective. They relieve symptoms in 60% and heal histologically mild esophagitis in over 40% of patients. Their safety profile is excellent (Table 1, Chapter 44). Better results are achieved if the esophagitis is mild, if higher and more frequent doses of H$_2$-antagonists are used or if treatment continues for longer periods (up to 12 weeks). Resolution of symptoms, however, does not correlate well with healing of esophagitis. Similarly, some patients with severe esophagitis (ulceration or Barrett's epithelium) have minimal symptoms. When initial therapy is beneficial, maintenance may be necessary if/when symptoms recur and cannot be controlled by nonpharmacologic means. The lowest dose possible should be used to control symptoms and prevent complications.

Prokinetic Agents

Cisapride, a 5-hydroxytryptamine (5-HT$_4$) agonist, can relieve symptoms and treat mild esophagitis at a dose of 10 mg PO TID AC and QHS (or 20 mg BID). It offers no advantage over H$_2$-antagonists. The first-generation prokinetic agents, the dopamine antagonists (**metoclopramide** and **domperidone**), are less expensive, but the incidence of side effects is higher. The addition of cisapride to an H$_2$-antagonist will improve the response in those who do not respond to H$_2$-antagonist therapy alone, but such dual therapy provides no advantage over proton pump inhibitors alone.

Table 1: Drugs Used in Gastroesophageal Reflux Disease

Drug	Dosage		Adverse Effects	Comments	Cost*
Antacids					
Numerous aluminum hydroxide – magnesium hydroxide combinations	30 mL (regular strength) 1 h PC and QHS		Constipation, diarrhea.	↓ bioavailability of digoxin, tetracycline, quinolone antibiotics; separate dosing by 2 h.	$$
Alginates Gaviscon, Rafton	10–20 mL or 2–4 tablets (chewed) PC and QHS, followed by glass of water		Flatulence, eructation.	Alginates and some antacids contain significant amounts of sodium.	$–$$
H₂-antagonists	**Treatment**	**Maintenance**	See below.	Comparable in efficacy to antacids.	
Nonprescription					
famotidine Pepcid AC, others	10 mg BID				$–$$
ranitidine Zantac-75	75 mg BID				$–$$
Prescription					
cimetidine Tagamet, generics	600 mg BID	600 mg BID	Diarrhea, constipation, headache, fatigue, confusion (most likely in elderly and those with poor renal function), cardiac effects, rash.	Cimetidine ↓ cytochrome P-450 metabolism of several agents (e.g., warfarin, phenytoin, theophylline) – use another H₂-antagonist; ranitidine has minor effect.	$
ranitidine Zantac, generics	150 mg BID	150 mg BID			$$
famotidine Pepcid, generics	20 mg BID	20 mg BID	Cimetidine: gynecomastia, impotence (rare).		$$
nizatidine Axid	150 mg BID	150 mg BID			$$$

	Recommended Adult Dosage	Selected Adverse Effects	Comments	Cost*
Prokinetic Agents ➤				
cisapride Prepulsid	10 mg TID AC and QHS or 20 mg BID	Diarrhea, abdominal discomfort (cramps, distention), headache.	Administration with azole antifungals and macrolide antibiotics contraindicated. Metoclopramide or domperidone may be used (less expensive than cisapride but ↑ side effects). ↓ dose of cisapride in hepatic dysfunction.	$$$$
Proton Pump Inhibitors				
omeprazole Losec	20–40 mg/day†	Abdominal pain, nausea, headache.	Omeprazole may interfere with cytochrome P-450 metabolized agents (e.g., diazepam, warfarin, phenytoin).	$$$$–$$$$$
lansoprazole Prevacid	30 mg/day			$$$$
pantoprazole Pantoloc	40 mg/day			$$$$

† Not to exceed 20 mg/d in hepatic impairment.

➤ Dosage adjustment may be required in renal impairment – see Appendix I.

* Cost of 30-day supply – includes drug cost only.

Legend: $ < $20 $$ $20–40 $$$ $40–60 $$$$ $60–80 $$$$$ > $80

Table 2: **Efficacy of Drugs Used to Treat GERD**

	Acute treatment		Prevention of recurrences
	Symptoms	Esophagitis	
Antacids	+	−	−
Alginates/antacids	+	−	−
Metoclopramide, domperidone	+	−	−
H$_2$-antagonists	++	+	±
Cisapride	++	+	+
Proton pump inhibitors	+++	+++	+++

+ *Drug of proven value (controlled trials).*
− *Not established (negative trial or not tested).*

Proton Pump Inhibitors

Marked suppression of acid secretion eliminates acid reflux episodes and selectively heals esophagitis in most patients (60% by 4 weeks, 80% by 8 weeks). Occasionally a higher dose (e.g., omeprazole 40 mg per day) is necessary in those with continued symptoms. Proton pump inhibitors can heal ulceration but do not reverse Barrett's epithelium. Their use short term is quite safe. Choice between the available proton pump inhibitors should be driven by cost rather than subtle differences in pharmacokinetics.

Maintenance Therapy for Moderate to Severe GERD

The recurrence rate following successful therapy for erosive/ severe esophagitis is extremely high (75 to 90%). Proton pump inhibitors maintain remission more effectively than H$_2$-antagonists. Some cases require omeprazole 40 mg per day. Maintenance therapy for such severe disease appears to be long term. Cost and safety are concerns with chronic use of proton pump inhibitors. The lowest dose possible should be used. Using half the regular dose (e.g., omeprazole 10 mg per day) may have a role but requires evaluation of effectiveness. In patients who are infected with *Helicobacter pylori*, prolonged acid suppression during maintenance therapy may accelerate the natural history of these bacteria leading to chronic atrophic gastritis, a potential forerunner of gastric carcinoma. Currently it is unknown if *H. pylori* should be eradicated in such cases. Until any relation- ship is confirmed, there is no indication to detect or treat *H. pylori* gastritis in those destined for long-term therapy with proton pump inhibitors. The informed patient should be involved in any decision concerning lifelong maintenance therapy.

Antireflux Surgery

Antireflux surgery is effective for reflux control in 80% of well-selected patients. Indications include intractable reflux esophagitis (particularly in a young person) and major complications (aspiration, recurrent stricture or major bleeding). Laparoscopic approaches may become a reasonable, cost-effective treatment, but will require comparison to outcome analysis of long-term therapy with potent acid-suppressing agents.

Pharmacoeconomic Considerations

Jeffrey A. Johnson, PhD

A number of pharmacoeconomic evaluations of therapeutic choices for GERD have been conducted. In general, these evaluations indicate that proton pump inhibitors are more cost-effective than H_2-antagonists, for grades II to IV esophagitis. For example, a recent evaluation commissioned by CCOHTA indicated that, even though the acquisition cost of an 8-week course of omeprazole was almost three times that of an 8-week course of ranitidine, omeprazole was more cost-effective because downstream costs were avoided due to higher healing and lower recurrence rates. The study concluded that substituting maintenance ranitidine therapy with intermittent omeprazole therapy would result in savings of $52,000 and an extra 3,410 weeks of time free from GERD per 1,000 patients treated per year. Maintenance omeprazole would be even more effective, resulting in 6,220 extra weeks free from GERD, but at an additional cost of $348,000 per 1,000 patients treated per year, when compared to maintenance ranitidine therapy.

An important consideration in evaluating these economic studies is that they have been based on clinical trial results so some costs (e.g., endoscopy) may be driven more by the trial protocol than usual practice. In addition, most trials used limited time horizons (i.e., 1 year) and often only considered surgical intervention as a final therapeutic option. In some cases, such as in grades III and IV GERD, surgery at an earlier stage may be more cost-effective (see Sridhar S et al). Furthermore, the economic evaluations did not always differentiate between grades, often grouping grades II to IV, even though healing and recurrence rates may differ.

Suggested Reading

O'Brien B, Goerre R, Hunt R, Wilkinson J, Levine M, Willan A. *Cost-effectiveness of alternative therapies for the long-term management of gastroesophageal reflux disease*. Ottawa, ON: Canadian Coordinating Office on Health Technology Assessment (CCOHTA). 1996.

Sridhar S, Huang J, O'Brien BJ, Hunt RH. Clinical economics review: cost-effectiveness of treatment alternatives for gastro-esophageal reflux disease. *Alimentary Pharmacology and Therapeutics* 1996;10:865–773.

Suggested Reading List

Beck IT, Champion MC, Lemire S, Thomson ABR. The second Canadian consensus conference on the treatment of patients with gastroesophageal reflux disease. *Can J Gastroenterol* 1997;11(suppl B).

Bell NJU, Hunt RH. Role of gastric acid suppression in the treatment of gastro-oesophageal reflux disease. *Gut* 1992;33:118–124.

Hetzel DJ. Controlled clinical trials of omeprazole in the long-term management of reflux disease. *Digestion* 1992;51: 35–42.

Ramirez B, Richter JE. Promotility drugs in the treatment of gastro-oesophageal reflux disease. *Aliment Pharmacol Ther* 1993;7:5–20.

Richter JE. Surgery for reflux disease – reflections of a gastroenterologist. *N Engl J Med* 1992;326:825–827.

Sontag SJ. Rolling review: gastro-oesophageal reflux disease. *Aliment Pharmacol Ther* 1993;7:293–312.

CHAPTER 43

Inflammatory Bowel Disease

Brian G. Feagan, MD, FRCPC

The idiopathic inflammatory bowel diseases (IBD) consist of
Crohn's disease (CD), ulcerative colitis (UC) and ulcerative
proctitis (UP). CD may involve any part of the gastrointestinal
tract, while UC is restricted to the colon. UP is a variant of UC,
which involves less than 30 cm of the distal colon.

Investigations

- History:
  - diarrhea, abdominal pain, rectal bleeding and weight loss
    are the most important symptoms
  - presence of nocturnal diarrhea usually indicates "organic"
    pathology
  - extraintestinal manifestations (e.g., aphthous ulcers,
    arthritis, erythema nodosum, iritis, perianal disease, fever)
  - genetics: increased risk with family history, Ashkenazi
    Jews
  - previous endoscopic/radiologic test results
  - previous medical/surgical treatment

- Physical examination: abdominal tenderness, presence of
  abdominal mass, malnutrition, perianal disease (fistulae,
  abscess)
  - growth failure in children (chart height and weight, Tanner
    stage)
  - extraintestinal manifestations

- Precise diagnosis:
  - biopsy/histopathology, small bowel x-rays
  - presence of small bowel involvement, granulomata is
    pathognomonic for CD

- 10% of cases cannot be classified and are termed
  indeterminate colitis

- A definitive diagnosis is important since:
  - colectomy cures UC; CD recurs following surgery
  - differential responses to drug therapy (especially
    aminosalicylates)

- Precise anatomic localization is necessary for selecting drug
  therapy and planning surgery

- Laboratory tests:
  - measures of inflammation (WBC, Hgb, ESR, albumin)
  - stool cultures

Goals of Therapy

- To relieve symptoms and improve patients' quality of life
- To improve nutritional status and growth (children/adolescents)
- To prevent disease recurrence
- To prevent development of colon cancer (UC)

Therapeutic Choices (Table 1)

Therapy is determined by site and extent of disease, and the severity of symptoms.

Pharmacologic Choices

Management of IBD includes the use of aminosalicylates, corticosteroids, immunosuppressives, antibiotics, antidiarrheals and opioid analgesics.

Aminosalicylates

Preparations containing **5-aminosalicylic acid** (5-ASA) are formulated to release the drug at specific sites in the GI tract, since efficacy is dependent on luminal concentration. Salofalk, Mesasal and Pentasa release 5-ASA into the small bowel. Sulfasalazine, olsalazine and Asacol release 5-ASA primarily into the colon.

5-ASA has only modest efficacy in active CD (40% efficacy for induction of remission vs 30% with placebo) and is generally used in mild cases. Although clinical trials have evaluated only sulfasalazine and Pentasa for this indication, the other preparations are often used interchangeably.

Sulfasalazine has the least favorable adverse effect profile; however, many of these effects are minor and dose-related. The majority of these events (> 90%) are related to the sulfapyridine moiety which is not present in 5-ASA preparations. Oligospermia, reversible on withdrawal of sulfasalazine, has been reported. 5-ASA can be substituted, as male infertility has not been associated with its use.

Corticosteroids

Patients with a moderately severe exacerbation of CD are treated initially with **prednisone** 40 to 60 mg per day. In those with severe disease, hospitalization and **IV steroids** (e.g., hydrocortisone) may be necessary. Patients who respond to IV therapy are switched to prednisone once stabilized. The prednisone dose is then tapered as improvement occurs (total duration of therapy is 12 to 16 weeks).

Long-term use of corticosteroids is restricted to those unresponsive to other drugs. Patients must be made aware of potential side effects, and informed consent obtained. Osteoporosis is a concern with long-term therapy. Adequate calcium intake, smoking cessation, exercise and, in selected individuals, treatment with vitamin D and bisphosphonates are useful interventions. In addition, use of glucocorticoids is associated with avascular necrosis of the femoral head.

Budesonide is rapidly inactivated in the liver resulting in lower systemic bioavailability and a reduced effect on the hypothalamic-pituitary-adrenal axis. It is available as an oral controlled-release capsule for the treatment of terminal ileal/right sided colonic CD, and as an enema for use in UC. In clinical trials, response rates for oral budesonide are marginally less than those observed with prednisone for active CD (50 to 60% vs 70%); Cushing's syndrome occurs less frequently. Budesonide enemas are as effective as other steroid enemas, have a lower incidence of side effects, but are more costly.

Immunosuppressives

Azathioprine, **6-mercaptopurine (6-MP)**, or **methotrexate** are used in some refractory patients with CD to control symptoms or reduce the dose of prednisone. All immunosuppressive drugs have important side effects which must be considered (e.g., bone marrow suppression and cytopenias). Hypersensitivity pneumonitis and hepatotoxicity are associated with methotrexate. Pancreatitis occurs in approximately 3% of patients treated with azathioprine or 6-MP.

Antibiotics

Short courses (2 to 4 weeks) of **metronidazole** are useful in treating CD with perianal fistulae. It has a potent disulfiram-like effect if alcohol is ingested and neuropathy may occur with long-term use. The use of metronidazole during pregnancy should be avoided.

Antidiarrheals

Antidiarrheals should be used with caution and avoided in severe disease because of the risk of toxic megacolon. Diphenoxylate with atropine (Lomotil) is a combination of an opiate and an anticholinergic drug which can cause CNS side effects. Loperamide (Imodium) acts on both cholinergic and opiate receptors, but has a lower incidence of adverse effects than diphenoxylate.

Table 1: Drugs Used in the Treatment of Inflammatory Bowel Disease

Drug	Dosage		Comments	Cost*
Corticosteroids				
Injectable				
hydrocortisone – Solu-Cortef	300–400 mg/d IV		Adverse effects: acne, glucose intolerance, weight gain, hypertension, hypokalemia, osteoporosis, aseptic necrosis of femoral head, adrenal insufficiency with sudden cessation.	$$$
methylprednisolone – Solu-Medrol	300–400 mg/d IV		No advantage over hydrocortisone.	$$$$$
Oral				
prednisone – Deltasone, generics	30–60 mg/d PO (Q am)		Useful in moderately severe and severe UC and CD. No role in maintenance therapy.	$
budesonide – Entocort	9 mg/d PO (acute exacerbation) 3–6 mg/d PO (maintenance)		Controlled-release capsule for treating CD in the ileum and/or ascending colon. Rapidly metabolized, somewhat fewer adverse effects than conventional corticosteroids.	$$
Topical				
hydrocortisone – Cortenema, Cortifoam	80–100 mg QHS		Enemas effective in ulcerative proctitis (UP).	$$
betamethasone – Betnesol	5 mg QHS		Topical therapy, in general, has less severe adverse effects than systemic therapy.	$$
budesonide – Entocort	2 mg QHS			$$
tixocortol – Rectovalone	250 mg QHS			$$
Aminosalicylates				
Oral	Active (UC)	Maintenance (UC)		
sulfasalazine Salazopyrin, generics	≥ 4 g/d divided	2–3 g/d divided	All aminosalicylates are equally effective in UC. Sulfasalazine 4–8 g/d has shown moderate benefit in CD. Dose-related adverse effects of sulfasalazine: nausea, vomiting, diarrhea, anorexia, headache. Hypersensitivity reactions (rash, fever), aplastic anemia, oligospermia (reversible).	$
olsalazine Dipentum	> 1 g/d divided	1 g/d divided	Olsalazine: ↑ diarrhea, may be minimized by gradually increasing the dose.	$

Drug	Dose	Dose	Comments	Cost*
5-aminosalicylic acid			The value of 5-ASA as maintenance therapy in CD is controversial. Best evidence for Asacol 2.4 g/d and Pentasa 3 g/d. Pentasa has shown moderate benefit in active CD.	
Asacol	>1.6 g/d divided	0.8–1.6 g/d divided		$
Mesasal	>1.5 g/d divided	1–1.5 g/d divided		$
Pentasa	>2 g/d divided	1.5–2 g/d divided		$-$$
Salofalk	3–4 g/d divided	1–2 g/d divided		$
Topical			Enemas and suppositories effective in UP.	
Salofalk, Quintasa	Enema: 1–4 g/d			$$$
	Suppositories: 0.5–1 g/d			$
Immunosuppressives				
azathioprine ● Imuran	2.5 mg/kg/d PO		Common adverse effects with all: nausea, stomatitis, GI discomfort, diarrhea, anorexia.	$$
6-mercaptopurine ● Purinethol	100 mg/d PO		Major adverse effects with azathioprine and 6-MP: blood dyscrasias and hepatotoxicity.	$$
methotrexate ● Various	25 mg IM Q wk		Methotrexate is potentially hepatotoxic. Oral methotrexate has not shown efficacy in controlled trials.	$$$$
cyclosporine ● Sandimmune	4 mg/kg/d IV		Cyclosporine is nephrotoxic and causes hypertension, seizures.	$250

Legend: $ <$2 $$ $2–5 $$$ $5–10 $$$$ $10–20 $$$$$ > $20

● *Dosage adjustment may be required in renal impairment – see Appendix I.*

* *Cost of 1-day supply – includes drug cost only.*

Opioid Analgesics

Opioids depress GI motility, and chronic use may lead to narcotic bowel syndrome. The risk for habituation is also high, and in some individuals their use may worsen symptoms.

Codeine is useful for pain control and to decrease the number of bowel movements. The use of morphine or meperidine should be avoided; restrict use to a small number of severe patients.

Crohn's Disease

Therapeutic Choices (Figure 1)

Nonpharmacologic Choices

- Encourage the patient to stop smoking (limited evidence suggests smoking worsens CD).
- Nutritious diet; do not arbitrarily limit food groups. The goal is to ensure an adequate caloric intake. Nutritional supplements or parenteral nutrition may be necessary in selected patients who are malnourished.
- Surgery may be necessary to treat strictures, abscesses, fistulae or for patients refractory to medical management. Recurrence after surgery is almost universal, so conservative surgical management is favored.
- Psychological and social support is important, especially for adolescents.

Pharmacologic Choices (Table 1)

See previous general discussion of pharmacologic choices in IBD.

- **Corticosteroid** therapy is most effective for the induction of remission (70% response rate). Prednisone (40 to 60 mg/day) is the most commonly used drug.
- Chronic low-dose steroid therapy is *ineffective* for the maintenance of remission. However, some patients experience chronically active disease and may require continuous low-dose prednisone (10 to 15 mg/day) to suppress their symptoms.
- 5-ASA 4 g/day (Pentasa) or 6 to 8 g/day of sulfasalazine is only marginally effective for the induction of remission (approximately 40% response rate vs 30% with placebo) – mild cases only.
- The value of 5-ASA as a maintenance therapy for CD (in distinction to its use in UC) is controversial. Only a modest effect (20% 1-year reduction in relapse rate) is likely. (Consider for patients at high risk for relapse based on previously documented aggressive clinical course and requirement for previous surgery.)

Figure 1: **Management of Crohn's Disease**

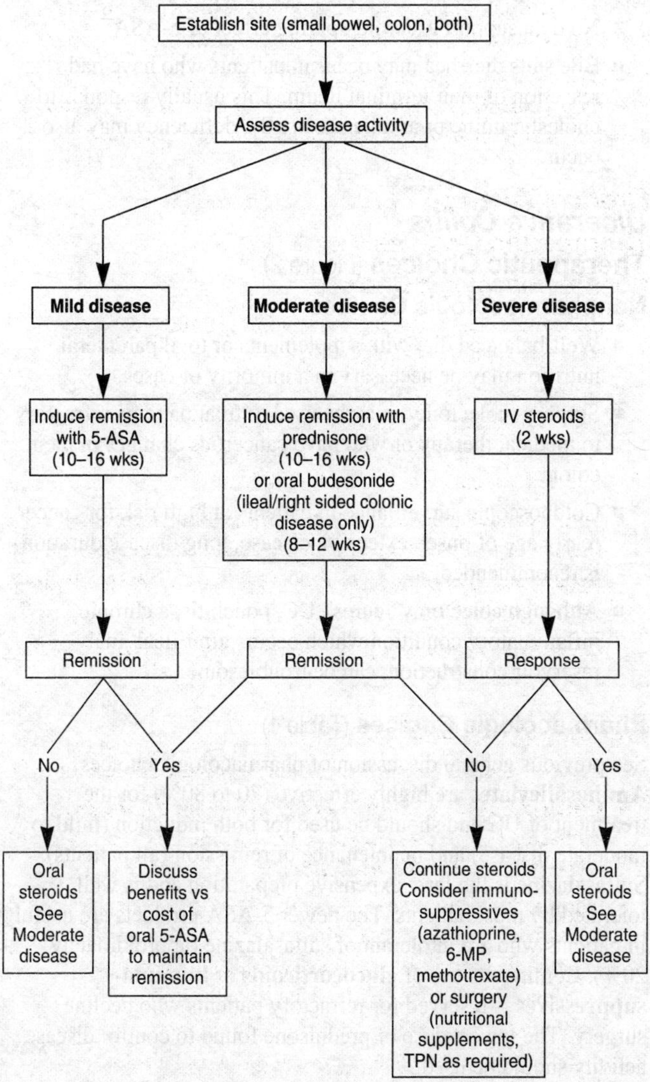

```
┌─────────────────────────────────────────────┐
│ Establish site (small bowel, colon, both)    │
└─────────────────────────────────────────────┘
                      │
                      ▼
┌─────────────────────────────────────────────┐
│          Assess disease activity             │
└─────────────────────────────────────────────┘
```

Mild disease	Moderate disease	Severe disease
Induce remission with 5-ASA (10–16 wks)	Induce remission with prednisone (10–16 wks) or oral budesonide (ileal/right sided colonic disease only) (8–12 wks)	IV steroids (2 wks)
Remission	Remission	Response

Mild disease / Remission — No: Oral steroids See Moderate disease

Mild disease / Remission — Yes: Discuss benefits vs cost of oral 5-ASA to maintain remission

Severe disease / Response — No: Continue steroids Consider immuno-suppressives (azathioprine, 6-MP, methotrexate) or surgery (nutritional supplements, TPN as required)

Severe disease / Response — Yes: Oral steroids See Moderate disease

- Patients who receive purine antimetabolites or methotrexate should use effective contraception since these drugs may be teratogenic.
- In pregnancy, methotrexate is absolutely contraindicated and purine antimetabolites are often discontinued (although this is controversial). Aminosalicylates and corticosteroids are safe and their use in pregnancy may continue if indicated.

Therapeutic Tips

- 5-ASA preparations rarely worsen symptoms.
- No data support a steroid-sparing effect of 5-ASA.
- Bile salts diarrhea may occur in patients who have had resection of their terminal ileum. This usually responds to cholestyramine or antidiarrheals. B_{12} deficiency may also occur.

Ulcerative Colitis
Therapeutic Choices (Figure 2)
Nonpharmacologic Choices

- Well-balanced diet with supplements or total parenteral nutrition may be necessary in a minority of cases.
- Surgery (colectomy) may be used to treat patients refractory to medical therapy or who have cancerous changes in their colon.
- Colonoscopic surveillance in patients at high risk for cancer (early age of onset, extensive disease, long disease duration) is recommended.
- Although colectomy "cures" UC, pouchitis, a chronic inflammatory condition which occurs after ileal-anal reservoir construction, can be troublesome.

Pharmacologic Choices (Table 1)

See previous general discussion of pharmacologic choices. **Aminosalicylates** are highly effective (70 to 80%) for the treatment of UC and should be used for both induction (mild to moderate disease) and maintenance of remission (all patients). Sulfasalazine is the least expensive preparation and is well tolerated by most patients. The newer 5-ASA products are useful in patients who are intolerant of sulfasalazine (approximately 20%). Continuous use of **glucocorticoids** or **immuno-suppressives** is reserved for refractory patients who decline surgery. The lowest dose of prednisone found to control disease activity should be used.

The efficacy of the **purine antimetabolites** in UC is less well established than in CD. **Methotrexate** has not proven to be effective for treatment of UC. The use of high dose **cyclosporine** in patients with severe UC should be considered investigational.

Therapeutic Tips

- Extreme caution should be used in prescribing narcotics and anticholinergic drugs in patients with active UC due to the

Figure 2: **Management of Ulcerative Colitis**

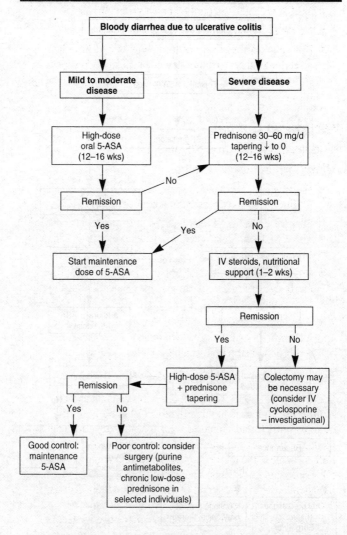

risk of toxic megacolon. Use only when all other alternatives have failed.

- **NB:** Since there is an increased incidence of colorectal carcinoma in patients with long-standing UC, colonoscopy should be performed to detect dysplastic changes in the colonic mucosa, beginning 10 years after diagnosis.

- Weak evidence suggests that folate supplementation may reduce the risk of colon cancer.

- Patients with severe colitis often will not tolerate tube feeds, due to diarrhea.

Figure 3: **Management of Ulcerative Proctitis**

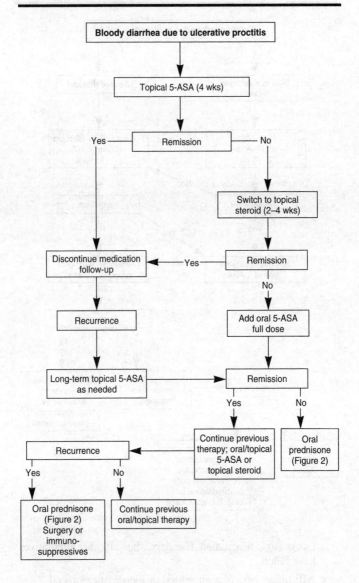

Ulcerative Proctitis
Therapeutic Choices (Figure 3)
Pharmacologic Choices (Table 1)

Given the limited extent of the inflammation (rectum/sigmoid colon), the focus is on topical therapy. **5-ASA** preparations (suppositories, enemas) administered at bedtime are the initial treatment of choice. Alternatively, topical **corticosteroids** can be used. If a response is not achieved with one of these strategies, switching to the other is advised.

If remission is not induced within 2 to 4 weeks, oral 5-ASA can be added. A patient unresponsive to these measures should be switched to prednisone, or rarely, IV steroids.

Patients brought into remission easily with a first episode (i.e., within 4 to 8 weeks) may have all medications discontinued. Follow-up is essential; patients with recurring symptoms should receive chronic topical maintenance therapy with 5-ASA.

Patients brought into remission with difficulty should be continued on long-term oral or topical 5-ASA preparations, or steroid enemas, without attempting discontinuation of therapy. Some patients require chronic treatment with low-dose prednisone. Colectomy may be necessary in a few cases, despite the limited extent of the disease.

Therapeutic Tips

- Topical therapy is preferred.
- A repeat sigmoidoscopy should be performed to ensure that the inflammation has not progressed to more extensive colitis.

Suggested Reading List

Feagan B, McDonald JWD, Rochon J, Fedorak R, Irvine EJ, Sutherland L, et al. Methotrexate for the treatment of Crohn's disease. *N Engl J Med* 1995;332:292–297.

Hanauer SB. Drug therapy: Inflammatory bowel disease. *N Engl J Med* 1996;334:841–848.

Lichtiger S, Present DH, Kornbluth A, Gelernt I, Bauer J, Galler G, et al. Cyclosporine in severe ulcerative colitis refractory to steroid therapy. *N Engl J Med* 1994;330:1841–1845.

Moore TL. Living with inflammatory bowel disease: Can you tell me about medication? *Can J Gastroenterol* 1992;6:235–239.

Pearson DC, May GR, Fick GH, Sutherland LR. Azathioprine and 6-mercaptopurine in Crohn's disease. A meta analysis. *Ann Intern Med* 1995;123(2):132–142.

Sutherland LR, May GR, Shaffer EA. Sulfasalazine revisited: a meta analysis of 5-aminosalicylic acid in the treatment of ulcerative colitis. *Ann Intern Med* 1993;118:540.

CHAPTER 44

Peptic Ulcer Disease and Upper Gastrointestinal Bleeding

Richard H. Hunt, FRCP, FRCP Ed, FRCPC, FACG

Peptic Ulcer Disease

The acid-related disorders include dyspepsia, gastroesophageal reflux disease (Chapter 42), duodenal and gastric ulcer, and NSAID-related gastroduodenal ulcer. It is now recognized that several of these conditions are complications of *Helicobacter pylori* infection.

Goals of Therapy

- To alleviate symptoms
- To accelerate healing of duodenal and gastric ulcer
- To prevent complications
- To prevent recurrence of ulceration
- To cure the disease

Investigations

- History to determine characteristic features including site, character and frequency of symptoms
  - determine periodicity of symptoms and their relationship to meals
  - identify aggravating factors (e.g., acid or fruit drinks)
  - determine ASA or NSAID use. NSAID ulceration and associated bleeding may occur in the absence of symptoms
- Physical examination is usually unhelpful although tenderness in the epigastrum may be present
  - exclude other abdominal conditions
  - examine stool for overt bleeding or test for fecal occult blood
- Consider referring for investigation patients with:
  - new onset of symptoms
  - age over 45 years
  - severe frequent and/or persistent symptoms
  - "alarm" symptoms (e.g., anorexia, vomiting, weight loss, anemia)
  - failed medical therapy
  - recurrent symptoms if previously not investigated endoscopically or radiologically

- **Upper GI endoscopy** is the best primary investigation for the above indications and has greater sensitivity and specificity than an upper GI barium series. Perform endoscopy to:
  - evaluate radiologic abnormalities, obtain biopsies to exclude malignancy, and confirm healing of gastric ulcer
  - obtain biopsy for determining the presence of *H. pylori* infection by rapid urease test or histology (at least 2 biopsies should be taken)
- **Upper GI barium** series may be useful when endoscopy is not available. Avoid when investigating patients with acute bleeding
- **Nonendoscopic tests for *H. pylori*** infection include serological assays and breath tests for urease activity
  - ^{14}C or ^{13}C urea breath tests (CUBT) and hospital-based serology tests (ELISA) have high sensitivity and specificity. Office-based serology tests are variable and can be less sensitive[1]
  - follow-up is essential for complicated or refractory ulcers. CUBT is the most appropriate test for confirming post-treatment eradication. Serology cannot detect active infection and should not be used since antibody titers take 6 months or more to drop by 50% and pre- and post-treatment serum must be tested together
  - both the rapid urease biopsy test and CUBT may be affected by the use of proton pump inhibitors, bismuth or antibiotics that suppress *H. pylori*, resulting in a false-negative result. These drugs should be stopped 1 week before testing

Therapeutic Choices (Figure 1)

Nonpharmacologic Choices

- Patients should avoid any foods that aggravate their symptoms.
- Smoking should be avoided since it reduces lower esophageal sphincter pressure, reduces mucosal blood flow and lowers mucosal defenses. Smoking increases the likelihood of ulcer recurrence in patients infected with *H. pylori*.
- Stress, traditionally considered to play a role in peptic ulcer disease (PUD), has never been shown in controlled trials to do so. However, stress is known to affect the immune system and may influence the inflammatory response to *H. pylori* in those infected. This needs to be explored.

---

[1] *Am J Med 1996;100(5A):35S–39S.*

Figure 1: **Management of Suspected Peptic Ulcers**

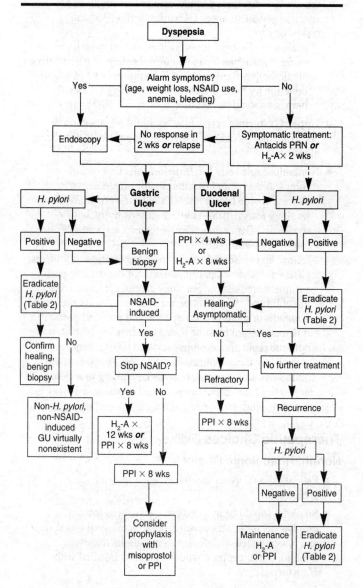

Abbreviations: GU = gastric ulcer; H₂-A = H₂-antagonist; PPI = proton pump inhibitor.
Adapted from: Shaffer EA. Peptic Ulcer Disease. In: Gray J, ed. Therapeutic Choices.
Ottawa: Canadian Pharmaceutical Association, 1995:311.

Pharmacologic Choices (Table 1)

Antacids have been shown in controlled trials to heal peptic ulcer; however, large and frequent doses are required. Now they are seldom used for anything more than symptom relief.

H$_2$-antagonists may be used as initial therapy for patients with dyspepsia, providing no alarm symptoms are present. There is no marked difference among available H$_2$-antagonists. They provide similar pain relief and have similar ulcer-healing profiles, despite slight differences in molar potency and antisecretory effects. About 75% of duodenal ulcers heal within 4 weeks and about 85% after 8 weeks. Gastric ulcers generally take longer to heal and similar healing rates require 8 and 12 weeks respectively.

Proton pump inhibitors (PPI) include omeprazole, lansoprazole and pantoprazole. They provide significantly faster symptom relief and significantly higher healing rates than H$_2$-antagonists in duodenal and gastric ulcer. Approximately 80% of duodenal ulcers will heal after 2 weeks and over 90% after 4 weeks treatment. Gastric ulcers again take longer to respond, with 80% healed after 4 weeks and 90% within 8 weeks.

H. pylori Eradication Therapy

H. pylori infection is recognized as the causative agent in 80 to 85% of DU and 60 to 80% of GU, especially when NSAIDs are not being taken. Effective eradication of *H. pylori* infection virtually abolishes ulcer recurrence, thus effecting cure of the ulcer diathesis. Reinfection rates are about 1% per year. Several Canadian studies have shown that cure of *H. pylori* infection in ulcer patients is more cost-effective than long-term maintenance therapy with an H$_2$-antagonist.

Three *H. pylori* eradication regimens are now recognized as the most effective, and have been endorsed by the Canadian Consensus Conference on *Helicobacter pylori* Infection (Table 2). These treatments, when complied with, provide eradication rates in excess of 80% by intention to treat (ITT) analysis. Compliance is often better with PPI-based regimens. Avoid regimens containing metronidazole in areas with known metronidazole resistance, such as inner city areas, and in young females and patients who have previously taken the drug.

In the event of treatment failure, patients should be referred to a gastroenterologist who will usually consider changing the regimen to avoid metronidazole resistance (seen in 25 to over 40% of patients in some Canadian studies).

Treatments under evaluation include ranitidine bismuth citrate (Pylorid) combined with clarithromycin and either amoxicillin or metronidazole, and the classic bismuth triple therapy (Table 2) combined with a PPI.

Table 1: Drugs Used in Peptic Ulcer Disease

Drug	Dosage		Adverse Effects	Drug Interactions	Cost*
Antacids Numerous aluminum hydroxide–magnesium hydroxide combinations	30 mL (regular strength) 1 h PC and HS		Constipation, diarrhea.	Antacids ↓ bioavailability of digoxin, tetracycline, quinolone antibiotics; separate dosing by 2 h.	$–$$
H$_2$-antagonists	**Treatment†**	**Maintenance‡**			
cimetidine Tagamet, generics	800 mg QHS	400 mg PM	Diarrhea, constipation, headache, fatigue, confusion (most likely in elderly and those with poor renal function); cardiac effects, rash. Cimetidine: gynecomastia, impotence (rare).	**Cimetidine** ↓ cytochrome P-450 metabolism of several agents (e.g., warfarin, phenytoin, theophylline) — use another H$_2$-antagonist; **ranitidine** has minor effect.	$
ranitidine Zantac, generics	300 mg QHS	150 mg PM			$$
famotidine Pepcid, generics	40 mg QHS	20 mg PM			$$
nizatidine Axid	300 mg QHS	150 mg PM			$$$
Proton Pump Inhibitors					
omeprazole Losec	Treatment: 20 mg/d Refractory: 40 mg/d × 8 wks NSAID-induced: 40 mg/d × 8 wks		Abdominal pain, nausea, headache.	May interfere with cytochrome P-450 metabolized agents (e.g., warfarin, phenytoin, theophylline).	$$$$ (20 mg × 30 d)
lansoprazole Prevacid	Treatment: 15 mg/d 2–4 wks for DU 4–8 wks for GU		Diarrhea, headache, constipation, abnormal laboratory tests.	Metabolized via the cytochrome P-450 system. No significant interactions with warfarin, antipyrine, indomethacin, ASA, phenytoin, prednisone, antacids, diazepam.	$$

Drug	Dose	Adverse Effects	Drug Interactions/Comments	Cost*
pantoprazole Pantoloc	Treatment: 40 mg/d 2–4 wks for DU 4–8 wks for GU	Diarrhea, headache, dizziness, pruritus.	Metabolized via the cytochrome P-450 system. No interactions with antipyrine, diazepam, phenytoin, nifedipine, theophylline, warfarin, digoxin, oral contraceptives or antacids.	$$$$
misoprostol Cytotec	Treatment: 200 µg QID	Diarrhea (dose-related), abdominal cramps, flatulence. **Contraindicated in pregnancy** – abortifacient.		$$$
sucralfate⬤ Sulcrate, generics	Treatment: 2 g BID Maintenance: 1 g BID	Constipation, aluminum absorption. (Avoid in renal failure.)	Intraluminal drug binding may ↓ absorption of antibiotics, ketoconazole, warfarin, digoxin, NSAIDs, theophylline; separate dosing by 2 h.	$

* Cost of 30-day (treatment dosages) supply – includes drug cost only.
  Legend: $ < $20 $$ $20–40 $$$ $40–60 $$$$ $60–80
  Adapted from: Shaffer EA. Peptic Ulcer Disease. In: Gray J, ed. Therapeutic Choices. Ottawa: Canadian Pharmaceutical Association, 1995:314.

† Split treatment dose for gastric ulcer.
‡ Dose given in the evening.
π Not to exceed 20 mg/d in hepatic impairment.
⬤ Dosage adjustment may be required in renal impairment – see Appendix I.

Table 2: *H. pylori* Eradication Regimens

Regimen	Dosage	Treatment Period	Cost*
PPI†	BID	7 days	$$$$
clarithromycin	500 mg BID		
amoxicillin	1 g BID		
PPI†	BID	7 days	$$$$
clarithromycin	500 mg BID		
metronidazole	500 mg BID		
bismuth subsalicylate	2 tabs QID	14 days	$
metronidazole	250 mg QID		
tetracycline ☙	500 mg QID		

† *Proton pump inhibitor = lansoprazole 30 mg BID or omeprazole 20 mg BID or pantoprazole 40 mg BID.*
* *Cost per treatment period – includes drug cost only.*
Legend: $ < $20 $$ $20–40 $$$ $40–60 $$$$ $60–80
☙ *Dosage adjustment may be required in renal impairment – see Appendix I.*

NSAID-associated Ulcers

ASA and NSAIDs may cause gastrointestinal mucosal damage, erosions, ulcers and delay ulcer healing when specific treatments are given. They may cause pre-existing ulcers to bleed.

For NSAID-induced ulcers (Figure 1), the NSAID should be discontinued and *H. pylori* treated, if present. If NSAID use must be continued, a PPI should be considered.

Preventive therapy is appropriate for high-risk patients (e.g., history of ulcer disease, cotherapy with anticoagulants or corticosteroids) taking NSAIDs who cannot stop the drug or reduce the dose. **Misoprostol,** a cytoprotective agent, will protect from both GU and DU, and reduce ulcer complications. Adverse effects include abdominal cramping and loose stools, which may limit compliance in the elderly, especially as QID dosing is required. Use of lower doses is better tolerated but may diminish efficacy. **PPIs** will reduce the risk of both GU and DU. However, studies have not been undertaken to show that they reduce ulcer complications. **H$_2$-antagonists** will reduce the risk of DU but high doses (e.g., famotidine 40 mg BID) are required for GU prevention.

Long-term Maintenance Therapy

H$_2$-antagonists and proton pump inhibitors have reduced ulcer recurrence and the need for surgery over the past 20 years. However, with the acceptance of *H. pylori* as the key factor in ulcerogenesis, long-term maintenance therapy is only required for the small number of patients in whom eradication therapy has failed or those with a history of peptic ulcer who are taking

NSAIDs long term. Studies are underway to determine whether eradication of *H. pylori* infection, when present in patients taking NSAIDs, will reduce or abolish the risk of taking these drugs.

Upper Gastrointestinal Bleeding

Bleeding from the upper GI tract may be acute or chronic and arise from a lesion in the esophagus, stomach or duodenum. Commonly encountered lesions include esophageal varices, esophageal ulceration, esophageal carcinoma, gastric erosions or ulcer, gastric malignancy and duodenal erosions or ulcer. Less common conditions include Mallory-Weiss lesions, vascular abnormalities and unusual malignancies.

Goals of Therapy

- To resuscitate the patient and restore circulating blood volume
- To assess the severity of blood loss
- To determine the site of blood loss
- To arrest active bleeding
- To prevent recurrence of bleeding through specific therapy

Investigations

- **History** to obtain information about presentation (e.g., hematemesis and/or melena or bloody stools). The volume and color of blood can be helpful in considering magnitude and location of blood loss. Determine the presence of symptoms suggestive of anemia or compromised circulation (e.g., collapse, syncope, dyspnea or chest pain). It is important to determine any history of ASA or NSAID ingestion
- **Physical examination** to determine cardiovascular status, including hypotension and tachycardia, which reflect hypovolemia. A nasogastric tube should be passed and aspiration undertaken to confirm upper GI bleeding. However, it is possible to have serious bleeding from the duodenum and a negative gastric aspirate
- **Routine blood tests** include CBC, PT, PTT, serum electrolytes and BUN
- An **ECG** may be required in unstable and elderly patients
- **Endoscopy** should be undertaken once the patient is stable (i.e., systolic blood pressure > 100 mm Hg and pulse rate < 100). Provides accurate diagnosis and helpful prognostic information in about 90% of patients. Iced water lavage

may be required for good visualization but does not arrest ongoing hemorrhage. If a peptic ulcer is seen, the presence of a visible vessel, oozing blood or a sentinel clot in the base of the ulcer are strong predictors of a further bleed. These are also indications for making an endoscopic intervention to arrest bleeding using injection, thermal or banding techniques

■ **Radiologic investigations** are confined to radionuclide scanning after the injection of labeled red cells or angiography. Barium studies should not be undertaken in the acute stage, since barium will occlude the view for any subsequent endoscopic, scanning or angiographic studies and takes several days to clear the gut

Therapeutic Choices

Peptic Ulcers

No pharmacologic agents have been shown to alter the acute outcome of upper gastrointestinal bleeding, despite the widespread use of H_2-antagonists for this condition.

Nonpharmacologic Choices

Nonpharmacologic treatments are usually undertaken at the time of endoscopy. The most common approach is to inject **saline, epinephrine** or **sclerosing agents** (e.g., ethanolamine or polidocanol). Injection of clotting factors remains experimental, and the use of tissue adhesives (e.g., Krazy Glue) becomes expensive if the glue adheres to the endoscope.

Thermal techniques are widely used and include the heater probe, electrocautery or laser therapy. These techniques arrest active bleeding, reduce rebleeding and have been shown to reduce mortality.

Pharmacologic Choices

Acid suppression has been studied most, but even IV **proton pump inhibitors** do not reduce transfusion requirements, rebleeding or mortality. No benefit has been seen from reducing splanchnic blood flow with **vasopressin**, **somatostatin** or its analogue, **octreotide**. However, it is logical to start treatment with an antisecretory drug when PU has been diagnosed. Successful eradication of *H. pylori* in infected patients virtually abolishes the risk of ulcer rebleeding in contrast to untreated patients who have a 30 to 40% risk of further bleeding in the subsequent year. Therefore, long-term antisecretory maintenance treatment is not required in ulcer patients who are successfully cured of infection.

Bleeding Stress Ulcer

Superficial gastric erosions predominantly affecting the fundus of the stomach were common with severe trauma, sepsis, burns and head injuries. They are much less common now because of improvements in resuscitation and prevention of shock. Patients with these conditions are still at high risk if they require ventilation or are seriously ill and need support for long periods.

Prophylaxis is more effective than treatment and should be considered for critically ill patients, especially those with a coagulopathy or requiring ventilation. IV H_2-antagonists are commonly used, despite some evidence to suggest that nosocomial infections are more common than with **sucralfate**. Antacid therapy has been superceded by these two approaches.

Esophageal Varices
Nonpharmacologic Choices

Principal approaches are nonpharmacologic and involve **endoscopic sclerotherapy** or **band ligation**. Sclerotherapy is most widely used, with ethanolamine, absolute alcohol, polidocanol, or sodium tetradecyl sulfate being of equal efficacy. Recently, band ligation has become increasingly popular. It is as effective as injection techniques and may be associated with fewer complications (e.g., esophageal ulceration or stricture).

Either injection or banding is effective in arresting active hemorrhage, but no benefit has been shown for prophylactic treatment of patients with varices that have never bled.

Two other approaches rely on establishing a shunt between the portal and systemic circulations. **Transjugular intrahepatic portosystemic shunting** (TIPS) avoids open surgery by the passage of a guidewire through the jugular vein to the hepatic vein under radiologic screening. A small stent is then advanced over the guidewire to provide the shunt. This is effective in reducing the portal pressure and variceal bleeding, but hepatic encephalopathy may occur and long-term results are not well established. The second approach is **surgical**: a portocaval shunt may be performed or esophageal transection undertaken with devascularization of the esophagus and proximal stomach.

Pharmacologic Choices

Pharmacologic treatments are used to reduce portal pressure and inhibit gastric acid secretion, which is considered logical after injection sclerotherapy or banding. These approaches have not been shown to improve survival.

Octreotide, an analogue of somatostatin, is given as a 50 μg bolus injection followed by infusion of 25 to 50 μg/hour for at least 24 hours after bleeding stops, and up to 2 days. Alternatively, **vasopressin** may be given IV in a dose of 0.4 units/min for 2 hours or 20 units in 20 mL 5% dextrose over 20 minutes, and maintained at 0.4 units/min for up to 2 days. Vasopressin may cause ischemic complications, including myocardial infarction or peripheral ischemia, which may be partly avoided by giving nitroglycerin.

Beta-blockers have been widely studied and are of use prophylactically in preventing an initial bleed or reducing the risk of recurrent bleeding. Hence, they are indicated following a bleed and in patients with large varices who may never have bled. A recent meta-analysis concluded that beta-blockers reduced the incidence of rebleeding by 21%, mortality by 5.4% and death from bleeding by 7.4%.[2]

Pharmacoeconomic Considerations

Jeffrey A. Johnson, PhD

The cost-effectiveness of the therapeutic choices for ulcer therapy have been extensively evaluated in Canada and other countries. In general, the results of available studies are comparable, with *H. pylori* eradication regimens being clearly the dominant and the most cost-effective strategy when compared to treating only the acute ulcer episode or using maintenance H_2-antagonists to prevent ulcer recurrence. Of the various eradication regimens, bismuth triple therapy plus H_2-antagonist regimens are less expensive than omeprazole-antibiotic regimens, but may also be less effective in terms of the length of disease-free period (O'Brien et al., 1996). Important aspects of the different regimens that should be considered are the local metronidazole resistance rates, compliance, and eradication rates. Where metronidazole resistance rates are low, the relative cost-effectiveness of bismuth triple therapy would increase; compliance is a concern, however, with patients taking up to 18 tablets a day for 2 weeks. When metronidazole resistance is high, or where poor compliance with the complicated bismuth triple therapy plus H_2-antagonist regimen is anticipated, omeprazole-antibiotic regimens would be even more cost-effective.

Suggested Reading

O'Brien G, Goeree R, Mohamed AH, Hunt R. Cost-effectiveness of Helicobacter pylori eradication for the long-term management of duodenal ulcer in Canada. Arch Intern Med 1995;155:1958–1964.

O'Brien B, Goeree R, Hunt R, Wilkinson J, Levine M, Willan A. Cost-effectiveness of alternative therapies for the long-term management of peptic ulcer disease. Ottawa: Canadian Coordinating Office for Health Technology Assessment (CCOHTA), 1996.

Vakil N, Fennerty MB. Cost-effectiveness of treatment regimens for the eradication of Helicobacter pylori in duodenal ulcer. Am J Gastroenterol 1996;91:239.

---

[2] *Hepatology* 1997;21:63–70.

Suggested Reading List

Brunner G, Luna P, Thiesemann C. Drugs for pH control in upper gastrointestinal bleeding. *Aliment Pharmacol Ther* 1995;9(Suppl 1):47–50.

Cook DJ. Risk factors for gastrointestinal bleeding in critically ill patients. *N Engl J Med* 1994;330:377–381.

Cutler AF. Testing for Helicobacter pylori in clinical practice. *Am J Med* 1996;100(5A):35S–39S.

Huang JQ, Hunt RH. Review: eradication of Helicobacter pylori. Problems and recommendations. *Gastroenterol Hepatol* 1997;12(8):590–598.

Huang JQ, Hunt RH. A clinician's view of strategies for preventing NSAID-induced gastrointestinal ulcers. *Inflammopharmacology* 1996;4:17–30.

Hunt RH. Diagnosis and treatment of gastrointestinal bleeding: When, with what and by whom? *Eur J Gastroenterol Hepatol* 1990;2:69–110.

CHAPTER 45

Benign Prostatic Hyperplasia

Richard W. Norman, MD, FRCSC

Goals of Therapy

- To improve or abolish symptoms
- To reduce the risk of surgical intervention
- To prevent the sequelae of long-term bladder outlet obstruction (urinary tract infections, bladder stones, hydronephrosis)

Investigations

- Thorough history with special attention to:
  - obstructive (weak/interrupted stream, dribbling, hesitancy, straining) and nonobstructive (nocturia, frequency, urgency) symptoms
  - onset and progression of symptoms and degree of inconvenience
  - details of urethral infection, injury or instrumentation
  - episodes of urinary tract infection, hematuria or urinary retention
- Physical examination:
  - abdomen (bladder distension, flank tenderness)
  - external genitalia (phimosis, meatal stenosis, urethral mass/induration)
  - digital rectal examination (DRE) (documentation of prostate size, consistency, symmetry and tenderness)
- Laboratory tests:
  - urinalysis (and urine culture if pyuria)
  - serum creatinine
  - prostate specific antigen (PSA) (optional and controversial but generally recommended when a diagnosis of prostate cancer would alter treatment in otherwise healthy men between 50 and 70 years of age)
  - symptom score (recommended)
- Other diagnostic tests occasionally required when the history is not clear, there are abnormalities of the physical examination or laboratory tests, or the response to treatment is unsatisfactory:
  - cystoscopy
  - urodynamic studies
  - renal/bladder/transrectal ultrasonography
  - IV pyelography

Figure 1: **Management of Benign Prostatic Hyperplasia**

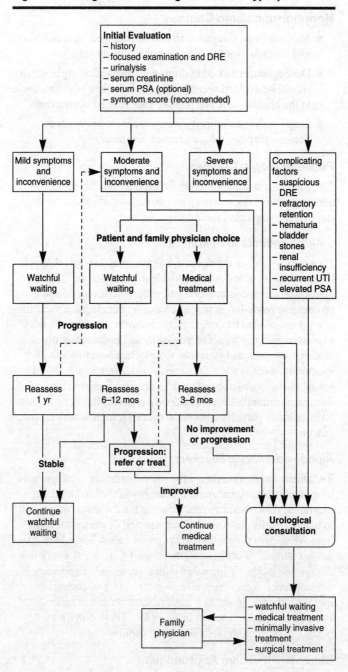

Abbreviations: DRE = digital rectal examination; PSA = prostate specific antigen.

Therapeutic Choices (Figure 1)

Nonpharmacologic Choices

- Minimal or no symptoms should be managed by reassurance and watchful waiting (i.e., regular reassessment).
- Decongestants and other drugs with alpha adrenergic activity should be avoided because they can stimulate smooth muscle in the bladder neck and prostate and increase obstruction.
- Drugs with anticholinergic activity should be avoided because they can reduce detrusor contractility.

Pharmacologic Choices

The 5 alpha-reductase inhibitor, finasteride, and the alpha$_1$ adrenergic blockers, terazosin and doxazosin, are all useful in improving symptoms (Table 1).

5 Alpha-reductase Inhibitors

Finasteride inhibits the enzyme 5 alpha-reductase, which blocks the metabolism of testosterone to dihydrotestosterone. The net effect is a decrease in intraprostatic dihydrotestosterone and a progressive reduction in prostatic volume. This reduces the static component of bladder outlet obstruction over a period of weeks to months and may be accompanied by an improvement in urinary flow rates and symptom scores. Because of its site specificity, there is a low incidence of side effects (e.g., 3 to 4% sexual dysfunction) and little risk of drug interactions. Finasteride decreases serum PSA levels by approximately 50% in men with BPH and may partially suppress serum PSA in men with prostate cancer.

Alpha$_1$-adrenergic Blockers

Terazosin and **doxazosin** are the most commonly used agents to block alpha$_1$ adrenergic muscular activity in the bladder neck, prostate and prostatic capsule, reducing the dynamic component to bladder outlet obstruction. Over a period of weeks, this may improve urinary flow rates and symptom scores. Since both drugs cause systemic vasodilatation, they must be started at a very low dosage and gradually increased until symptomatic improvement or intolerance occurs. Side effects in 10 to 15% of patients include asthenia, headaches, nasal congestion and dizziness. Postural hypotension occurs in about 4%. These drugs may potentiate other antihypertensive medications.

Minimally Invasive Approaches

- Long-term catheter drainage is appropriate for patients who are not candidates for any other intervention.

Other options under investigation include:

- Urethral stents
  - both temporary and permanent are used in investigative protocols.
- Thermotherapy
  - intraurethral thermotherapy shows promise, but long-term assessment of efficacy is lacking.
- Transurethral needle ablation (TUNA) of the prostate
  - intraprostatic placement of needle electrode via urethral route allows heating and necrosis of tissue, but confirmation of long-term benefits is lacking.

Surgical Approaches

While transurethral resection of the prostate (TURP) and retropubic prostatectomy are traditional means of dealing with an enlarged and obstructing prostate gland, evidence is accumulating that transurethral incision of the prostate and laser prostatectomy are useful in some patients.

- Transurethral resection
  - most effective treatment for symptomatic BPH and one against which other treatments should be compared.
  - may cause long-term side effects such as impotence, retrograde ejaculation and urethral strictures.
- Retropubic prostatectomy
  - required when the prostate is very enlarged or other bladder pathology requires concomitant attention; similar success and side effects to TURP.
- Transurethral incision of the prostate (TUIP)
  - useful for small prostates; associated with a lower incidence of retrograde ejaculation than TURP.
- Laser prostatectomy
  - technology allows transurethral coagulation or vaporization of the prostate on an outpatient basis; short-term data encouraging, but long-term data needed.

Therapeutic Tips

- Patients with minimum symptoms that do not interfere with their normal activities should be managed by watchful waiting and regular follow-up.
- Patients starting to develop progressive symptoms or moderate inconvenience are candidates for pharmacologic intervention.
- Side effects of alpha$_1$-adrenergic blockers can be reduced by taking at bedtime.

Table 1: Drugs Used in Benign Prostatic Hyperplasia

Drug	Dosage	Adverse Effects	Comments	Cost*
5α-Reductase Inhibitors				
finasteride Proscar	5 mg daily	Sexual dysfunction (3-4%). Decreased PSA.	Maximal response seen in 6 months or more.	$$$$
α₁-Adrenergic Blockers				
terazosin Hytrin	1-10 mg QHS	Postural hypotension (4%). In 10-15% of patients: asthenia, headaches, nasal congestion, dizziness.	Dose titrated weekly to desired response. Maximal response seen in 2-4 weeks or more.	$$-$$$
doxazosin Cardura	1-12 mg QHS		Drug interactions. May potentiate other antihypertensives.	$$-$$$$

* Cost of 30-day supply – includes drug cost only.
Legend: $ < $15 $$ $15-30 $$$ $30-45 $$$$ > $45

- Preliminary evaluation of combination therapy with both classes of drugs shows no additive benefit.
- There is evidence that finasteride is most effective in men with large prostates and may not be appropriate for men with small prostates.
- Drug therapy should be continued indefinitely since symptoms recur when medication is stopped.
- Long-term benefits and risks of medical management are unknown.

Pharmacoeconomic Considerations

Jeffrey A. Johnson, PhD

The clinical and economic impact of different treatment options for BPH were recently reviewed and evaluated by the Canadian Coordinating Office for Health Technology Assessment (CCOHTA). The focus of the evaluation was finasteride, compared to TURP and watchful waiting. The results of this review indicated that the relative cost effectiveness of the treatment options is dependent on two main factors: life expectancy and severity of symptoms. For men with mild symptoms, watchful waiting is considered the most cost-effective option. For patients with moderate or severe symptoms, and life expectancy less than 3 years, finasteride is the less expensive option. For patients with life expectancy longer than 4 years, finasteride provides a favorable cost-effectiveness ratio only in patients with moderate symptoms, when compared to surgery or watchful waiting. For patients with severe symptoms, however, using finasteride is likely more expensive than surgery in the long run, and with poorer results.

Unfortunately, no studies are available that evaluate the economic impact of alpha-blockers in the management of BPH. While recent clinical studies suggest that finasteride is most effective in men with large prostates, alpha-blockers work in men with small or large prostates. Alpha-blockers are more effective than finasteride during the first year of treatment, but only finasteride has been shown to induce regression of the gland and offer increased efficacy over time.

Overall, it is likely that the economic cost of BPH treatment will continue to increase due to increased use of both drug therapies. The magnitude of the increase will depend on the degree to which medical therapy substitutes, rather than simply delays, surgical intervention. This will depend on what percentage of men begin long-term therapy, and at what age. At present, the answers to these questions are not available.

Suggested Reading

Baladi, J-F Cost-effectiveness and cost-utility analyses of finasteride therapy for the treatment of benign prostatic hyperplasia. Ottawa, ON: Canadian Coordinating Office for Health Technology Assessment, 1995.

Eri LM, Tveter KJ. Treatment of benign prostatic hyperplasia. A pharmaco-economic perspective. Drugs & Aging 1997;10:107–118.

Suggested Reading List

Agency for Health Care Policy and Research. Benign prostatic hyperplasia: diagnosis and treatment. Rockville, MD: United States Department of Health and Human Services, 1994. Publication No. 94-0582.

Boyle P, Gould AL, Roehrborn CG. Prostate volume predicts outcome of treatment of benign prostatic hyperplasia with finasteride: meta-analysis of randomized clinical trials. *Urology* 1996;48:398–405.

Lepor H, Williford WO, Barry MJ, et al. The efficacy of terazosin, finasteride, or both in benign prostatic hyperplasia. *N Eng J Med* 1996;335:533–538.

Nickel JC, Fradet Y, Boake RC, et al. Efficacy and safety of finasteride therapy for benign prostatic hyperplasia: results of a 2-year randomized controlled trial (the PROSPECT study). *Can Med Assoc J* 1996;155:1251–1259.

Nickel JC, Norman RW. BPH – A physician's guide to care and counselling. Montreal: Grosvenor House, 1993.

Norman RW, Nickel JC, Fish D, et al. "Prostate-related symptoms" in Canadian men 50 years of age or older: prevalence and relationship among symptoms. *Br J Urol* 1994;74:542–550.

CHAPTER 46

Urinary Incontinence and Enuresis

S.A. Awad, MB, ChB, FRCSC and R.D. Schwarz, MD, FRCSC

Incontinence

Goals of Therapy

- To achieve symptomatic relief of urinary symptoms
- To increase functional capacity of the bladder

Definitions

Overflow incontinence is the leakage of urine due to an over-distended bladder, commonly caused by outlet obstruction (e.g., prostatic hyperplasia) or neurogenic causes (e.g., multiple sclerosis).

Stress incontinence is loss of urine due to an increase in intra-abdominal pressure (e.g., cough, exercise). It is more common in women. Weakness in pelvic musculature (e.g., due to childbirth) is the primary cause.

Urge incontinence is leakage of moderate to large amounts of urine due to inability to delay voiding when an urge is perceived. Causes include bladder wall hyperactivity or instability and CNS disorders (e.g., parkinsonism, stroke).

Functional incontinence is loss of urine because of the inability to get to a toilet. Some causes include physical or cognitive disabilities and environmental barriers. It may also occur in those with a normal neuromuscular anatomy whose mechanism of voiding is functionally disturbed.

Developmental or maturational incontinence is the involuntary loss of urine in people with no uropathy or neuropathy whose control has not yet fully developed.

Investigations

- History and physical examination:
  - to determine type of incontinence
  - to rule out fistula (in women), neurologic lesions, congenital anomalies, bladder infection or other forms of cystitis, bladder cancer, gynecologic disorders, previous pelvic radiation

Figure 1: **Management of Stress Incontinence in Women**

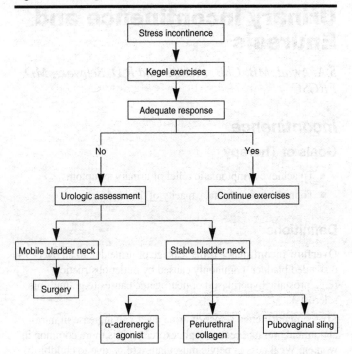

– to identify reversible/correctable causes in the elderly (e.g., medications, constipation, inadequate or restricted access to washrooms, delirium, depression)

- Laboratory tests:
  – urinalysis, urine culture and possibly cystoscopy

- A time/volume voiding diary or a cystometrogram helps to demonstrate reduced bladder capacity in urge incontinence. The latter also establishes diminished bladder compliance or instability

Stress Incontinence (Figure 1)

Therapeutic Choices

Nonpharmacologic Choices

- **Kegel exercise**s should be the initial therapy. The exercises involve tightening followed by relaxation of pelvic floor (perineal) muscles 10 to 15 times consecutively, 3 to 4 times a day.

- Bladder neck suspension **surgery** to correct bladder neck prolapse may be indicated.

Pharmacologic Choices (Table 1)

Pharmacotherapy has a limited role. Alpha-adrenergic agents are used in females with no significant bladder neck prolapse or in patients with mild stress incontinence after surgery (e.g., bladder neck suspension). These agents may also be beneficial in males with postprostatectomy incontinence. **Phenylpropanolamine** seems to be more effective than pseudoephedrine possibly because of its prolonged action.

It has been postulated that **estrogen** supplementation in post-menopausal women may improve urethral mucosa coaptation and increase vascularity and tone. A meta-analysis revealed a favorable effect of estrogen on incontinence in postmenopausal women.

Therapeutic Tips

- If drug therapy is effective, patients will usually improve in 1 to 2 weeks.

Urge Incontinence

Therapeutic Choices

Nonpharmacologic Choices

- A voiding routine should be established in the elderly.

Pharmacologic Choices (Table 1)

Pharmacotherapy is the first-line treatment for urge incontinence with no underlying cause (e.g., in idiopathic detrusor overactivity, more common in females). Drug therapy also seems to be effective in patients with partial neurologic lesions (e.g., multiple sclerosis) but not in complete lesions (e.g., following spinal cord injury); and in chronic cystitis not secondary to bacterial infection. Drugs with **anticholinergic plus smooth muscle relaxant** effects are most effective. They act by increasing the functional capacity of the bladder, partially blocking the detrusor reflex or increasing bladder compliance. Side effects can frequently limit treatment.

Therapeutic Tips

- A satisfactory response is achieved in only about 50 to 60% of patients, even with careful screening and accurate diagnosis.
- Several weeks are required to achieve maximum effect. If no subjective improvement occurs after 4 to 6 weeks, the drug should be discontinued.

Enuresis

Goals of Therapy

- To manage symptoms
- To reassure the family and to provide advice

Definitions

Daytime wetting in children under 7 years of age is usually related to delayed neurologic maturation of the conscious sensation of bladder fullness and cortical inhibition of detrusor contractions. The episodic wetting is sometimes associated with squatting or urgency.

Nocturnal enuresis refers to sleep wetting. The causes are still being debated, and treatments are empirical.

Investigations

- History and physical examination to exclude:
  - *acute cystitis:* sudden change of voiding pattern, confirmed with urinalysis and culture and sensitivity
  - *posterior urethral valves* in boys: an obstructive voiding pattern
  - *urethral or vaginal ectopic ureter* in girls: void normally but are always damp or wet
  - *occult neuropathy:* usually have bowel dysfunction and show abnormal perineal sensation and/or anal sphincter reflexes
  - *female epispadias or cecoureterocele* (rare): determined by introital exam
  - *stool holders* with urinary symptoms: bladder symptoms improve with proper bowel management (often a "hidden" symptom)
- Diagnostic imaging is **not** indicated in wetters with negative history and physical. Urodynamic evaluation or imaging may be considered in children unresponsive to or intolerant of drug therapy

Therapeutic Choices (Figure 2)

Treatment, if any, is based on the child's social and developmental indications. Often the knowledge that enuresis is a common problem coupled with an understanding that the child is not "ill" or "at risk" reassures the parent that no treatment is required. Older children may have legitimate psychosocial indications for treatment.

Figure 2: **Management of Daytime and Sleep Wetting in Children**

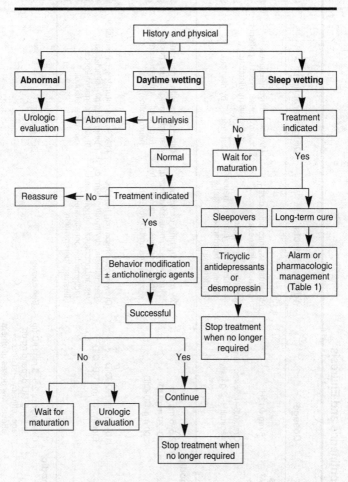

Nonpharmacologic Choices

- **Behavior modification** using a time-void schedule with rewards for successful toileting may be tried.
- **Alarms** (e.g., Palco or Nitone) serve as a learning tool that, with time and effort, can free the child entirely of symptoms.

Pharmacologic Choices (Table 1)

If treatment is appropriate for day wetting, a combination of pharmacologic and behavior modification techniques may be used. The anticholinergic/antispasmodic drugs can be tried at very low doses and titrated up to efficacy without side effects. Occasionally, the child will not respond to this plan or will have

Table 1: **Drug Therapy of Urinary Incontinence and Enuresis**

Type of Incontinence	Drug	Dosage	Adverse Effects	Drug Interactions	Cost*
Stress	**Alpha-adrenergic Agonists** *phenylpropanolamine* – Entex LA[†]	75 mg Q12H	Nervousness, insomnia, dizziness, restlessness.	MAOIs, antihypertensives, neuroleptics; avoid in patients on thyroid medications.	$$
	Conjugated Estrogens[‡] Premarin, generics	Oral: 0.3–1.25 mg daily Vaginal: 1–2 g daily	Breakthrough bleeding, sodium/water retention, nausea, vomiting, headache, breast tenderness.	Clearance ↑ by rifampin.	$ $–$$
Urge	**Anticholinergic/Antispasmodic[π]** *oxybutynin* – Ditropan, generics *dicyclomine* – Bentylol, Formulex *flavoxate* – Urispas	2.5–5 mg TID 10–20 mg TID 200 mg TID–QID	Dry mouth, flushing, drowsiness, blurred vision, nausea/vomiting, constipation (less frequent with dicyclomine and flavoxate).	Other drugs with significant anticholinergic side effects (e.g., cyclic antidepressants, neuroleptics).	$–$$ $[#] $$$
	Tricyclic Antidepressants *imipramine* Tofranil, generics	10–25 mg TID–QID Elderly: 10 mg TID–QID	Drowsiness, insomnia, tremors/ paresthesia, dry mouth, blurred vision, orthostatic hypotension, tachycardia, constipation, flushing, perspiration.	MAOIs, barbiturates, carbamazepine, rifampin, cimetidine, fluoxetine, neuroleptics, clonidine, alcohol.	$
Enuresis	**Anticholinergic/Antispasmodic[π]** *oxybutynin* – Ditropan, generics *dicyclomine* – Bentylol, Formulex *flavoxate* – Urispas	Oxybutynin: 2.5–5 mg BID up to 5 mg TID depending on age, efficacy and side effects; low doses of others	See above.	See above.	$–$$

Tricyclic Antidepressants
imipramine
Tofranil, generics

8–12 yrs: 25 mg HS
> 12 yrs: 50 mg HS

See above.

See above.

$

Antidiuretic
desmopressin
DDAVP

2–4 sprays HS

Water intoxication, seizures.

$$$$$

---

† Contains guaifenesin also.
‡ In women with an intact uterus: systemic estrogens should be given with a progestin; chronic use of vaginal estrogens may require concurrent progestin use (Chapter 68).
π Listed in decreasing order of potency and side effects.

\# Cost of liquid formulation significantly higher than tablets.
* Cost of 30-day therapy – includes drug cost only.
Legend: $ < $20 $$ $20–40 $$$ $40–60 $$$$ $60–80 $$$$$ > $80

unpleasant side effects. Urodynamic evaluation or imaging may be useful in modifying management.

In children with strictly nocturnal enuresis, management options include tricyclic antidepressants (e.g., imipramine), desmopressin or alarm programs. The tricyclic antidepressants or desmopressin can be used to protect the child for sleepovers but neither provide a "cure."

Therapeutic Tips

- If the child is not embarrassed or does not feel social pressure, no treatment may be necessary.
- No single option is best for every child; decision making requires the child's input, interest and commitment.

Suggested Reading List

Fantl JA, Cardozo L, McClish DK, et al. Estrogen therapy in the management of urinary incontinence in postmenopausal women: a meta-analysis. First report of the Hormones and Urogenital Therapy Committee. *Obstet Gynecol* 1994;83: 12–18.

Gajewski JB, Awad SA. Oxybutynin versus propantheline in patients with multiple sclerosis and detrusor hyperreflexia. *J Urol* 1986;135:966–968.

Thruoff JW, Bunke B, Ebner A, et al. Randomized, double-blind, multicenter trial on treatment of frequency, urgency and incontinence related to detrusor hyperactivity: oxybutynin versus propantheline versus placebo. *J Urol* 1991;145: 813–817.

Wein AJ, Barrett D. Physiology of micturition and urodynamics. In: Kelalis PP, King LR and Belman AB, eds. *Clinical pediatric urology*. 3rd ed. Philadelphia: W.B. Saunders, 1992.

CHAPTER 47

Fibromyalgia

Andrew Chalmers, MD, FRCPC

Fibromyalgia is characterized by diffuse musculoskeletal pain accompanied by increased tenderness at specific sites known as "tender points" (Figure 2).

Goals of Therapy

- To differentiate and treat conditions that also present as diffuse aches and pains but have specific pharmacologic therapies (e.g., polymyalgia rheumatica)
- To reduce pain and fatigue, improve quality of life, educate and promote self-management for conditions that require significant nonpharmacologic therapy and for which drug therapy is of limited benefit

Investigations (Figure 1)

Figure 1: **Investigation of Diffuse Aches and Pains**

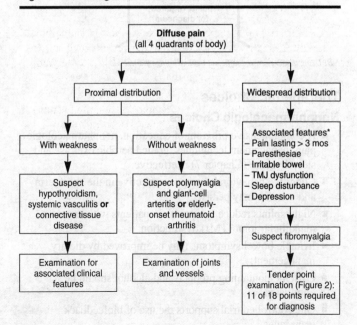

NB: Lab tests are generally negative (unless fibromyalgia is associated with specific connective tissue diseases).

Figure 2: **Tender Point Examination**

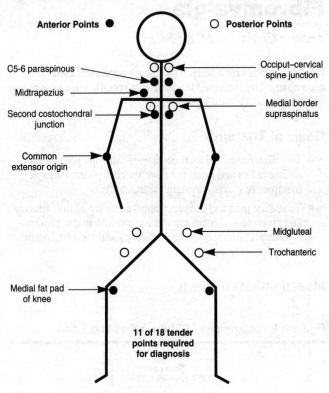

Anterior Points ●   ○ **Posterior Points**

C5-6 paraspinous

Occiput–cervical spine junction

Midtrapezius

Medial border supraspinatus

Second costochondral junction

Common extensor origin

Midgluteal

Trochanteric

Medial fat pad of knee

11 of 18 tender points required for diagnosis

NB: Using thumb pressure sufficient to blanch fingernail.

Therapeutic Choices

Nonpharmacologic Choices

- A comprehensive program of education, nonpharmacologic pain management techniques, graded aerobic exercise and sleep hygiene (Chapter 7) is effective.
- Cognitive behavioral therapy is effective in the short term and benefits may persist.
- Night splints reduce symptoms in patients with temporo-mandibular joint (TMJ) dysfunction.
- Irritable bowel symptoms may be improved by dietary management.
- Caffeine-containing products and alcohol should be eliminated.
- One controlled trial supports the use of biofeedback techniques.[1]

---

[1] *J Rheumatol 1987;14:820–825.*

Table 1: Drugs Used in Fibromyalgia

Drug	Dosage	Adverse Effects	Drug Interactions	Cost*
Tricyclic Medications				
amitriptyline Elavil, generics	10–20 mg 2–3 h before bedtime	Dry mouth, weight gain, night-mares, insomnia, hypersomnia.	MAO inhibitors, alcohol, CNS depressants, anticholinergics.	$
cyclobenzaprine Flexeril				$$–$$$
Cyclopyrrolones				
zopiclone Imovane	7.5 mg QHS (begin with 3.75 mg in the elderly)	Bitter taste, drowsiness.	Alcohol, CNS depressants, antidepressants.	$$
ibuprofen Actiprofen, Advil, Motrin, generics	200 mg QHS	Epigastric pain, gastric erosion, aggravation of ulcer.	For complete list of drug interactions, see Chapter 50.	$
Muscle Relaxant/Analgesic Combinations				
methocarbamol plus *ASA* (Robaxisal) or *acetaminophen* (Robaxacet)	2 tablets QHS	Drowsiness, nausea, dizziness.	CNS depressants.	$$$

* Cost of 30-day supply – includes drug cost only.
Legend: $ < $10 $$ $10–20 $$$ > $20

- Heat, massage and physiotherapy may provide transient benefit during flares. Ultrasound and TENS may help (or occasionally aggravate) symptoms, but should not be used chronically.

Pharmacologic Choices (Table 1)

- Concomitant depression when present should be actively treated.
- Low doses of **tricyclic medications** (e.g., amitriptyline, cyclobenzaprine) combined with low doses of **ibuprofen** at bedtime improve sleep disturbance and, in a few patients, reduce pain. Short-term efficacy of tricyclics has been confirmed in a small percentage of patients, but long-term efficacy could not be demonstrated.[2] Predictors of response were not determined.
- Although **zopiclone** would theoretically be of benefit and is used, no evidence has been published as to its efficacy.

Muscle relaxant/analgesic combinations (e.g., **methocarbamol with ASA or acetaminophen**) are useful, but they should **not** be used with other medications. Preparations containing either narcotic analgesics or benzodiazepines are not advised.

Therapeutic Tips

- Patients with arthritis may develop concomitant fibromyalgia, which should be treated separately. NSAIDs are usually ineffective for fibromyalgia; benzodiazepines and corticosteroids should also be avoided.
- Tricyclics should be prescribed 2 to 3 hours before bedtime to minimize hangover effects.
- If tricyclics are not tolerated, zopiclone may be tried.[3]
- Important and sustained clinical improvement occurs only in a minority of patients.

Suggested Reading List

Bennet RM. The fibromyalgia syndrome: myofascial pain and chronic fatigue syndrome. In: Kelly WN, Harris ED, Sledge CB, eds. *Textbook of rheumatology*. Philadelphia: WB Saunders, 1993:471–476.

Carette S. What have clinical trials taught us about the treatment of fibromyalgia? *J Musculoskeletal Pain* 1996;3:133–140.

Spencer B. *Fibromyalgia: fighting back*. Toronto: LRH Publications, 1992.

---

[2] *Arthritis Rheum 1994;37:32–40.*
[3] *Scand J Rheumatol 1991;20:288–293.*

CHAPTER 48

Acute Low Back Pain and Sciatica

R.B. Dunlop, MD, FRCSC

Goals of Therapy

- To improve function
- To decrease disability
- To improve symptoms (pain)
- To prevent recurrences

Investigations (Table 1)

- Careful history with attention to:
  - risk factors: age, heavy/awkward work, smoking, obesity
  - onset, cause of flare-ups
  - factors causing improvement or worsening
  - any major neurologic symptoms
  - previous systemic diseases
  - medications
- Physical examination:
  - range of motion (what causes the pain)
  - careful neurologic examination – for signs of root compression
  - straight-leg raising – for signs of root irritation
- Radiographic investigations: plain x-ray, bone scan, magnetic resonance imaging (MRI) scan, myelogram with specialized investigation for specific findings (can be organized in parallel with a therapy program)
- Laboratory tests: directed by history and physical findings
- **NB:** Investigation for sciatica should be considered earlier than that for simple back pain.

Therapeutic Choices (Figure 1)

Nonpharmacologic Choices

- 2 to 3 days of **back rest** is indicated in an acute episode.
- A well-organized and monitored **active exercise program**, combined with reassurance of the natural history of back pain, is appropriate. Symptoms should be monitored and the program altered if required.
- A surgeon should be consulted if symptoms continue or if radiographic investigation suggests a surgical lesion.

Table 1: **Clinical Presentations of Back-related Disease**

Low back pain (Figure 1)	Buttock radiation common. History to rule out systemic disease (e.g., malignancy, diabetes). Bone scan to exclude tumor, infection, fracture.
Sciatica (Figure 1)	Leg pain exceeds back pain. CT/myelogram demonstrates root compression. 90% improve spontaneously. Exercise program confirms improvement and increases confidence. History and physical to exclude cauda equina syndrome.
Cauda equina syndrome	Rare complication of disc herniation. Low back pain, sciatica, saddle sensory disturbance, bowel and bladder dysfunction, paraparesis and/or paraplegia. Requires urgent investigation and surgical opinion.
Neurogenic claudication (spinal stenosis) (Figure 1)	Differs from vascular claudication, requiring spinal flexion or sitting for relief. Common in older population with facet osteoarthritis. 1/3 of patients will improve spontaneously. NSAIDs often helpful. Surgical opinion if increased walking limitation.

Pharmacologic Choices
Opioid Analgesics
In the first few days a potent analgesic that diminishes anxiety (e.g., meperidine or morphine) may be appropriate. Longer-term analgesia has been achieved with codeine. Opioid analgesics can be habit-forming and constipating (Chapter 13).

Nonsteroidal Anti-inflammatory Drugs (NSAIDs)
Back pain is frequently caused by an arthritic-type pain arising from the facet joints (which are synovial joints). NSAIDs would be expected to improve this type of pain. (See Chapter 50 for information on NSAIDs.)

Skeletal Muscle Relaxants
Carbamic esters (e.g., cyclobenzaprine) and benzodiazepines, frequently used in back pain, seem to have little indication after the first few days of back rest. Once the patient is up, skeletal muscle tone will increase.

Antidepressants
Antidepressants have been used to potentiate analgesia and to help with sleep disorder and mood elevation in a reactive depression secondary to back pain. Small doses seem to be effective.

Figure 1: **Management of Acute Low Back Pain**

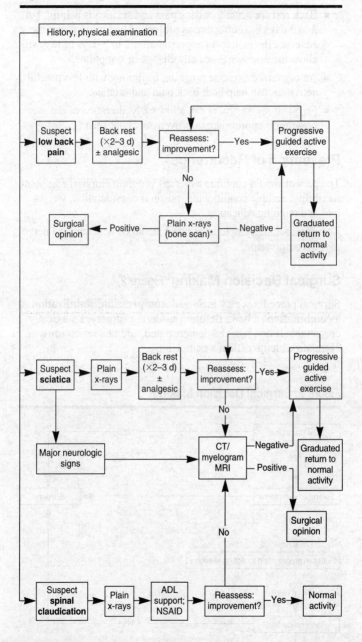

* *Becoming more helpful.*

Abbreviations: CT = computed tomography; MRI = magnetic resonance imaging;
ADL = activities of daily living.

Therapeutic Tips

- Back rest for acute low back pain and sciatica is helpful, but 2 to 3 days is as effective as prolonged bed rest without the adverse effects. Repeat appraisal after 2 to 3 days of rest will allow the assessor to see any change in symptoms.
- An organized exercise program, beginning with less painful activities, can help both back pain and sciatica.
- Frequent reassessment can allow early alteration of the program if appropriate improvement is not seen.

Prevention of Recurrence

The patient should continue a therapy program emphasizing point flexibility, aerobic conditioning, postural consideration, weight loss and ongoing education.

Recurrent sciatic symptoms are best managed with surgical nerve root decompression.

Surgical Decision Making (Figure 2)

Surgical procedures may include **decompression, stabilization** or a **combination** of both. Before considering surgery, a surgically correctable lesion must be demonstrated, and that lesion **must** correlate with the patient's complaint.

Figure 2: **Surgical Decision Making**

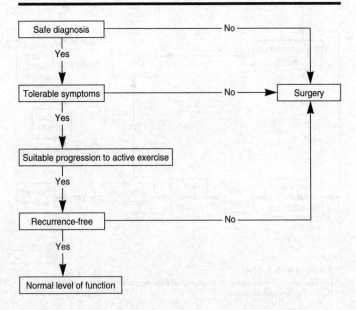

NB: Like any other treatment choice, surgery is either indicated or not indicated; it is not a last resort.

Once a surgical lesion has been identified, the choice of surgery or other conservative treatment is based on the diagnosis, the degree of symptoms, the ability to rehabilitate, and the frequency or degree of recurrence of symptoms.

Suggested Reading List

Dunlop RB. Back pain and sciatica: What intervention is appropriate? *Can J Diagn* 1991;3:47–60.

Fondyce WE, Lansky D, et al. Pain measurement and pain behavior. *Pain* 1984;18:53–69.

Gillette RD. A practical approach to the patient with back pain. *Am Fam Physician* 1996;53:670-676.

Hoppenfeld S. *Physical examination of the spine and extremities.* New York: Appleton-Century-Crofts, 1987.

Mayer TC, Catchel RJ. Functional restoration for spinal disorder. In: *The sports medicine approach.* Philadelphia: Lea & Febiger, 1988.

The Quebec Task Force on Spinal Disorders. Scientific-approach to the assessment and management of activity-related spinal disorders. *Spine* 1987;12(Suppl 7):1–59.

CHAPTER 49

Hyperuricemia and Gout

Gunnar Kraag, MD, FRCPC

Goals of Therapy

- To terminate the acute attack of arthritis
- To prevent recurrence
- To prevent or reverse complications
- To deal with associated disorders

Stages in Gouty Arthritis

The 4 stages of gouty arthritis are asymptomatic hyperuricemia, acute arthritis, the intercritical period and chronic tophaceous gout.

Asymptomatic Hyperuricemia

Hyperuricemia is not a specific disease nor is it an indication for therapy. It may be secondary to a specific disorder or the ingestion of certain drugs (Table 1). A number of associated conditions (Table 2) deserve treatment. Asymptomatic hyperuricemia ends with the first attack of acute arthritis or nephrolithiasis, usually after more than 25 years of sustained hyperuricemia.

Table 1: **Drugs Causing Hyperuricemia**

Low-dose salicylates	Phenylbutazone (low dose)
Diuretics	Ethambutol
Alcohol	Pyrazinamide
Cyclosporine	Nicotinic acid
Levodopa	IV nitroglycerin

Table 2: **Conditions Associated With Hyperuricemia**

Obesity	Atherosclerosis
Hypertension	Ischemic heart disease
Hyperlipidemia	Alcohol consumption
Myeloproliferative disorders and some cancers	Intrinsic renal disease
	Diabetes

Figure 1: **Treatment of Acute Gout**

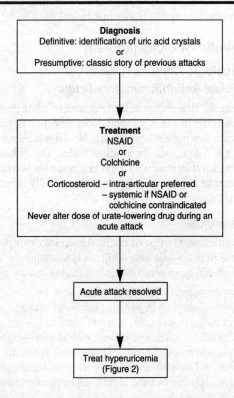

Diagnosis
Definitive: identification of uric acid crystals
or
Presumptive: classic story of previous attacks

Treatment
NSAID
or
Colchicine
or
Corticosteroid – intra-articular preferred
– systemic if NSAID or
colchicine contraindicated
Never alter dose of urate-lowering drug during an
acute attack

Acute attack resolved

Treat hyperuricemia
(Figure 2)

Acute Gouty Arthritis

Investigations

- History and physical examination:
  - abrupt onset of excruciating joint pain and inflammation of affected joint
  - may be any joint but lower limbs more commonly affected
  - 50% of first attacks occur in the metatarsophalangeal joint of the great toe, which is affected in 90% of patients over time
  - 10% of attacks can be polyarticular
  - mild attacks may resolve over 1–2 days but can take up to several weeks to completely settle
  - precipitants of acute attacks include trauma, acute illness, surgery, alcohol (beer and wine) and drugs (Table 1)
- Laboratory investigations including
  - serum uric acid may or may not be elevated; several determinations should be made

– 24-hour urine uric acid excretion dictates choice of therapy
– definitive diagnosis by identification of intracellular
  monosodium urate crystals in synovial fluid

Therapeutic Choices (Figure 1)

Pharmacologic Choices (Table 3)
Nonsteroidal Anti-inflammatory Drugs

NSAIDs are the first choice in the treatment of acute gout. All
NSAIDs are effective in equivalent doses; selection depends on
the physician's or patient's preference. NSAIDs are used in full
doses for 4 to 5 days until the attack subsides. The author uses
indomethacin if tolerated, with naproxen being the second choice.
Phenylbutazone has been replaced by other equally effective but
safer NSAIDs.

Corticosteroids

The intra-articular injection of corticosteroid into a single large
joint at time of diagnostic arthrocentesis is ideal therapy and
usually results in rapid control of inflammation and symptoms.

Systemic corticosteroid therapy (prednisone or IV
methylprednisolone) can be used for refractory attacks,
particularly polyarticular gout, or when other agents are
contraindicated. Simultaneous low-dose colchicine or NSAID
will help prevent rebound when systemic corticosteroids are
discontinued. A single IM injection of adrenocorticotropic
hormone (ACTH) can be used as an alternative to corticosteroids.

The side effects of corticosteroids are well known but rarely a
problem in the short courses of therapy used in acute gout.

Colchicine

Colchicine relieves pain within 24 hours in 90% of patients.
However, its role is limited due to its toxicity and its questionable
value as a diagnostic guide because other conditions including
pseudogout, tendonitis and rheumatoid arthritis can respond to
this therapy.

The use of IV colchicine is controversial; many countries and
institutions have banned it. It is used when NSAIDs, colchicine
or steroids cannot be given by mouth (e.g., postoperatively).
Because of its potential toxicities and the precautions required
with its use, IV colchicine should be administered with great care
or by a specialist.

Therapeutic Tips

- The earlier therapy is introduced, the quicker the attack will
  be resolved.

- Uric acid-lowering agents should never be started or stopped during an acute attack because symptoms may be exacerbated or prolonged.
- The use of colchicine in the treatment of acute gout should generally be discouraged. (Low-dose colchicine is effective for prophylaxis and is not associated with the toxicities of high-dose colchicine used in acute gout.)
- Dietary restriction of purines rarely causes a fall of plasma urate of > 60 μmol/L.

Intercritical Period and Prophylaxis

The intercritical period is asymptomatic. After the initial attack, the interval between subsequent attacks may vary from a few days to many years.

Therapeutic Choices

Nonpharmacologic Choices

- Dietary indiscretions can precipitate attacks and should be avoided. These include fasting, overindulgence in purine-rich foods (kidney, liver, anchovies, sardines) and specific foods, beer or wines that precipitate attacks.
- Reduction in purine intake achieves only modest decreases in serum urate and uric acid excretion. Currently used drugs make strict monitoring of purine intake unnecessary.
- Weight reduction is important in treating associated conditions (e.g., diabetes, obesity, hyperlipidemia), but strenuous diets may increase uric acid and precipitate an acute gouty attack.
- Alcohol should only be used in moderation. Binge drinking should be avoided.

Pharmacologic Choices (Figure 2, Table 3)

Colchicine, 1 mg per day, is very effective in preventing recurrent attacks. If it cannot be used, a low-dose **NSAID** (e.g., indomethacin 25 mg BID or naproxen 250 mg BID) may be substituted. If no attacks have occurred for 1 year, the drug can be stopped, but the patient must be warned about the possibility of an acute attack.

Antihyperuricemic Drugs

Whether or when to begin long-term antihyperuricemic therapy is controversial. One view is that the first attack is a late event in the gouty diathesis; even if further attacks do not occur, it cannot be assumed that renal damage will not. Thus, therapy should be initiated. The other view is that, because recurrence may be

Figure 2: **Treatment of Hyperuricemia**

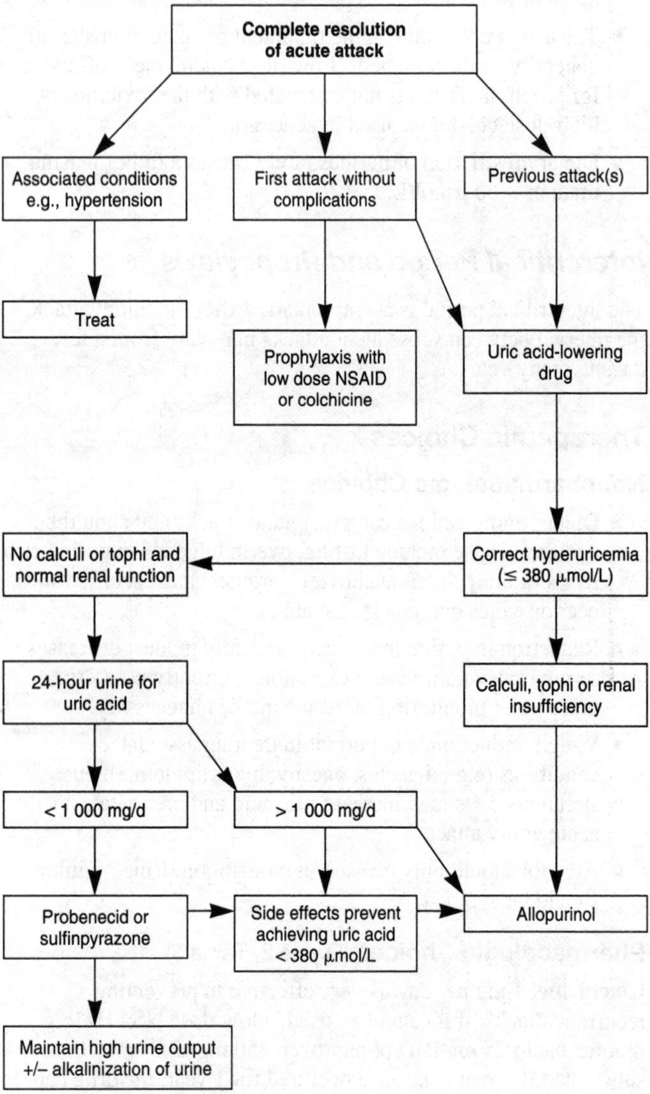

delayed for many years and chronic tophaceous gout develops only in a minority, therapy can be delayed until recurrence or detection of tophi. The author treats after the first documented attack of gout.

The aim of antihyperuricemic therapy is to reduce the serum urate concentration to below 380 μmol/L, the saturation point of monosodium urate in the extracellular fluid.

Table 3: Drug Therapy of Gout

Drug	Dosage	Adverse Effects	Drug Interactions	Comments	Cost*
NSAIDs					
indomethacin ➤ Indocid, generics	Acute attack: 75 mg STAT, then 50 mg Q6H × 2 d then 50 mg Q8H × 1 d then 25 mg Q8H × 1 d Prophylaxis: 25 mg BID	(For all NSAIDs) GI disturbances; other adverse effects uncommon with short-term therapy. For side effects with long-term use, see Chapter 50.	(For all NSAIDs, see Chapter 50.)	Both agents: Suppositories may be used if oral route inadvisable.	$
naproxen ➤ Naprosyn, generics	Acute attack: 750 mg STAT, then 500 mg BID × 4–5 d Prophylaxis: 250 mg BID				$
Colchicine generics	Acute attack: 0.5–0.6 mg Q1H until relief or side effects occur; max. 10–12 doses Prophylaxis: 0.5–1.8 mg/d; usual: 1 mg/d	Very common: abdominal pain and cramps, diarrhea, nausea and vomiting. Rare: neuropathy, myopathy, bone marrow depression.		Poor benefit/toxicity ratio. May be given IV: consult specialized references. Dosage should be ↓ in elderly and in renal impairment.	$

(cont'd)

Table 3: **Drug Therapy of Gout** (cont'd)

Drug	Dosage	Adverse Effects	Drug Interactions	Comments	Cost*
Corticosteroids†					
triamcinolone hexacetonide Aristospan	Acute attack: Large joints: 10–20 mg IA Small joints: 2–6 mg IA	Not usually significant after single IA injections.			$
methylprednisolone acetate Depo-Medrol	Acute attack: Large joints: 20–80 mg IA Medium joints: 10–40 mg IA Small joints: 4–10 mg IA	Not usually significant after single IA injections.			$
methylprednisolone sodium succinate Solu-Medrol	Acute attack: 50–100 mg IV × 1 dose	Not usually significant after single injection.		Use when prednisone cannot be used PO.	$$
prednisone Deltasone, generics	Acute attack: 30 mg daily × 5 d Effective dose range: 20–50 mg/d	Except for GI disturbances and glucose intolerance, not usually significant in short-term use. Long-term effects are numerous.	Barbiturates, phenytoin and rifampin ↓ steroid effect.	Doses below 20 mg/d tend to be ineffective. Simultaneous low-dose colchicine or NSAID helps prevent rebound when steroid stopped.	$
ACTH Acthar	Acute attack: 40 mg IM × 1 dose	Not usually significant after single injection.			‡

Uricosurics

probenecid 🔵 Benemid, generic	Starting dose: 250 mg BID; titrate gradually; max: 3 g/d	**Both agents:** May precipitate acute attack during initial phase of therapy; renal calculi, hypersensitivity reactions, GI irritation.	**Both agents:** Liberal fluid intake and alkalinizing the urine can help prevent stones. Severe toxicity is rare.	$$–$$$
		Salicylates ↓ effect of probenecid. Dapsone concentration ↑ by probenecid. Methotrexate plasma levels ↑ by probenecid. Heparin activity ↑ by probenecid.		
sulfinpyrazone 🔵 Anturan, generics	Starting dose: 50 mg BID with meals; titrate gradually; max: 800 mg/d	Salicylates may ↑ bleeding time, ↓ uricosuric effect of sulfinpyrazone. Action of oral hypoglycemics, insulin and anticoagulants ↑ by sulfinpyrazone.		$

Xanthine Oxidase Inhibitors

allopurinol 🔵 Purinol, Zyloprim, generics	Starting dose: 100 mg daily Usual: 300 mg/d titrated to levels: Max. 800 mg/d → Maintenance dose in renal impairment[π] Chemotherapy/irradiation: 600–800 mg/d × 2–3 d before therapy Children with malignancies or enzyme deficiencies: 10 mg/kg/d	Skin rash, GI upset, hepatotoxicity, fever, severe hypersensitivity syndrome, xanthine stones (rare). May precipitate attack during initial phase of therapy.	May need to ↑ dose or combine with uricosuric agents in chronic tophaceous gout. To prevent acute attacks on initiation of therapy, give prophylactic NSAID or colchicine for 2–3 wks.	$
		Half-life of azathioprine and 6-mercaptopurine ↑ by allopurinol. May ↑ toxicity of cyclophosphamide. With ampicillin and amoxicillin ↑ incidence of rashes. Allopurinol inhibits hepatic metabolism of warfarin.		

[†] Author's preferences for acute gout—other options exist.

🔵 Dosage adjustment may be required in renal impairment – see Appendix I.

[π] Maintenance dose of allopurinol must be adjusted downward in renal impairment. If CrCl is 20–10 mL/min, the dosage is 100 mg/d; if CrCl is < 5 mL/min, the dosage is 100 mg Q2–3 d.

[‡] Available through the Special Access Program (formerly the Emergency Drug Release Program), Therapeutic Products Directorate, Health Canada.

* Cost of 30-day supply – includes drug cost only.

Legend: $ < $10 $$ $10–20 $$$ $20–30 $$$$ > 30

Abbreviations: IA = intra-articular.

Allopurinol, a xanthine oxidase inhibitor, inhibits the production of uric acid. Clinically very effective, it has become one of the most frequently prescribed drugs for hyperuricemia. To avoid unnecessary risks and costs, allopurinol should be reserved for patients with the following indications:

– presence of tophi
– history of renal calculi of any type
– 24-hour urinary uric acid excretion > 1 000 mg
– hypoxanthine-guanine phosphoribosyl transferase (HGPRT) deficiency or phosphoribosyl pyrophosphate (PRPP) synthetase overactivity (both ↑ uric acid production)
– renal insufficiency
– uric acid nephropathy
– prophylaxis of hyperuricemia secondary to cytotoxic agents
– allergy to uricosurics

The overall incidence of side effects with allopurinol is about 15 to 20%, but only half of patients with side effects must discontinue therapy. Severe toxicity can occur; the allopurinol hypersensitivity syndrome characterized by fever, rash and severe involvement of the kidney and liver can result in death.

Higher doses of allopurinol and combination with uricosuric agents are occasionally required to speed mobilization of extensive urate deposits in chronic tophaceous gout.

Allopurinol is used before chemotherapy or irradiation and in severe enzyme deficiencies to prevent acute gouty nephropathy.

Uricosuric agents (probenecid and **sulfinpyrazone)** are effective in 70 to 80% of patients, are safe and do not influence purine metabolism as allopurinol does. They are used in patients < 60 years of age with normal renal function, a 24-hour urine uric acid < 1 000 mg and no history of renal calculi. They are ineffective when the glomerular filtration rate is below 30 mL/min. Salicylates at any dose block the uricosuric effect of both drugs and must not be used concomitantly.

Both agents have similar efficacy, but probenecid is better tolerated than sulfinpyrazone.

Therapeutic Tips

- Asymptomatic hyperuricemia (i.e., before the initial attack of gouty arthritis) should not be treated. A definite diagnosis of gout must be made.
- Patients started on antihyperuricemic therapy should receive an anti-inflammatory agent for the first 2 to 3 weeks to lower the risk of an acute attack.

- The dose of the antihyperuricemic agent should be titrated against the uric acid levels.
- The dosage of allopurinol should be adjusted according to the creatinine clearance.
- Compliance may be improved by carefully explaining treatment objectives (e.g., allopurinol has no pain-relieving properties and must be used continuously).
- Risk of damage beyond the musculoskeletal system is low: 1% annual incidence of calculi and interstitial renal damage is likely after 10 years of inadequately treated gout.

Chronic Tophaceous Gout

The best treatment for chronic tophaceous gout is prevention by aggressive management of acute gout and correction of hyperuricemia. Once joint and bone destruction has occurred, it cannot be reversed, and chronic gouty nephropathy often results.

The aims of therapy are to control pain and inflammation (usually with NSAIDs) and to decrease serum uric acid levels. The disappearance of tophaceous deposits can be dramatic but may take several years.

Suggested Reading List

Emmerson BT. The management of gout. *N Engl J Med* 1996; 334:445–451.

Kelly WN, Harris ED, Ruddy S, et al. *Textbook of rheumatology*. 4th ed. Philadelphia: W.B. Saunders, 1993: Chapters 31, 50 and 76.

Star VL, Hochberg MC. Prevention and management of gout. *Drugs* 1993;45:212–222.

CHAPTER 50

Rheumatoid Arthritis

*Thomas W. Paton, PharmD and
Mary Bell, MD, FRCPC*

Goals of Therapy

- To minimize symptoms (pain)
- To preserve joint function
- To prevent disease progression and deformity
- To optimize patient's lifestyle

Investigations

- A thorough history with emphasis on:
  - duration of morning stiffness
  - presence of fatigue and anorexia
  - distribution/duration of painful and swollen joints
- Physical examination:
  - number of painful and swollen joints
  - range of joint motion
  - presence of extra-articular manifestations
- Laboratory tests:
  - CBC, platelet count, ESR, serum creatinine, urinalysis
  - rheumatoid factor titer, antinuclear antibody titer
- X-ray films of affected joints

Therapeutic Choices (Figure 1)

Nonpharmacologic Choices

- Education (patients and family).
- Balance of rest and activity.
- Articular rest (including splinting).
- Exercise (e.g., range of motion), aerobic exercise.
- External application of heat (warm water, hot baths, hydrotherapy) or cold.
- Emotional support (patient and family).
- Nutrition.
- Surgery.

Pharmacologic Choices

Nonsteroidal Anti-inflammatory Drugs (Table 1, Figure 1)

NSAIDs may be used before or concomitant with disease-modifying antirheumatic drugs (DMARDs). There is **no** single

Figure 1: **Management of Rheumatoid Arthritis**

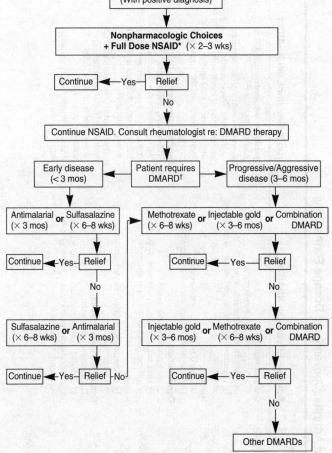

* *Try up to 2 different NSAIDs over a period of up to 6 weeks.*
† *Systemic or intra-articular corticosteroids may be required between courses of DMARDs.*

best NSAID; **all** are equally effective (consider the lowest cost drug). There is little advantage in using higher priced modified-release dosage forms, as many conventional dosage forms can be used once daily or BID in patients with compliance problems. **Phenylbutazone** and **oxyphenbutazone** should be avoided.

There is great variability in individual patient response to NSAIDs. Selection should be guided by the prescriber's familiarity with the agent. At full anti-inflammatory dosages,

Table 1: NSAIDs Used in Rheumatoid Arthritis (Conventional Dosage Forms Only)

NSAID	Dosage* (mg/d)	Adverse Effects (all NSAIDs)	Drug Interactions (all NSAIDs)	Cost†
ASA (enteric coated) Entrophen, generics	2 600–3 900	**Gastrointestinal** VC: Dyspepsia, nausea/vomiting.	**Oral Anticoagulants** – use with caution (monitor PT).	$
choline magnesium trisalicylate Trilisate	2 000–3 000	UC: Gastric and duodenal ulcers. R: Gastric hemorrhage, perforation, small bowel	**Diuretics** – reduction in natriuretic and diuretic effect; avoid	$$
diclofenac Voltaren, generics	75–150	ulceration. **Renal**	combination of triamterene and indomethacin; may lead to	$–$$
diflunisal Dolobid, generics	500–1 000	UC: Fluid retention, hyperkalemia. R: Acute renal failure, interstitial nephritis.	hyperkalemia with K+-sparing diuretics.	$–$$
etodolac Ultradol	400–600	**Dermatologic** C: Nonspecific rash/pruritus.	**Antihypertensives (Diuretics, β-Blockers,**	$$$–$$$$
fenoprofen Nalfon	1 200–3 200	R: Urticaria, erythema multiforme, fixed drug eruptions, Stevens-Johnson syndrome.	**ACE Inhibitors)** – possible reduction in hypertensive effect; may require additional antihyper-	$$–$$$$
flurbiprofen Ansaid, Froben, generics	150–200	**Hepatic** R: Cholestasis, hepatitis, Reye's syndrome (primarily ASA).	tensive therapy.	$$
ibuprofen Motrin, generics	1 200–2 400	**Central Nervous System** C: Dizziness, headache.	**Methotrexate** – reduced clearance with ASA (avoid combination); less risk with other NSAIDs	$
indomethacin Indocid, generics	50–200	C: Tinnitus: salicylates; (UC with other NSAIDs).	(monitor carefully).	$–$$
ketoprofen Orudis, Rhodis, generics	150–200	UC: Disorientation, confusion, memory loss. R: Aseptic meningitis.	**Lithium** – lithium toxicity (monitor lithium levels).	$
nabumetone Relafen	1 000–2 000			$$$–$$$$

Oral Hypoglycemics –
NSAIDs may lead to transient changes in blood glucose (monitor initially).

Hematologic
VC: Antiplatelet effect (not with nonacetylated salicylates).
R: Agranulocytosis/aplastic anemia (indomethacin), thrombocytopenia.

Pulmonary
R: Asthma (patients with ASA hypersensitivity), pulmonary alveolitis.

Drug	Dosage	Cost
naproxen Naprosyn, generics	500–1 000	$
oxaprozin Daypro	1 200–1 800	$$$–$$$$
piroxicam Feldene, generics	10–20	$
salsalate Disalcid	1 500–3 000	$$
sulindac Clinoril, generics	200–400	$–$$
tenoxicam Mobiflex, generic	10–20	$$
tiaprofenic acid Surgam, Tiafen, generic	600	$$
tolmetin Tolectin, generic	1 200–1 800	$$–$$$

● *Dosage adjustment may be required in renal impairment – see Appendix I.*
* *In hepatic disease, reduce dosage.*
Abbreviations: VC (very common > 10%); C (common 5–10%); UC (uncommon 1–4%); R (rare < 1%).

† *Cost of 30-day supply – includes drug cost only.*

Legend: $ < $ 20 $$ $20–40 $$$ $40–60 $$$$ > $60

maximal effect may take 2 to 3 weeks. In elderly patients, the dose adjustments may be necessitated by changes in renal or hepatic function or cardiovascular disease. All NSAIDs should be used cautiously in patients with pre-existing renal disease. Evidence does not support the use of one NSAID over another at this time.

Nonacetylated salicylates (e.g., choline magnesium trisalicylate) may be considered in patients with ASA hypersensitivity.

No one NSAID is clearly less gastrotoxic than another. The use of enteric-coated products will minimize the risk of gastric lesions. Consider cytoprotective therapy with **misoprostol** (200 μg BID or TID) in high-risk patients (> 60 years of age, female or with recent peptic ulcer or GI hemorrhage). The fixed-dose combination of **misoprostol/diclofenac** (Arthrotec) is a cost-effective alternative for those patients responsive to diclofenac where cytoprotection is needed. Early results of reduced gastro-toxicity with nabumetone and etodolac require confirmation in long-term studies. There is no added benefit in combining two NSAIDs, but there is evidence of increased risk of gastric lesions.

Data on the use of NSAIDs in pregnancy are inadequate to estimate risk; however, it is generally accepted that they be avoided in the third trimester. In contrast, except for indomethacin, NSAIDs are considered safe in lactation.

Disease-modifying Antirheumatic Drugs (DMARDs)
(Table 2)

These second-line or slow-acting antirheumatic agents should only be used in patients with active inflammatory disease because of the associated toxicity, cost and monitoring (all require intensive monitoring for response and side effects). DMARD therapy should begin only after consultation with a rheuma-tologist. Therapy is associated with a delay in response (6 to 8 weeks with methotrexate, 3 to 6 months with IM gold and other agents).

◻ Chloroquine and Hydroxychloroquine

These may be considered first in a patient with early disease (less than 3 to 6 months). They have low toxicity and good efficacy.

◻ Auranofin

Auranofin (oral gold) has modest efficacy and significant GI side effects and cannot be recommended as a first-line DMARD therapy.

◻ Methotrexate, IM Gold and Sulfasalazine

These agents are useful in patients in whom antimalarials have failed or who have early progressive disease. Response can be

Table 2: Disease-modifying Antirheumatic Drugs

Drug	Dosage	Adverse Effects	Drug Interactions	Cost*
Antimalarials† *chloroquine* Aralen, generic	250 mg/d	UC: Nausea, abdominal cramps, diarrhea.	Penicillamine: avoid – ↑ toxicity of penicillamine.	Chloroquine $
hydroxychloroquine Plaquenil	200–400 mg/d	R: Retinopathy, keratopathy, corneal opacities, tinnitus, nerve damage, rash, neuromyopathy, blood dyscrasias.		Hydroxy-chloroquine $$
methotrexate†🌑 Rheumatrex, generic	Initial: 7.5 mg/wk Max.: 20 mg/wk	UC: GI side effects, bone marrow suppression, stomatitis, hepatic damage. R: Pulmonary toxicity. **NB:** need for routine use of folinic or folic acid to prevent toxicity unclear.	Salicylates, probenecid: avoid. NSAIDs: monitor methotrexate effects.	$
Gold Salts†🌑 Injectable *sodium aurothiomalate* Myochrysine *sodium aurothioglucose* Solganal	10 mg and 25 mg test doses 1 wk apart; 50 mg/wk to 1 g total, then maintenance dose	**Injectable** C: rash, mucocutaneous reactions. UC: proteinuria. R: blood dyscrasias, hepato-toxicity, pulmonary fibrosis, GI toxicity, nephrotic syndrome; vasomotor (nitritoid) reactions (not reported with auranofin).	None known.	Myochrysine $$$$$ Solganal‡ $$$

(cont'd)

Table 2: Disease-modifying Antirheumatic Drugs *(cont'd)*

Drug	Dosage	Adverse Effects	Drug Interactions	Cost*
sulfasalazine Salazopyrin, generics	2 000–3 000 mg/d	VC: nausea, vomiting, anorexia, gastric distress, headache. UC: rash, pruritus, hemolytic anemia, leukopenia. R: aplastic anemia, thrombocytopenia, agranulocytosis.	↓ absorption of digoxin and folic acid. Avoid probenecid and methotrexate.	$

Abbreviations: VC (very common > 10%); C (common 5–10%); UC (uncommon 1–4%); R (rare < 1%).

† *Avoid in patients with hepatic impairment.*

✱ *Dosage adjustment may be required in renal impairment – see Appendix I.*

‡ *Supplied in 10 mL vials; cost is for 4 doses (4 mL) only. Full vial is $$$$$.*

* *Cost of 4-wk supply – includes drug cost only.*

Legend: $ < $15 $$ $15–30 $$$ $30–45 $$$$ $45–60 $$$$$ > $60

seen within 6 to 8 weeks with **methotrexate** and **sulfasalazine** therapy; response with **gold** may take 3 to 6 months.

❏ Azathioprine, Chlorambucil, Cyclophosphamide and Penicillamine

These are currently considered only when patients have failed to respond to other DMARDs. **Penicillamine** has moderate efficacy and moderate to severe toxicity relative to **gold** and **methotrexate**. **Azathioprine** has moderate toxicity with efficacy in late disease. **Chlorambucil** and **cyclophosphamide** are seldom used due to toxicity.

❏ Corticosteroids

Systemic oral corticosteroids are used as bridge therapy between courses of DMARDs. While there is a trend towards the use of oral corticosteroids early in aggressive RA, there is currently no clinical support for this approach. Pulse-dose IV therapy should only be used under the supervision of a rheumatologist. Intra-articular steroids are used intermittently with isolated problem joints.

❏ Other Agents

Cyclosporine, gamma-linoleic acid and **thalidomide** are under study.

At varying times both **analgesics** and **corticosteroids** may be useful (systemic or intra-articular). **Topical analgesics** may provide local and temporary relief, but systemic absorption is possible, which may lead to toxicity.

Highly selective cyclo-oxygenase inhibitors and nitric oxide-releasing NSAID derivatives are under study.

Suggested Reading List

American College of Rheumatology Ad Hoc Committee on Clinical Guidelines. Guidelines for the management of rheumatoid arthritis. *Arthritis Rheum* 1996;39:713–722.

American College of Rheumatology Ad Hoc Committee on Clinical Guidelines. Guidelines for monitoring drug therapy in rheumatoid arthritis. *Arthritis Rheum* 1996;39:723–731.

Tannenbaum H, Davis P, Russell A, et al. An evidence-based approach to prescribing NSAIDs in musculoskeletal disease: a Canadian consensus. *Can Med Assoc J* 1996;155:77–88.

Van der Heide A, Jacobs JW, Bijlsma JW, et al. The effectiveness of early treatment with second-line antirheumatic drugs. A randomized controlled trial. *Ann Intern Med* 1996;12418: 699–707.

Wallace JL. NSAID gastroenteropathy: past, present and future. *Can J Gastroenterol* 1996;10:451–459.

CHAPTER 51

Osteoarthritis

Paul M. Peloso, MD, MSc, FRCPC

Definition

Osteoarthritis (OA), formerly known as degenerative joint disease, encompasses a wide array of rheumatic conditions that share a common final pathway. It can be generalized (affecting spine, knees, hips, hands or feet), localized (affecting only one joint) or nodal (affecting primarily the hands). OA is endemic, increases with age, affects women slightly more often than men and is the leading cause of disability in Canada. Joint pain, crepitus and deformity, with or without swelling, characterize the disease.

Goals of Therapy

- To reduce or eliminate the joint pain
- To increase patient and joint mobility
- To increase muscle tone around the joint
- To prevent progression and heal the underlying damaged cartilage

Investigations

- History with attention to:
  - pattern of pain (worse with use and better with rest)
  - duration of stiffness (gelling) – usually < 30 minutes
  - ruling out associated inflammatory conditions although these may coexist
  - identifying pre-existing conditions leading to early OA: developmental abnormalities (e.g., slipped capital epiphysis), congenital abnormalities (e.g., benign hypermobility syndrome), occupational factors
  - use of drugs (e.g., prednisone, alcohol) that can lead to avascular necrosis and secondary OA
- Physical examination to confirm deranged joint: limited range of motion, pain, deformity with or without swelling, bony enlargement, misalignment, crepitus
- X-rays to confirm nonuniform joint space narrowing (symmetrical loss suggests an underlying inflammatory condition), osteophytes (new bone), subchondral cyst formation (or geodes) and bony sclerosis; if chondrocalcinosis is suspected on x-ray, diabetes, hemochromatosis, hypo-phosphatemia and hypothyroidism should be ruled out

- Bone scan – rarely helpful
- CT scan – rarely helpful
- Magnetic resonance imaging – when avascular necrosis is suspected; not routinely indicated
- Joint fluid analysis – high WBC and turbidity suggest other causes

Therapeutic Choices (Table 1)

Prevention

Obesity, mechanical stresses and **occupational** or **sports-related trauma** should be modified. Early and aggressive treatment of **inflammatory arthritis**, **metabolic abnormalities** and **congenital abnormalities** may prevent secondary OA. A good intake of vitamin D (400 to 800 IU daily) and calcium (1 000 to 1 500 mg daily) may also delay progression, at least for the knee.

Nonpharmacologic Choices

The following should be tried prior to most pharmacologic therapies but may be considered at any stage of joint problems. Best results may be obtained using a combined approach.

- **Exercise** (stretching, low-impact aerobics, swimming, stationary cycling or walking) does not cause acute episodes and results in improved muscle strength, sense of well-being and functional status. The program should be tailored to the individual and undertaken 3 times a week for at least 20 minutes.
- **Physical therapies** (i.e., TENS, laser, ultrasound, acupuncture and thermal therapy) may be tried. The most efficacious appear to be TENS and laser.
- Correctly fitted and used **aids** are helpful. A **cane** reduces forces through a hip or knee by up to 60%. **Braces or shoe lifts** can help an unstable joint if misalignment or a leg length discrepancy exists. For the neck, a **double ruff collar** worn at night, and for the back, **abdominal and lumbar strengthening**, may be helpful.
- **Taping the patella** medially with a broad elasticized tape when the knee is relaxed in slight flexion is beneficial in all patterns of knee OA.
- **Education** (in a group setting), a **positive and supportive attitude** and **regular telephone calls** from nursing staff have been shown to improve pain control.

Table 1: Treatment Choices for Osteoarthritis

Joint	Physical Therapy	Pharmacologic Therapy*	Surgery
Knee	Quadriceps exercise Walk, swim, bike Weight loss Canes Orthoses for angulation and instability	Corticosteroid injection if effusion present Acetaminophen Capsaicin cream Low-dose NSAID or nonacetylated salicylate Full-dose NSAID (+ misoprostol) Hyaluronan	Lavage Chondral holes Osteotomy Arthroplasty
Hip	Exercise for range of motion, strength Cane Orthoses for leg length abnormalities	Acetaminophen Low-dose NSAID or nonacetylated salicylate Full-dose NSAID (+ misoprostol) Corticosteroid injection	Osteotomy Arthroplasty
CMC	Ultrasound CMC splints	Topical NSAIDs† Capsaicin cream Corticosteroid injection	Trapezectomy Plastic joint spacer
DIP PIP	Heat, cold, wax	Topical NSAIDs† Capsaicin cream Corticosteroid injection	Prosthetic surgery

* Use in a step-wise approach. Physical therapies should always be recommended and may be used in combination with medical therapy. Surgery is usually tried when other techniques have failed to provide adequate relief. See Table 2 for further information.
† Topical NSAIDs are not available in Canada but are used in Europe. Topical diclofenac is under investigation. Topical diclofenac is available in Europe. Some pharmacists will compound extemporaneous preparations.
Abbreviations: CMC = carpometacarpal; DIP = distal interphalangeal; PIP = proximal interphalangeal.

† Topical NSAIDs are not available in Canada but are used in Europe. Topical diclofenac is under investigation. Topical diclofenac is under investigation. Some pharmacists will compound extemporaneous preparations.

Pharmacologic Choices (Table 2)
Oral and Topical Agents

Acetaminophen is often combined successfully with non-pharmacologic approaches. **Acetaminophen**, **ibuprofen** and **naproxen** have been shown to provide equivalent pain relief. In acute exacerbations, codeine, 30 to 60 mg QID, may be necessary for 1 to 2 weeks. **Codeine** is an alternative in individuals unresponsive to acetaminophen and for whom NSAIDs are contraindicated or not tolerated.

Topical 0.025% **capsaicin** cream is efficacious in knee OA and possibly other joints. Topical NSAIDs, popular in Europe, are only beginning clinical trials in Canada although some pharmacists formulate their own solutions.

The 1995 American College of Rheumatology (ACR) guidelines on the treatment of both hip and knee OA suggest that NSAIDs be considered only when nonpharmacologic, and both oral and topical analgesia have failed. The ACR guidelines favor the use of low dose ibuprofen or the nonacetylated salicylates such as **salsalate** first, and if these are not effective, full dose NSAIDs are indicated. NSAID benefits do not seem to be offset by their toxicity to the gastrointestinal tract and kidneys, and tendency to exacerbate hypertension and congestive heart failure. In patients at high risk of gastrointestinal bleeding, co-therapy with misoprostol is recommended. The possibility that newer NSAIDs that are more selective for cyclo-oxygenase enzyme II will reduce toxicity to the gut and kidneys remains to be established. If they do, NSAIDs may have greater utility earlier in the treatment of OA. Whether NSAIDs accelerate OA is also controversial, but is another argument for limiting NSAID use.

There is considerable public interest in **glucosamine sulfate** in the treatment of OA. It appears efficacious when compared to ibuprofen and naproxen, but a lack of studies evaluating long-term side effects limits enthusiasm for widespread use.

Joint Injection (For Accessible Joints)

Corticosteroid joint injections are used when signs of inflammation exist and may follow or complement oral and topical therapies. They may be most beneficial when crystalline arthritis coexists but may be efficacious even when signs of inflammation are not present. Corticosteroids may act by reducing metalloproteinases that digest cartilage. Benefits can last up to 6 months, but 4 to 6 weeks is about average. No more than 3 to 4 injections of corticosteroid should be given in any one joint per year. Judicious use of rest *postinjection* is advised, but should not exceed 3 days because the loss of muscle bulk and strength is counterproductive. Very rarely, a synovitis is induced following injection.

Table 2: Pharmacologic Agents Used in Osteoarthritis

Drug	Dosage	Comments	Cost*
acetaminophen ❓ Tylenol, generics	650 mg Q4H – 1 000 mg Q6H	May cause hepatitis if taken in excess or by patients with liver disease.	$
NSAIDs ❓ (e.g., *ibuprofen* Motrin, generics)	200 mg TID up to 800 mg TID × 10 d	For comparison of available NSAIDs, see Chapter 50.	$ for ibuprofen
Nonacetylated salicylates			
choline magnesium trisalicylate Trilisate	1 g BID–TID	Gastrointestinal effects seen in 3% of patients.	$$$
salsalate Disalcid	1 g TID–1.5 g BID	Tinnitus and gastrointestinal effects are common side effects.	$$$
capsaicin Zostrix	Apply to joint area TID–QID May require 14–28 d for optimal effect	Shown efficacious in knee OA. Continued application necessary for effect; transient burning on application. Avoid contact with eyes, open lesions.	$$$
methylprednisolone acetate (intra-articular) Depo-Medrol	Knee: 40–60 mg Hip: 80 mg CMC: 10 mg DIP/PIP: 10 mg Max: 3 injections/joint/year	Joint activity should be minimized for 3 d following injection. Benefits last 4–6 wks.	$$–$$$$
hyaluronans Neovisc Suplasyn Synvisc	1 injection/wk × 3–5 wks	Transient pain and swelling on injection; contains avian protein: avoid in patients with related hypersensitivities.	per 3 injections: $156 $198 $291
sterile saline lavage	0.5 to 2 L/lavage		

❓ *Dosage adjustment may be required in renal impairment – see Appendix I.*
Abbreviations: CMC = carpometacarpal; DIP = distal interphalangeal; PIP = proximal interphalangeal.

* Cost of 1 week's therapy – includes drug cost only.
Legend: $ < $2 $$ $2–5 $$$ $5–10 $$$$ > $10

Hyaluronan and its derivatives, proteinaceous derivatives of cartilage, are useful in mild to moderate cases of knee OA, and are indicated prior to NSAIDs. Three injections separated by 1-week intervals show benefits lasting up to 6 months. These courses may be repeated. There are no direct comparisons of the different hyaluronan derivatives. About 2% of people injected experience a sterile joint effusion postinjection.

Joint lavage with a large-bore needle (14 or 16 gauge) and large volumes of **sterile saline** (500 mL to 2 L) may work by removing joint debris and inflammatory molecules.

Radioactive yttrium-90[1] provides a chemical synovectomy; it appears to work best in patients who have responded well to intra-articular steroids.

Surgical Choices

The main indication is pain unresponsive to other measures. The common dictum to be followed is, "can't sleep, can't walk, can't work."

Arthroscopic techniques include joint débridement, abrasion arthroplasty to smooth the joint surface, and drilling out portions of osteochondral bone. These loose joint particles may act as a proinflammatory nidus, and burr holes reduce subchondral hypertension. Proper trials are lacking for these approaches, but they continue to have wide support in the surgical community.

Open approaches are osteotomy of the distal femur or proximal tibia to redistribute forces through healthier cartilage. This delays the need for total joint replacement but does not provide a permanent solution.

Total joint replacement appears to be best for more sedentary, nonobese and older individuals because subsequent demands on the prosthesis are lessened. Repeat operations are required in approximately 10 to 15% of patients over a 20-year span, because of either prosthetic loosening or secondary infection.

Suggested Reading List

Hochberg MC, Altman RD, Brandt KD, et al. Guidelines for the management of osteoarthritis. *Arthritis and Rheumatism* 1995;38:1535–1546.

Osteoarthritis. In: Klippel JH, Dieppe PA, eds. *Rheumatology*. Toronto: Mosby, 1994.

---

[1] *May be obtained from Atomic Energy of Canada via your nuclear medicine diagnostic imaging department.*

CHAPTER 52

Osteoporosis

David A. Hanley, MD, FRCPC

Goals of Therapy

- Prevention of fractures, disability and loss of independence
- Preservation or enhancement of bone mass

Investigations

- History:
  - height as a young adult (compare with current *measured* height)
  - chronic or acute back pain; development of dorsal kyphosis
  - menstrual history: menarche, occurrence of episodes of oligomenorrhea or amenorrhea (excluding pregnancies), age of menopause (high risk if menopause prior to age 45, or surgical menopause), use of postmenopausal ovarian hormone therapy
  - hypogonadism in males
  - diet: calcium intake, anorexia nervosa, weight loss after age 25, use of calcium or vitamin D supplements, lactose intolerance
  - lifestyle issues: inactivity or prolonged periods of bed rest, smoking history, alcohol intake, excessive caffeine intake
  - medications: glucocorticoids, excessive thyroid hormone replacement, long-term heparin therapy, anticonvulsants, sedatives
  - past medical history: previous fractures; increased propensity to fall; endocrine diseases: hyperthyroidism, hyperparathyroidism, hypogonadism, Cushing's syndrome; renal diseases; organ transplantation; gastrointestinal disease: gastric surgery, malabsorption; chemotherapy for malignancy
  - family history of osteoporotic fracture (particularly hip)
- Physical examination:
  - kyphosis
  - muscle weakness (inability to rise from a chair)
  - impaired visual acuity, other disability causing a tendency to fall
- Laboratory investigations:
  - all should be normal: complete blood count, calcium, alkaline phosphatase (may be elevated in acute recovery from fracture), creatinine. Consider TSH and serum protein electrophoresis

Figure 1: **Use of Bone Density and Risk Factors in Osteoporosis Management**

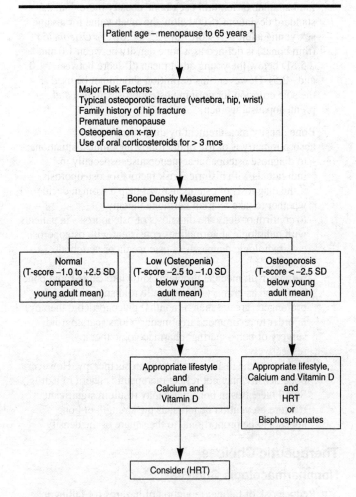

```
┌─────────────────────────────────┐
│ Patient age – menopause to 65 years * │
└─────────────────────────────────┘
                  │
┌─────────────────────────────────────────────────┐
│ Major Risk Factors:                              │
│ Typical osteoporotic fracture (vertebra, hip, wrist) │
│ Family history of hip fracture                   │
│ Premature menopause                              │
│ Osteopenia on x-ray                              │
│ Use of oral corticosteroids for > 3 mos          │
└─────────────────────────────────────────────────┘
                  │
         ┌────────────────────────┐
         │ Bone Density Measurement │
         └────────────────────────┘
```

| Normal (T-score –1.0 to +2.5 SD compared to young adult mean) | Low (Osteopenia) (T-score –2.5 to –1.0 SD below young adult mean) | Osteoporosis (T-score < –2.5 SD below young adult mean) |

| Appropriate lifestyle and Calcium and Vitamin D | Appropriate lifestyle, Calcium and Vitamin D and HRT or Bisphosphonates |

Consider (HRT)

** After age 65, many experts would recommend treatment with HRT or a
bisphosphonate if the patient was taking corticosteroids, regardless of bone density.
Abbreviations: SD = standard deviation(s); HRT = hormone replacement therapy.*

- other more specific markers of calcium or bone metabolism are not appropriate routinely
- Diagnostic imaging:
  - x-rays are unreliable in diagnosing osteopenia (thin bones) and should only be used for detecting fractures
  - bone scans can be used to identify new fracture activity in patients with back pain and no obvious new fracture on x-ray

- Bone density measurements (Figure 1)
  Osteoporosis in the postmenopausal female is defined as a lumbar spine or femoral neck bone density more than 2.5 standard deviations (SD) below the mean value for a same sex young adult ("T-score" of –2.5 or lower). *Osteopenia* (thin bones) is defined as a bone density between 1.0 and 2.5 SD below the young adult mean (T-score between –1.0 and –2.5). However, this definition should not be used as the sole criterion for defining osteoporosis in men and premenopausal women.

  Bone density measurement by dual energy x-ray absorptiometry is of use in the following clinical situations:
  – to diagnose osteopenia at menopause, especially in individuals with historical risk factors for osteoporosis, if the diagnosis of osteopenia will help a woman decide whether to take ovarian hormone therapy
  – to confirm or deny the diagnosis of osteoporosis in patients with radiologic abnormalities consistent with osteoporosis, e.g., radiologic diagnosis of osteopenia or vertebral fractures
  – patients with medical problems known to cause rapid bone loss, such as primary hyperparathyroidism or high dose prolonged (greater than 3 months) glucocorticoid therapy, in order to recommend treatment options (parathyroid surgery or bone-sparing pharmacologic therapy, respectively)
  – to monitor the response to osteoporosis therapy. However, bone density may not reflect therapeutic benefit of a drug. Small increases in bone mass may result in significant fracture prevention benefits, as the strength of bone appears to be proportional to the square of the density

Therapeutic Choices

Nonpharmacologic Choices

- Reduce risk of falling: reduction of hazards for falling in the home, elimination of drugs implicated in falls, e.g., benzodiazepines; exercise to improve strength and coordination.
- Adequate dietary calcium: dairy products; canned fish with bones (sardines, salmon); certain vegetables (broccoli, kale, beans, lentils); almonds.
- Stop smoking, reduce alcohol and caffeine intake.

Pharmacologic Choices (Table 1)

Therapies for osteoporosis can be classified as those which prevent bone resorption (antiresorptive) and those which stimulate bone formation. At present, all three of the approved drugs (estrogen, alendronate, and cyclical etidronate) are anti-resorptive in their action. By acting to reduce both the *depth* and *rate* of bone resorption, while the mandatory coupled bone formation proceeds normally, these agents cause an initial increase in bone mass. This increase eventually plateaus, as the overall rate of bone turnover is markedly reduced. In contrast, **bone formation agents** like sodium fluoride have been shown to cause a steady gain in bone density for the duration of their use, as much as 30 percent over 4 years.

Antiresorptive Agents
Estrogen (+/-) Progesterone

Estrogen, with progesterone (if the patient has not had a hysterectomy), is first choice for both prevention of osteoporosis in the postmenopause, and the treatment of established osteoporosis in older postmenopausal women. However, most clinicians would now rank the bisphosphonates equally with estrogen for women over age 65. The risks and benefits of estrogen therapy are discussed in Chapter 68.

Bisphosphonates

These agents are analogues of pyrophosphate, a naturally occurring inhibitor of crystallization. Different bisphosphonates vary in potency and action on bone.

Etidronate and alendronate are approved for osteoporosis treatment. Clodronate and pamidronate have also been used in the treatment of osteoporosis in small clinical trials of short duration.

Bisphosphonates bind to bone mineral and inhibit osteoclast activity. Normal bone mineralization is inhibited (osteomalacia), when etidronate is given continuously in higher than recommended doses. Other bisphosphonates have not caused mineralization defects because their higher potency allows for the antiresorptive effects to be obtained at a much lower dose than the levels required to inhibit mineralization.

Etidronate taken for 2 weeks every 3 months increases bone density and prevents vertebral fractures. Data indicate safety and efficacy for up to 7 years of cyclical etidronate therapy.

Didrocal provides 14 days of 400 mg of etidronate followed by 76 days of 500 mg of elemental calcium as calcium carbonate. Calcium supplements are avoided during the 2-week cycle of etidronate.

Alendronate increases bone mass throughout the skeleton and reduces the risk of all fractures (including hip) by at least 50%.

Safety or efficacy data for treatment beyond 3 years is not available. However, more long-term data will be available by the time the patients now starting alendronate have been treated for 3 years.

Table 1: Drugs Used in Management of Osteoporosis

Drug	Dosage	Comments	Cost*
Nutritional Supplements			
calcium	1 000–1 500 mg/d of elemental calcium	Recommend supplements if unable to achieve intake by diet alone. The Osteoporosis Society of Canada prefers name brands of calcium carbonate or citrate. Constipation and nausea are common side effects.	$
vitamin D Drisdol, Ostoforte Multivitamins containing vitamin D	400–1 000 IU/d of cholecalciferol (vitamin D_3) or ergocalciferol (vitamin D_2)	Increases calcium absorption. Higher doses (e.g., 50 000 IU/week) may be needed in some individuals. Possible side effects are hypercalcemia, hypercalciuria, renal calcification and renal stones. Most multivitamin supplements contain 400 IU vitamin D and are the agents most commonly used.	$
Ovarian Hormone Therapy			
Estrogens	(Starting dose in brackets)		
conjugated equine estrogen Premarin	0.625 mg/d (0.3 mg × 2–3 mos)		$
conjugated estrone sulfate C.E.S.	0.625 mg/d (0.3 mg × 2–3 mos)	Synthetic estrogens are better tolerated than equine source.	$
estrone sulfate (estropipate) Ogen	0.625 mg/d (0.3 mg × 2–3 mos)		$
estradiol-17β micronized Estrace	1–2 mg/d (0.5 mg × 2–3 mos)		$
estradiol-17β transdermal Estraderm, Vivelle	50–100 μg/d (25 μg × 2–3 mos)	Patch is recommended if upper GI disease, liver disease, clotting problems or high triglyceride levels.	$$

Progestins

Drug	Dose	Comments	Cost
medroxyprogesterone acetate (MPA) Provera, generics	(Dose for 12–14 d/mo) 2.5, 5 and 10 mg	Halve dose if taken daily for 30 days. Start with 10 mg MPA or equivalent if 0–3 yrs postmenopause; 5 mg if 4–10 yrs postmenopause; 2.5 mg if > 10 yrs. Often better tolerated.	$
micronized oral progesterone Prometrium	100, 200 and 300 mg HS	More beneficial lipid effects.	$$
norethindrone Micronor	0.35 and 0.7 mg	May produce less bleeding and breast stimulation.	$–$$

Combination estrogen and progestin

Drug	Dose	Comments	Cost
estradiol 50 µg plus	4 patches over 1st 2 wks, then		$$
estradiol 50 µg/norethindrone 0.25 µg transdermal Estracomb	4 patches over last 2 wks		

Bisphosphonates

Drug	Dose	Comments	Cost
alendronate 🍷 Fosamax	10 mg/d plus calcium at a different time of day	All are poorly absorbed and must be taken on an empty stomach with water only. Side effects are minimal (GI symptoms, altered taste, nighttime leg cramps). Rarely, allergic reactions. Esophageal ulceration is a rare side effect of alendronate; patient must remain upright after taking the pill. Safety in impaired renal function (CrCl < 35 mL/min) is unknown.	$$$$
etidronate 🍷 Didronel, Didrocal	Cyclic: 400 mg/d × 14 d Q 3 mos, then calcium × 76 days		$$

(cont'd)

Table 1: Drugs Used in Management of Osteoporosis *(cont'd)*

Drug	Dosage	Comments	Cost*
Drugs not yet approved for osteoporosis			
calcitonin, salmon Calcimar	50–100 MRC units SC/d or Q 2nd day or 5 d/wk	Should be restricted to patients who fail conventional therapy. Analgesic effect in addition to antiresorptive effect. Dose is not standardized. Adverse effects: nausea, facial flushing, metallic taste, hypersensitivity (rare).	$$$$$
sodium fluoride, enteric coated Fluotic	20–40 mg daily PO	Gastrointestinal disturbances and arthralgia occur in up to 30% as early as 1 mo after starting therapy. Stop the drug and re-start at a lower dose. Duration of therapy should not exceed 2–4 yrs.	$–$$
calcitriol Rocaltrol	0.25–0.5 µg/d PO	Monitor calcium intake and serum calcium because usual recommendations for dietary calcium supplementation could cause hypercalcemia. Otherwise, well tolerated and safe.	$$–$$$
clodronate ● Bonefos, Ostac	Cyclic: 400 mg/d × 1 mo, followed by 2 mos off	See bisphosphonates.	$$

* *Cost of 30-day supply – includes drug cost only.*
Legend: $ *< $15* $$ *$15–30* $$$ *$30–45* $$$$ *$45–60* $$$$$ *>$60*

Which Bisphosphonate?

The dose schedule of etidronate (only 2 weeks every 3 months) and its lower cost are attractive to some patients.

Alendronate, taken continuously, appears to show a more rapid improvement in bone density. The gains in spinal bone density at 3 years with alendronate are marginally greater than those reported with cyclical etidronate (8% vs. 5 to 6%). Alendronate significantly increases bone density at all measured sites including the assessment of total body bone mineral which has not yet been demonstrated with etidronate.

Alendronate is the only osteoporosis therapy which has been clearly shown to prevent hip fractures (50% risk reduction) in a randomized controlled clinical trial. Postmarketing studies of cyclical etidronate therapy of osteoporosis in the UK also indicate a reduction in the rate of hip fracture.

There have been no comparative trials of bisphosphonates. Both drugs appear to be effective therapies for osteoporosis.

Calcitonin

Calcitonin is a potent depressor of osteoclast activity and has been shown to increase bone mass, particularly in osteoporotic patients with a high rate of bone turnover. It is an exceedingly safe agent that must be given parenterally (SC), and is expensive. Salmon calcitonin (Calcimar) is longer acting and perhaps more potent than human calcitonin, but the latter may be less prone to cause the development of resistance to the hormone.

Calcitonin has not yet been convincingly shown to be effective in fracture prevention. It has the advantage of demonstrated analgesic properties in addition to its antiresorptive effect.

The nasal spray (not yet approved in Canada) is less well absorbed; the minimal effective dose is probably 200 units daily.

Calcitriol (Rocaltrol)

A recent prospective, single blind, multicentre trial of calcitriol found a fracture prevention benefit with 0.25 μg twice daily, compared to patients receiving only calcium supplementation (1 g per day).

Androgens

Hypogonadism is a major diagnostic consideration for males with osteoporosis. Treatment with testosterone is indicated.

Anabolic steroids have been prescribed for women with osteo-porosis in selected cases, particularly elderly patients with low muscle mass. These drugs cause modest increases in bone mass, then prevent further bone loss. Some of the skeletal benefits in studies of osteoporotic elderly women may result from their effects on improved muscle mass.

Side effects include abnormal liver enzyme elevation, cholestasis, and more seriously, hepatoma or peliosis hepatis, as well as virilization, fluid retention and adverse effects on the lipid profile (reduced HDL, increased LDL cholesterol).

In the few Canadian osteoporosis clinics which prescribe androgens for osteoporosis, 50 mg nandrolone decanoate IM every 3 to 6 weeks for 1 to 2 years seems to be reasonably well tolerated and moderately effective.

Bone Formation Agents

These therapies have not received regulatory agency approval for the treatment of osteoporosis in Canada.

Sodium Fluoride

Fluoride is the most potent stimulator of bone formation currently available, seemingly without stimulating a concomitant increase in bone resorption. In clinical trials of fluoride, there is a progressive increase in bone mass of 5 to 10 percent per year, most pronounced in the spine.

There is concern that the increased bone mass seen in the clinical trials of fluoride does not correlate with bone strength, and may be associated with an increased risk of nonvertebral fractures.[1] Therefore, fluoride therapy of osteoporosis should be considered investigational. However, recent trials of "slow-release" fluoride therapy given cyclically (12 months on, 2 months off), coupled with calcium citrate supplementation have shown a fracture prevention benefit.[2,3] The slow-release tablets, not available in Canada, do not appear to allow the blood concentration of fluoride to reach toxic levels which interfere with the mineralization process. The enteric-coated form of sodium fluoride which is available in Canada may have more prolonged absorption and fewer side effects than plain sodium fluoride. However, it does not have the same absorption profile as the slow-release formulation.

Fluoride may have a future role in treating individuals who present with low bone mass, in order to build bone strength and prevent fractures, but more study is needed.

Conclusion

Postmenopausal estrogen/progesterone therapy remains the first choice for prevention of osteoporosis for women in the first

[1] N Engl J Med 1990;322:802–809.
[2] Ann Intern Med 1995;123:401–408.
[3] J Bone Miner Res 1996;11:160–168.

10 years postmenopause and for treatment of established osteoporosis. After age 60, one of the two approved bisphosphonate therapies would be equal to ovarian hormone therapy.

Therapeutic Tips

- A person over the age of 50 years with a vertebral compression fracture, wrist fracture, or hip fracture should be considered to have osteoporosis until proven otherwise. These individuals should be tested with bone densitometry, if available.

- It is clear that in all age groups, adequate calcium and vitamin D nutrition preserves or enhances bone mass, and prevents fractures in the elderly.

- For the prevention of osteoporosis in the early post-menopause, estrogen (with progesterone if the woman has not had a hysterectomy) is the treatment of choice. In the US, a low dose of alendronate (5 mg daily) has been approved as an alternative.

- For patients with established osteoporosis (a fragility fracture and bone density in the "osteoporosis" range), ovarian hormone therapy or bisphosphonate therapy should be offered first.

Suggested Reading List

Scientific Advisory Board of the Osteoporosis Society of Canada. Prevention and management of osteoporosis: Consensus Statements of the Scientific Advisory Board of the Osteoporosis Society of Canada. *Can Med Assoc J* 1996; 155:921-965.

Writing Group for the PEPI Trial: Effects of hormone therapy on bone mineral density: results from the Postmenopausal Estrogen/Progestin Interventions (PEPI) trial. *JAMA* 1996;276:1389-1396.

CHAPTER 53

Paget's Disease of Bone

Samuel E. York, MD, FRCPC

Paget's disease of bone (osteitis deformans) produces abnormal
bone architecture from excessive bone breakdown by osteoclasts
and excessive bone formation by osteoblasts. The etiology is
unknown, although infection by a slow virus is suspected. It is
characterized by thick cortices, coarse trabeculations, increased
blood supply and distortion of one or many bones, especially the
skull, pelvis, vertebrae and long bones. It may be asymptomatic,
but pain and distorted bones are common features. Neurologic
compression syndromes (due to bone entrapment of nerves) and
high output congestive heart failure (from increased bone blood
flow) are less common.

Goals of Therapy

- To decrease pain
- To decrease disease activity

Investigations

- Thorough history with attention to the description of bone
  pain; patients often have pain at rest relieved by movement
  (in contrast to arthritic patients who have pain on movement
  and pain that is relieved by rest). Patients with pagetic
  pseudofractures (usually in the tibia or femur) have pain at
  the site of the lesion, aggravated by movement and relieved
  by rest, and are at risk of fracture.
- Physical examination, especially for:
  - bowing, thickness and warmth of long bones
  - enlargement, deformity of skull
- Laboratory tests:
  - serum alkaline phosphatase (elevated) with normal liver
    function tests
  - serum calcium and phosphorus (usually normal)
  - urinary hydroxyproline or pyridinoline cross links (rarely
    necessary)
- Diagnostic imaging:
  - x-rays are usually characteristic
  - a technetium diphosphonate bone scan is sensitive but not
    specific for Paget's disease; it is useful to establish the
    extent of disease and to determine areas for radiologic
    examination
- Bone biopsy is only necessary if the diagnosis is doubtful

Figure 1: **Treatment of Paget's Disease of Bone**

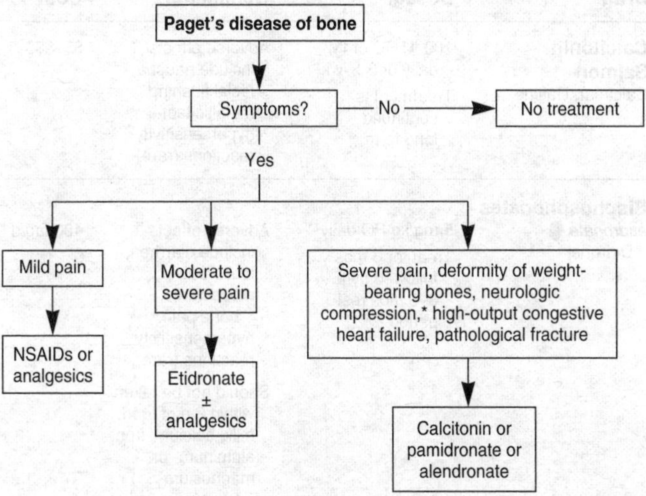

* *May require surgery.*

Therapeutic Choices (Figure 1)

Pharmacologic Choices (Table 1)

There is no proof that treatment prevents deformity or dysfunction. Second-generation bisphosphonates, especially IV pamidronate, can normalize the alkaline phosphatase. Long-term studies are not available to determine whether normalization will result in improved outcome, such as prevention of deformities, but it may delay their development. There is no uniform agreement on which medication to use initially, but bisphosphonates are usually given first (except as noted in Figure 1).

Bisphosphonates

Etidronate is useful for treating Paget's disease. Most symptomatic patients can be treated with oral etidronate; it may be preferred due to its oral dosing convenience in patients with less severe disease and no fractures. Therapy should not exceed 6 months to avoid impairment of mineralization and should be followed by an etidronate-free period of at least 90 days. Larger than recommended doses are not advised.

Patients on etidronate may develop spontaneous or pathological fractures, especially of lytic weight-bearing bones. If fractures occur, etidronate should be discontinued and the patient treated with a second-generation bisphosphonate or calcitonin.

Table 1: **Drugs Used in Paget's Disease of Bone**

Drug	Dosage	Comments	Cost*
Calcitonin Salmon Calcimar, Caltine	100 IU SC or IM daily or 3 ×/wk[†] Treatment is continued long term	Adverse effects include nausea, facial flushing, metallic taste, hypersensitivity reactions (rare).	$$–$$$
Bisphosphonates *etidronate* 🦴 Didronel	5 mg/kg PO daily[†] Treat for 6 mos followed by a 3–6 mos rest period	Adverse effects include diarrhea, loose bowel movements, ↑ bone pain, hypersensitivity reactions (rare). Should not be taken within 2 h of food, milk, calcium, iron, aluminum- or magnesium-containing substances.	400 mg/d $
alendronate 🦴 Fosamax	40 mg/d × 6 mos	Diarrhea, constipation, abdominal pain, and occasional esophagitis. Must be taken with a full glass of water on an empty stomach while erect (and stay erect) at least ½ h before any kind of food.	$$$
pamidronate 🦴 Aredia	30 mg IV over 3 h at 1 week intervals × 3 d	Adverse effects includes mild low grade fever, and transient hypocalcemia.	$$$$$

[†] *With adjuvant oral calcium, 1 g/d.*
🦴 *Dosage adjustment may be required in renal impairment – see Appendix I.*
* *Cost of 30-day supply – includes drug cost only.*
Legend: $ < $100 $$ $100–200 $$$ $200–300 $$$$ $300–400 $$$$$ > $400

The newer generation of bisphosphonates do not interfere with mineralization and will probably replace etidronate. These include the following:

Pamidronate (IV) is approved for treatment of moderate to severe Paget's disease of bone. Various dosing schedules are used. It is very effective, resulting in relief of pain in 70 to 90% of patients and normalization of serum alkaline phosphatase in up to 90% of patients. Its effect is long lasting, often 12 months or more. It is well tolerated with minimal side effects, and may well become the treatment of choice in the future.

Alendronate is available in oral form, and is effective, although gastrointestinal symptoms occur occasionally. It has not been used for as long as etidronate. Other bisphosphonates (e.g., **tiludronate** and **clodronate**) are being studied and show promise.

Calcitonin

Injectable calcitonin salmon is used currently. It is effective and decreases bone pain. However, antibodies may develop resulting in a loss of effectiveness. Recent experience with IV pamidronate (see above) suggests that this medication is more effective than calcitonin.

Others

Ipraflavone appears promising. **Plicamycin (mithramycin)** has serious side effects and is now rarely used. **Gallium nitrate** is effective but often associated with nephrotoxicity.

Monitoring Therapy

Serum alkaline phosphatase is adequate to follow treatment progress. With the ability of newer bisphosphonates to normalize serum alkaline phosphatase, this probably should be the new goal.

Therapeutic Tips

- Patients may become resistant to calcitonin treatment and to first-generation bisphosphonates, but current experience suggests the second-generation bisphosphonates continue to be effective.
- Pain relief may still occur despite the lack of decrease in alkaline phosphatase.
- Patients with painful disease usually respond to IV pamidronate or calcitonin.
- Patients with associated degenerative joint disease often benefit from joint replacement or osteotomy.
- Patients with Paget's disease of adjacent bones who are scheduled for elective joint replacement should be treated with calcitonin for 3 to 6 months, or a short course of IV pamidronate.
- Increasing pain and alkaline phosphatase during treatment suggests fracture or sarcomatous changes. Radiographs should be taken.

Suggested Reading List

Kanis JA. *Pathophysiology and treatment of Paget's disease of bone.* London: Martin Dunitz, 1991.

Delmas PD, Meunier PJ. The management of Paget's disease of bone. *N Engl J Med* 1997;336:558–566.

Hamdy RC. Clinical features and pharmacologic treatment of Paget's disease. *Endocrinol Metab Clin North Am* 1995;24:421–436.

Merkow RL, Lane JM. Paget's disease of bone. *Endocrinol Metab Clin North Am* 1990;19:177–204.

CHAPTER 54

Sports Injuries

James Kissick, MD, CCFP, Dip Sport Med

The majority of sports injuries encountered by physicians involve the soft tissues: strains, sprains and contusions.

Goals of Therapy

- To reduce acute symptoms (pain, inflammation) and recurrences
- To correct contributing factors (e.g., malalignment, muscle weakness)
- To return the athlete's weight-bearing capability, flexibility, range of motion, strength and proprioception to normal
- To enable the athlete to participate comfortably and fully in all pre-injury activities

Therapeutic Choices

For management of specific injuries, see Table 1.

General Approaches

Acute treatment is best summarized by the RICE protocol:
- **R**est of the injured part.
- **I**ce: Wrap an ice bag, cold pack or package of frozen peas in a damp, thin cloth and apply to the injured area for 15 minutes at a time, at least QID for the first 48 hours (or longer if swelling continues).
- **C**ompression with an elastic bandage if there is swelling such as in an ankle sprain.
- **E**levation: Try to elevate the injured part above the level of the heart.

Further treatment (e.g., modalities such as ultrasound) facilitates healing and allows participants to return safely to their activities.

NSAIDs or **ASA** (if not contraindicated) can decrease swelling and discomfort but should be used for short periods only.

Aggravation of the injury must be avoided, but alternative activities should be encouraged (e.g., the runner with a stress fracture of the fibula should not run but can swim or run in deep water).

Table 1: Management of Specific Sports Injuries

Injury	Investigations	Therapeutic Choices
Patellofemoral Syndrome Anterior knee pain resulting from patellofemoral articulation dysfunction (also known as patellofemoral pain syndrome or anterior knee pain syndrome).	**History** of anterior knee pain, worse with prolonged flexion, running. **Physical examination:** patellar malalignment, pain with patellar pressure, painful quads setting. **X-rays** (including skyline view of patella) if trauma or bony pathology is a concern.	**Relief of acute symptoms:** Rest from aggravating activities (emphasize alternative activities); ice, both PRN and postactivity; physiotherapy (ultrasound, etc.). **Correction of contributing factors:** *Foot overpronation:* appropriate shoes with straight to slightly curved last, good medial arch and support. If severe, may require custom foot orthotic. *Patellar lateral tracking due to vastus medialis obliquus (VMO) weakness:* VMO strengthening (e.g., closed kinetic chain exercises such as quarter squats, wall sits). Electrical muscle stimulation and/or biofeedback can assist. *Improve flexibility:* quadriceps, hamstrings, gastrocnemius, ilio-tibial band stretches *Taping techniques* (e.g., McConnell[1]) to correct patellar malposition *Correction of training errors:* in runners, more gradual distance increases, fewer hills. Decrease jumping, squats; avoid resisted leg extensions to ≥ 90° flexion. *Patellar stabilizing brace:* neoprene or elastic, with supporting buttress. Use with activities or more regularly if subluxation. *Surgery:* e.g., lateral release of tight retinacula, patellar tendon transfer (Elmslie-Trillat procedure)[2] is rarely required and should be a last resort.
Ankle Sprain Partial or complete tear to ankle-stabilizing ligaments, most commonly lateral (anterior and posterior talofibular, calcaneo-fibular). **Grade I:** No laxity, bears weight without pain, minimal swelling.	**History** of acute inversion (eversion less common). **Physical examination:** tenderness (most marked over injured ligament), swelling, pain with passive inversion and plantar flexion, positive drawer test in Grade III sprains.	**Grade I & II Sprains** Initial RICE protocol. Gradual ↑ weight bearing; may use tape/brace as support. Begin as soon as pain and stability allow (facilitates healing and proprioception). Early range of motion exercises. Stretching in dorsiflexion and plantar flexion. Strengthening: dorsiflexors, plantar flexors, then invertors and evertors.

Grade II: Swelling, painful weight bearing, possible slight laxity. **Grade III:** Unstable, significant laxity, complete disruption of at least two ligaments.	**X-rays** PRN[3]	Proprioceptive retraining. Progressive ↑ activities: walk → jog → run → run backward → curves → zig-zags. **Grade III Sprains** **Varying opinions:** Below-knee cast for 6 wks, cast for 3 wks then brace, brace only. If grossly unstable, may need surgical repair. Should be referred for orthopedic consultation. **NB:** Don't forget to check for associated injury more proximally in the leg.
Lower Leg Pain **"Shin Splints"** Inflammation of the tibialis posterior or anterior at its origin or of the tibial periosteum.	**History** of shin pain, usually in inexperienced and/or inadequately stretched or strengthened athletes. **Physical examination:** tenderness, usually diffuse, at medial border of tibia and adjacent muscle. **X-rays** normal; may need bone scan to differentiate from stress fracture.	Rest from aggravating activities (e.g., running). Alternative activities: cycling, swimming, pool running (running in deep water with flotation belt). Ice. Muscle stretching and strengthening. Correction of predisposing anatomic factors (i.e., with foot orthotics) and training errors. Gradual return to running or activity.
Stress fractures of the tibia/fibula Failure of bone due to repetitive over-load, resulting in microfractures.	**History** of well-localized shin pain with pounding activities. **Physical examination:** localized bony tenderness. **X-rays** usually negative until at least 2 wks after onset; may see periosteal thickening. Bone scan will show discrete increased uptake at stress fracture site.	No pounding activities until pain-free and nontender (usually 6–8 wks). Alternative activities: cycling, swimming, pool running. Flexibility and strength work. Long Air Cast-type brace often provides more comfort and possibly earlier return to pounding activities (if pain-free in Air Cast). Correction of anatomic factors, training errors.

(cont'd)

Table 1: **Management of Specific Sports Injuries** (cont'd)

Injury	Investigations	Therapeutic Choices
Stress fractures of the tibia/fibula (cont'd)	**NB:** Beware of anterior midshaft tibial stress fractures ("the dreaded black line"). On x-ray, appear as a horizontal fissure extending into the cortex of the tibia. These are slow to heal and often go on to nonunion.	Gradual return to running when pain-free and nontender: Wk 1: Run every other d, 1/2 usual distance, 1 min off usual mile pace. Wk 2: Usual run frequency, 3/4 usual distance, 1 min off mile pace. Wk 3: Usual frequency, 3/4 distance, 30 s off mile pace. Wk 4: Usual frequency, full distance, 30 s off mile pace[4]. Anterior midshaft tibial stress fractures should be assessed by orthopedic surgeon; may need immobilization.
Lateral Epicondylitis "Tennis Elbow" Degenerative tears (+/– inflammation) of the common extensor tendon at its origin at the lateral epicondyle of the humerus.	**History** of pain at the lateral elbow, usually due to overuse and/or faulty mechanics. **Physical examination:** tenderness at lateral epicondyle area, painful resisted wrist extension. **X-ray** if any concern (i.e., bony pathology).	Rest from aggravating activities. Tennis elbow "counter-force" brace. Ice, ice massage with "ice cup." Physiotherapy, stretching. Strengthening exercises as improvement occurs. **Correction of faulty mechanics:** *poor strokes, especially backhand (leading with the elbow), correct grip size, string tension to maximum 50–55 lbs, lighter racquet, avoid heavy duty or wet balls.* Suggest consultation with teaching pro. Gradual return to activity. If above unsuccessful, consider corticosteroid injection (e.g., triamcinolone acetonide 20 mg) to common extensor origin area at lateral epicondyle (maximum 3 injections, at least 1 mo apart). If still unsuccessful, consider surgery (usually release of part of common extensor origin and fascia).

Plantar fasciitis
Microtears of the plantar fascia and inflammation of the periosteum at its calcaneal origin (heel bone).

History of pain at plantar aspect of calcaneus, worse upon arising in the morning, getting up after a prolonged sit, and with running or prolonged walking.

Physical examination: pes planus or cavus, overpronation with walking. Tender at plantar fascial origin at the heel.

X-ray not usually needed, may show "spur" as a result of more chronic fasciitis.

Limit overpronation, cushion heel. Footwear important; running shoe best. Should wear for all weight bearing. Arch supports, heel pads or cups may be necessary. Custom foot orthotics needed in some cases.

Rest from aggravating activities (e.g., bike instead of run).

Ice or ice massage.

Roll foot on soup can before weight bearing in morning.

Stretches: gastrocnemius, soleus, plantar fascia, foot intrinsics.

Night splint to prevent ankle plantar flexion while sleeping; decreases fascial shortening and morning pain.[5]

Corticosteroid injection if not improving with above (e.g., triamcinolone acetate 20 mg mixed with 0.5 mL xylocaine 1% to tender area).

Surgery rarely required.

[1] *Aust J Phys Ther 1986;32:215.*
[2] *Am J Sports Med 1984;12:104.*
[3] *JAMA 1993;269:1127–1132.*
[4] *The team physician's handbook. Philadelphia: Hanley and Belfus, 1990:446.*
[5] *Clin J Sport Med 1996;6:158.*

As the injury heals, it is crucial to regain and, in most cases, improve flexibility and muscle strength. Return to activity should not occur until full strength is obtained. Before the patient resumes activity, any factors that may have contributed to the injury (improper shoes, poor protective equipment) should be corrected, and sport-specific skills regained.

Suggested Reading List

Hershman EB, Mailly T. Stress fractures. *Clin Sports Med* 1990;9:1.

Mellion MB, Walsh WM, Shelton Gl, eds. *The team physician's handbook*. Philadelphia: Hanley and Belfus, 1990.

Reid DC. *Sports injury assessment and rehabilitation*. New York: Churchill Livingstone, 1992.

Stiell IG, Greenberg GH, McKnight RD, et al. Decision rules for the use of radiography in acute injuries: refinement and prospective validation. *JAMA* 1993;269:1127–1132.

CHAPTER 55

Acne

Rob Miller, MD, FRCPC

Definition

A multifactorial disease caused by increased sebaceous gland activity at puberty due to hormonal effects, overgrowth of *Propionibacterium acnes* on skin surface and/or immature keratinization of follicular epithelium and subsequent follicular occlusion.

Acne can be subclassified into different clinical patterns in which one type may predominate:

- Comedogenic acne (closed and open comedones – "whiteheads and blackheads")
- Papulopustular acne (papules and pustules – "pimples")
- Nodulocystic acne (a deeper, more inflammatory form)

Each type can lead to scarring, although it is much more commonly associated with the nodulocystic variety.

Goals of Therapy

- To minimize the symptoms and cosmetic disfigurement
- To prevent recurrence
- To prevent scarring

Investigations

- History, including:
  - use/abuse of cosmetic agents including hair gels, mousses, pomades
  - topical (including OTC) and oral medications used in acne treatment and duration of use
  - medications that may positively or negatively affect acne (e.g., oral contraceptives, steroids)
- Laboratory tests: if isotretinoin is to be used, baseline and follow-up pregnancy tests, liver function tests, fasting serum triglyceride and cholesterol levels

Therapeutic Choices

Nonpharmacologic Choices

- A balanced diet is good for overall health, but there is no evidence that acne is caused by specific foods.

Figure 1: **Management of Acne**

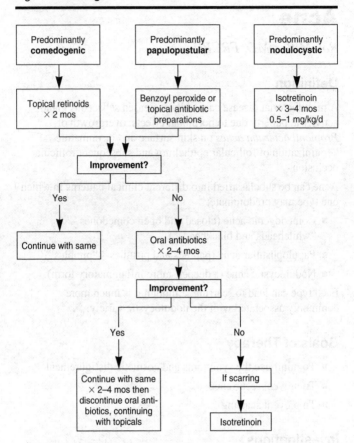

- Squeezing pimples may increase the risk of scarring.
- Avoid excessive cosmetic use and use only non-comedogenic, water-based products.

Pharmacologic Choices (Figure 1)

Topical Agents (Table 1)

Benzoyl peroxide is a peeling agent that also has some anti-bacterial action; it is used mainly in papulopustular acne.

Retinoids (topical isotretinoin, tretinoin) are used predominantly in comedogenic acne.

NB: Topical tretinoin and benzoyl peroxide have been reported to cause cancer in experimental animal studies. The clinical significance of these reports in humans is unknown.

Antibiotics (erythromycin, clindamycin) are used to decrease colonization of skin with *P. acnes*, mainly in papulopustular acne.

Other agents include nicotinic acid, combinations of topical retinoids and antibiotics, and sulfur, salicylic acid, resorcinol, abrasive cleansers, etc. (which have largely been displaced by newer topical agents).

Table 1: **Topical Acne Preparations**

Drug	Comments
Benzoyl Peroxide PanOxyl, Oxyderm, Acetoxyl, Benzac AC, Benzac W, Benoxyl, Desquam-X, Dermoxyl, Benzagel, Solugel, others	Depending on brand, may be available in 2.5% to 20% concentrations and in creams, lotions, gels (water, acetone or alcohol-based); concentrations ≤ 5% are available OTC
	May bleach fabric
Retinoids *tretinoin* StieVA-A, Vitamin A Acid, Retin-A, Retisol-A, Vitinoin	Depending on brand, available in 0.01%, 0.025%, 0.05%, 0.1% concentrations and in creams, gels, solutions
isotretinoin Isotrex	Retisol-A also contains sunscreen
tazarotene Tazorac	0.1% gel. Place in acne therapy remains to be established.
Retinoid Analogs *adapalene* Differin	0.1% gel for mild to moderate comedonal acne
Antibiotics *erythromycin* Erysol (gel), Sans-Acne (solution), Staticin (lotion), T-Stat (lotion, pads) *clindamycin* Dalacin T (solution); can also add 2% clindamycin to Duonalc or Dilusol	
Combinations *benzoyl peroxide + erythromycin* Benzamycin *tretinoin + erythromycin* Stievamycin *neomycin + methylprednisolone* Neo-Medrol Acne Lotion	
Miscellaneous *nicotinamide* Papulex *salicylic acid 2%* Acnex, Salac, others	Many combination products (salicylic acid + sulfur) Available OTC

Systemic Agents (Table 2)
Antibiotics

Tetracycline is the most commonly prescribed oral agent; 1 g per day reduces the number of *P. acnes* and may exert an anti-inflammatory effect by inhibiting leukocyte chemotaxis. When control is achieved the dosage can often be reduced to 250 to 500 mg per day for maintenance.

Tetracycline during the first trimester of pregnancy is unlikely to cause teeth discoloration or other teratogenic effects, but it is nevertheless contraindicated during all trimesters of pregnancy. It may exacerbate azotemia in patients with pre-existing renal disease.

Minocycline has the advantages of fewer side effects and once daily dosing. Information to date on interactions with oral contraceptives is insufficient to conclude whether the risk of pregnancy is increased, decreased or unaffected.

Erythromycin is an alternative to tetracycline due to its excellent safety profile. Side effects are mainly gastrointestinal (dose related).

Isotretinoin

Isotretinoin is indicated in the treatment of severe nodulocystic and/or inflammatory acne vulgaris. Patients with other forms of acne for whom the risk of scarring is great and who have not responded to maximal topical and oral antibiotic therapy should be considered for this drug.

Divided doses of 0.5 to 1 mg/kg/day are prescribed for 16 to 20 weeks in the majority of patients. Some may require longer treatment times and higher doses. Truncal involvement resolves more slowly than facial. Relapses occur more frequently if lower dosages (e.g., 0.1 mg/kg) are used. If relapses occur, the recommendation is to wait 8 weeks after completion of the first course before reinstituting therapy.

Because of its **teratogenic effects**, use in females of childbearing age requires appropriate contraception as well as baseline and once monthly pregnancy tests.

Others

Spironolactone, with its anti-androgen effects, has been used both topically and orally to treat acne although it is not yet approved for this indication. **Oral contraceptives** are not approved for treating acne. **Estrogen** and **conjugated estrogens** are used primarily for the androgen excess associated with an estrogen deficiency for selected patients (alopecia, acne, hirsutism and in some instances seborrhea). **Zinc** is of unproven value. **Cyproterone acetate**, an anti-androgen, has been used successfully for female androgen-excess disorders (e.g., hirsutism, alopecia and acne) but it is not approved in Canada for treating acne.

Physical Therapy

- Comedone extraction (care must be taken to avoid unnecessary manipulation).
- Intralesional steroids for inflamed cysts.

Table 2: Commonly Prescribed Systemic Drugs Used in Acne Therapy

Drug	Dosage	Adverse Effects	Drug Interactions	Cost*
Antibiotics 🎗️ tetracycline Tetracyn, generics	**Tetracycline:** 500 mg BID initial 250–500 mg/d maintenance	GI effects; overgrowth of Candida; photosensitivity; pseudotumor cerebri; may exacerbate azotemia.	GI absorption of tetracycline may be impaired by iron, bismuth, aluminum, calcium, magnesium, in drugs and foods (e.g., dairy products). Separate doses by 2 h.	1 g/d $
minocycline Minocin, generics	**Minocycline:** 100 mg/d initial 50 mg/d maintenance	Dizziness, vertigo, ataxia (dose-related) with minocycline; abnormal cutaneous pigmentation with minocycline.		100 mg/d $$
doxycycline Doryx, Vibra-Tabs, generics	**Doxycycline:** 100 mg/d initial and maintenance	Contraindicated in pregnant women, children under 8.		100 mg/d $-$$
erythromycin Eryc, Erythromid, PCE, EES, Ilosone, generics	500 mg BID initial 250–500 mg/d maintenance	GI effects: nausea, vomiting, epigastric distress, diarrhea. Estolate-induced cholestatic jaundice.	May ↑ blood levels of theophylline, cyclosporine, carbamazepine, warfarin, digitalis, ergotamine, methylprednisolone. Concurrent use with astemizole, terfenadine or cisapride is contraindicated.	1 g/d base $ EC caps $$ PCE $$$
isotretinoin Accutane	0.5–1.0 mg/kg/d for 16–20 wks	Teratogenicity; ocular effects (conjunctivitis, ↓ night vision); bone effects (rarely premature epiphyseal closure); ↑ triglyceride and cholesterol levels (25–50% of patients); ↑ liver function tests in 10% of patients; pseudotumor cerebri; mucocutaneous effects; myalgias (15%); reversible hair loss.	NB: No adverse interaction known between retinoids and oral contraceptives.	40 mg/d $$$

* Cost of 30-day supply – includes drug cost only.
Legend: $ < $20 $$ $20–50 $$$ $50–100 $$$$ $100–150

🎗️ *Dosage adjustment may be required in renal impairment – see Appendix 1.*

- Liquid nitrogen (occasionally helpful for papulopustular lesions).
- Ultraviolet light therapy.
- Chemical peels (of value in treating comedogenic and papulopustular acne not responding to medical therapy).
- Dermabrasion/facial peels/resurfacing laser for acne scars.

Therapeutic Tips

- Start with one topical preparation at a time and apply initially only QHS; increase to BID if well tolerated.
- Lower concentrations and creams of benzoyl peroxide and retinoids are, in general, less irritating than the higher concentrations and gel formulations.
- Advise patients to apply preparation over general affected area and not just to individual lesions.
- Warn patients of irritation around mucous membranes and irritation that may be aggravated by sun exposure.
- Advise patients that improvement is slow and may not be seen before 6 to 8 weeks.
- If inflamed cysts are present, do not incise as this causes scarring; they may be managed by intralesional steroid injections after aspiration (0.1 to 0.5 mg triamcinolone acetonide into each cyst).
- If no improvement after 2 months of topical therapy, add oral antibiotic to regimen.
- Patients on long-term antibiotic therapy may develop gram-negative folliculitis (Chapter 65).
- If using isotretinoin, stop all other topical and oral acne therapy as they provide no added benefit. Patients should also be advised to stop taking vitamin supplements containing vitamin A.

Suggested Reading List

Leyden JJ. Therapy for acne vulgaris. *N Engl J Med* 1997;336:1156–1162.

Strauss J. Sebaceous glands. In: Fitzpatrick T, Eisen A, Wolff K, et al, eds. *Dermatology in general medicine*. Toronto: McGraw-Hill, 1993:708–726.

Wolverton S, Wilkin J. *Systemic drugs for skin diseases*. Toronto: W.B. Saunders, 1991.

CHAPTER 56

Rosacea

Donald Rosenthal, MD, FRCPC

Goals of Therapy

- To decrease symptoms and signs: burning, redness, flushing, papules and pustules
- To prevent recurrence

Investigations

- Thorough history with special attention to central facial flushing, crops of papules and pustules, red face, red eyes, recurrent external eye infections/irritation and thickening/deformity of the distal nose. Increasing numbers of persistent tiny red facial lines (telangiectasia)
- Family history of similar changes in adult life
- Physical examination:
  - telangiectasia, acneiform papules and pustules
  - rhinophyma
  - evidence of chronic recurrent eye changes (e.g., blepharitis, conjunctivitis)
- Other causes of red face and flushing should be ruled out (e.g., seborrheic dermatitis, contact dermatitis, photosensitivity reactions, lupus erythematosus, perioral dermatitis)

Therapeutic Choices

Nonpharmacologic Choices

- Avoid facial exposure to sun, either direct or reflected, via appropriate hats, sunscreens and lifestyle alterations.
- The use of potent or prolonged facial corticosteroid medications should be avoided.
- Where possible flushing stimuli should be minimized (e.g., alcohol, extremes of heat or cold, psychological stress).

Laser Therapy

- Telangiectasia and rhinophyma may be significantly improved by appropriate laser treatment.

Pharmacologic Choices (Table 1)

Table 1: **Drugs Used in Rosacea**

Drug	Dosage	Adverse Effects	Drug Interactions	Comments	Cost*
Oral Antibiotics *tetracycline* ♥ Tetracyn, generics	1 g daily for 4 wks; maintenance: lowest dose that will control symptoms	GI effects; overgrowth of Candida; photosensitivity; may ↑ azotemia; pseudotumor cerebri; contraindicated in pregnant women.	Calcium, aluminum, magnesium, iron, bismuth → ↓ tetracycline absorption. Separate dosing by 2 h.	Most cost-effective treatment. Can be given on empty stomach with clear fluids as bolus dose once daily. Improvement indicated by reduction in number of active papules and pustules and improved eye symptoms. Telangiectasia will remain and fade slowly in intensity.	$
minocycline Minocin, generics	200 mg daily for 4–6 wks; maintenance: lowest dose that will control symptoms	See tetracycline. Also dizziness; vertigo; ataxia (dose-related); abnormal cutaneous pigmentation; rarely LE-like syndrome; hepatic dysfunction.		Can be tried if tetracycline fails after compliant 4–6 wks trial.	$$$$
erythromycin Erythromid, EES, Eryc, Ilosone, PCE, generics	0.5–1 g daily in divided doses for 4–6 wks; maintenance: lowest dose that will control symptoms	Nausea; vomiting; epigastric distress; diarrhea; cholestatic jaundice (more common with estolate).	Concurrent use with cisapride, astemizole or terfenadine is contraindicated. May ↑ blood levels of digitalis, theophylline, warfarin, carbamazepine, cyclosporine, ergotamine, methylprednisolone.	Less effective than tetracyclines. Can be tried if patient intolerant of tetracyclines.	$

Topic Therapy			
Topical Therapy			
metronidazole Metrocream, Metrogel, Noritate	0.75% gel or 1% cream applied as thin film BID; maintenance: as needed to control symptoms	Watery eyes (if applied too closely); redness; dryness; burning/irritation.	Of significant benefit. Best alternative to oral tetracyclines particularly for papules and pustules component. Can be used in combination with oral tetracyclines.	$$
benzoyl peroxide Solugel, PanOxyl, Acetoxyl, others	2.5–5% in water-based gel BID; maintenance: as needed to control symptoms	Skin irritation.	May bleach fabric or hair.	$
erythromycin Erysol, Sans-Acne, Staticin, T-Stat	2–4% lotion or gel BID	Skin irritation and dryness.		$$
tetracycline	4% in Duonalc lotion BID; maintenance: as needed to control symptoms	Irritation; burning; yellow discoloration of skin.	Less effective than oral tetracyclines.	$$†
clindamycin Dalacin T	1% in lotion base BID; maintenance: as needed to control symptoms	Irritation; burning; redness; GI disturbances (rare); pseudomembranous colitis (extremely rare).	Less effective than oral tetracyclines.	$$
hydrocortisone	1% lotion with or without 5–10% precipitated sulfur BID; maintenance: as needed to control symptoms		Prolonged topical steroid use should be avoided. Hydrocortisone may reduce some inflammation. Sulfur may dry/decrease papules and pustules.	$–$$†

Legend: $ < $10 $$ $10–20 $$$ $20–50 $$$$ > $50
† *Compounding fees are additional.*

● *Dosage adjustment may be required in renal impairment – see Appendix I.*
* *Cost of 30-day therapy – includes drug cost only.*

Therapeutic Tips

- Rosacea fluctuates in severity but is a chronic process. Therapy should address this. Patient understanding is mandatory. Long periods of remission may occur.
- Improvement is measured by:
  - a significant reduction in number of active papules/pustules.
  - improvement in eye symptoms and signs.
- Smoothing of skin is the therapeutic challenge.
- Telangiectasia and flushing "red face" will remain indefinitely to some extent.

Suggested Reading List

Bleicher PA, Charles JH, Sober AJ. Topical metronidazole for rosacea. *Arch Dermatol* 1987;123:609–613.

Gamborg NP. A double-blind study of 1% metronidazole cream versus systemic oxytetracycline therapy for rosacea. *Br J Dermatol* 1983;109:63–65.

Marks R. The problem of rosacea. *Br Med J* 1976;1:94.

Sibenge S, Gawkrodger DJ. Rosacea. *J Am Acad Dermatol* 1992;26:590–593.

CHAPTER 57

Sunburn

Lyn Guenther, MD, FRCPC

Sunburn is caused by excessive exposure to ultraviolet (UV) radiation. It is characterized by **erythema**, with onset 2 to 6 hours after exposure to a threshold dose of UV radiation; it peaks at 15 to 36 hours and regresses by 72 to 96 hours. **Edema** and **pain** may be present. **Blistering** in severe cases may take a week or more to resolve. Nausea, abdominal cramping, fever, chills and headache may also occur. **Desquamation** with resolution results from cellular injury and death.

Any person, even black, will burn with large doses of UV radiation. Blue- or green-eyed, lighter-skinned individuals who tan poorly and freckle burn more readily. The trunk, neck and head burn at a lower dose of UV radiation than the upper limbs, which burn more readily than the lower limbs.

Characteristics of Ultraviolet Radiation

UV radiation consists of:

- UVC (200 to 290 nm):
  - filtered by the ozone layer, does not reach the earth
  - emitted by welding arcs, bactericidal and mercury arc lamps
- UVB (290 to 320 nm):
  - the primary cause of sunburn from sunlight
  - 1 000 times more erythemogenic than UVA
  - substantially absorbed by the ozone layer
  - does not penetrate glass
- UVA (320 to 400 nm):
  - responsible for most phototoxic reactions to drugs
  - penetrates the skin more deeply than UVB
  - negligibly absorbed by the ozone layer
  - causes 10% of solar erythema
  - can pass through glass

A 1% decrease in ozone results in a 1.5% increase in UVB, leading to a 2 to 6% increase in basal and squamous cell cancers and a 0.3 to 2% increase in melanomas. For every 300 meters above sea level, UV radiation increases by 4%. Radiation effects are enhanced by reflective surfaces (e.g., sand, snow and water). Up to 80% of UV radiation penetrates clouds. Increased humidity decreases the threshold for erythema to UV radiation. In 1992, Environment Canada developed the UV index, which forecasts the intensity of UV rays. It is estimated that a fair-skinned person will burn in less than 15 minutes with a UV index over 9, in approximately 20 minutes with an index of 7 to 9, and approximately 30 minutes with an index of 4 to 7.

Prevention of Sunburn

Prevention is critical since repeated sun exposure and sunburns are associated with skin cancer and premature skin aging. One severe sunburn during childhood can double the risk of skin cancer later in life. UV radiation can also suppress the immune system and habitual exposure can cause cataracts.

Nonpharmacologic Choices

- Cosmetic tanning should be avoided. Pigmentation does not occur without damage and death of epidermal cells.

- Tanning salons should be avoided. UVA-induced tanning may only produce a sun protective factor (SPF[1]) of 2 to 4.

- Outdoor activities at peak UV irradiance times (10:00 a.m. to 3:00 p.m.) should be avoided.

- Umbrellas may reduce UV radiation by about 70%; however, they do not protect against reflected radiation.

- Protective clothing (pants, long-sleeved shirts, gloves) and sunglasses should be worn. Loosely woven, white or wet clothing offers less protection.

- Wide-brimmed hats (at least 7.5 cm) of tightly woven fabric (not straw) should be worn to protect the face, ears and neck.

- Sun exposure should be minimized while one is taking phototoxic medications or using certain local agents (Table 1), which can interact with UV/visible light to cause a dose-related sunburn.

Pharmacologic Choices

No sunscreen offers complete protection from the sun.

Topical Sunscreens

Sunscreens should be used to protect the skin and not to prolong sun exposure. They should provide protection against both UVB and UVA, and have an SPF of at least 30. The SPF of sunscreens is measured under ideal laboratory conditions and may be considerably less when applied thinly and used outdoors. Topical sunscreens should be applied generously (2 mg/cm^2) to all exposed surfaces including lips, tops of ears and dorsal aspect of feet. Reapplication does not extend the period of protection. A person who burns in 10 minutes will burn in 300 minutes using

---

[1] $SPF = \dfrac{\textit{least amount of UVB energy to produce erythema with sunscreen}}{\textit{least amount of UVB energy to produce erythema without sunscreen}}$

Table 1: **Agents That May Cause Phototoxic Reactions***

Systemic Drugs	Local Agents
Amiodarone	Cadmium sulfide
Antibiotics	Yellow pigment in tattoos
Ceftazidime	Coal tar derivatives
Griseofulvin	Acridine
Quinolones	Anthracene
Ciprofloxacin	Fluoranthene
Nalidixic acid	Naphthalene
Norfloxacin	Phenanthrene
Ofloxacin	Pyridine
Sulfonamides	Thiophene
Tetracyclines	Dyes
Demeclocycline	Acriflavine
Doxycycline	Anthraquinone
Tetracycline	Eosin
Antineoplastics	Methylene blue
Dacarbazine	Rose bengal
5-fluorouracil	Toluidine blue
Vinblastine	Furocoumarins
Diuretics	Psoralen from plants
Furosemide	Leguminoseae family
Hydrochlorothiazide	Moraceae family
Hematoporphyrin	Figs
NSAIDs	Rutaceae family
Diclofenac	Bergamot orange
Ibuprofen	Gas plant
Indomethacin	Lemon
Ketoprofen	Lime
Naproxen	Umbellifereae family
Piroxicam	Angelica
Sulindac	Anise
Tiaprofenic acid	Bishop's weed
Psoralens	Celery
Methoxsalen	Cow parsley
Trioxsalen	Dill
Quinidine	Fennel
Quinine	Giant hogweed
Retinoids	Wild parsnip
Acitretin	Wild carrot
Isotretinoin	5-methoxypsoralen
Sulfonylureas	Bergamot oil
Tolbutamide	Methoxsalen
	Tretinoin

* *Radiation in the UVA range causes most drug-related phototoxic reactions.*

a sunscreen with an SPF of 30, no matter how many times it is applied. This person will develop erythema in < 300 minutes if the sunscreen is not reapplied after swimming, towelling or sweating.

Chemical Sunscreens (Table 2)

Commercial products usually contain more than one active ingredient. They should be applied 15 to 60 minutes before UV exposure to allow active ingredients to bind to the skin. They can be used in children older than 6 months of age. Chronic sunscreen use has not been associated with vitamin D deficiency. Only a few minutes of sun daily, to the back of one hand, results in sufficient vitamin D production. In addition, adequate amounts of vitamin D can be absorbed from cereal, dairy products and fish.

Physical Sunscreens

Titanium dioxide, zinc oxide, kaolin, talc (magnesium silicate), ferric chloride, melanin and **red veterinary petrolatum** protect against UVA and UVB and can be used in people of all ages including infants. They reflect and scatter UV and visible light. Recent data have shown that titanium dioxide and zinc oxide can also absorb UVA wavelengths up to 400 nm. Physical sunscreens are generally thicker, less cosmetically elegant and may rub off easily or melt with the sun's heat. Although they have less risk of sensitization, their occlusive effect may cause miliaria and folliculitis. Micronized titanium dioxide is relatively transparent to visible light but scatters UV light well.

Oral Sunscreens

There is no effective oral sunscreen. Oral beta-carotene, anti-malarials, vitamin A, vitamin E and oral PABA *do not* provide effective protection against sunburn. Vitamin C or E in a topical sunscreen may however enhance photoprotection.

Treatment of Sunburn

No effective treatment is available. The following may provide relief if given at the time of sunburn or shortly after.

Nonpharmacologic Choices

Cool baths or **wet compresses** for 20 minutes several times a day provide some relief. **Moisturizers** help with dryness and peeling.

Pharmacologic Choices

Topical vitamin E (alpha tocopherol) applied 2 minutes after UV exposure may decrease erythema and edema. The effect is diminished if applied later post-irradiation and is probably insignificant if applied after 5 hours.[1]

Indomethacin 25 mg or **ibuprofen** 400 mg Q6H for 4 doses, starting at time of insult, may decrease erythema and reduce the degree of epidermal injury.

Potent topical corticosteroids transiently decrease erythema by causing vasoconstriction but do not reduce epidermal damage. They may soothe stinging and itching. Their effect is additive when used with indomethacin or ibuprofen.[2]

Acetaminophen may relieve pain.

---

[1] *Oxidative Stress in Dermatology. New York: Marcel Dekker Inc., 1993:67–80.*
[2] *Dermatology 1992;184:54–58.*

Table 2: **Chemical Sunscreens**

Active Ingredient	Comments
UVB Absorbers **Para-aminobenzoic acid (PABA) esters** Padimate O (octyl dimethyl PABA) Padimate A (amyl dimethylamino benzoate) Lisadimate (glyceryl aminobenzoate or glyceryl PABA)	Adhere well to skin. May cause contact/photocontact dermatitis. May cross react with sulfonamides, thiazides, sulfonylurea hypoglycemics, ester anesthetics, paraphenylenediamine, aniline, azodye A, picric acid, saccharin. PABA may stain fabrics yellow upon sun exposure.
Salicylates Homosalate (homomenthyl salicylate) Octyl salicylate Triethanolamine salicylate	Rarely cause contact dermatitis. Do not adhere well to skin; easily removed by perspiration or swimming.
Cinnamates Octyl methoxycinnamate (Parsol MCX) 2-ethoxyethyl p-methoxycinnamate (Cinoxate)	Do not adhere well to skin. May cross react with balsam of Peru, coca leaves, benzyl and methyl cinnamate, cinnamic alcohol, cinnamic aldehyde, cinnamon oil.
Benzylidene camphor derivative 4-methylbenzylidene camphor	Maximum absorption at 300 nm. Photostabilizes dibenzoylmethanes.
UVA Absorbers **Benzophenones** Oxybenzone Sulisobenzone Dioxybenzone	Broad-spectrum UVA/UVB protection. Oxybenzone may cause contact/photocontact dermatitis. Dioxybenzone may cause contact urticaria/contact dermatitis.
Anthranilates Menthyl anthranilate	Rarely cause sensitization.
Dibenzoylmethanes Avobenzone or t-butylmethoxy-dibenzoylmethane (Parsol 1789)	Broad UVA absorption. Better protection against UVA than benzophenones, anthranilates and Mexoryl SX. Photodegradable.
Benzylidene camphor derivative Terephthalylidene dicamphor sulfonic acid (Mexoryl SX)	Good photostability. Maximum absorption at 345 nm.

Therapeutic Tips

- Systemic corticosteroids have little effect in treating sunburn; oral antihistamines have no effect.
- Topical anesthetic sprays are associated with a risk of sensitization and should be avoided.

- After a sunburn, the skin should not be exposed to the sun for at least a week.
- Blistering sunburns may require treatment in a burn unit.
- **Waterproof** sunscreens maintain efficacy after 80 minutes of water immersion.
- **Water-resistant** sunscreens maintain efficacy after 40 minutes of water immersion.
- **Sweat-resistant** sunscreens maintain efficacy after 30 minutes of continuous heavy perspiration.

Suggested Reading List

Buescher LS. Sunscreens and photoprotection. *Otolaryngol Clin North Am* 1993;26(1):13–22.

Dromgoole SH, Maibach HI. Sunscreening agent intolerance: contact and photocontact sensitization and contact urticaria. *J Am Acad Dermatol* 1990;22:1068–1078.

Gonzalez E, Gonzalez S. Drug photosensitivity, idiopathic photodermatoses, and sunscreens. *J Am Acad Dermatol* 1996;35:871–885.

Gould JW, Mercurio MG, Elmets CA. Cutaneous photosensitivity diseases induced by exogenous agents. *J Am Acad Dermatol* 1995;33:551–573.

Panthak MA. Sunscreens: topical and systemic approaches for protection of human skin against harmful effects of solar radiation. *J Am Acad Dermatol* 1982;7:285–312.

CHAPTER 58

Basal Cell Carcinoma

Robert D.L. Tremaine, MD, FRCPC

General Information

- Accounts for 75% of all malignant skin tumors
- Most common in fair-skinned, blond or red-haired people
- UV light is the most common cause
- Frequency increases with age
- Also caused by ionizing radiation, scars or trauma, arsenic and genetic predisposition
- Can cause marked local tissue destruction and even rare metastases so early detection and treatment is important
- Metastases with small lesions are extremely rare because, in general, tumor cells cannot proliferate without the surrounding connective tissue stroma; therefore, systemic work-up is generally **not** indicated
- Every 1% decrease in ozone leads to a 2% increase in UVB light reaching the earth's surface and a 3 to 6% increase in skin cancer rates

Clinical Variants

Nodular basal cell carcinoma
- classic erythematous or flesh-colored papule with telangiectasia and rolled pearly borders

Pigmented basal cell carcinoma
- similar features to nodular basal cell carcinoma but with brown pigmentation
- often mistaken for nevi

Superficial multicentric basal cell carcinoma
- scaling erythematous persistent plaques often with a thread-like pearly border
- usually on the trunk
- often mistaken for inflammatory lesions

Sclerosing basal cell carcinoma
- flat or depressed shiny indurated plaques that extend well beyond the clinically visible margins

Fibroepithelioma
- one or several raised or pedunculated nodules covered with smooth reddened skin

Table 1: Therapeutic Choices for Basal Cell Carcinoma (BCC)

Treatment Option	Advantages	Disadvantages
Electrodesiccation and curettage (ED&C) – lesion is curetted 3 times in succession followed by electrodesiccation, leaving a shallow crust to heal by secondary intention.	Very simple and quick. Very high cure rates for small lesions. Excellent cosmetic results with very little normal tissue damage.	Not as useful for lesions over 2 cm as recurrence rates are higher. Not useful for sclerosing BCC or other lesions with very indistinct borders.
Surgical excision – lesion is excised in traditional fashion with primary closure or the use of flaps or grafts.	Simple procedure for most physicians. High cure rates. Good cosmetic results; vary with location.	Higher recurrence rates around lesions with indistinct borders (i.e., sclerosing BCC). Higher infection rates than with ED&C. Often leaves large defect that may require specialized surgery.
Mohs' microsurgery – specialized procedure where surgeons and pathologists cooperate to ensure lesion is completely excised. Slices of tumor are examined immediately by pathologist using special staining techniques or frozen sections; the team can immediately determine if residual tumor is left and at exactly which margin the problem exists.	Very high cure rates even with large tumors, sclerosing BCC or lesions in difficult anatomic sites (e.g., eyelids, ear canals, nasolabial folds).	Very time-consuming. Very expensive. Closure of defects may be difficult. Not readily available in every centre.
Carbon dioxide laser – complete laser ablation or vaporization of a basal cell.	Useful for large lesions; procedure provides complete hemostasis, which allows good visualization of the surgical field. Healing is by secondary intention, which alleviates the necessity for grafting, flaps, etc. Scar: soft, supple, generally cosmetically acceptable. Low infection rates.	Not always readily available. Somewhat slower healing time. Recurrences more common in lesions with indistinct borders. Pathologic specimens cannot be sent using only this procedure.

Treatment	Advantages	Disadvantages
Radiotherapy – multiple modalities used including superficial x-ray therapy, Grenz rays, electron beam therapy and, more recently, brachytherapy.	Useful for large lesions, those in difficult areas or those with indistinct borders because large areas can be done. Very good in elderly patients or in those at poor surgical risk. High cure rates. Relatively easy for the patient.	Not always readily available. Slow healing time (at least 6 wks). Potentially poor cosmetic results though they may often be very good.
Cryotherapy – generally accomplished using liquid nitrogen spray that allows a deep freeze.	Very quick and simple for the patient. Potentially outstanding cosmetic results. Very good for superficial multicentric BCC or for lesions on the eyelids but not for lesions with indistinct borders.	Unless biopsy previously performed, histologic confirmation of pathology is not available. Not useful for large or deep lesions. Cure rates are not as high as for other modalities. Procedure may be painful.
Photodynamic therapy[1] – a photosensitizing medication (usually a hematoporphyrin derivative) is injected IV or applied topically (aminolevulenic acid) in an ointment base. It preferentially accumulates in tumor cells; the tumor is then exposed to red light or intense visible light which leads to the production of singlet oxygen that is cytotoxic to tumor cells.	Completely removes the need for surgery. Minimal surrounding tissue damage so cosmetic results are excellent. Cure rates can be very high, although results vary in the literature. Very useful for patients with multiple BCCs. Relatively painless and nontraumatic.	Not readily available and still in experimental stages. Expensive.
Systemic therapies – most drug treatments have been tried in patients with multiple BCCs in whom new lesions constantly develop; therapies tried include: oral retinoids (isotretinoin), interferon alfa (intralesionally), 5-fluorouracil, topical methotrexate and cisplatin.	May, in some instances, help prevent new lesion formation and therefore decrease the number of surgeries required. May shrink tumor size and make it more amenable to surgical intervention.	Low cure rates. Significant side effects associated with each drug.

[1] *Arch Surg 1989;124:211–217.*

Therapeutic Choices (Table 1)

Therapeutic Tips

- Treatment depends on type of lesion, size of tumor and anatomic site.

- **Prevention** should be the primary focus as accumulated sun and sunburns are the primary cause (Chapter 57). Sun avoidance, protective clothing and hats must be emphasized. Sunscreen application should become a daily routine for patients who have had basal cell carcinoma. SPF 30 should be the minimum UVB protection used and proper UVA protection with products containing Parsol 1789 or titanium dioxide, as a physical sunblock, must be emphasized.

- Therapy is almost always surgical or other physical modalities; in general, cure rates are over 90%, but larger lesions (i.e., over 2 cm) may have higher recurrence rates.

Suggested Reading List

Grimwood RE, Siegle RJ, Ferris CF, et al. The biology of basal cell carcinomas – a revisit and recent developments. *J Dermatol Surg Oncol* 1986;12:805–808.

Kripke ML. Impact of ozone depletion on skin cancers. *J Dermatol Surg Oncol* 1988;14:853–857.

Marks R. Nonmelanotic skin cancer and solar keratoses. *Int J Dermatol* 1987;26:201–205.

Rosenthal DI, Glatstein E. Clinical applications of photodynamic therapy. *Ann Intern Med* 1994;26:405–409.

Wilson BD, Mang TS, Stoil H, et al. Photodynamic therapy for the treatment of basal cell carcinoma. *Arch Dermatol* 1992;128:1597–1601.

CHAPTER 59

Burns

David Warren, MD, FRCPC

Goals of Therapy

- Provide early management of serious burns to reduce associated morbidity and mortality
- Triage patients for inpatient, referral and outpatient care
- Optimize cosmetic results and minimize functional morbidity of burns
- Provide appropriate analgesia, burn wound management and follow up

Investigations

- A thorough history of the burn injury with special attention to:
  - burning agent, its temperature, duration of exposure
  - fire in open or enclosed space, explosion, fall, electrical or chemical exposure
  - past medical history, medications and tetanus status
- Physical examination:
  - general physical examination with attention initially to airway, breathing and circulation
  - head to toe examination to assess for other systemic or musculoskeletal injuries
  - presence of headache, irritability, nausea, confusion, agitation and uncoordination which may indicate **carbon monoxide poisoning**
  - assess for **pulmonary complications**. Upper airway edema may occur from direct thermal injury especially with steam. Smoke inhalation doubles the mortality risk of a burn from systemic and direct toxicant effects to the airway. Indicators would include fire in an enclosed space, inhalation of noxious fumes, facial burns, pharyngeal burns, carbonaceous sputum, hoarseness, elevated carboxy-hemoglobin > 5%, abnormal pulmonary function. Pulmonary edema may be an early or late finding
  - assess **depth of wound** (Table 1)
  - assess the **extent of the burn** quantified as the percentage of total body surface area (BSA). The palm size of the victim is approximately 1% BSA, or estimate following the rule of nines (Figure 1)

- some burns due to their extent or potential morbidity should be considered for **referral to a burn centre** or specialized care (Table 2). Transfer should be facilitated by contact between physicians. All pertinent documentation, tests, flow sheets and transfer records should accompany the patient
- Laboratory tests in moderate and severe burns:
  - CBC, electrolytes, glucose, BUN, creatinine, blood type and clotting studies
  - ethanol and drug toxicology if warranted
  - carboxyhemoglobin level and other toxins in suspected inhalation injuries
  - urinalysis and if blood positive or > 30% BSA burn, urine myoglobin
  - arterial blood gas and chest radiograph, often normal early with findings 6 to 24 hours later

Table 1: **Burn Depth Classification**

Degree	Class	Description	Example	Healing Time
1st	Superficial	involves epidermis: skin red and painful	sunburn	7 days
2nd	Superficial partial thickness	epidermis and upper dermis: blisters, underlying skin red and moist, very painful	scald with water	10–21 days
	Deep partial thickness	epidermis and deep dermis: some hair follicle and sweat gland damage, blisters to charring	flame, oil	> 14 days, some scarring
3rd	Full thickness	epidermis through dermis to subcutaneous fat: skin pale, painless, leathery	flame, hot metal	scars–will not heal, surgery ± grafts

Therapeutic Choices

Nonpharmacologic Choices
Initial First Aid Management

- Remove the victim from the source of injury, taking care to limit risk to rescuers in electrical and chemical burn injuries.
- Remove any burning clothing or hot material.
- Assess airway, breathing and circulation (ABC).

Figure 1: **Rule of Nines Estimation of Body Surface Area for Child and Adult**

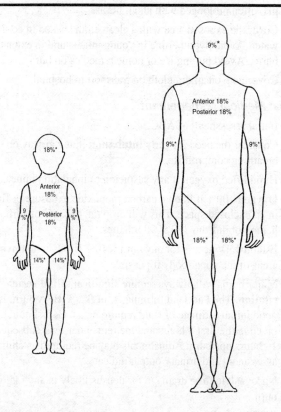

* Includes both anterior and posterior aspects.

Table 2: **Criteria for Referral or Transfer to a Burn Centre**

- Partial thickness burn > 10% BSA if patient under 10 years or over 50 years of age
- Partial thickness burns > 20% BSA in other age groups
- Partial and full thickness burns involving the face, eyes, ears, hands, feet, perineum, or overlying major joints
- Full thickness burns > 5% BSA
- Significant chemical burns
- Inhalation injuries
- Patients with pre-existing illness likely to complicate recovery
- Patients with concomitant trauma should be treated initially in an appropriate trauma setting and subsequently transferred to a burn centre
- Children should be treated in facilities with appropriate capabilities and equipment
- Patients with special psycho-social needs and/or rehabilitative support (child abuse, mental health needs, drug addiction)

- In chemical exposures copiously irrigate burn region with lukewarm water until testing demonstrates a normal tissue pH, often prolonged with alkali burns.
- Cover the exposed area with a clean cloth soaked in cool water. Avoid hypothermia in young infants and in extensive burns. Avoid putting ice or home remedies on burn.
- Cover with clean dry cloth on transport to hospital.

Initial Medical Management

- Initial assessment of ABC.
- Consider the need for early **intubation** if any airway or breathing compromise.
- Humidified oxygen if any suspicion of inhalation injury.
- **Oxygen** 100% if known carbon monoxide exposure or fire in an enclosed space. This will drop the half-life of carboxy-hemoglobin from 330 to 90 minutes.
- Establish IV access for any burn > 10% BSA, in noninvolved areas of the upper body if possible.
- Major burns will always require significant **fluid resuscitation**. The Parkland formula, 4 mL/kg/% BSA burn, is a good initial estimate of fluid requirements. Half should be given in the first 8 hours and the remainder over subsequent 16 hours postburn. Adjustments may be required as clinical assessment and urinary output indicate.
- **Nasogastric tube** drainage for ileus is likely in any major burn.
- **Bladder catheterization** to monitor appropriate urinary output, minimum 1 mL/kg/h.
- Elevate any encircling limb burn and closely assess for neurovascular status. Chest burns should be assessed for restriction of normal excursion and pulmonary compromise. Surgical escharotomy considered as required.
- Ensure adequate **tetanus prophylaxis**; 0.5 mL tetanus toxoid in previously immunized patient with additional 250 units human immune globulin if previously unimmunized.

Burn Wound Management

- Removal of any attached clothing and loose tissue.
- Gentle washing of the burn surface with sterile water or normal saline.
- Débridement of open blisters and loose tissue.
- Neosporin ointment can be used as an emulsifying agent to remove tar.

- The application of **topical antibiotic** agents will lower the incidence of wound infections. Often not used with superficial burns, they have a more significant role with deeper, more extensive injuries (Table 3).
- Topical antibiotics are applied using sterile technique to approximately 2 mm twice daily or as required if rubbed off. Cleanse the wound prior to reapplication.
- Semi-closed **dressings** permit ambulatory management while maintaining hygiene, limiting mobilization, and preventing tampering with the wound.
  - innermost dressing layer is porous mesh gauze impregnated with nonpetroleum-based water soluble lubricant.
  - second layer is bulky, fluffed coarse mesh gauze to absorb exudate and protect the wound.
  - outer layer of semi-elastic coarse mesh will provide even moderate pressure to keep the dressing in place but should not be constrictive.
  - alternative for superficial partial thickness wounds, semisynthetic occlusive dressings (e.g., Biobrane, DuoDerm, Tegaderm) in flat partial thickness burns.
- Dressing changes:
  - semi-closed dressings; every other day, daily, or twice daily dependent on the wound, antibiotic use and the patient.
  - semisynthetic occlusive dressings; removal, cleansing, and redressing is required if fluid collects beneath, otherwise removal at 7 to 10 days.
- Open therapy is often used on the head, neck and perineum, which are areas difficult to dress and prone to maceration.

Pharmacologic Choices

- Avoid prophylactic oral and IV antibiotics in all but exceptional circumstances to avoid development of resistant infections.
- **Topical antibiotics** application is discussed above. Various agents have been used with specific indications and limitations (Table 3).

Nonsteroidal Anti-inflammatory Drugs (NSAIDs)

- Have been used to manage pain in minor burns and suppress the inflammatory response in major burns. Standard soft tissue analgesic dosing on a regular basis can be used.

Table 3: Topical Antibiotics Used in the Treatment of Burns

Drug	Application[†]	Adverse Effects	Comments	Cost*
bacitracin Baciguent, Bacitin, generics	OD, BID open or semi-closed	Poor eschar penetration, moderate antibacterial spectrum	Transparent, easy to apply, cosmetically acceptable	$–$$
silver sulfadiazine 1% Dermazin, Flamazine, SSD	BID–QID open or semi-closed	Only fair penetration, sulfonamide sensitivity (rash), leukopenia	Broad antibacterial spectrum, painless, washable	$$$$–$$$$$
povidone-iodine 1% Betadine, Proviodine	BID open or semi-closed	Poor penetration, tissue staining, painful, iodine absorption	Broad antibacterial action	$$$

[†] Approximately 5 g per 1% BSA burn per application.
* Cost of 7-day supply based on 5% BSA burn – includes drug cost only.
Legend: $ < $20 $$ $20–50 $$$ $50–80 $$$$ $80–110 $$$$$ > $110

Opioid Analgesics

- Potent analgesia with small aliquots of morphine (0.05 to 0.1 mg/kg IV) or meperidine (0.5 to 1 mg/kg IV) are often required initially to manage pain.
- Care should be taken not to suppress the signs of other injuries initially with analgesia.
- Children especially require analgesia to manage their burns.
- Longer term and outpatient analgesia can be achieved with oral codeine.

Therapeutic Tips

- Avoid contamination of the wound; infection is the major threat to burn outcome.
- Advise patients regarding signs of infection; any evidence of infection should be reviewed quickly and treatment altered as appropriate.
- Outpatient follow-up schedule may be daily initially and extended as dressing requirements and healing progress.
- Electrical burns often have more extensive damage below the surface than is initially identified and should be followed appropriately.

Suggested Reading List

American Burn Association. Guidelines for service standards and severity of classification in the treatment of burn injury. *American College of Surgery Bulletin* 1984;69:24.

Baxter CR, Waeckerle JF. Emergency treatment of burn injury. *Ann Emerg Med* 1988;17:1305–1315.

Griglak MJ. Thermal injury. *Emerg Med Clin North Am* 1992; 10(2):369.

Schwartz LR. Thermal injury. In: Tintinalli JE, Ruiz E, Krome RL, et al, eds. *Emergency Medicine: A Comprehensive Study Guide*. 4th ed. New York: McGraw-Hill, 1996:893–899.

Braen RG. Thermal injury. In: Rosen P, Baker FJ, Barkin RM, et al, eds. *Emergency Medicine Concepts and Clinical Practice*. 3rd ed. St. Louis: CV Mosby, 1988:573–584.

CHAPTER 60

Decubitus Ulcers

W. Alastair McLeod, MD, FRCPC

Goals of Therapy

- Prophylaxis
- To promote wound healing once ulceration occurs
- To treat infection and prevent systemic sepsis
- To enhance the rehabilitation process

Classification of Pressure Ulcers

Stage 1	Redness of the skin
Stage 2	Blistering or partial thickness skin loss resulting in abrasion or shallow ulcer
Stage 3	Full thickness skin loss with extension into subcutaneous fat
Stage 4	Extension into deep subcutaneous tissue, muscle or bone

This classification cannot be used in reverse to evaluate healing (i.e., a stage 3 ulcer does not become a stage 2 ulcer).

Therapeutic Choices for Prophylaxis

Once decubitus ulceration occurs, treatment is prolonged, frustrating and frequently interferes with the patient's and caregiver's quality of life. Protocols have been developed (including the Norton scale [Figure 1] and the Braden scale) to identify high-risk patients, who require immediate implementation of measures to prevent pressure ulceration. The same factors used for predictive purposes are important in assessing the probability of healing the ulcer.

Figure 1: **Norton Scale for Identification of High-risk Patients**

Physical Condition	Mental State	Activity	Mobility	Incontinence
Good (4)	Alert (4)	Ambulant (4)	Full (4)	None (4)
Fair (3)	Apathetic (3)	Walks with help (3)	Slightly limited (3)	Occasional (3)
Poor (2)	Confused (2)	Chairbound (2)	Very limited (2)	Usually urine (2)
Very bad (1)	Stuporous (1)	Bedbound (1)	Immobile (1)	Double (1)

Score: ≤ 12: High risk of decubitus ulcers.   < 14: Vulnerable to decubitus ulcers.

Measures to relieve pressure include:

- turning and positioning the patient.
- use of surfaces such as sheepskin fleeces, padding mattresses on top of a standard mattress and foam mattresses.
- air support beds are available. Due to their high cost, they are most appropriately used in the short-term setting before ulceration develops in very high risk patients. Comparative studies do not support their cost-effectiveness.

Moisture is a significant factor in the development of decubitus ulcers; urine or stool also aggravate developing ulcers.

Although the US Public Health Service has published clinical practice guidelines on decubitus ulcer prophylaxis, most were based on common sense rather than on high-quality research, indicating the lack of scientific literature in this area.[1]

Therapeutic Choices for Treatment

The US Public Health Service has also published guidelines for the treatment of pressure ulcers.[2] The guidelines include treatment algorithms, a clinicians quick reference guide and a consumers guide.

It is important to recognize that many pressure ulcers do not heal during the patient's remaining lifetime and one should not present unrealistic expectations to patients and their families or unrealistic demands on the caregiver if the patient is at home.[3]

The rehabilitation prospects of the patient are a major determining factor in the intensity of efforts to heal the ulcer and coincide with the prospects of healing the ulcer. Nutrition is a major determinant in healing, and dietary advice should be sought. Correction of anemia and maximization of oxygenation are important, but the role of dietary supplements such as zinc and vitamins is not well established.

Pressure Relief

It has been said that *"you can put anything on a decubitus ulcer – except the patient."* Pressure-relieving systems are the same for treatment as for prophylaxis, but for long-term treatment, expensive air beds are less attractive.

[1] *Pressure ulcers in adults: Prediction and prevention. Clinical practice guideline #3. Rockville, MD: Agency for Health Care Policy and Research, US Department of Health and Human Services, 1992. Publication #92–0047.*

[2] *Pressure ulcer treatment. Clinical practice guideline #15. Rockville, MD: Agency for Health Policy and Research, US Department of Health and Human Services, 1996. Publication #95–0654.*

[3] *Advances in Wound Care 1994;7(3):40–46.*

Infection

Infection in decubitus ulcers is common, and cultures are frequently polymicrobial. Bacteremia and sepsis syndrome are frequent, with *B. fragilis, P. mirabilis* and *S. aureus* the most common organisms cultured. Cultures from ulcers do not correlate well with blood cultures. Positive blood cultures should be treated with appropriate antibiotics. Swabs from the surface of infected ulcers may not reveal the true pathogens involved in deep tissue invasion; thus, cultures from the deep part of the wound are important, taken during débridement or by needle aspiration.

If osteomyelitis is present, a culture from the bone is desirable as the organisms cultured from the wound or blood may not correlate with those from bone biopsy.

Local Wound Care

Débridement

Surgical: Important in ulcer management, particularly for stage 3 and 4 ulcers or if there is a thick black leathery sphacelus. Bacteremia can occur during débridement.

Enzymatic: Fibrinolysin-desoxyribonuclease ointment or sutilains ointment have been advocated as chemical débridement therapy; some investigators recommend mixing them with hydrogels. There is no literature to support this approach, but occasionally it might be useful.

Synthetic Dressings (Table 1)

In choosing a dressing material and regimen for local wound care from the many available dressings, material and labor costs are important considerations, and those applying the dressing may be more familiar/comfortable with one type of dressing over another. Comparative studies do not exist but the prospect of wound healing is more dependent on the patient's status than on the dressing type. At the present time there is no reason to believe that *"newer/more expensive is better."*

Other Dressings

Saline-soaked wet to dry dressings are used in the early stages of ulceration to remove necrotic debris or following surgical débridement. In the later stages of wound healing they interfere with re-epithelialization and should be withdrawn when a clean granulating base is established, usually after about 2 weeks. **Continuous moist saline compresses** can be used, but they increase maceration and are very time consuming and labor intensive.

Table 1: **Some Synthetic Dressing Materials***

Dressing Type	Comments
Semipermeable adhesive films – OpSite, Tegaderm	Not suitable if significant exudation.
Hydrocolloid gels – DuoDerm, Comfeel, Reston, Cutinova-Hydro	Melt on pressure areas leaking exudate and gel; most useful on non-pressure areas.
Hydrogels – IntraSite Gel, Second Skin, Comformagel	Well tolerated. Provide some débride-ment – require more elaborate dressings.
Alginates – Fibracol, Algoderm	Absorb exudate. Simple to use, do not melt.
Foam dressings – Allevyn	Provide absorption without melting and draining. May be used with hydrogels.
Zinc dressings – Mezinc	Not useful if there is much drainage. May be some irritation.
Absorption dressings – Debrisan	Relatively expensive when used to fill a large wound; difficult to keep in wound.
Silicone dressings – Mepitel	Allow dressing changes to remove exu-date without disturbing wound surface.

* *This table is not inclusive of all available dressing materials. An annual product list is published by Springhouse Corporation: Anon. 1996–1997 Wound Care Resource Guide. Advances in Wound Care 1996;9 (5Pt2): 1–64. Specific product and manufacturer information is also available at their website http://www.woundcarenet.com.*

Acetic acid compresses may be useful in *Pseudomonas*-infected wounds.

Hydrogen peroxide, hypochlorite solutions (e.g., **Dakin's, Hygeol**) and silver nitrate are no longer recommended as they are toxic to tissue and interfere with wound healing.

Topical Antibiotics

Mupirocin or fusidic acid may be useful in shallow early ulcerations that are colonized or very superficially infected. Mupirocin has been recognized as a potential sensitizer. Other antibiotic mixtures, particularly those containing neomycin, are not recommended due to the risk of sensitization.

Silver sulfadiazine may be useful in wounds infected with *Pseudomonas*. The risk of sulfonamide adverse effects appears to be small. Some literature suggests silver sulfadiazine interferes with wound healing but a larger volume of literature suggests it does not. Silver sulfadiazine may produce increased wound exudation, which can alarm caregivers.

Benzoyl peroxide 20% dressings have been used for many years; the mechanisms of action are believed to be antibacterial and promotion of granulation tissue.

458 Skin Disorders

Suggested Reading List

Agency for Health Care Policy and Research. *Treatment of pressure ulcers. Clinical practice guideline #15.* Rockville, MD: US Department of Health and Human Services, 1994. AHCPR Publication #95–0652.

Agency for Health Care Policy and Research. *Treating pressure sores. Consumer version clinical practice guideline #15.* Rockville, MD: US Department of Health and Human Services, 1994. AHCPR Publication #95–0654.

Agency for Health Care Policy and Research. *Pressure ulcers in adults: prediction and prevention. Clinical practice guideline #3.* Rockville, MD: US Department of Health and Human Services, 1992. AHCPR Publication #92–0047.

Ryan JT. Wound dressing. *Dermatol Clin* 1993;11:207–213.

Xakellis GC, Frantz RA, Ortega M, et al. A Comparison of patients' risk for pressure ulcer development with nursing use of preventative interventions. *J Am Geriatr Soc* 1992; 40:1250–1254.

CHAPTER 61

Psoriasis

J. Barrie Ross, MB, BS, FRCPC

Goals of Therapy

- To increase patient's understanding of psoriasis and expectations of management
- To decrease or heal lesions
- To relieve symptoms
- To prevent recurrences

Investigations

- Complete history including the pattern of onset, possible provocative factors, pattern of the course and remission, family history and social history
  - in particular a history of recurrent infections (sore throat, dental, bladder), diabetes, alcohol consumption, obesity, arthritis
- Physical examination:
  - skin: distribution and character of lesions
  - initial: general examination of body systems, with focus on teeth, throat and sinuses, chest and bladder
  - repeat: mainly skin assessment; annual general physical assessment if not performed elsewhere or on presentation of new phase of disorder
- Laboratory tests (as indicated by history and physical examination)
  - CBC and differential; hepatic and renal chemistry
  - throat swab, AST, streptozyme test, other serology as required
  - urinalysis, cells and culture
  - dental assessment

Therapeutic Choices (Figure 1)

Nonpharmacologic Choices

- General health and well-being should be maximized.
- Diet, exercise, smoking, alcohol ingestion and mental health should be addressed.
- Factors adversely affecting the disease should be controlled (i.e., trauma, recurrent infections [teeth, upper respiratory tract], alcohol abuse, diabetes, obesity).

Figure 1: **Management of Psoriasis**

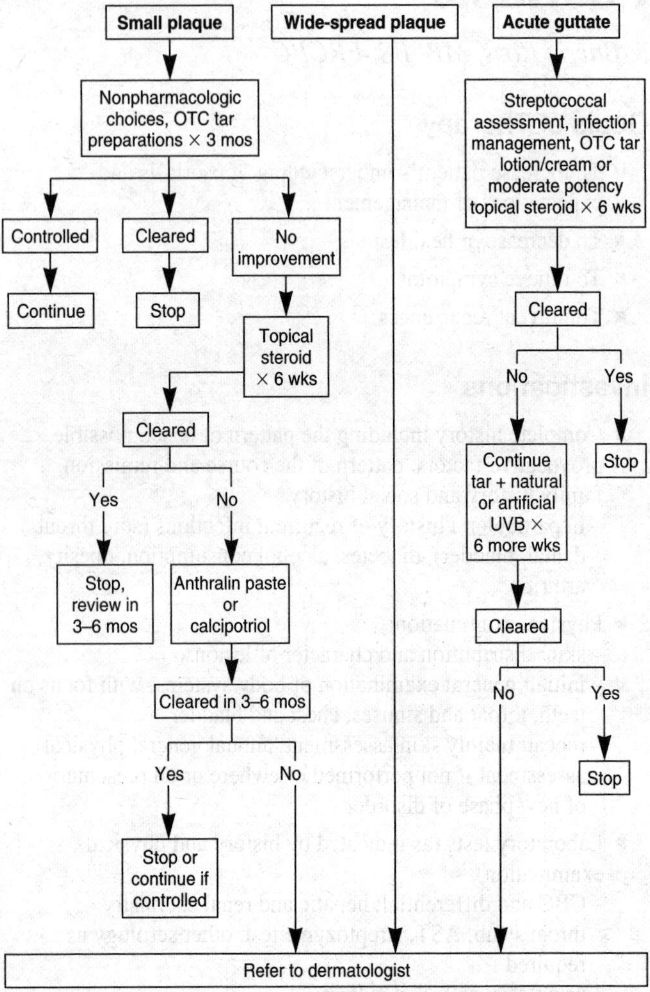

Pharmacologic Choices and Phototherapy
Topical Therapy

Many patients with mild involvement can be managed with topical therapy (Table 1) alone using a single agent or rotational therapy.

Phototherapy

Natural sunshine: Exposure to sunlight is beneficial. Precautions are necessary to prevent burning due to phototoxic action if tar is used.

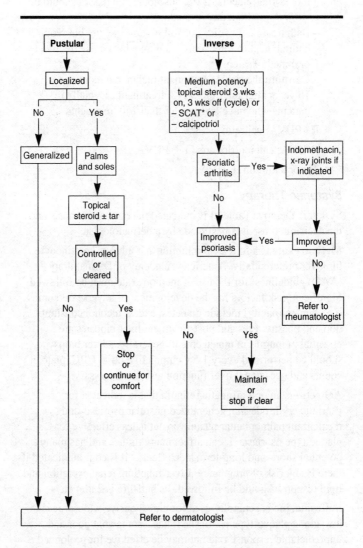

* Short contact anthralin therapy.

Ultraviolet B light (UVB) is usually institutionally based. It should be monitored by a dermatologist because of possible long-term effects.

Ultraviolet A light (UVA) is combined with topical or systemic agents.

- PUVA: psoralens (oral or topical methoxsalen) with UVA
  – Oral methoxsalen has a variety of side effects including nausea and nervousness. PUVA therapy requires full

monitoring. Special UVA-absorbing sunglasses should be worn throughout day of treatment.
- Bath treatment avoids general organ exposure but requires bathtub next to light source and may not be as effective as oral methoxsalen.
- **Caution:** the risk of malignant melanoma increases 15 years after the first PUVA treatment especially in patients who have had greater than 250 treatments.[1]

- Re-PUVA: acitretin + PUVA.
- D-UVA: calcipotriol cream + PUVA.
- Tar or anthralin + UVA.

Systemic Therapy

Systemic therapy (Table 2) is indicated in resistant psoriasis and the decision to use it is best made by a dermatologist.

Methotrexate is a folic acid inhibitor that inhibits keratinocyte turnover preferentially. American Academy of Dermatology (AAD) guidelines[2] for the use of methotrexate must be followed. Significant risk factors for the development of adverse outcomes (i.e., hepatotoxicity) include diabetes, excess alcohol consumption and obesity. Pre- and post-treatment liver biopsies are essential in long-term management: generally, a liver biopsy should be performed every 1.5 g cumulative dose. CBC, platelet counts and occasional liver function tests are necessary.

Acitretin is an oral aromatic retinoid that is indicated for psoriatic erythroderma, generalized pustular psoriasis and recalcitrant palmoplantar pustulosis but is less effective for plaque-type psoriasis. It can affect many tissues and has many potential short- and long-term side effects.[3] It is contraindicated if there is any risk of pregnancy. Liver function, renal excretion and lipid response should be followed. Its half-life is 2 to 4 days.

Sulfasalazine is generally used for unresponsive widespread low-grade plaque-type psoriasis. It has a somewhat poor and unpredictable response rate but may be effective for prolonged periods in some patients. Liver function monitoring is required. The drug is inexpensive.

Hydroxyurea is slow in onset and withdrawal. Since bone marrow depression is the principal adverse effect, any drugs causing potential blood loss (e.g., NSAIDs) should be used with care. Full laboratory monitoring is required with long-term use.

---

[1] *N Engl J Med 1997;336:1041–1045.*
[2] *J Am Acad Dermatol 1992;26:661–679.*
[3] *J Am Acad Dermatol 1992;26:661–679.*

Table 1: Topical Therapy of Psoriasis

Drug	Dosage	Adverse Effects	Comments	Cost*
Tar Various extemporaneous preparations (e.g., Whites Tar Paste)	Once daily	Allergies (can substitute wood tars).	Usually used as coal tar (crude coal tar, tar distillate or coal tar liquid). Generally the cleaner and more aesthetic tars are less effective. Enhanced by sunlight or UVB effect. Mode of action unknown; interferes with cell replication.	$
crude coal tar and allantoin Tegrin	Once daily			$$
Anthralin (e.g., 0.1% anthralin in 1/2 Lassar's Paste)	Once daily	Stains skin temporarily. Stains clothing permanently.	Most effective in paste base for body and pomade base for scalp. Concurrent UVB shortens course of therapy but not essential. Affected area should be covered with dressing for best effect. Reduces cell turnover rate.	$–$$
Corticosteroids Numerous (e.g., betamethasone ointment 0.1%)	Once daily	Local atrophy, tachyphylaxis. Systemic absorption occurs if very potent agent is used over wide area.	Only fluorinated corticosteroids are generally effective. High-potency agents should be used for no longer than 6 wks. Low-potency agents should be used on face, flexures, genitalia.	$–$$$
Nonsteroidals *calcipotriol* Dovonex	BID	Local irritation (possibly due to hyperkeratosis). Hypercalcemia can occur if used on wide area.	Vitamin D_3 analogue with slow onset but no tachyphylaxis. Recent reports indicate safe use in children with dose related to size and age.† Health Canada approval is awaited.	$$$$$

(cont'd)

Table 1: Topical Therapy of Psoriasis (cont'd)

Drug	Dosage	Adverse Effects	Comments	Cost*
Retinoids *tazarotene 0.1%, 0.05%* Tazorac	Once daily	Most common adverse effects include skin irritation, pruritus, burning sensation, erythema, skin pain. All are dose related.	Onset of action within 1 wk and effects may persist for up to 12 wks after stopping therapy. Should not be used by women who are pregnant or may become pregnant.	$$$$
Rotational Therapy	As appropriate		Total agent changed to a different one if resistance develops or after a planned period. Local application can rotate through wide range of therapies.	Varies

† For additional information on use of calcipotriol in children see: J Am Acad Dermatol 1997;36:203–208 and Brit J Dermatol 1996;135:390–393.
* Cost of 30-day supply based on 20% of 70 kg adult affected with psoriasis – does not include dispensing or compounding fee. See also Table 3.
Legend: $ < $10 $$ $10–50 $$$ $50–125 $$$$ $125–200 $$$$$ > $200

Table 2: Systemic Agents Used in Psoriasis

Drug	Dosage	Adverse Effects	Drug Interactions	Cost*
methotrexate † 🌻 Rheumatrex, generics	Starting dose of 25 mg once weekly for 70 kg adult and reduced as required Can be divided to 3 doses Q12H once weekly	Nausea, ↓ platelets, generalized marrow suppression, hepatic fibrosis.	Ethanol, acitretin – ↑ hepatotoxicity. Probenecid/salicylates/NSAIDs – ↓ renal excretion of methotrexate. Cyclosporine – ↓ elimination of both drugs. Sulfonamides – ↑ methotrexate-induced bone marrow suppression.	$
acitretin ‡ Soriatane	25–50 mg/d increased to a maximum of 75 mg/d	Dry lips in all, dry eyes and mucosa, xerotic eczema, hair loss, arthralgia (5%), headache, hyperlipidemia.	Anticoagulants – ↓ anticoagulant effect. Carbamazepine – ↓ effect of acitretin. Methotrexate – ↑ hepatotoxicity.	$$–$$$
sulfasalazine ‡ Salazopyrin, generics	500 mg TID–QID initially then adjusted to response	Dose-related adverse effects: GI irritation, headache, abdominal pain. ↓ sperm count (reversible). Methemoglobinemia, drug rash, hemolytic anemia, (adverse effects more frequent with slow acetylators).	Anticoagulants – ↑ anticoagulant effect. Cyclosporine – ↓ cyclosporine levels. Digoxin – ↓ digoxin absorption. Hypoglycemics – ↑ hypoglycemic effect. Methotrexate – ↑ methotrexate toxicity.	$

(cont'd)

Table 2: Systemic Agents Used in Psoriasis (cont'd)

Drug	Dosage	Adverse Effects	Drug Interactions	Cost*
hydroxyurea ‡ ● Hydrea	0.5–1.5 g/d divided TID-QID adjusted to blood count	Marrow depression, GI irritation, maculopapular eruption.	Fluorouracil – ↑ neurotoxicity. Allopurinol, colchicine, probenecid, sulfinpyrazone – ↑ blood uric acid; dosage adjustment of antigout agents may be required.	$–$$
cyclosporine ‡ ● Sandimmune	3.5–5 mg/kg/d	Renal dysfunction, hypertension, hirsutism, tremor, GI irritation.	Ketoconazole, erythromycin, corticosteroids, calcium channel blockers – ↑ cyclosporine levels. Phenytoin, rifampin, carbamazepine, sulfonamides → ↓ cyclosporine levels.	$$$$$

● *Dosage adjustment may be required in renal impairment – see Appendix I.*
† *Should be initiated with specialist's advice and preferably followed by same or at least with regularly planned directive advice.*
‡ *Should preferably be initiated with specialist's advice and continued with occasional long-term directive advice.*
* *Cost of 30-day supply – includes drug cost only. See also Table 3.*
Legend: $ < $50 $$ $50–150 $$$ $150–300 $$$$ $300–450 $$$$$ > $450

The response to **cyclosporine** is variable. It can be effective if other managements have failed and is particularly useful for widespread inflammatory psoriasis. The same guidelines as for transplant patients should be followed.[4] Routine cyclosporine blood levels should be done as well as creatinine and BUN twice weekly for the first 2 to 3 months then every month. BP should be taken frequently.

Table 3: **Estimated Cost of One Year of Treatment**

Treatment	(US $ 1993)
Outpatient Goeckerman	$3914.90
PUVA	$2604.83
Outpatient UVB	$1966.80
Methotrexate	$1381.41
Hydroxyurea	$1131.08
Cyclosporine	$6648.38

Adapted with permission from J Am Acad Dermatol 1993;28:422–425.

Therapeutic Tips

- The nature of psoriasis should be described to the patient on first visit when diagnosis is made.
- The patient's understanding of the condition should be reviewed occasionally.
- Do not suggest that all psoriasis must be cleared in a minimally affected patient.
- Remember the All-or-None Law: psoriasis should be completely cleared in extensive disease if long-term remission is desired.
- As a guide for estimating the amount of topical agent to prescribe, 30 g of ointment will cover the body of a 70 kg adult once; creams and lotions will go further. Also helpful in estimating quantity is the "Rule of Hand": 4 hand areas = 2 FTU (finger tip units) = 1 g.
- If potent topical steroids have been applied continuously for 6 weeks or longer, resting the skin by applying bland local therapy for 4 to 6 weeks may be required before nonsteroidal remedies such as tar and anthralin can be effective.

---

[4] *J Am Acad Dermatol 1992;26:661–679.*

Suggested Reading List

Champion RH, Burton JL, Ebling FJG, eds. *Textbook of dermatology*. 5th ed. Oxford: Blackwell Scientific Publications, 1992:1416–1440.

Fitzpatrick TB, Eisen AZ, Wolff K, et al. *Dermatology in general medicine*. 4th ed. New York: McGraw Hill, 1993:508–511.

Guidelines for care for psoriasis. *J Am Acad Dermatol* 1993;28:632–637.

Lebwohl M, Zanolli M, eds. Psoriasis. *Dermatologic Clinics* 1995;13:717–955.

CHAPTER 62

Atopic Dermatitis

Robert S. Lester, MD, FRCPC

Atopic dermatitis is an inflammatory skin disease marked by intense pruritus and a tendency to lichenification of the skin. There is a natural tendency in many but not all patients to improve with age.

Goals of Therapy

- To increase patient/parent understanding of the course of atopic dermatitis and reasonable expectations of management
- To relieve pruritus and decrease or heal lesions
- To minimize and/or manage recurrences

Investigations

- Complete history with special emphasis on family history of atopic disorders including atopic dermatitis, allergic rhinitis and asthma
- Physical examination: primary sites may vary with age of patients
  - infant stage (birth to 2 years): face and lateral aspects of lower legs
  - childhood phase (2 to 12 years): lichenification in flexural areas
  - adult phase: hand dermatitis; eyelid dermatitis; localized areas of lichenification (e.g., anogenital area)

In all phases, the eruption may become more generalized and inflammation and pruritus may become incapacitating with disturbance of sleep and agitation.

Table 1 lists the associated findings in patients with atopic dermatitis.

Table 1: **Associated Findings**

Dry skin and xerosis	Hyperlinear palmar creases
Ichthyosis vulgaris	Dennie-Morgan infraorbital folds
Keratosis pilaris	Anterior subcapsular cataracts
Pityriasis alba	Keratoconus

Therapeutic Choices

Refer to Table 2 for general management.

- **Lubrication**
  - attention to dryness of the skin is an important aspect of treatment of atopic dermatitis.
  - use agents such as nondrying soaps, nonperfumed oils or oatmeal baths.
  - apply lubricating ointments after bathing (e.g., petrolatum)
  - encourage use of humidifiers.

- **Antihistamines**
  - primary action of antihistamines may be sedative.
  - sedative antihistamines such as hydroxyzine or diphenhydramine are more effective than the nonsedative types (Chapter 63).

- **Topical steroids**
  - the mainstay of management is the use of topical steroids twice daily.
  - topical steroids are now available in a wide range of potencies (Table 3). The same drug may show different potency depending on the delivery vehicle used. In general, greater potency occurs when the drug is delivered as an ointment as compared to a cream or lotion.
  - the choice of agent depends on the age, location and extent of skin lesions (Table 4).
  - the lowest potency steroid that is effective should be used. Short courses of higher potency topical steroids can be used in all cases of resistant disease.
  - several factors may influence response to topical steroids (Table 5).
  - topical steroids are usually trouble free and highly effective especially when used for brief periods, on limited areas, and without occlusion. More potent topical steroids are associated with increased risks of side effects. Percutaneous absorption varies with the site of application. Least absorption occurs on the palms and soles with maximum absorption occurring in intertriginous areas. Children, as a result of their surface area to weight ratio, absorb relatively more topically applied corticosteroid and

Table 2: General Management of Atopic Dermatitis

Address psychosocial issues	Antihistamines
Modify diet (where indicated)	Topical corticosteroids
Avoid aggravating factors	Antimicrobials (when indicated)
Avoid primary irritants and allergens	Systemic therapy (severe, generalized)
Lubrication	

Table 3: **Potency Classification of Topical Corticosteroids**

Topical Corticosteroid	Cost*
Very potent [†]	
betamethasone dipropionate 0.05% in propylene glycol base Diprolene Glycol, Topilene	$$
clobetasol propionate 0.05% Dermasone, Dermovate, generics	$$
halobetasol propionate 0.5% Ultravate	$$$
Potent [†]	
amcinonide 0.1% Cyclocort	$$
betamethasone dipropionate 0.05% Diprosone, Topisone, others	$
desoximetasone 0.25% Topicort	$$
fluocinonide 0.05% Lidex, Lyderm, Tiamol, others	$
halcinonide 0.1% Halog	$$
triamcinolone acetonide 0.5% Aristocort C	$$$$
Moderately potent [†]	
beclomethasone dipropionate 0.025% Propaderm	$$
betamethasone benzoate 0.025% Beben	$$
betamethasone valerate 0.05%, 0.1% Betnovate, Celestoderm V, others	$
clobetasone butyrate 0.05% Eumovate, generics	$$
desonide 0.05% Desocort, Tridesilon, generics	$
diflucortolone valerate 0.1% Nerisone	$$
fluocinolone acetonide 0.01%, 0.025% Synalar, Fluoderm	$$
hydrocortisone valerate 0.2% Westcort	$
mometasone furoate 0.1% Elocom	$$
triamcinolone acetonide 0.1% Kenalog, Aristocort R, others	$
Weak [†]	
flumethasone pivalate 0.03% Locacorten	$$
hydrocortisone 0.5%, 1%, 2.5% Aquacort, Cortate, generics	$
hydrocortisone acetate 0.1%, 1% Corticreme, Hyderm, others	$
methylprednisolone acetate 0.25% Medrol Veriderm	$

[†] *These classifications are broad guidelines and within any class there may be a range of potencies.*

* *Cost of 15 g – includes drug cost only.*

Legend: $ < $5 $$ $5–10 $$$ $10–15 $$$$ > $15

are at increased risk for developing systemic adverse effects. Adverse effects attributed to topical steroid use are summarized in Table 6.

Table 4: **Choice of Topical Corticosteroid**

Factor		Choice of Steroid
Age	Infant	Weak
	Child	Weak to moderate
	Adult	Moderate to very potent
Site	Face	Weak
	Intertriginous	Weak
	Trunk and extremities	Moderate to potent
	Palms and soles	Potent to very potent
Extent	Localized	Moderate to very potent
	Generalized	Weak to moderate

Table 5: **Factors Influencing Response to Topical Steroids**

Potency of steroid chosen	Frequency of application
Concentration of steroid	Occlusion
Amount of steroid applied	Vehicle chosen

Table 6: **Adverse Effects to Topical Corticosteroids**

I. **Systemic**
   Hypothalamic-pituitary adrenal axis suppression
   Iatrogenic Cushing syndrome
   Growth retardation (children)

II. **Local**
   A. Catabolic Effects
      Degeneration of dermal collagen
      Epidermal and dermal atrophy
      Telangiectasia
      Purpura and ecchymosis
      Striae
      Disturbances in wound healing
      Steroid acne
      Steroid rosacea
      Steroid perioral dermatitis
      Hypertrichosis
      Infection
   B. Modification of Local Response
      Tinea incognito
      Glaucoma and cataracts
      Hypopigmentation
   C. Allergic contact dermatitis

Therapeutic Tips

- Do not underestimate the importance of explanation of the natural course and reasonable expectations of therapy on the first visit.

- Relief of pruritus is essential in the management of atopic dermatitis.

- Use the least potent topical steroid which will control symptoms.

- When symptoms are in remission substitute lubrication for medication.

- If unresponsive to therapy, check for occult staphylococcus infection and treat with appropriate antibiotics.

- Do not rely on skin testing. As many as 80% of patients with atopic dermatitis react on skin testing to more than one of a large number of environmental allergens including a multitude of foods. History is more important than testing, and in most patients, dietary manipulation may be unsuitable.

Suggested Reading List

Krafchik BR. Eczematous Dermatitis. In: Schachner LA, Hansen RC, eds. *Paediatric Dermatology.* 2nd ed. New York: Churchill Livingston, 1995:1(15):685–721.

Lester RS. Atopic Dermatitis. In: Rakel RE, ed. *Conn's Current Therapy.* Toronto: WB Saunders, 1994:803–808.

Lester RS. Corticosteroids. *Clin Dermatol* 1989;7(3):80–97.

CHAPTER 63

Pruritus

Laura A. Finlayson, MD, FRCPC

Goals of Therapy

- To determine etiology of pruritus in each patient (commonly a skin disease)
- To rule out underlying systemic disease (found in about 20% of pruritic patients without skin disorders)
- To decrease or abolish the itching sensation

Investigations

- A complete history including:
  - nature, location, duration, severity of pruritus
  - skin rash or dryness
  - past history or symptoms to suggest renal, hepatic, hematopoietic, lymphoreticular or endocrine disease
  - hygiene practices, topical contacts to the skin
  - weight loss or night sweats
  - prescription, over-the-counter and illicit drug use, particularly opiates
- Physical examination with assessment for presence of skin rash or dryness, dermatographism, uremic pigmentation, jaundice, plethora, lymphadenopathy, hepatosplenomegaly
- Laboratory investigations are indicated only if a primary dermatological cause for the pruritus has been excluded and include CBC with differential, fasting serum glucose, liver function tests, renal function tests, chest x-ray
- Depending on the index of suspicion, further investigations may be required to identify underlying systemic disease (Figure 1)

Therapeutic Choices

Pruritus is a symptom, not a disease. Once the underlying cause is diagnosed, appropriate management can be prescribed (Figure 1, Table 1).

Nonpharmacologic Choices

- **Skin hydration:** Dry skin frequently causes or exacerbates pruritus. Overbathing, hot water, harsh soaps and bubble bath preparations dry and irritate the skin and should be avoided. However, a daily tepid bath or shower for 5 to 10 minutes,

Figure 1: **Management of Pruritus**

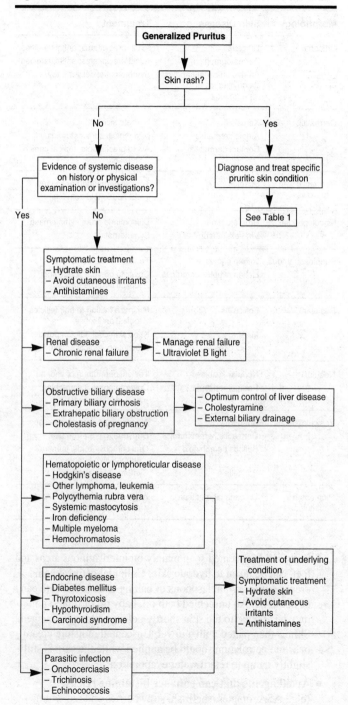

Table 1: **Pruritic Skin Diseases**

Morphology	Skin Disease	Treatment
Urticarial	Urticaria	Avoid precipitants; antihistamines.
	Dermatographism	Avoid precipitants; antihistamines.
	Pruritic urticarial papules and plaques of pregnancy	Symptomatic; deliver baby.
Dermatitic	Xerosis	Hydrate skin.
	Atopic dermatitis	Mild topical corticosteroids.
	Contact dermatitis	Avoid precipitants; topical corticosteroids.
Dermatitic with burrows	Scabies	Topical permethrin or lindane. Treat household contacts.
Maculopapular	Drug eruption	Discontinue drug; symptomatic.
	Viral exanthem	Symptomatic.
Papulosquamous	Lichen planus	Topical or oral corticosteroids.
	Lichen simplex chronicus	Cover to prevent scratching; topical corticosteroids.
Pustular	Folliculitis	Minimize friction to hair follicles; topical antibiotics.
	Miliaria	Keep skin cool; talcum powder.
	Insect bites	Prevention; topical antipruritics.
Nodular	Nodular scabies	Topical permethrin or lindane.
	Prurigo nodularis	Cover to prevent scratching; topical corticosteroids.
Vesiculobullous	Sunburn	Aluminum acetate compresses.
	Dermatitis herpetiformis	Dapsone; gluten-free diet.
	Bullous pemphigoid	Oral corticosteroids, immuno-suppressive agents.
	Varicella	Symptomatic; acyclovir.
Pigmented macules	Urticaria pigmentosa	Antihistamines; avoid ASA, opiates, rubbing skin.

using mild unscented soap mainly on intertriginous areas and feet, can be taken to hydrate skin. Colloidal oatmeal bath preparations or 4 tablespoons of baking soda in the bath can be soothing. An unscented bath oil, baby oil or mineral oil may be applied to the skin shortly before bathing is finished. Skin is then patted with a towel. Unscented moisture cream or white petrolatum should be applied while the skin is still slightly damp to retard water evaporation.

■ **Avoid agents that can enhance histamine release** (e.g., ASA, opiates, shellfish, strawberries and red wine).

- **Minimize friction and irritation to the skin.** Clothing should be soft and loose. Wool and synthetic clothing should be avoided. Washing detergent should be well rinsed from clothing, and antistatic agents in the dryer should be avoided. Avoid fragranced products.

- **Minimize scratching.** Generalized pruritus produces a powerful, almost uncontrollable stimulus to scratch the skin. The scratch-itch cycle is self-perpetuating. Rubbing is preferable to scratching. Fingernails should be kept short. Cool tap water compresses can be applied for acute localized itch.

- **Avoid vasodilatory stimuli** (e.g., excessive exercise, high environmental temperature and humidity, hot showers or baths, spicy foods, caffeine and alcohol).

- **Ensure adequate sleep.** Pruritus is frequently worse at night, mostly because lack of distracting stimuli allows one to focus on the itch. Antipruritic topical lotion, applied just before bedtime, use of light bedclothes, and a sedative or sedating antihistamine may be helpful.

Pharmacologic Choices
Topical Antipruritics

Menthol 0.25 to 0.5%, **camphor** 0.25 to 0.5% or **phenol** 0.25 to 0.5% in a light nonperfumed lotion, applied TID or PRN, is soothing. Phenol is contraindicated in pregnancy. **Pramoxine hydrochloride** 1% is a topical anesthetic with low sensitizing potential that may provide short-term relief. Topical benzocaine and other "caine" topical anesthetics and topical diphenhydramine and phenol should be avoided because they can sensitize the skin. **Doxepin** 5% cream is a topical formulation of a tricyclic anti-depressant which relieves pruritus in some patients. **Crotamiton,** a scabicide, may also be used for its nonspecific antipruritic properties. **Calamine** lotion is helpful for acute conditions such as contact dermatitis but will dry the skin excessively with long-term use.

Antihistamines (Table 2)

Histamine is directly involved in many but not all cases of pruritus; therefore, antihistamines may have a variable effect, providing profound to minimal relief. They are most effective in urticaria. Histamine$_1$ (H$_1$) blockers are the agents of choice because H$_2$ receptors are not directly involved in itch.

Choosing an antihistamine: Patient responses to various agents will vary. The following factors should be considered.

Precautions and contraindications: Antihistamines are contraindicated in patients with glaucoma, stenosing peptic ulcer, urinary retention and those taking MAO inhibitors.

Table 2: Antihistamines

Drug	Dosage (adult)	Sedative Effects	Anticholinergic Effects	Comments	Cost*
Alkylamines					
brompheniramine maleate Dimetane	4–8 mg TID–QID or 12 mg Extentab Q12H	++	++	Each of these agents has a longer-acting slow-release form which should not be chewed, crushed or dissolved.	$–$$
chlorpheniramine maleate† Chlor-Tripolon, generics	4 mg Q6H or 8 mg Repetabs Q12H	++	++		$–$$
dexchlorpheniramine maleate Polaramine	2 mg TID–QID or 6 mg Repetabs Q12H	++	++		$$$
Ethanolamines					
clemastine fumarate Tavist	2–6 mg/d in divided doses	+++	++++	This group is particularly useful in acute allergic reactions. High incidence of sedative and anticholinergic effects. Limit long-term use.	$–$$$
diphenhydramine HCl Benadryl, generics	25–50 mg Q6H	++++	++++		$–$$
Ethylenediamines					
tripelennamine HCl Pyribenzamine	50 mg QID	+++	+/0	Ethylenediamine, a stabilizer in topical products, is a common sensitizer and can cause severe dermatitis. Aminophylline, a complex of theophylline and ethylenediamine, is contraindicated in a sensitized asthmatic patient. Occasionally may cause paradoxical excitation in children.	$
Phenothiazines					
promethazine HCl Phenergan, generics	10 mg QID	++++	++++	Extrapyramidal symptoms, photosensitivity.	$$
trimeprazine tartrate Panectyl	2.5–5 mg TID	+++	++++		$–$$

Drug	Dose			Comments	Cost*
Piperazines					
hydroxyzine HCl Atarax, generics	25–75 mg TID–QID	++	++	Hydroxyzine: useful in both acute and chronic allergic conditions. Some anxiolytic and antiemetic properties. Occasionally may cause paradoxical excitation in children.	$–$$$$
cetirizine HCl†‡♥ Reactine	10 mg/d	+/0	+/0	Cetirizine: long acting and inhibits the late phase reaction of allergy. A metabolite of hydroxyzine. Headache and fatigue in up to 10%.	$$
Piperidines					
First generation					
azatadine maleate Optimine	1–2 mg BID	+++	+++	All long acting except cyproheptadine. Cyproheptadine and azatadine may stimulate appetite and have some antiserotonin effects.	$–$$
*cyproheptadine HCl*π Periactin, generics	4–8 mg TID	+++	++	Astemizole and terfenadine:	$$–$$$$
Second generation				– prescription drug status.	
astemizole‡π Hismanal	10 mg/d	+/0	+/0	– particularly useful in chronic allergic states. – contraindicated in patients taking macrolide antibiotics and systemic azole antifungals as combination may result in serious cardiac arrhythmias.#	$
loratadine‡π Claritin	10 mg/d	+/0	+/0	– do not combine with grapefruit juice.	$$
terfenadine‡ Seldane, generics	60 mg BID	+/0	+/0	– do not exceed recommended dose. – headache and fatigue may occur.	$$

† Long-acting antihistamines – terfenadine, astemizole, chlorpheniramine, astemizole, loratadine, cetirizine.
‡ Nonsedating antihistamines – terfenadine, astemizole, cetirizine, loratadine.
π Dosage adjustment may be required in hepatic impairment.
Consult product monograph for complete list of drug interactions.

♥ Dosage adjustment may be required in renal impairment – see Appendix I.
* Cost of 7-day supply – includes drug cost only.
Legend: $ <$5 $$ $5–10 $$$ $10–15 $$$$ >$15

Administration of astemizole or terfenadine with macrolide antibiotics or systemic azole antifungals (e.g., ketoconazole) is contraindicated as it can result in serious cardiac arrhythmias. Antihistamines should be avoided in epileptic or pregnant patients and those with heart disease.

Drug interactions (see above): All antihistamines, particularly the sedating ones, should be avoided in patients taking drugs that will depress the central nervous system, including alcohol. Concurrent use with tricyclic antidepressants can cause increased toxicity.

Adverse effect profile: Consider the risk and implications of the various side effects (particularly drowsiness and anticholinergic effects) for each patient (Table 2).

Individual patient factors: Antihistamines, particularly the sedating ones, are more likely to cause drowsiness, confusion, hypotension, syncope and dizziness in the **elderly. Children** may show paradoxical excitation rather than sedation.

If a patient is **allergic** to an antihistamine, consider them allergic to other drugs in the same class.

Occupation: Working adults and school children can function better and more safely with nonsedating antihistamines (i.e., astemizole, terfenadine, loratadine, cetirizine) during the day.

Underlying condition: Acute or severe pruritus and skin conditions other than urticaria often respond better to the older antihistamines as the sedative properties may contribute directly to relief of the pruritus. Antihistamines are more effective at preventing histamine release than combating the effects of previously released histamine. Therefore, in chronic pruritic conditions antihistamines should be administered regularly for at least a week rather than intermittently when itch is most severe.

Response to initial treatment: Antihistamines are classified by chemical structure (Table 2). If a patient does not respond to an antihistamine from one class, change to an agent from another class. At times, prescribing two antihistamines from different classes at the same time is useful, but it is rarely necessary to prescribe more than two.

Other Systemic Pharmacologic Treatments

Ketotifen, a selective H_1 antihistamine that also stabilizes mast cells and inhibits mediator release, is used primarily in asthma prophylaxis but can be useful in urticaria and mastocytosis.

Doxepin, an antidepressant with potent antihistaminic properties, is useful in some cases of chronic urticaria.[1] It has anticholinergic effects and is contraindicated in patients with congestive heart failure and in those taking MAOIs.

---

[1] *J Am Acad Dermatol 1986;14:375–392.*

Patients who scratch uncontrollably at night may benefit from a small dose of **diazepam, chlordiazepoxide** or **lorazepam** at bedtime. Large doses of sedating antihistamines, administered at the same time, should be avoided.

Cholestyramine and colestipol HCl resins are effective for pruritus related to cholestatic liver disease (Chapter 41). These agents have also been used successfully in uremic pruritus and polycythemia rubra vera.

Phototherapy

Phototherapy with ultraviolet B (UVB) wavelength (290–320 nm) is an effective treatment for uremic pruritus. Eight to 10 treatments usually result in symptomatic improvement. Maintenance therapy may be administered as required. UVB phototherapy is often effective for pruritus of other etiology, particularly primary dermatoses.

Therapeutic Tips

- Histamine$_2$ antagonists (e.g., cimetidine) should not be used unless the H$_1$ receptors are blocked with an H$_1$ antihistamine. H$_2$-antagonists alone can exacerbate pruritus by interfering with a negative feedback mechanism.
- Topical steroids should be avoided in the absence of clinically evident skin disease.
- Testing should be done for dermatographism or pressure sensitivity because symptomatic dermatographism or subclinical urticaria is a common cause of pruritus that can be suppressed with antihistamines.
- Careful follow-up is required. The itching of scabies, urticaria and drug eruptions may precede onset of skin manifestations. Likewise, symptoms of a systemic disease may eventually develop in a patient with apparent idiopathic pruritus.
- Topical agents may be kept in a refrigerator because the physical cooling enhances their antipruritic effect.
- Sustained-release preparations should be swallowed whole, not crushed or dissolved.

Suggested Reading List

Advenier C, Queille-Roussel C. Rational use of antihistamines in allergic dermatological conditions. *Drugs* 1989;38(4): 634–644.

Denman ST. A review of pruritus. *J Am Acad Dermatol* 1986;14: 375–392.

Goldsmith P, Dowd PM. The new H$_1$ antihistamines. *Dermatol Therapy* 1993;11(1):87–95.

CHAPTER 64

Scabies and Pediculosis

Neil H. Shear, MD, FRCPC and
Suzann R. Kronovic, BSc

Scabies and pediculosis are common infestations that cause
significant discomfort and are associated with large outbreaks
in institutions (e.g., long-term care facilities, schools).

Goals of Therapy

- To eradicate causative organisms and eggs
- To control symptoms (itching, secondary bacterial infection)
- To prevent spread to contacts

Investigations (Table 1)

- History of exposure and itching
- Physical examination for excoriated papules, characteristic
  distribution and to identify organism

Table 1: **Clinical Features of Pediculosis and Scabies**

Type	Organism	Clinical Features
Pediculosis capitis	Pediculus humanus capitis (head louse)	Child with itchy occiput or neck; nits and lice visible in hair.
		Contact from other children.
Pediculosis corporis	Pediculus humanus corporis (body louse)	The louse lives on the clothing in folds and seams, not on the body; lesions are usually on the flanks, in the axillae and around the waist and neck.
Pediculosis pubis	Phthirus pubis (crab louse)	Itching in pubic hair.
		Any short hair on the body may be affected (e.g., eyelashes in children).
Scabies	Sarcoptes scabiei	Lesions on finger webs, wrists, waist, anterior axillary folds, areolae, genitals, edge of palms and soles.
		Scalp rarely affected in adults but commonly affected in babies.
		Mite visualized as a pinpoint at the end of a burrow, removed with a needle point and seen under the microscope.

Figure 1: **Scabies or Lice**

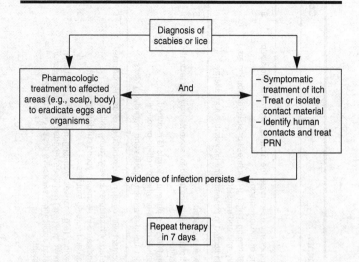

Therapeutic Choices (Figure 1)

Nonpharmacologic Choices

These measures will prevent reinfestation and spread.

- Remove **nits** daily for up to 30 days. Reports of apparent resistance to therapy are increasing, and nits can lie dormant for up to 30 days.

- **Treatment of room:** Isolate pillows, soft toys and articles that could have been exposed in a sealed plastic bag for 14 days. Head lice can remain alive, away from the body, for several days. Body lice can survive up to 10 days. Ideally, children with treated pediculosis capitis should be moved to another room for a few days.

- **Vacuuming** the floor of the patient's room is recommended.

- **Bedding, clothing, towels** and personal articles (e.g., hats) may be treated by:
  - washing in hot water (50°C for 30 minutes).
  - dry cleaning.
  - spraying with R & C II Spray.[1]
  - isolating intimate clothing and, for patients with scabies, isolating shoes in a plastic bag for 14 days.

- **Combs and brushes:** soak in a combination of pediculicide shampoo and water, or alcohol, or 2% Lysol solution for 1 hour. Alternatively, immerse them in 65°C water for 5 to 10 minutes.

---

[1] Not indicated for use in humans.

Table 2: Drugs Used for Scabies and Pediculosis

Drug	Directions	Comments	Cost*
Pediculicides			
permethrin 1% Nix Creme Rinse	Wash hair with regular shampoo, towel dry, then apply permethrin to thoroughly saturate the hair; leave on for 10 min and then rinse. May repeat after 7 d if live lice are observed.	May temporarily exacerbate the pruritus, erythema and scalp edema of lice infestation. Burning/stinging, tingling, numbness or scalp discomfort are usually mild and transient. Contraindicated in patients with chrysanthemum allergy.	$
pyrethrins with piperonyl butoxide Shampoo: Para Special Lice and Nit, R & C, Pronto Lice Killing Shampoo Kit Aerosol spray: Para Special Spray	Shampoo: Apply to thoroughly saturate dry hair and thoroughly massage scalp; leave on for 10 min, then rinse. Repeat treatment in 7 d. Aerosol: Saturate area (5–10 squirts); wash off after 30 min.	Few adverse effects. The petroleum distillates used for solvents may cause contact dermatitis. Contraindicated in patients allergic to ragweed, chrysanthemums or other pyrethrin products. Pronto kit includes a comb, gloves and magnifying glass.	$
lindane 1% (gamma benzene hexachloride) Shampoo: Hexit, generics Lotion: generics	Shampoo: Apply in sufficient quantities to thoroughly saturate dry hair, and massage for 4 min; add water, a little at a time, to produce lather; massage again for 4 min; rinse. Lotion: Apply to affected area, then dress in clean clothes. Leave on for 8–12 h, then thoroughly wash off. Treatment may be repeated if required (**only once**).	Avoid contact with eyes, nose, mouth, mucous membranes. Associated with seizures in very young children. Contraindicated in neonates, young children, pregnant women and nursing mothers. Neurotoxicity (e.g., nausea, vomiting, headache, irritability, insomnia, seizures) has been reported after oral ingestion, repeated application, excessive doses or prolonged treatment.	$

Scabicides

permethrin 5%† Cream: Nix Dermal Cream Lotion: Kwellada-P	Massage into all skin areas, from **the top of the head** to the soles of the feet; every bit of skin must be treated, including the fingernails, waist and genitalia; leave on for 8–14 h without interruption, then wash off (shower may be the best way).	Drug of choice for scabies; it is as effective as lindane without neurotoxicity. Pruritus, erythema, numbness, tingling and rash. Contraindicated in patients allergic to chrysanthemums.	\$\$
crotamiton 10% Eurax cream	Apply to all skin areas‡‡ daily for 2–5 d; wash off 48 h after last application.		\$
lindane (see above) – (lotion; shampoo not recommended)	Apply to all skin areas‡‡ (once); should be left on for 8–12 h. Reapply in 7 d if necessary.	Used for persons allergic to permethrin. See lindane above.	\$
sulfur 5–10% ointment ‡	Apply to all skin areas‡‡ at bedtime daily for 5–7 d.	Not popular because it is malodorous, absorbed percutaneously and stains clothing. Extemporaneously compounded.‡	\$
esdepallethrin Scabene (aerosol spray)	Apply to all skin areas;‡‡ should be left on for 12 h then washed off with soap and water; towels or other protective coverings should be used on floors; alternatively, apply while standing in tub/shower to ↓ mess.	A useful therapy for hard to reach places (e.g., mid-scapular).	\$\$

† Lower strengths are not effective as scabicides.
‡ May be commercially available through wholesale distributors in some areas.
‡‡ As described for permethrin.

* Cost of 1 unit (tube or bottle) of product – includes drug cost only. **NB:** All products are available without prescription; retail mark-ups may vary.
Legend:　　$ < $10　　$$ $10–20

- Identify and examine **potential human contacts** to prevent a cycle of reinfection. *All* contacts of scabies, even if asymptomatic, require treatment.

Pharmacologic Choices (Table 2)

Therapeutic Tips

- Insufficient treatment of itch and fear of infestation may cause patients with scabies to overuse scabicides, resulting in skin irritation and unnecessary repeated therapy.

- Patients should be re-examined 7 days after the first treatment. Evidence of persistent infestation demands a second course of therapy.

- Scabetics should be treated from the top of the head **not** the top of the neck.

- In patients with scabies, itching can persist for weeks after mites are eradicated. Medium-potency topical corticosteroids (e.g., betamethasone valerate 0.1% cream) and oral antihistamines (e.g., diphenhydramine) are helpful.

- In patients with pediculosis capitis, treatment may fail if hair is not thoroughly soaked with permethrin. Two bottles are often needed for thick or long hair.

- Lice can exist in an intermediate stage and may not be cleared after 1 treatment. It is usually necessary to repeat therapy in 7 days.

- Crusted scabies in immunocompromised or debilitated patients should be treated with chlorhexidine gluconate wash followed by permethrin 5% cream. Oral **ivermectin** (off-label use) can be used as a single dose therapy (200 μg/kg).

Suggested Reading List

Aubin F, Humbert P. Ivermectin for crusted (Norwegian) scabies. *N Engl J Med* 1995;332:612.

Canadian Pediatric Society Statement. Head lice infestations: a persistent itchy "pest." *Paediatric Child Health* 1996; 1:237–241.

Orkin M, Maibach HI. Scabies treatment: current considerations. *Curr Probl Dermatol* 1996;24:151–156.

Taplin D, Meinking TL. Pyrethrins and pyrethroids in dermatology. *Arch Dermatol* 1990;126:213–221.

CHAPTER 65

Superficial Bacterial Skin Infections

Vincent C. Ho, BSc(Pharm), MD, FRCPC

Definitions

Impetigo: Superficial skin infection caused mainly by *Staphylococcus aureus*, group A beta-hemolytic streptococci or a combination of both.

Bullous impetigo: Bullous form of impetigo caused by *S. aureus* phage group II. The organism elaborates an exfoliating toxin causing superficial skin blistering. In young children, immuno-compromised hosts and patients with renal disease, high blood levels of this toxin may lead to generalized skin peeling, the staphylococcal scalded skin syndrome (SSSS).

Folliculitis: Superficial infection of the hair follicle most commonly caused by *S. aureus*. *Pseudomonas* folliculitis is associated with hot tub use. Gram-negative folliculitis caused by enterobacteriaceae most often occurs in those on long-term antibiotics for acne. Pseudofolliculitis is inflammation of the hair follicle secondary to friction, irritation or occlusion.

Furuncle (boil): Infection of a hair follicle with involvement of subcutaneous tissues, most often caused by *S. aureus*.

Carbuncle: Deep-seated infection of several hair follicles by *S. aureus*.

Erythrasma: Infection of the stratum corneum with *Coryne-bacterium minutissimum* that manifests as brown patches in intertriginous areas.

Therapeutic Choices (Figures 1 and 2)

Nonpharmacologic Choices

- Remove impetigo crusts, which harbor bacteria, by saline compresses or washing with soap and water.
- Occlusion, friction, heat and moisture are predisposing factors for bacterial skin infections. Mild cases may be treated with topical drying agents (e.g., aluminum chloride hexahydrate solution) or topical antiseptics (e.g., chlorhexidine, hexachlorophene, triclosan or povidone-iodine). Occlusive skin care products and clothing should be avoided.
- Incision and drainage of a large and fluctuant furuncle or carbuncle will relieve much of the pressure and pain.

Figure 1: **Management of Impetigo**

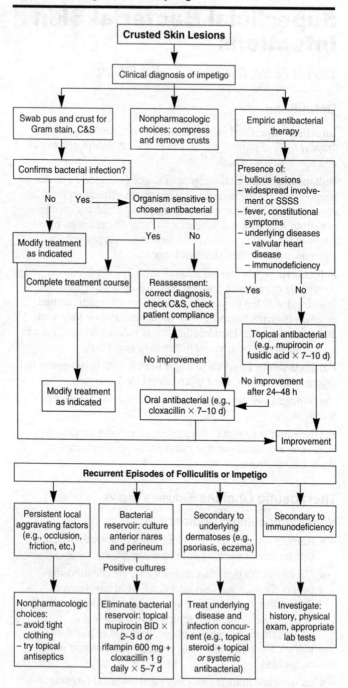

Abbreviations: SSSS = Staphylococcal scalded skin syndrome.

Figure 2: **Management of Folliculitis**

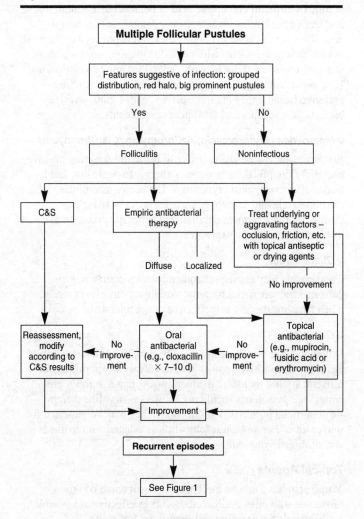

With effective antibacterials now available; however, there is less need for this surgical procedure.

- Antiseptics reduce the frequency of cross-infections among household contacts and recurrent skin infections in susceptible patients.

Pharmacologic Choices
Systemic Agents (Table 1)
□ *Beta-lactams*

Penicillinase-resistant penicillins (cloxacillin, flucloxacillin, nafcillin) are the drugs of choice for pyodermas because of their efficacy, low incidence of side effects and cost. The combination of **amoxicillin and clavulanic acid** (a beta-lactamase inhibitor) is effective but has no advantage over penicillinase-resistant penicillins for the usual pyodermas. **Cephalosporins** may be used as alternatives in patients with penicillin allergy; however, there is a 10% cross-reactivity between penicillins and cephalosporins. First-generation cephalosporins (cefadroxil, cephalexin) are preferred because they are more active against gram-positive bacteria than second- and third-generation agents.

❑ Macrolides (Erythromycin, Azithromycin, Clarithromycin)

Erythromycin is a good alternative to penicillin for gram-positive bacterial skin infections in patients allergic to penicillin, and it is also effective against erythrasma. The newer macrolides, clarithromycin and azithromycin, offer once- or twice-daily dosing, shorter treatment duration and better gastrointestinal tolerance but are more expensive.

❑ Clindamycin

Clindamycin may cause pseudomembranous colitis; it is not indicated for superficial bacterial skin infections except rarely, when first-line therapy is ineffective or not tolerated.

❑ Quinolones

Quinolones are broad-spectrum antibacterials, but their activity against gram-positive aerobes is relatively weak; ciprofloxacin-resistant strains, including methicillin-resistant *S. aureus*, are emerging. Quinolones should not be used as first-line therapy for superficial bacterial skin infections; they may be indicated for rare cases of *Pseudomonas* folliculitis associated with marked constitutional symptoms.

Topical Agents (Table 2)

Mupirocin has a unique mechanism of action and no cross-resistance with other antibacterials; it is as effective as systemic antibacterials for impetigo and superficial folliculitis.

Fusidic acid is available in systemic and topical form; its efficacy for superficial pyodermas is similar to mupirocin.

Bacitracin and **gramicidin** are active against gram-positive bacteria in vitro, but efficacy for established skin infections is not proven. **Polymyxin B** is active against gram-negative bacteria in vitro; it is often combined with bacitracin or neomycin, but its clinical efficacy is not proven.

The aminoglycosides **neomycin, framycetin** and **gentamicin** are active against gram-negative organisms, staphylococci and streptococci; they are probably less effective than systemic antibiotics for the treatment of established skin infections.

Table 1: Oral Antibacterials Used in Superficial Bacterial Skin Infections

Drug	Dosage (A: Adult, C: Children)	Antibacterial Spectrum	Major Adverse Effects[†]	Significant Drug Interactions[†]	Cost*
Penicillinase-Resistant Penicillins					
cloxacillin Orbenin, generics	Cloxacillin: A: 250–500 mg Q6H C: 12.5–25 mg/kg Q6H	Gram-positive bacteria: penicillinase-producing *S. aureus*, streptococci.	Hypersensitivity reactions (ranging from minor rashes to anaphylactic shock).		$
flucloxacillin Fluclox	Flucloxacillin: A: 250–500 mg Q6H C: 25–50 mg/kg/d in 4 divided doses				$$
Cephalosporins					
cephalexin Keflex, generics	Cephalexin: A: 250–500 mg Q6H C: 25–50 mg/kg/d in 4 divided doses	Gram-positive bacteria: *S. aureus*, streptococci. Gram-negative bacteria: *E. coli*, *Klebsiella*, *P. mirabilis*.	Hypersensitivity reactions (some cross-reactivity with penicillins).		$
cefadroxil Duricef	Cefadroxil: A: 1 g daily				$$

(cont'd)

Table 1: Oral Antibacterials Used in Superficial Bacterial Skin Infections *(cont'd)*

Drug	Dosage (A: Adult, C: Children)	Antibacterial Spectrum	Major Adverse Effects[†]	Significant Drug Interactions[†]	Cost*
Macrolides *erythromycin* E-Mycin, Erythromid, EES, Eryc, PCE, Ilosone, generics	Erythromycin: A: 250 mg Q6H C: 30–50 mg/kg/d in 4 divided doses	Gram-positive bacteria. *C. minutissimum.*	GI irritation (common), nausea and vomiting. Cholestatic jaundice with erythromycin estolate (rare).	Macrolide interactions:[‡] May ↑ serum levels of warfarin (E), triazolam (E), carbamazepine (E,C), astemizole (E), terfenadine (E,C), theophylline (E,C), cyclosporine (E).	$
clarithromycin 🕭 Biaxin	Clarithromycin: A: 250 mg Q12H C: not established			May ↓ zidovudine levels (C).	$$
clindamycin Dalacin-C	A: 150 mg Q6H C: (> 1 mo) 10–30 mg/kg/d in 3 or 4 divided doses	Aerobic and anaerobic gram-positive bacteria.	Pseudomembranous colitis.[π]		$$

[†] *Only the most important adverse effects/drug interactions are listed; consult product monograph for complete list.*

[‡] *Interactions have been documented with erythromycin (E), clarithromycin (C), or both (E,C); however, close monitoring is advised as other macrolides may not be safer alternatives.*

[π] *Most commonly associated with clindamycin but any antibiotic may cause this complication.*

🕭 *Dosage adjustment may be required in renal impairment – see Appendix I.*

* *Cost of 10-day supply – includes drug cost only.*

Legend: $ < $15 $$ $15–30 $$$ $30–45 $$$$ > $45

Table 2: Topical Antibacterials Used in Superficial Bacterial Skin Infections

Drug	Dosage	Antibacterial Spectrum	Adverse Effects	Cost*
mupirocin Bactroban	BID–TID	Gram-positive	Stinging, allergic contact dermatitis (rare).	$$†
fusidic acid Fucidin	BID–TID	Gram-positive	Allergic contact dermatitis (rare).	$$
bacitracin Baciguent, generics	BID–TID	Gram-positive	Allergic contact dermatitis, anaphylactic reactions following topical application (rare).	$†
polymyxin B Polysporin cream (with gramicidin), Polysporin ointment (with bacitracin), generics	BID–TID	Gram-negative	Nephrotoxicity when used extensively, allergic contact dermatitis.	$†
neomycin Neosporin (with polymyxin B and bacitracin), Myciguent	BID–TID	S. aureus, strep, gram-negative	Allergic contact dermatitis, especially when applied to eczematous skin.	$$
framycetin Soframycin, Sofra-tulle dressing	BID–TID	S. aureus, strep, gram-negative	Allergic contact dermatitis, cross-reaction with neomycin.	$ (ointment) $$ (10×10 cm dressing, 10s)
gentamicin Garamycin, generics	BID–TID	S. aureus, strep, gram-negative	Allergic contact dermatitis.	$$
silver sulfadiazine Dermazin, Flamazine, SSD	BID–TID	S. aureus, gram-negative, Pseudomonas	Allergic contact dermatitis, leukopenia when applied to large area of burned skin.	$

† Available OTC – retail mark-up not included in these costs.
* Cost of 15g tube – includes drug cost only.
Legend: $ < $5 $$ $5 $$ $5–10

Commonly used for prophylaxis and treatment of infection in serious burn victims, **silver sulfadiazine** is active against staphylococci and gram-negative organisms, including *Pseudomonas*.

Therapeutic Tips

- Impetigo and folliculitis may be treated with either topical (mupirocin or fusidic acid) or systemic antibacterials. Systemic antibacterials of choice are the beta-lactams (penicillinase-resistant penicillins or cephalosporins, e.g., cloxacillin or cephalexin). Alternative agents include erythromycin, clarithromycin or clindamycin. Systemic therapy should be used when there is widespread disease, fever or constitutional symptoms or when the patient has valvular heart disease or is immunocompromised.

- Bullous impetigo, furuncles or carbuncles should be treated with systemic antibacterials.

- Systemic antibacterials should be combined with topical measures such as cleaning or compresses to remove crusts that harbor bacteria.

- Avoid topical antibacterials that may cause cross-resistance with systemic antibiotics (e.g., gentamicin).

- Avoid prolonged use of topical antibacterials (> 2 weeks) to prevent development of bacterial resistance.

- Avoid manipulation of furuncles on the central face as this may lead to cavernous sinus thrombosis or brain abscess.

- Recurrent furunculosis or impetigo may be due to bacterial carriage in the nose or perineum (see Figure 1 for treatment suggestions).

- Recurrent furunculosis in the groin or axillae may be due to hidradenitis suppurativa; dermatologic consultation is suggested.

Suggested Reading List

Booth JH, Benrimoj SI. Mupirocin in the treatment of impetigo. *Int J Dermatol* 1992;31:1–9.

Gentry LO. Therapy with newer oral beta-lactam and quinolone agents for infections of the skin and skin structures: a review. *Clin Infect Dis* 1991;14:285–297.

Liu C. An overview of antimicrobial therapy. *Comprehen Ther* 1992;18:35–42.

Turnidge J, Grayson ML. Optimum treatment of staphylococcal infections. *Drugs* 1993;45:353–366.

CHAPTER 66

Contraception

Gillian Graves, MD, FRCSC

Goals of Therapy

- To prevent fertilization. Effective contraceptive control and education reduces the rates of maternal and child mortality, as well as population growth
- To tailor the method to an individual's specific needs, lifestyle, age, parity and desire for future fertility

Therapeutic Choices

Assessment of Consumer Needs

No single method of contraception is ideal for all individuals. The preferred methods in young women are reversible, have high safety profiles and low failure rates. They should not interfere with other physiologic processes, such as vaginal lubrication, spontaneity, or pleasure of either partner. Cost should be affordable.

Nonpharmacologic Choices (Table 1)

Pharmacologic Choices (Table 1)

Oral Contraceptives (Table 2)

Lowest failure rate outside of surgical sterilization.

Method of choice for most young couples, especially for teens if combined with condoms (required for STD protection).

Oral contraceptives (OCs) containing synthetic estrogen and progestogen have undergone several modifications resulting in dose reduction and the synthesis of newer and more potent steroids. This has been done to increase safety and reliability, and decrease adverse effects that reduce compliance.

"Minipills" (with progestin only) inhibit ovulation and alter cervical mucus and uterine physiology.

Triphasic pills claim better cycle control and reduced side effects.

Products containing **"new progestins"** (e.g., desogestrel, gestodene) are less androgenic and may in theory have less atherogenic risk; however, long-term studies are required to quantitate any potential changes in cardiovascular risk profile for users of third-generation OCs compared to older progestins.

Cardiovascular adverse events including venous thrombo-embolism (VTE) and acute myocardial infarction (AMI) are uncommon among OC users. Compared to nonusers, the calculated risk of VTE is 3.5-fold higher with sub-50 μg ethinyl estradiol (EE) OCs. The very low attributable or absolute risks of VTE associated with third-generation OCs (incidence: 2 extra cases per 10 000 or relative risk [RR] 1.3 to 2.4) are of insignificant public health or clinical importance. The stroke risks are extremely small and do not differ between generations of progestins. AMI risk is decreased with third-generation OCs compared to second generation (RR 0.3). All cardiovascular risks are appreciably higher in pregnancy compared to those on any sub-50 μg EE OC.

In the nonsmoking normotensive woman under the age of 35, the risk of cardiovascular disease is so small that there is no health impact related to the choice of second vs third generation of progestin. Clinicians make thoughtful decisions about which OC to prescribe based on monitoring and controlling an individual's other risk markers for cardiovascular disease, such as obesity (higher risk of VTE: consider second-generation OCs and weight reduction) and smoking (higher risk of AMI and arterial disease: consider third-generation OCs and smoking cessation/reduction).

Injectable Contraceptives

Medroxyprogesterone Acetate (Depo-Provera)

- an injectable contraceptive used worldwide for many years
- extremely safe, effective (99.7%), and private
- dose is 150 mg IM every 3 months
- injection schedule of four times a year facilitates compliance
- produces amenorrhea in the majority of women, but some experience irregular bleeding and progestational side effects such as bloating, weight gain/loss and mood swings
- an excellent product for women who should avoid high estrogen doses, such as migraine sufferers
- can be used in the postabortal state (5 days postpartum), or during lactation (6 weeks postpartum)
- duration of action may be up to a year until regular menses returns
- increasing the interval between injections increases the risk of pregnancy
- condoms required for STD protection
- more prospective data needed to document the long-term effect on bone mineral content with prolonged use
- long-term use is not associated with an increase in breast cancer

Table 1: **Available Contraceptive Methods**

Contraceptive Method	Contra-indications	Adverse Effects	Drug Interactions	Comments	Cost*
Coital Timing	Relative: irregular menses	None	None	Requires high motivation; depends on identification of mucous and temperature patterns to identify fertile time; very difficult if there is an irregular cycle or ovulation defects. High pregnancy rates.	
Condom	Relative: hypersensitivity to latex	Common: hypersensitivity to latex in either partner	None	Protects against STD including HIV (latex only); best for infrequent intercourse; high failure rate of 10–14%. Use with spermicide.	$0.50–0.70/ condom
Diaphragm/Sponge	Relative: hypersensitivity, inability to insert Absolute: inability to achieve proper fit, marked uterine prolapse, large cystocele/rectocele, vaginal deformity	Common: hypersensitivity to diaphragm and/or spermicide	None	Best for infrequent intercourse. High failure rate of 10–14%. Use with spermicide.	$33.00/ diaphragm, $6.00/4 sponges
Cervical Cap	Relative: abnormal cervical cytology, chronic cervicitis, recurrent salpingitis Absolute: cervical deformity (i.e., inability to obtain suitable fit)	Common: vaginal discharge, vaginal odor, cervical or fornices ulceration, hypersensitivity (cap or spermicide)	None	Use with spermicide. Protects against STD including HIV.	$35.00/cap

(cont'd)

Table 1: **Available Contraceptive Methods** (cont'd)

Contraceptive Method	Contra-indications	Adverse Effects	Drug Interactions	Comments	Cost*
Spermicide	Relative: hypersensitivity	Common: hypersensitivity	None	Use with condom, diaphragm or cervical cap.	$10.00/unit spermicide
IUD	Absolute: pregnancy; undiagnosed vaginal bleeding, stenosed cervix, nulliparity, copper allergy	Major: salpingitis, uterine perforation, cervical perforation, endometrial embedding menorrhagia, pain, infection, ectopic pregnancy	None	Excellent for spacing children in a stable relationship, failure rate 1–5% in 1st yr, risk of PID and tubal infections is too high for nullipara. Immediate risks are insertional infection or perforation. Late risks are infection and ectopic pregnancy.	$50.00 for copper IUD – lasts 3–5 yrs
Vasectomy	None	None	None	Method of choice for couples with completed family. Failure rate < 2%. Reversible with more surgery if < 10 yrs since procedure.	Cost-insured service in Canada. Cost of reversal surgery $3 000–$5 000
Tubal Ligation	None	Ectopic rates post tubal ligation were 7.3 per 1 000. (Highest follow-up rate in young women < 30 yrs)	None	Method of choice for couples with completed family. Low failure rate – 18.5 per 1 000 procedures at 10 yrs follow-up. Reversible only if salpingectomy not performed and sufficient length of undamaged tubal remnants remain.	Cost-insured service in Canada. Cost of reversal surgery $3 000–$5 000

Oral Contraceptives	Relative: estrogen hypersensitivity, classic migraine, gallbladder disease, brittle diabetes Absolute: history of coronary artery disease, hypercholesterolemia, recent history of thromboembolism, recent history of stroke, end-stage renal disease, proliferative retinopathy, symptomatic mitral valve prolapse, estrogen-dependent carcinoma or tumor, smoker > 35 yrs old, current jaundice or pregnancy	Major: rare thromboembolism, stroke, retinal artery thrombosis, myocardial infarction, benign liver tumor, cholelithiasis, hypertension Common: breakthrough bleeding/spotting, amenorrhea, nausea/vomiting, weight gain, bloating, chloasma, breast tenderness, depression, headaches	Antibiotics: reports of failure of OCs in women taking ampicillin, tetracycline, erythromycin, co-trimoxazole or nitrofurantoin. Rifampin is the only antibiotic consistently shown to reduce estrogen levels. Patients with diarrhea or breakthrough bleeding may be at higher risk. There is controversy as to whether barrier is also required at the time of antibiotic use	Lowest failure rate outside of surgical sterilization. Method of choice for most young couples, especially for teens, if combined with condoms. Lower dose estrogen products have increased safety and decreased side effects. Condoms needed for STD protection.	$20/mo
Medroxyprogesterone Acetate Depo-Provera	Thrombophlebitis, thromboembolic disorders, cerebral apoplexy or patients with a past history of these conditions. Known sensitivity to medroxyprogesterone acetate or to the vehicle or vaginal bleeding or urinary tract bleeding. Liver dysfunction or disease. Pregnancy. Undiagnosed breast pathology	Breast tenderness, galactorrhea. Occasionally nervousness, insomnia, somnolence, fatigue, depression, dizziness and headache. Thromboembolic disorders (thrombophlebitis and pulmonary embolism). Skin sensitivity reactions. Hyperpyrexia, change in weight, moon face	Aminoglutethimide may significantly depress the bioavailability of medroxyprogesterone	Injectable contraceptive that is extremely safe and effective (99.7%). Excellent for women who should avoid high estrogen doses, such as migraine sufferers. Condoms needed for STD protection.	$38.00 for 150 mg Q3 mos

(cont'd)

Table 1: **Available Contraceptive Methods** (cont'd)

Contraceptive Method	Contra-indications	Adverse Effects	Drug Interactions	Comments	Cost*
Levonorgestrel Implant Norplant	Active thromboembolic disorders; undiagnosed abnormal genital bleeding; known or suspected pregnancy; acute liver disease; benign or malignant liver tumors; known or suspected carcinoma of the breast	Changes in uterine bleeding or amenorrhea. Pain or itching near the implant site, infection at implant site, removal difficulties. Headache, nervousness, nausea, dizziness, adnexal enlargement, dermatitis, acne, change of appetite, mastalgia, weight gain, hirsutism, hypertrichosis and scalp hair loss	Phenytoin and carbamazepine may reduce efficacy and result in pregnancy. Warn patients of the possibility of decreased efficacy with the use of any related drugs	Efficacy close to that of tubal ligation. Expensive up-front cost. Condoms needed for STD protection.	$522.00/5 yrs
Emergency Postcoital Contraception ethinyl estradiol and levonorgestrel Ovral	See oral contraceptives	See oral contraceptives	See oral contraceptives	May prevent pregnancy when taken up to 72 hours after a single episode of unprotected intercourse. Method has a 98% success rate when used correctly.	

Approximate cost per unit (condom, tube, canister, package) – includes drug or contraceptive cost only. Mark-up is not included.

Table 2: **Oral Contraceptives**

Composition	Product
50 µg Estrogen	
EE 50 µg / ethynodiol diacetate 1 mg	Demulen 50
EE 50 µg / d-norgestrel 0.25 mg	Ovral
mestranol 50 µg / norethindrone 1 mg	Norinyl 1/50, Ortho-Novum 1/50
Sub-50 µg Estrogen Monophasic	
EE 35 µg / norethindrone 1 mg	Brevicon 1/35, Ortho 1/35, Select 1/35
EE 35 µg / norethindrone 0.5 mg	Brevicon 0.5/35, Ortho 0.5/35
EE 35 µg / norgestimate 0.25 mg	Cyclen
EE 30 µg / desogestrel 0.15 mg	Marvelon, Ortho-Cept
EE 30 µg / ethynodiol diacetate 2 mg	Demulen 30
EE 30 µg / levonorgestrel 0.15 mg	Min-Ovral
EE 30 µg / norethindrone acetate 1.5 mg	Loestrin 1.5/30
EE 20 µg / norethindrone acetate 1 mg	Minestrin 1/20
EE 20 µg / levonorgestrel 0.1 mg	Alesse
Biphasic	
EE 35 µg × 21 d / norethindrone 0.5 mg × 10 d, 1 mg × 11 d	Ortho 10/11
Triphasic	
EE 35 µg × 21 d / norethindrone 0.5 mg × 7 d, 0.75 mg × 7 d, 1 mg × 7 d	Ortho 7/7/7
EE 35 µg × 21 d / norethindrone 0.5 mg × 7 d, 1 mg × 9 d, 0.5 mg × 5 d	Synphasic
EE 35 µg × 21 d / norgestimate 0.18 mg × 7 d, 0.215 mg × 7 d, 0.25 mg × 7 d	Tri-Cyclen
EE 30 µg × 6 d, 40 µg × 5 d, 30 µg × 10 d / levonorgestrel 0.05 mg × 6 d, 0.075 mg × 5 d, 0.125 mg × 10 d	Triphasil, Triquilar
Progestin only	
norethindrone 0.35 mg	Micronor

Abbreviations: EE = ethinyl estradiol.

Levonorgestrel (Norplant)

- efficacy close to tubal ligation
- progestin-containing rods are implanted in the subcutaneous tissue of the upper, inner arm
- may cause dysfunctional or breakthrough bleeding
- occasionally can be difficult to remove the rods
- similar adverse effects and benefits as injectable medroxyprogesterone acetate
- expensive up-front costs
- condoms required for STD protection

Emergency Postcoital Contraception

- Ethinyl estradiol and levonorgestrel (e.g., 2 tablets of Ovral) with an antinauseant, followed by a second identical dose 12 hours later. Prevents pregnancy when taken up to 72 hours after a single episode of unprotected intercourse. This is followed by menstrual bleeding within 21 days after treatment when successful.

- This method has a 98% success rate (failure rate 0.16 to 5%) when used correctly. Counseling is necessary in the event of treatment failure.

Contraception While Breast-feeding

- Barrier plus spermicides can provide lubrication to the hypoestrogenic vagina but not as effective for contraception as other methods.

- IUD can be inserted 4 to 6 weeks postpartum once involution has occurred and the uterus is firm enough to decrease the risk of insertional perforation. Need to ensure good fundal placement with larger uterine cavity, since efficacy of current copper T devices requires the IUD arms to be near the fundus.

- Progestin-only OCs can be used during lactation, without increasing thromboembolic rates in the puerperium. Must be taken every day at the same time without missing a pill, in order to minimize spotting and maintain contraceptive efficacy.

- Low-dose combination OCs can be used once the milk supply is well established. There is some decrease in milk quantity; however, no negative effect on the infant has been described.

Therapeutic Tips

- Age – In the past, OCs were not given to women older than age 35 since earlier publications had indicated an increased rate of myocardial infarction. Recent data have shown that smoking and other cardiovascular risk factors contribute to the myocardial risk in these women. In nonsmoking selected women with no other risk factors, low dose OCs may be considered for contraception or control of dysfunctional uterine bleeding up to the menopause.

- OCs help control anemia and regulate cycles.

- Acne is considered an androgen-dependent condition. OCs with androgenic progestins (e.g., norethindrone acetate) would not be the first choice for individuals with acne vulgaris (theoretical advantage of new progestins). However,

OC estrogenicity affects sex hormone binding globulin, which may be more important than the choice of progestin in hirsutism and acne.

- Noncontraceptive health benefits attributed to OC use include a decrease in: the frequency of endometrial cancer, fibroids, endometriosis pain, benign breast disease, functional ovarian cysts, ectopic pregnancy, dysmenorrhea and PID.

Suggested Reading List

Anon. Pill scares and public responsibility. *Lancet* 1996;347:1707.

Farmer RDT, Lawrenson RA, Thompson CF, Kennedy JG, Hambleton IR. Population-based study of risk of venous thromboembolism associated with various oral contraceptives. *Lancet* 1997;349:83–88.

Lefebvre G, Lea RH, Boroditsky R, Fisher W, Belisle S, Sand M. The benefits of awareness study: an evaluation of a targetted, user-friendly education among oral contraceptive users. *J SOGC* 1996;18:1111–1121.

Peterson HB, Xia Z, Hughes JM, Wilcox LS, Tylor LR, Trussel J. US Collaborative Review of Sterilization Working Group. The risk of ectopic pregnancy after tubal sterilization. *N Engl J Med* 1997;336:762–767.

Silvestre L, Bouali Y, Ulmann A. Postcoital contraception: myth or reality? *Lancet* 1991;6:39–41.

CHAPTER 67

Dysmenorrhea

Glenn H. Gill, MD, CCFP, FRCSC

Definition

Dysmenorrhea is menstrual pain, which affects over 50% of menstruating women to some degree, 10% of whom are incapacitated for 1 to 3 days per month. It is most common from age 20 to 25.

Goals of Therapy

- To decrease or abolish menstrual pain that interferes with everyday activities
- To rule out organic causes of pain that may require alternative therapies

Investigations

- A thorough history to differentiate primary from secondary dysmenorrhea (Table 1). In primary dysmenorrhea:
  - pain starts within 1 to 4 hours of onset of menses and lasts at most 1 to 3 days
  - pain is described as crampy, located in the lower abdomen and present with each period
  - other symptoms of prostaglandin excess may be present (i.e., nausea, vomiting, diarrhea, backache, thigh pain, headache, dizziness)

Table 1: **Characteristics of Dysmenorrhea**

Primary	Secondary
– absence of identifiable pelvic pathology – occurs in ovulatory cycles – onset within 2 yrs after menarche – pain due to myometrial contractions induced by prostaglandin production in the secretory endometrium	– associated with pelvic pathology (e.g., endometriosis, adenomyosis, uterine myomas, endometrial polyps, intrauterine device, pelvic inflammatory disease, obstructed outflow, congenital mullerian malformations). Diagnostic clues include infertility, dyspareunia, premenstrual or intermenstrual bleeding, pain onset before menses
	– onset at menarche or after age 25 suggests a possible pelvic abnormality
	– component of pain may be due to endometrial prostaglandins; therefore partial response to therapy for primary dysmenorrhea may be seen

Figure 1: **Management of Dysmenorrhea**

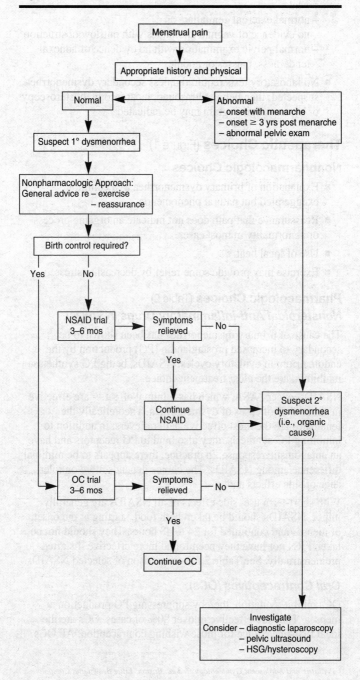

Abbreviations: OC = oral contraceptive, HSG = hysterosalpingogram.

- Physical examination for primary dysmenorrhea should reveal:
  - normal external genitalia
  - no evidence of vaginal anomalies with outflow obstruction
  - normal pelvic examination with no evidence of adnexal tenderness, masses or nodules
- No laboratory tests required unless secondary dysmenorrhea suspected; then pelvic ultrasound, laparoscopy, hysteroscopy or hysterosalpingogram may be indicated

Therapeutic Choices (Figure 1)

Nonpharmacologic Choices

- Explanation of primary dysmenorrhea as a common, exaggerated but natural phenomenon.
- Reassurance that pain does not indicate an organic process or abnormality in most cases.
- Use of local heat.
- Exercise may provide some relief by decreasing stress.

Pharmacologic Choices (Table 2)

Nonsteroidal Anti-inflammatory Drugs (NSAIDs)

The cause of primary dysmenorrhea has been shown to be secondary to increased prostaglandin (PG) production by the endometrium in ovulatory cycles. NSAIDs, being PG synthetase inhibitors, are the clear treatment choice.

NSAIDs, except ASA, which has minimal effect,[1,2] are effective in about 80% of cases of dysmenorrhea. Theoretically the fenamates are the most effective pain relievers; in addition to inhibiting PG synthesis, they also bind to PG receptors and have an antagonistic response. In practice, there appears to be minimal difference among NSAIDs. The choice depends more on tolerance of side effects and cost.

With short-term use, side effects of all NSAIDs are generally minor. NSAIDs should be taken with food, starting at the onset of menses and continued for 24 to 48 hours. They should not be taken PRN nor have they been found more effective if started premenstrually. See Table 2 for comparison of selected NSAIDs.

Oral Contraceptives (OCs)

OCs inhibit ovulation, thereby suppressing PG production at menses. They are effective in over 80% of cases. OCs are the ideal first-line choice for those wishing contraception. All OCs

[1] *Pediatric and Adolescent Gynaecology. 3rd ed. Boston: Little Brown and Company, 1990:295.*
[2] *J Pediatr 1981;98:97.*

Table 2: Drugs Used for Dysmenorrhea

Drug	Dosage	Contraindications	Adverse Effects	Efficacy (Clinical Pain Relief)	Cost*
PG Synthetase Inhibitors (NSAIDs) (See Chapter 50 for more information on adverse effects and drug interactions of NSAIDs.)					
Indoleacetic Acid ⚫ *indomethacin* Indocid, generics	25 mg TID to 6×/d	For **all agents:** Hypersensitivity to ASA, active peptic ulcer disease, gastritis, inflammatory bowel disease, existing renal disease, clotting disorders.	For **all agents:** Very common (> 10%): dyspepsia, nausea/ vomiting.	70–80%	$
Fenamates ⚫ *mefenamic acid* Ponstan, generics	250–500 mg QID		Common (5–10%): nonspecific rash/ pruritus, dizziness, headache.	86–94%	$$–$$$
Propionic Acid Derivatives ⚫ *ibuprofen* Motrin, generics	400 mg QID			66–90%	$
naproxen sodium Anaprox, generics	275 mg QID				$$
ketoprofen Orudis, Rhodis, generics	50 mg TID				$
flurbiprofen Ansaid, Froben, generics	50 mg QID				$$

(cont'd)

Table 2: **Drugs Used for Dysmenorrhea** (cont'd)

Drug	Dosage	Contraindications	Adverse Effects	Efficacy (Clinical Pain Relief)	Cost*
Miscellaneous 🍁					
piroxicam Feldene, generics	10–40 mg/d			≈ 80%	$–$$
diclofenac sodium Voltaren, generics	50–75 mg/d			≈ 80%	$
Other					
Oral Contraceptives Numerous products	According to product monograph	See Chapter 66 for contraindications and adverse effects.			$$$$†

🍁 *Dosage adjustment may be required in renal impairment – see Appendix 1.*

* *Cost of 2-day/cycle supply – includes drug cost only.*
† *Cost of one pack of oral contraceptives – includes drug cost only.*
Legend: $ < $2 $$ $2–4 $$$ $4–10 $$$$ $10–15

are effective, although in theory monophasic OCs with a more androgenic progestational component are ideal (e.g., levonorgestrel, dl-norgestrel) (Chapter 66).

Therapeutic Tips

- A therapeutic trial of 3 to 6 months of either an NSAID or OC is usually sufficient to demonstrate effectiveness.

- Pharmacotherapy fails in 20% of patients. These patients usually have secondary dysmenorrhea and require prompt investigation. Diagnostic laparoscopy is the most useful test to differentiate primary from secondary dysmenorrhea. Therapy can then be directed and may involve surgery, such as laser ablation of endometriosis or uterosacral nerve ablation.

- In a small percentage of patients in whom pharmacotherapy fails, extensive investigation will not identify a specific cause. In these patients psychogenic factors should not be overlooked.

- Calcium channel blockers, magnesium, clonidine, transcutaneous electrical nerve stimulation (TENS), acupuncture and chiropractor spinal manipulation have been studied. None has shown greater efficacy than NSAIDs or OCs.

Suggested Reading List

Daywood MY. Dysmenorrhea. In: Speroff L, Simpson JL, Sciarra JJ, eds. *Sciarra gynecology and obstetrics.* Vol 5. Philadelphia: JB Lippincott, 1991:1–12.

Emans SJH, Goldstein DP. *Pediatric and adolescent gynecology.* 3rd ed. Boston: Little, Brown, and Company, 1990:291–299.

Fraser IS. Prostaglandins, prostaglandin inhibitors and their roles in gynecological disorders. *Bailliere's Clinical Obstetrics and Gynecology International Practice and Research* 1992;6:829–857.

Rapkin AJ. Pelvic pain and dysmenorrhea. In: Berek JS, Adashi EY, Hillard PA. *Novak's Textbook of Gynecology.* 12th ed. Baltimore: Williams & Wilkins, 1996:399–428.

CHAPTER 68

Menopause

John Collins, MD, FRCPC

Definition

Menopause is the cessation of menstrual periods and occurs when the ovaries stop producing estrogen. This change takes place naturally when ovarian follicles are depleted at approximately 51 years of age, or following surgical removal of the ovaries, with or without hysterectomy.

Goals of Therapy

- To reduce symptoms due to estrogen depletion, including hot flushes, sleeplessness, lethargy, depression and symptoms arising from urogenital atrophy
- To prevent disorders that may be less frequent with estrogen therapy, including osteoporotic fractures, myocardial infarction and colonic cancer
- To avoid causing disorders that may be more frequent with estrogen therapy, including endometrial and breast cancer

Investigations

- Confirm cessation of ovarian activity (Figure 1)
  - if 6 months have elapsed since the last menstrual bleeding, ovarian failure is virtually certain
  - if in doubt, or if symptoms are present while menses continue, two serum FSH values 1 week apart in excess of 30 IU/L will detect incipient ovarian failure (an ovulatory rise in FSH lasts only 2 to 3 days and cannot affect both estimates)
- Health maintenance screening
  - initial examination should include blood pressure measurements, breast examination and cervical cytology
  - mammography is indicated for all women over 50 years of age. It should be considered for younger women who have a higher than average risk
  - lipid screening and bone densitometry may be considered in women with a family history or a strong personal risk profile for heart disease or osteoporosis

Therapeutic Choices (Figure 1, Tables 1 and 2)

Nonpharmacologic Choices

Not all women with menopausal symptoms seek medical attention. Many rely on **lifestyle changes**, including exercise and reductions in caffeine and alcohol intake. **Herbal remedies** are also widely used; their effects are unlikely to be due to their minuscule content of estrogen and their beneficial effects remain unproven. Increasing **calcium** intake to 1 g daily and taking **vitamin D** is a useful approach to minimize bone loss.

Pharmacologic Choices

Preparations (Table 1)

Estrogen preparations are essential to manage symptoms and prevent disease. The efficacy of pharmaceutical estrogen preparations correlates with the amount of estradiol that binds to target organ receptors. Therefore, the therapeutic ratios of benefits and side effects among the various preparations are similar when they are used in pharmacologically equivalent doses.

Progesterone preparations (progestins) are necessary among estrogen users who have not had a hysterectomy. Progestins prevent the unrestrained endometrial growth that increases the risk of endometrial cancer.

Dosage Regimens

Cyclic administration emulates estrogen and progesterone secretion in normal menstrual cycles. In this treatment regimen, estrogen is given daily. Progestin is given on the 1st to the 14th days of the calendar month. Most women will have withdrawal bleeding shortly after completing the progesterone phase. The daily estrogen regimen has replaced the regimen in which estrogen is given for the first 21–25 days of the calendar month because some women develop symptoms during the days without estrogen.

Continuous combined therapy avoids withdrawal bleeding, but unpredictable spotting or light bleeding occurs in most women during the first year of treatment. Estrogen and progestin are given daily without breaks in the regimen.

Dosage

Regardless of the product selected, the dose should be the lowest capable of controlling symptoms or known to prevent disease. In the case of conjugated estrogens 0.625 mg per day is a rational starting dose. The starting dose for progestins should be equivalent to 5 mg medroxyprogesterone acetate for sequential regimens and 2.5 mg for continuous regimens.

Figure 1: **Treatment of Menopause**

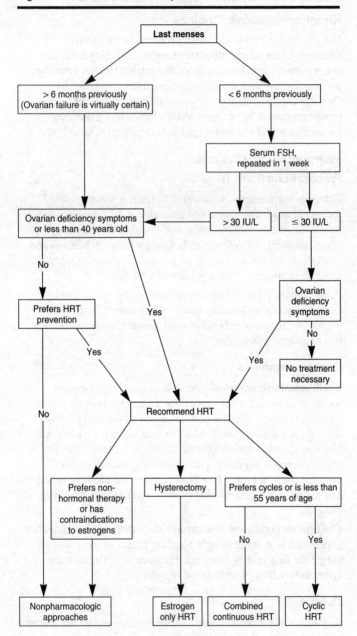

Abbreviations: HRT = hormone replacement therapy.

Table 1: Agents Used to Treat Perimenopause and Menopause

Drug	Usual Dosage	Adverse Effects	Comments	Cost*
Estrogens (Oral)		Bloating, headache, nausea, breast tenderness, dose-related bleeding.	Estrogen is given daily. To reduce risk of endometrial cancer give with progestin.	
conjugated equine estrogen Premarin	0.625–1.25 mg/d			$
estropipate Ogen	0.625–1.25 mg/d			$
estradiol (micronized) Estrace	1–2 mg/d			$
ethinyl estradiol Estinyl	0.02–0.05 mg/d			$
conjugated estrone sulfate generics	0.625–1.25 mg/d			$
Estrogens (Transdermal)		See above. Redness, skin irritation.	Less effect on hepatic protein synthesis than oral estrogens. Preferred application site is buttocks.	$$
estradiol-17β Estraderm, Vivelle Climara	0.025–0.1mg/d (1 patch 2×/wk) 0.05–0.1mg/d (1 patch 1×/wk)			
Estrogens (Vaginal) Cream		Systemic effects are caused by higher doses.	For all: Indicated when vaginal dryness and urogenital symptoms predominate.	
conjugated equine estrogen Premarin	Applied to introitus QHS × 1 wk, then 1×/wk			$
dienestrol Ortho Dienestrol				
estrone Oestrilin				

(cont'd)

Table 1: Agents Used to Treat Perimenopause and Menopause *(cont'd)*

Drug	Usual Dosage	Adverse Effects	Comments	Cost*
Ring *estradiol* Estring	7.5 µg/d continuously			$$
Progestins *medroxyprogesterone acetate* Provera	5–10 mg/d cyclically or 2.5–5 mg continuously	Bloating, irritability, weight gain, mood swings.	Progestin is given daily or on the 1st–14th day of the calendar month. Progestins normalize the endometrial response and decrease breakthrough bleeding. When given continuously prevent flow.	$–$$
norethindrone Micronor	0.35–0.7 mg/d continuously (contraceptive)			$
progesterone (micronized) Prometrium	200–300 mg/d QHS cyclically or 100–200 mg continuously			$$–$$$
Combination estrogen/progestin (Transdermal) Estracomb	estradiol 0.05 mg/d (4 patches over 1st 2 wks) estradiol 0.05 mg/d + norethindrone 0.25 mg/d (4 patches over last 2 wks)	As for cyclic estrogens, progestins above.		$$

* Cost of 1-month therapy as directed – includes drug cost only.
Legend: $ <$15 $$ $15–30 $$$ $30–45

Table 2: **Contraindications to Estrogen**

Recent treatment for breast cancer
Abnormal uterine bleeding
Active hepatic disease

Therapeutic Tips

- **Individual decision-making**
  Many physicians have a general policy of encouraging
  patients to take hormone replacement therapy (HRT) because
  this form of treatment appears to provide long-term benefits
  and increase both life span and quality of life. A uniform
  policy of this kind is doomed to failure, as shown by the fact
  that the majority of patients who start HRT subsequently
  stop. Physicians must recognize that each woman should
  make her own decisions concerning her life and health.
  Furthermore, each woman's health history is singularly
  unique, and provides a risk profile that leads to more, or less,
  benefit from HRT. As a result, an unswerving policy applied
  to all women is unlikely to meet the individual needs of
  many. Physicians should consider the needs and wants of
  each patient before recommending a course of therapy for
  menopause.

- **Premature ovarian failure**
  Less than 1% of North American women experience
  menopause before age 40. Premature ovarian failure
  is associated with an early rise in the incidence of
  cardiovascular disease and osteoporosis. The risk profile of
  patients who enter menopause prior to age 40 dictates that
  HRT should be prescribed for all such individuals. Treatment
  should continue until at least the age of 50, the age when
  other women are also in or nearing menopause.

- **Route of administration**
  Estrogen preparations may be taken orally, transdermally,
  vaginally, and parenterally. Although there is some indication that lipid bio-markers may show greater changes with
  different routes of administration, there is no evidence that
  route of administration has any bearing on the clinical outcomes of greatest interest, such as myocardial infarction.

- **Duration of use**
  Treatment of menopausal symptoms may require several
  years of hormonal treatment. Prevention of cardiovascular
  disease and osteoporosis may need much longer use. The
  rates of myocardial infarction and hip fracture do not reach
  appreciable levels until women are in their late sixties and
  seventies. Optimal prevention of these events is seen only
  among current users of HRT.

- **Unexplained bleeding**
  Estrogen therapy increases the risk of endometrial cancer in
  postmenopausal women who have a uterus. Therefore, any
  unexpected bleeding requires investigation. In most cases, a
  tissue diagnosis may be required.

Suggested Reading List

Menopause Consensus Conference Committee. The Canadian
    Menopause Consensus Conference. *J SOGC* 1994;16(5).

Cramer DW, Xu H, Harlow BL. Family history as a predictor of
    early menopause. *Fertil Steril* 1995;64:740–745.

Limouzin-Lamouthe MA, Mairon N, Joyce CRB, Le Gal M.
    Quality of life after menopause: influence of hormonal
    replacement therapy. *Am J Obstet Gynecol*
    1994;170:618–624.

CHAPTER 69

Erectile Dysfunction

S.K. Afridi, MBBS, FRCS(Ed), FRCSC, FRCS (Eng), FACS

Goals of Therapy

- To find the cause of impotence
- To restore potency

Investigations

- A thorough history with special attention to onset, performance anxiety, partner cooperation, diabetes, hypertension, neurologic disorders, trauma, vascular diseases and use of erectolytic agents, which include:
  - antihypertensives (beta-blockers, methyldopa, diuretics)
  - psychotropics
  - antiandrogens (spironolactone, ketoconazole, finasteride)
  - drugs of addiction (nicotine, alcohol, heroin, LSD, cocaine)
- Physical examination focusing on signs of endocrinopathies, neurologic disorders, peripheral vascular diseases and genital abnormalities
- Laboratory tests:
  - blood glucose, TSH, testosterone and prolactin
  - if testosterone levels abnormal, determine FSH and LH
  - if testosterone and LH are low, or if prolactin is high, refer to endocrinologist for consultation

Therapeutic Choices (Figures 1 and 2)

Nonpharmacologic Choices

- Smoking, alcohol and other substances potentially causing impotence should be discontinued.
- Psychotherapy (sex counseling, hypnosis) should be provided.
- Erectile band, penile implants, vacuum devices and, rarely, revascularization surgery may be tried when other methods are unsuitable or have failed.

Figure 1: **Management of Erectile Dysfunction**

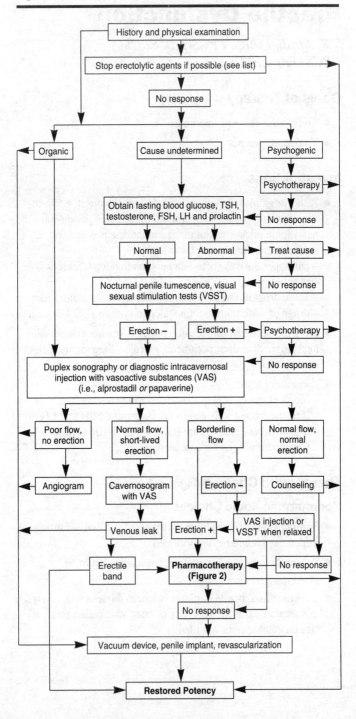

Pharmacologic Choices (Table 1, Figure 2)

Figure 2: **Therapeutic Choices in Erectile Dysfunction**

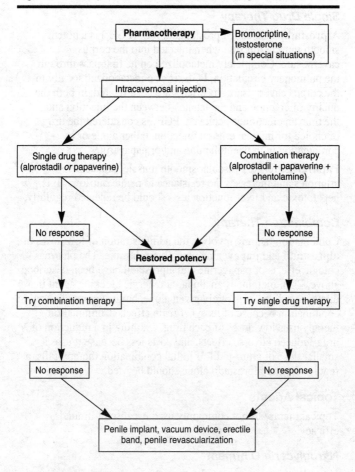

Intracavernosal Medications

Vasoactive substances are injected into the corpus cavernosum of the penis. Patients can be taught self-injection. After 1 or 2 sessions most become comfortable with this approach.

NB: Priapism – A prolonged erection for more than 4 to 6 hours is a potentially dangerous complication of intracavernosal injection therapy. Urgent consultation with a urologist should be sought. Priapism is usually reversible when the corporal bodies are washed with a diluted solution of phenylephrine and ephedrine; however, a beta$_2$-agonist should be tried first. Salbutamol 4 mg PO, followed by a second 4 mg dose 30 minutes later if required, has provided good results in the author's clinical practice. (Terbutaline is frequently used in place of salbutamol in the US.)[1]

Single Drug Therapy

Alprostadil, also called prostaglandin E_1 (PGE_1) is a potent smooth muscle relaxant when injected into the corpus cavernosum. Completely metabolized on its first pass through the pulmonary circulation, PGE_1 is also metabolized locally in the corpus cavernosum. Its effects are dose-related, in both the quality of erection and the latency between the injection and the time an erection is achieved. PGE_1 is considered the drug of choice for intracavernosal injection, either alone or in combination with phentolamine and/or papaverine.

Papaverine relaxes vascular smooth muscle, dilates penile arterioles and increases the resistance to penile outflow.[2] It is hepatotoxic and liver function tests should be repeated regularly.

Combination Therapy

Combination therapy involves the administration of low doses of **alprostadil** and **papaverine** plus **phentolamine**. The pharma-cologic effects of papaverine and alprostadil have been described above. Phentolamine is an alpha$_1$ adrenergic blocking agent that dilates arterioles. It is rarely given alone, but is commonly used in combination because of its synergistic effects. Combination therapy uses low doses of each drug, resulting in a reduction of drug-induced adverse effects, and costs less because it uses a smaller dose of alprostadil. If initial combination therapy fails, a regular dose of alprostadil alone should be tried.

Topical Agents

Topical therapy is not commonly used because of limited efficacy.

Nitroglycerin Ointment

Nitroglycerin relaxes vascular smooth muscles and dilates arterioles. It is applied as a 2% ointment over a 3 cm area of penile skin until erection occurs. Severe headaches have been reported in the partner because of vaginal absorption. This can be prevented by using a condom.

Minoxidil

Minoxidil, a vasodilator used to treat hypertension and alopecia, has been tested on the genital area. Some success has been reported when 1 mL of a 2% solution is applied over the entire penile skin.

---

[1] *J Urol 1989;141:1427–1429.*
[2] *J Urol 1987;138:187.*

Table 1: **Drugs for Erectile Dysfunction**

Drug	Dosage	Adverse Effects	Drug Interactions	Comments	Cost*
Intracavernosal					
alprostadil (PGE₁) Caverject	Begin with 2.5 μg and titrate upwards PRN. For erectile dysfunction of pure neurogenic etiology, begin with 1.25 μg and titrate upwards PRN. Max. dose 60 μg.	Severe penile pain (10%), priapism (rare), penile corporal fibrosis (rare).		Prepared product is stable for 48 h at room temperature and 7 days under refrigeration.	\$\$\$\$\$
papaverine Papaverine HCl	10–30 mg PRN by intracavernosal injection. 5–10 mg doses for neurogenic sexual dysfunction.	Penile corporal fibrosis, priapism (dose-related). Systemic effects: pallor, dizziness, facial flushing, sweating, hepatotoxicity.	Vasodilators: additive effect. Vasoconstrictors: reverse papaverine's effect.	Liver function tests required regularly.	\$\$
phentolamine Rogitine	0.5 mg PRN by intracavernosal injection.	Hypotension, fainting spells.	Sympathomimetics: may reverse the effect of phentolamine.	Rarely used alone.	\$\$
combination therapy (papaverine, PGE₁, phentolamine)	0.36 mL (mixture of papaverine 22.5 mg/mL, PGE₁ 8.33 μg/mL and phentolamine 0.8 mg/mL).	See papaverine, PGE₁, and phentolamine.	See papaverine, PGE₁, and phentolamine.	Extemporaneous preparation.	\$\$

(cont'd)

Table 1: Drugs for Erectile Dysfunction (cont'd)

Drug	Dosage	Adverse Effects	Drug Interactions	Comments	Cost*
Topical					
nitroglycerin 2% ointment Nitrol	Apply PRN over 3 cm area of penile skin.	Headaches in both partners, usually in female (due to vaginal absorption).		Limited efficacy.	$
minoxidil 2% solution Rogaine, generics	Apply 1 mL over entire penis.	Itching or skin rash.		Limited efficacy.	$
Oral					
bromocriptine Parlodel, generics	Start with 1.25–2.5 mg daily, titrate up to a total daily dose of 5–7.5 mg.	Gastrointestinal upset, cardiac arrhythmias, dyskinesias, psychiatric reactions (confusion, hallucinations), hypotension.	Ergot alkaloids, other vasoconstrictors: avoid, may cause hypertension. Phenothiazines: may ↓ bromocriptine efficacy and ↑ hypotensive effects. Antihypertensives: may ↑ hypotensive effect. Alcohol: avoid, may ↑ alcohol intolerance and ↑ severity and incidence of bromocriptine's side effects.	For hyperprolactinemia – associated sexual dysfunction. Start with low dose to decrease gastric intolerance.	5 mg/d $$$$

yohimbine Yocon, generics	4–6 mg TID for 4–6 wks.	Antidepressants, other mood-modifying agents: effect of these agents antagonized by yohimbine.	Hypotension, fainting spells.	Role in organic impotence questionable. May be effective in psychogenic impotence. If improvement after 4–6 wks, continue indefinitely.	$$$-$$$$
Intramuscular *testosterone* Depo-Testosterone Cypionate, Delatestryl, generics	200 mg IM Q3–4 wks	Oral anticoagulants: enhanced response.	Prostate cancer, gynecomastia, Na⁺ and water retention, hyperlipidemia, hepatotoxicity.	For testosterone-deficient sexual dysfunction. Monitor for potential development and enhancement of prostate cancer.	$

Cost of 30-day supply (intracavernosal and topical products, used twice a week) – includes drug cost only.
Legend: $ < $10 $$ $10–20 $$$ $20–30 $$$$ $30–40 $$$$$ > $40

Oral Medications

Bromocriptine

Bromocriptine is a dopaminergic agonist used in the treatment of hyperprolactinemia secondary to pituitary microadenomas. It is often effective in normalizing the prolactin level and improving sexual function. Hyperprolactinemia associated with macroadenomas may require surgery.

Yohimbine

The role of yohimbine in treating erectile dysfunction is controversial. On the basis of current literature, the American Urological Association panel on establishing guidelines for erectile dysfunction does not recommend yohimbine as a treatment option.[3] Yohimbine is a presynaptic alpha$_2$ adrenergic blocker that causes smooth muscle relaxation of arteriolar and sinusoidal musculature of the corpus cavernosum. Its role in organic impotence is questioned. Yohimbine probably has a placebo effect and may be effective in psychogenic impotence. If a dose of 4 to 6 mg TID for 4 to 6 weeks improves the patient, the drug should be continued indefinitely. Yohimbine is generally well tolerated with minimal side effects. However, it may cause hypotension and fainting spells. Yohimbine interacts with antidepressants and other mood modifying drugs and should not be administered to psychiatric patients.

Intramuscular Medications

Testosterone

Testosterone should not be given to patients with normal serum testosterone levels because of feedback inhibition of endogenous testosterone. IM administration of testosterone may improve erectile dysfunction in men with hypogonadism or low serum testosterone levels. Oral testosterone replacement is available but absorption is uncertain.

Future Therapeutic Choices

- **Intraurethral Alprostadil Pellets (MUSE)**
  Alprostadil is instilled into the distal urethra using a special device called a MUSE (medicated urethral system for erection). Alprostadil is delivered to the corporal bodies through the spongiocavernosal communication. In a recently conducted multicentre study in the US, these pellets were found to be effective in 64.9% of patients while placebo was effective in 18.6% of patients.

---

[3] *J Urol 1996;156:2007–2011.*

- **Sildenafil** can be taken daily and 1 to 2 hours before planned sexual intercourse. The drug is a selective inhibitor of type V cyclic guanosine monophosphate-specific phosphodiesterase, thus sparing nitric oxide for longer action.

- **Oral phentolamine** (Vasomax) has been tried and appears to have a positive response in 40 to 50% of patients with erectile dysfunction.

Suggested Reading List

Bennett AH. *Impotence: diagnosis and management of erectile dysfunction.* Philadelphia: W.B. Saunders, 1994.

Krane RJ, ed. Andrology, sexual dysfunction and infertility. *Curr Opin Urol* 1993;3:418–499.

Krane RJ, ed. Impotence. *Urol Clin North Am* 1988;15:90–91.

CHAPTER 70

Diabetes Mellitus

Stewart H. Van Vliet, MD, FRCPC

Goals of Therapy

- To control symptoms
- To attain optimum metabolic control of glucose, lipids and intermediate metabolites
- To prevent acute and long-term complications
- To achieve optimal longevity and quality of life

Classification

Type I: insulin-dependent diabetes mellitus (IDDM) characterized by pancreatic islet destruction and insulin deficiency.

Type II: non–insulin-dependent diabetes mellitus (NIDDM) characterized by insulin resistance.

Maturity-onset diabetes of the young (MODY): formerly a subset of Type II, now separate because of known genetics.

Gestational diabetes: first presenting in pregnancy, usually due to increased insulin resistance late in pregnancy, usually temporary but sometimes continues after pregnancy.

Secondary diabetes: caused by pancreatic trauma or damage, or by increased insulin resistance due to other diseases (e.g., Cushing's disease, acromegaly).

Diagnosis (Figures 1 and 2)

Therapeutic Choices

The Diabetes Control and Complications Trial and other studies show that tight blood glucose control is important to reduce complications and that ideal control is not achieved in the majority of patients. Table 1 provides targets for the average patient. The values presented are those accepted by the World Health Organization (WHO).

Nonpharmacologic Choices (Types I and II)

Nonpharmacologic approaches to the treatment of Type I diabetes are not enough. Insulin must be started immediately. In Type II, nonpharmacologic approaches should be the initial therapy unless the symptoms are severe.

Table 1: **Targets for Control of Diabetes***

Laboratory Values	Optimal	Acceptable	Compromised†
Plasma glucose			
Preprandial	4–7 mmol/L	≤ 10 mmol/L	> 10 mmol/L
2 h postprandial	5–10 mmol/L	≤ 12 mmol/L	> 12 mmol/L
HbA₁c‡ or equivalent (% of normal)	< 110	111–125	> 125

Can Med Assoc J 1992;147:700.

† *Acceptable only in special circumstances.*

‡ *HbA_{1c} = glycosylated subfraction of hemoglobin (i.e., degree of glycemia during the 4–6 wks before lab sample): should be measured at 2–6 mo intervals to assess and validate self-monitored blood glucose data.*

Figure 1: **Diagnosis of Diabetes**

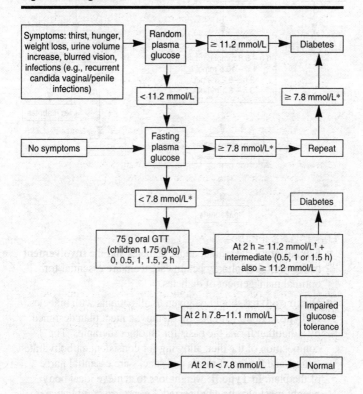

Abbreviations: GTT = glucose tolerance test.
Values are those accepted by the WHO.
*American Diabetes Association proposes a value of 6.9 mmol/L.
†American Diabetes Association accepts a value at 2 h of ≥ 11.2 mmol/L with no intermediate values.

Figure 2: **Screening for Gestational Diabetes**

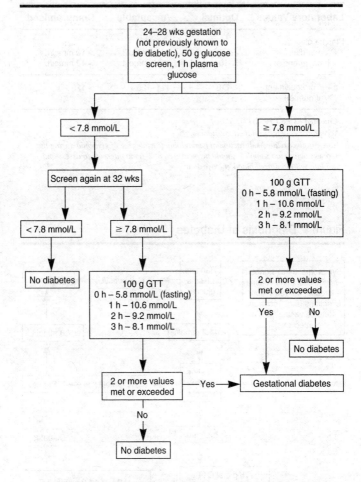

- **Education** of the patient about diabetes and the **involvement** of the multidisciplinary health care team are essential for optimal management of diabetes.

- **Dietary advice** should be given to all patients with diabetes. In **Type I**, along with insulin therapy, a meal plan designed by a dietitian forms the basis for all other therapies. The composition of the diet, allowing for consistent carbohydrate intake, and timing of meals and snacks are essential parts of the plan. In **Type II**, weight loss to achieve ideal body weight must also be emphasized. Long-term compliance is often poor, but continued involvement with the dietitian and reassessment of diet suitability help.

- **Regular exercise** is part of optimal diabetes management: it reduces weight, lowers glucose and lipid levels, decreases insulin resistance, reduces cardiovascular disease, lowers blood pressure and promotes general well-being. It is best immediately following meals when hypoglycemia is less likely. When exercising, **patients using insulin** should carefully plan meals and dosing to avoid hypoglycemia or hyperglycemia. Patients without complications can choose intense exercise, but some types (e.g., running with neuropathy, intense activity with myocardial ischemia, isometric exercise with retinopathy) may worsen complications and should be avoided.

- **Hypoglycemia recognition, treatment** (with oral sugar) and **prevention** (e.g., never miss meals or snacks, anticipate exercise with extra carbohydrate) are essential. (See discussion under Adverse Effects of Insulin.)

- **Self-monitored blood glucose** (SMBG) allows patients to monitor their control with meaningful measurements of glucose. The frequency of SMBG varies, but patients should keep a record of their results and be taught to make appropriate adjustments to their program based on results. SMBG technique should be assessed every 6 months against laboratory plasma glucose values, which are now equal with "lab-like" strips. Glucose urine testing is less useful because it does not differentiate hypoglycemia from mild hyperglycemia and is frequently misleading due to variations in renal threshold for glucose, urine output and bladder emptying.

- **Urine tests for ketones** are not routine. They are useful in initial diagnosis, in times of illness and in gestational diabetes and occasionally to indicate inadequate carbohydrate intake, nighttime hypoglycemia or more severe insulin deficiency.

Pharmacologic Choices for Type I Diabetes

Patients with Type I diabetes who are more than moderately ketotic, dehydrated, vomiting or severely nauseated or who live far from the treatment centre are usually admitted to hospital for acute treatment and education. Others can be treated as outpatients if a dietitian, nurse–educator and physician are available and patients have been taught a diet, insulin-injecting techniques and SMBG techniques.

Insulin

Patients with Type I diabetes should receive human insulin at the time of diagnosis to reduce symptoms and to emphasize the importance of prompt blood glucose reduction. Those in good control who are taking nonhuman insulin need not be switched. Table 2 lists available insulins and some of their characteristics.

Insulin lispro (Humalog) is the newest form of insulin. By producing more rapid and higher serum insulin concentrations with a shorter duration of activity (3.5 to 4.75 hours), insulin lispro decreases glucose excursion during and after meals with less chance for hypoglycemia. Due to its quick onset of action, insulin lispro should be given within 15 minutes of a meal.

Table 2: **Insulin Classification**

Type of Insulin*	Onset (h)	Duration (h)
Short-acting		
Insulin lispro (Humalog)	0.5–0.75	3.5–4.75
Regular (Humulin R, Iletin, Iletin II, Novolin ge)	0.5–1	6–8
Intermediate-acting		
NPH, Lente (Humulin N, Humulin L, Iletin, Iletin II, Novolin ge)	3	up to 24
Long-acting		
Ultralente (Humulin U, Novolin ge)	8	12–24
Combination – Premixed regular/NPH available in various proportions.		
Sources: bovine/porcine, porcine, human.		

Abbreviations: NPH = neutral protamine Hagedorn.
* Cost of insulins (drug cost only) ranges $10–35/vial.

Patients with Type I diabetes who are not ketoacidotic are treated with an initial insulin total daily dose of 0.5 units/kg of ideal body weight (IBW).

Short- and intermediate-acting insulin should be started immediately. Sliding scales of rapid-acting insulin have no ability to predict the eventual insulin requirement and often delay stabilization. Because once-a-day injections even with mixtures rarely suffice, either a twice-daily (split-mix) system (rapid-acting and intermediate-acting insulins, morning and supper) or a basal-bolus system (premeal rapid-acting insulin with a supper or bedtime intermediate-acting insulin) should be started as shown on opposite page.

With either approach, subsequent doses should be adjusted in response to blood glucose values. Adjustments by 10% of the total daily dose should establish control promptly without producing unexpected hypoglycemia.

In the first week, the goal is to achieve modestly elevated blood glucose levels (8 to 10 mmol/L) to avoid hypoglycemia when the patient resumes activity. A long-term blood glucose level of 5 to 8 mmol/L should be the goal in most patients.

System	Protocol
Split-Mix	**2/3** of total daily dose 30 min before breakfast (2/3 intermediate-acting, 1/3 rapid-acting).
	1/3 of total daily dose 30 min before supper (2/3 intermediate-acting, 1/3 rapid-acting).
Basal-Bolus	**30%** of total daily dose 30 min before breakfast (rapid-acting).
	20% of total daily dose 30 min before lunch (rapid-acting).
	25% of total daily dose 30 min before supper (rapid-acting).
	25% of total daily dose either 30 min before supper or at bedtime (intermediate-acting).

Insulin should not be adjusted if blood glucose values are randomly elevated (changes in diet or activity are most likely the cause). If elevated blood glucose is seen at the same time of each day, or if it shows the same temporal pattern of increase from day to day, the dose of the appropriate insulin should be increased to prevent high glucose levels.

Adverse Effects of Insulins

Hypoglycemia occurs more frequently when tight control is pursued. Except in a small number of patients, this does not justify undertreating. Hypoglycemic reactions are:

Mild: sweating, shaking, hunger, weakness and tachycardia. These are recognized and treated easily by the patient.

Severe: start as mild but if not treated, progress to additional neurologic symptoms (e.g., confusion, aggressiveness, disorientation, coma) that prevent the patient from taking appropriate measures.

Dangerous (hypoglycemia unawareness): the patient cannot recognize early signs and take corrective action; the level of control must be reconsidered to avoid recurrence.

Treatment of hypoglycemia includes:

Conscious: requires immediate ingestion of sugar, 10 to 15 g glucose (e.g., 125 to 250 mL unsweetened juice, 3 to 5 Lifesavers or 2 to 3 sugar cubes). Glucose or dextrose show faster absorption than fructose or other disaccharides in patients taking acarbose.

Compromised: one packet of Monogel, corn syrup or honey (15 g, or 1 tablespoon) in the cheek. These are viscous and less likely to be aspirated.

Unconscious: glucagon 1 mg IM or SC (repeated PRN) will increase blood glucose for 20 to 30 minutes, allowing the patient to swallow carbohydrate. Glucagon enhances glycogenolysis and may not be effective in malnourished patients. Glucose 25 g IV is reliable. Once blood glucose returns to normal, determine the cause of hypoglycemia to avoid recurrences.

Allergic reactions (including rashes, local redness and swelling, and systemic reactions) are rare with human-type insulin and infrequent with highly purified insulins. Switching from animal to human-type insulin usually resolves these reactions.

Local lipohypertrophy is currently seen only with overfrequent injections at a single site.

Insulin resistance due to antibody binding is rare with human-type insulin. True resistance to animal-source insulins (> 200 units/day) should prompt a switch to human-type (usually allowing a gradually decreasing dose). Obese patients experience insulin resistance, but it is not immunologic. Highly concentrated insulin (500 units/mL) is available to enable the injection of smaller volumes.

Diabetic Ketoacidosis

Diabetic ketoacidosis occurs with severe insulin deficiency and may be apparent at diagnosis or in patients with established diabetes (Type I *and* Type II) associated with acute infections, myocardial infarction, surgery and omission of insulin. It is characterized by dehydration, acidotic breathing, obtundation to the point of coma, marked ketonuria and ketonemia, metabolic acidosis with electrolyte abnormalities (hyponatremia, normal or elevated serum potassium despite net potassium depletion, and depressed serum bicarbonate), prerenal azotemia and markedly elevated glucose (sometimes only a modest increase in glucose, despite serious ketoacidosis).

Treatment includes hospitalization and immediate administration of **rapid-acting human insulin,** 5 to 10 units per hour by continuous IV infusion or IM hourly.

IV fluids and electrolytes should be administered (commonly 0.45% saline with the addition of potassium 20 to 40 mmol/L). Frequently, 1 to 2 L of 0.9% saline should be given in the first 2 hours, depending on the extent of dehydration, before switching to 0.45% saline. The infusion rate subsequently may be reduced to continue hydration despite polyuria.

Bicarbonate is administered if serum HCO_3^- is < 6 mmol or pH ≤ 7.1. One or two ampuls (i.e., 50 or 100 mmol) usually suffice. Patients with cardiovascular or peripheral vascular disease may not tolerate such severe acidosis and should be treated when acidosis is less severe.

Hourly monitoring of glucose and electrolytes guides the gradual reduction of insulin dosage and modification of fluid and electrolyte administration. When glucose levels fall to < 11 mmol/L (rate of fall usually 5 mmol/h), start 5% glucose IV 100 mL/h to provide calories and prevent hypoglycemia. For pediatric patients, adjust quantities to body weight.

Supportive measures (nasogastric tube, antibiotics, cardiac monitoring PRN) should continue until the patient is fully conscious and cooperative. Once the patient is able to begin oral feeding, a switch is made to SC insulin as per protocol previously described.

Pharmacologic Choices for Type II Diabetes

See Figure 3 for management of Type II diabetes.

Diabetogenic drugs (corticosteroids, estrogens, NSAIDs, thiazide diuretics and loop diuretics in high doses) should be discontinued and alternative therapy instituted. Alcohol should be stopped. The need for beta-blockers should be reassessed because of their potential to mask symptoms of hypoglycemia.

Oral Antidiabetic Agents (Table 3)

Oral agents are used if nonpharmacologic approaches are inadequate. **Acarbose** inhibits alpha-glucosidase, the enzyme responsible for the hydrolysis of sucrose into absorbable mono-saccharides. As a result, it delays glucose absorption, reduces postprandial hyperglycemia and decreases HbA_{1c} in Type II diabetes. Acarbose is approved as an adjunct to prescribed diet for the management of blood glucose levels in NIDDM patients who are not adequately controlled by diet alone. In contrast to the sulfonylureas and metformin, acarbose will not produce hypoglycemia.

Sulfonylureas and **metformin** are also effective in many patients. Sulfonylureas stimulate insulin release. Metformin's mechanism of action is still unclear. A 2-week trial with either a sulfonylurea or metformin is likely sufficient to determine response and adequacy of dose, although additional improvements may continue.

In choosing the best oral agent, either acarbose, a sulfonylurea or metformin can be selected. The specific drug is chosen by matching the patient and drug characteristics in Table 3. Doses can be increased to maximum recommended amounts.

Combination Oral Therapy (Table 4)

If one drug alone proves insufficient, add a second drug from another group until adequate control is achieved. There is no advantage to combining two sulfonylureas. Before adding a second drug, review drug compliance.

Insulin (Table 2)

Insulin is often used as second-line therapy in Type II diabetes when oral agents have failed; however, it is preferred initially in patients < 40 years, women contemplating pregnancy (tight control 1 to 2 months preconception and in early pregnancy prevents malformations), nonobese patients and those with

Table 3: Oral Antidiabetic Agents

Class of Drug	Dose	Duration of Action	Adverse Effects	Drug Interactions	Comments	Cost*
Sulfonylureas						
tolbutamide Orinase, generics	Initially, 500 mg BID–TID, 20–30 min before meals or with meals if GI upset (max. 3 g/d)	8 h	For all sulfonylureas: Hypoglycemia, nausea, epigastric fullness and heartburn, jaundice of both cholestatic and mixed types, allergic skin reactions, agranulocytosis, thrombocytopenia, hemolytic and aplastic anemia, headache.	For all sulfonylureas: *β-blockers* – may delay recovery from hypoglycemia and suppress hypoglycemic symptoms. *Rifampin* – ↑ tolbutamide, glyburide metabolism.	Alcohol-associated flushing.	$
chlorpropamide ⬤ Diabinese, generics	100–500 mg/d single dose with breakfast (max. 500–1 000 mg/d)	36 h		*Salicylates* – hypoglycemia may be potentiated when used concurrently with sulfonylureas. *Sulfonamides* – may inhibit tolbutamide metabolism or displace it from plasma protein binding sites.	Alcohol-associated flushing. Causes prolonged hypoglycemia, which may require several days of glucose support. Causes hyponatremia, fluid retention.	$
glyburide ⬤ Diaβeta, Euglucon, generics	2.5–5 mg/d single dose before or immediately after breakfast (max. 10 mg BID)	8–16 h		*Alcohol* – ↑ tolbutamide metabolism.	Causes prolonged hypoglycemia, which may require several days of glucose support.	$
gliclazide ⬤ Diamicron	80 mg/d, 15–30 min before meals (max. 160 mg BID)	8–16 h		*Monoamine oxidase inhibitors* – ↑ hypoglycemic effect.	Reduces platelet adhesiveness.	$$

Biguanides

metformin 🍴
Glucophage, generics

Initially, 500 mg BID–TID with meals (max. 2 000 mg/d)

8 h

Nausea, diarrhea, metallic taste, anorexia at high doses or initially with starting doses; lactic acidosis when used with significant renal/hepatic dysfunction.

Mechanism of action not clear. Delays and may ↓ glucose absorption.
Should not produce hypoglycemia when used alone.
May provide first-line therapy, particularly in obese patients with modestly ↑ blood glucose levels.

$–$$

α-glucosidase Inhibitors

acarbose
Prandase

Initially, 25 mg TID with meals increased to 50 mg TID. Some patients benefit from an increase to 100 mg TID

↑ GI effects (e.g., flatulence, abdominal distention, diarrhea) especially during first 2 mos, but ↓ with continued therapy; may cause weight loss.

Indicated as an initial treatment alone or as an adjunct to either a sulfonylurea or insulin or metformin.
↓ postprandial ↑ in blood glucose and insulin; ↓ fasting plasma triglyceride levels; ↓ HbA$_{1c}$

May ↓ bioavailability of metformin.

$$

Thiazolidinediones

troglitazone †
Rezulin

Initially, 200 mg once daily, increased PRN in 2–4 weeks to 400 mg once daily (max. dose 600 mg/d)

Generally well tolerated.
Reversible ↑ of AST or ALT > 3 times upper limit of normal (2.2% troglitazone-treated vs. 0.6% placebo-treated patients). Recommend liver function tests; monthly for first 6 mos, bimonthly for remainder of first yr, then periodically. Not recommended in acute liver disease.

May ↑ risk for hypoglycemia in combination with sulfonylureas or insulin. A reduction in the dose of sulfonylurea or insulin may be necessary.

Improves insulin resistance.
Simplifies attempts to improve glucose control by eliminating the need for massive insulin dosage with the concomitant weight gain that usually occurs.

†

Legend	$	$$	$$$	$$$$	> $50
	< $10	$10–25	$25–50		

† Will be marketed in 1998.

🍴 Dosage adjustment may be required in renal impairment – see Appendix I.
* Cost of 30-day supply – includes drug cost only.

Figure 3: **Treatment of Non–insulin-dependent Diabetes Mellitus (NIDDM)**

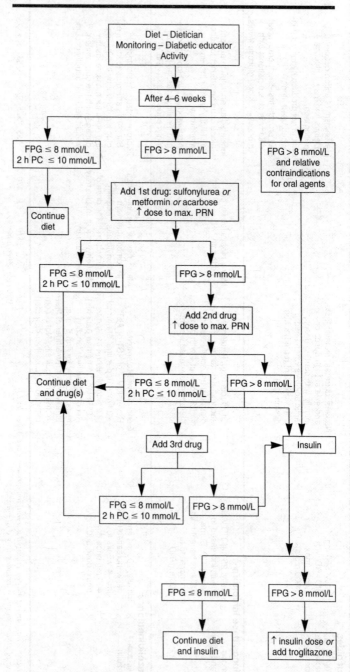

Abbreviations: FPG = fasting plasma glucose.

Table 4: **Combination Therapy**

Combination	Effect
Sulfonylurea + sulfonylurea	Not beneficial (i.e., not additive at maximum doses).
Sulfonylurea + metformin	↓↓ plasma glucose; ↓ sulfonylurea-induced weight gain; may ↓ peripheral insulin resistance; ↓ caloric intake.
Insulin + sulfonylurea	Rarely indicated. Occasionally, bedtime intermediate-acting insulin added to a daytime sulfonylurea regimen produces excellent fasting blood glucose levels (difficult to attain in NIDDM); usually a stopgap measure before switching the patient totally to insulin.
Insulin + metformin	May ↓ glucose absorption; improve postprandial glucose control; prevent weight gain.
Acarbose + any of the other drugs	Acarbose can be used in combination with all other groups of drugs – metformin may be less well absorbed/effective with concomitant α-glucosidase inhibition and may have more gastrointestinal side effects in this combination.
Troglitazone	Troglitazone improves tissue sensitivity to insulin. In Type II patients not responding to insulin, it can lower blood glucose and reduce the dose of insulin required. In some patients, it may be possible to discontinue insulin.

MODY, nonketotic severely hyperglycemic patients, alcoholic patients and patients with pre-existing complications.

The decision to switch to insulin therapy should not be delayed if other measures fail to control blood glucose.

Insulin daily dose is 0.3 to 0.5 units/kg actual body weight. Using actual body weight instead of IBW compensates for the increased insulin resistance in obese patients. The same twice-daily (split-mix) approach described for Type I therapy can be used in NIDDM. Frequently, a single daily dose (mix) can be used initially, although a dose of 70 to 80 units/day or higher should be split. In obese patients, insulin doses may be very high (> 100 units/day) due to resistance.

The introduction of **troglitazone** (Rezulin) offers an additional mode of treatment for Type II diabetic patients not adequately managed on insulin. Troglitazone improves sensitivity to insulin in muscle and adipose tissue and inhibits hepatic gluconeo-genesis. Troglitazone is indicated for the treatment of patients with Type II diabetes inadequately controlled with insulin therapy. As glycemic control is improved, it may be possible to reduce the dose of insulin or even completely eliminate insulin in some patients. **However, a reduction in insulin dosage should not come at the expense of optimal diabetes control.**

Therapeutic Tips

- A **review** should be made every 3 to 6 months of blood glucose records, frequency and treatment of hypoglycemic reactions, weight changes and diet, blood pressure and complications (retinopathy, urine protein, peripheral or autonomic neuropathy, peripheral pulses, feet and skin).

- When blood glucose control is inadequate, diet and compliance should be reviewed before adding an oral hypoglycemic or insulin.

- When initiating insulin or sulfonylurea treatment, a night snack is essential. A morning snack is not always needed. An afternoon snack should be considered.

- Insulin and sulfonylureas are usually best taken 20 to 30 minutes before a meal to lower postprandial glucose peaks and decrease the risk of hypoglycemia before the next meal. Acarbose and metformin should be taken with meals.

Pharmacoeconomic Considerations

Jeffrey A. Johnson, PhD

The lifetime costs and benefits of intensive insulin therapy as defined in the Diabetes Control and Complications Trial (DCCT) have been examined in only one study. For approximately 120 000 persons in the US who would meet DCCT eligibility criteria implementing intensive, rather than conventional, therapy would result in 611 000 years of life gained at an additional cost of $4.0 billion over the lifetime of the population. The incremental cost per year of life gained would be $28 661, i.e., intensive therapy would cost $28 661 more than conventional therapy to gain one additional year of life. Such cost-effectiveness is considered to be a good value when compared to other health care interventions. This value, however, may not be applicable to the entire population of diabetic patients because of the strict inclusion criteria used in the DCCT.

Another area of pharmacoeconomic consideration for diabetes therapy is the use of ACE inhibitors. An economic analysis of captopril in diabetic nephropathy indicated that in postponing the development and costs associated with end stage renal disease, captopril could result in savings of approximately

$2.4 billion in the US over a 10-year period. This includes savings in both direct medical and indirect societal costs (Appendix II).

Suggested Reading

The DCCT Research Group. Lifetime benefits and costs of intensive therapy as practiced in the Diabetes Control and Complications Trial. JAMA 1996;276: 1409–1415.

Rodby RA, Firth L, Lewis EJ. An economic analysis of captopril in the treatment of diabetic nephropathy. Diabetes Care 1996;19:1051–1061.

Suggested Reading List

American Diabetes Association. Position statement: continuous subcutaneous insulin infusion. *Diabetes Care* 1997;20 (Suppl 1):S50.

DCCT Research Group. Epidemiology of severe hypoglycemia in Diabetes Complications and Control Trial. *Am J Med* 1991;90:450–459.

Rifkin H, Porte D Jr, eds. *Ellenberg and Rifkin's Diabetes Mellitus: Theory and Practice.* 4th ed. New York: Elsevier, 1990.

UK Prospective Diabetes Study Group. UK prospective diabetes study 13: relative efficacy of randomly allocated diet, sulfonylurea, insulin, or metformin in patients newly diagnosed non-insulin dependent diabetes followed for three years. *BMJ* 1995;310:83–88.

UK Prospective Diabetes Study Group. UK prospective study 16: overview of 6 years' therapy of type II diabetes: a progressive disease. *Diabetes* 1995;44:1249–1258.

CHAPTER 71

Thyroid Disorders

C. Joyce, MD, FRCPC

Goals of Therapy

- To return the patient with hyperthyroidism or hypothyroidism to the euthyroid state
- To control symptoms of hyperthyroidism, hypothyroidism, and thyroiditis and provide the patient with an improved quality of life
- To evaluate the cause of thyroid enlargement (goitre) and determine if surgical or pharmacologic therapy is needed

Hyperthyroidism (Table 1)

Most common causes of hyperthyroidism are:

- Graves' disease (diffuse toxic goitre)
- Toxic adenoma
- Toxic multinodular goitre
- Transient thyroiditis – subacute (painful)
  – silent (painless)
  – postpartum
- Factitious (excessive ingestion of thyroid hormone tablets)

Graves' Disease

Graves' disease is mediated by the abnormal elaboration of an antibody (thyroid-stimulating antibody [TSAb] or thyroid-binding immunoglobulin [TBII]) that binds to thyroid-stimulating hormone (TSH) receptors on the thyroid follicular cells and causes unregulated thyroid gland stimulation. The consequence of this antibody–receptor interaction is a diffuse goitre with increased vascularity (resulting in a thyroid bruit).

Investigations

- A thorough history with attention to symptoms (heat intolerance, weight loss, tremor, diaphoresis, tachycardia, diarrhea and proximal muscle weakness)
- Physical examination (presence of goitre and exophthalmos in Graves' disease)
- Thyroid scan (demonstrates diffuse thyroid enlargement with increased trapping of the isotope)

Table 1: **Causes and Treatment of Hyperthyroidism**

Cause	Treatment
Graves' disease	Propylthiouracil or methimazole, beta-blocker, ^{131}I, surgery rarely.
Toxic adenoma	Propylthiouracil or methimazole, beta-blocker, ^{131}I, or surgery.
Toxic multinodular goitre	Propylthiouracil or methimazole, beta-blocker, followed by ^{131}I. Surgery only if gland is very large with obstructive features.
Transient thyroiditis	Beta-blocker to treat hyperthyroid phase, ASA or NSAID to treat subacute, painful form. Prednisone to control inflammatory symptoms in severe cases.
Factitious hyperthyroidism	Stop thyroxine. Temporary use of beta-blocker if symptoms are severe.

- 24-hour ^{131}I uptake (elevated, as measured in percent)
- Laboratory abnormalities
  - elevated serum total and free thyroxine (T_4)
  - elevated serum triiodothyronine (T_3)
  - low serum TSH due to negative feedback
  - positive thyroid autoantibodies

The combination of high free T_4, low TSH, diffuse thyroid enlargement and elevated 24-hour ^{131}I uptake in the gland is diagnostic of Graves' disease.

Therapeutic Choices

Nonpharmacologic Choices

Oral radioactive iodine (^{131}I) is the preferred definitive treatment for Graves' disease. It is cost-effective, safe and easy to administer. Subtotal thyroidectomy is generally reserved for young children, those intolerant of iodine and those with a coexisting nodule that is suspicious for malignancy. The main adverse effect of both ^{131}I and subtotal thyroidectomy is hypothyroidism, requiring oral thyroxine therapy.

Pharmacologic Choices
Propylthiouracil (PTU) and Methimazole (MMI)

Both drugs produce a smooth inhibition of T_4 and T_3 synthesis. PTU also reduces conversion of T_4 to T_3. They do not affect release of previously synthesized thyroid hormone; therefore, their pharmacologic effects take days to weeks to appear.

PTU and MMI do not "cure" patients. Hyperthyroidism recurs in the majority of patients after medication is stopped. A minority (20%) of patients may undergo spontaneous remission, but this is likely attributable to the natural history of the disease. Response to therapy is monitored clinically and by following free T_4 levels every 1 to 4 weeks (depending on initial severity). The dose can often be titrated down over time.

PTU and MMI are generally used in the following situations:
- for 1 to 2 years, to control hyperthyroidism, in patients reluctant to have definitive ^{131}I therapy. Treatment is then stopped to see if spontaneous remission has occurred. If remission has not occurred, ^{131}I is needed.
- for several weeks to months, to render the patient euthyroid, in preparation for definitive treatment (^{131}I or surgery). This approach is important if the patient is elderly and/or has underlying heart disease. (Stop PTU or MMI 5 to 7 days before ^{131}I therapy.)
- in children
- in pregnant women (see Hyperthyroidism in Special Circumstances)

The frequency of adverse effects is similar for both drugs. Although they occur infrequently, adverse effects are important and patients should be counseled prior to beginning treatment. The most frequent adverse effects are:
- GI upset (incidence not well documented). Usually mild, if not tolerable try switching to the other drug.
- rash (5% of patients) – maculopapular – can range from mild to severe and desquamative. In mild cases, discontinuing the drug alone is sufficient, followed by trying the alternate agent. In more severe cases, a short course of oral steroids may be needed, but prescribing the alternate medication is not recommended.
- elevated liver function tests – transient and usually asymptomatic. Not common (exact incidence unknown).
- neutropenia – rare (< 1% of users), but the most serious side effect. Usually reversible with discontinuation of the drug, but may present with serious bacterial sepsis. If neutropenia occurs with 1 of the drugs, *neither* of the 2 agents should be reintroduced.

Iodide (inorganic, cold)

Administration of inorganic iodide orally (Lugol's solution) or IV (iodinated contrast dye) reduces the release of already formed thyroid hormone. Iodide produces a transient, useful effect in the acute situation and is used for life-threatening hyperthyroidism (thyroid storm or thyrotoxic crisis). Either PTU or MMI must be administered first to prevent incorporation of the administered iodide into thyroid hormone, and worsening hyperthyroidism.

Beta-blockers

Beta-blockers inhibit the peripheral catecholamine-mediated manifestations of thyroid hormone action. They reduce tremor and tachycardia, the main catecholamine-mediated symptoms. Prior to starting a beta-blocker, patients should be evaluated for potential contraindications, such as asthma, peripheral vascular disease, or insulin-dependent diabetes.

Agents to Reduce Peripheral Conversion of T_4 to T_3

Glucocorticoids (used only in thyroid storm), **PTU** and **propranolol** reduce the peripheral conversion of T_4 to T_3. This may provide PTU and propranolol with a theoretical advantage over MMI and other beta-blockers, respectively.

Toxic Adenoma

Toxic adenoma is a solitary hyperfunctioning benign thyroid nodule.

Investigations

- Lab testing shows a high free T_4, low TSH and negative autoantibodies
- Scan shows a "hot" nodule, with suppression of the remainder of the gland
- 24-hour ^{131}I uptake is normal to slightly increased

Therapeutic Choices

Nonpharmacologic Choices

Definitive treatment consists of ^{131}I ablation of the nodule (in doses higher than needed for Graves' disease) in patients older than 40, or surgical removal in patients younger than 40.

Pharmacologic Choices

Treatment includes either PTU or MMI, and a beta-blocker. Spontaneous remissions are rare.

Toxic Multinodular Goitre

Usually a disease of older patients.

Investigations

- Lab testing shows high free T_4, low TSH
- Scan shows multiple hot and cold areas in a large, "lumpy" gland
- 24-hour ^{131}I uptake is often normal

Therapeutic Choices

Treat with PTU or MMI, and a beta-blocker followed by
^{131}I therapy. Surgery is only needed if the gland is very large
with obstructive features.

Transient Thyroiditis

Hyperthyroidism is caused by the release of preformed thyroid
hormone, *not* increased synthesis. The gland is "damaged", either
by a presumed viral infection in the subacute painful form, or a
presumed autoimmune process in the painless and postpartum
forms. The hyperthyroid phase is often followed by a transient
hypothyroid phase, then recovery of normal function, all over the
course of a few months.

Investigations

- The hallmark diagnostic test is a *low* 24-hour ^{131}I uptake in
  the face of a *high* free T_4 and suppressed TSH, in a patient
  with thyroid enlargement. The low ^{131}I uptake is due to the
  inability of the "sick" thyroid follicular cells to concentrate
  iodine
- In the hypothyroid phase, the 24-hour ^{131}I is often
  normal or high, as recovery of the gland is gradually
  occurring

Therapeutic Choices

Beta-blockers are used in the hyperthyroid phase. ASA or nonsteroidal anti-inflammatories (NSAIDs) are also used to treat the
subacute, painful form of transient thyroiditis. Prednisone may
be required to control the inflammatory symptoms in severe
cases.

Factitious Hyperthyroidism
Investigations

Diagnosed by the presence of hyperthyroidism in a patient who
has a small atrophic gland (compare with thyroiditis, where goitre
is usually present) and a low 24-hour ^{131}I uptake (caused by
negative feedback from excessive exogenous thyroid hormone
suppressing TSH).

Therapeutic Choices

Treatment consists of cessation of thyroxine ingestion. If symptoms are severe, the temporary use of a beta-blocker may be
required.

Hyperthyroidism in Special Circumstances

Pregnancy

Hyperthyroidism *during* pregnancy is most often due to Graves' disease. Toxic adenoma is the next most common cause. Hyperthyroidism *after* pregnancy is often due to postpartum thyroiditis or Graves' disease.

PTU, given at the lowest possible dose to keep T_4 at the upper end of normal, is the treatment of choice for hyperthyroidism in pregnancy. PTU crosses the placenta, and high doses can cause fetal goitre and hypothyroidism. **MMI should not be used in pregnancy because it has been associated with a scalp defect in the fetus (aplasia cutis).** Beta-blockers should be used only when necessary (based on clinical judgment). The lowest possible dose should be used, as high doses have been associated with intrauterine growth retardation. **Scanning or administration of isotopes (or cold iodide) is contraindicated in pregnancy, since iodine crosses the placenta.**

Thyrotoxic Crisis (Thyroid Storm)

Thyroid storm is severe hyperthyroidism associated with hyperthermia and cardiac instability. Treatment consists of:

- **PTU** 200 mg PO QID or **MMI** 20 mg PO QID.
- **propranolol** 20 mg PO BID – titrate dose cautiously based on cardiac status.
- **inorganic cold iodide** (i.e., 1 dose of IV contrast dye or oral Lugol's solution 2 drops QID for 2 to 3 days) given *after* PTU or MMI has been started.
- **dexamethasone** 2 mg Q6H or hydrocortisone 100 mg Q6H, for 2 to 3 days or until stable.

After administration of exogenous cold iodide, subsequent isotope studies or ^{131}I therapy must be postponed 2 to 3 months.

Hypothyroidism

Common causes of hypothyroidism are:

- Chronic autoimmune thyroiditis (Hashimoto's thyroiditis) – the most common cause of both an euthyroid goitre and hypothyroidism. This condition is associated with lymphocytic infiltration of the gland
- Post-^{131}I therapy
- Post-thyroidectomy
- Hypothyroid phase of subacute, painless, or postpartum thyroiditis
- Inherited enzyme defect
- Congenital (i.e., thyroid agenesis or dysgenesis)

Table 2: Drugs Used in Thyroid Disorders

Drug	Dosage	Adverse Drug Reactions	Drug Interactions	Comments	Cost*
radioactive iodine (^{131}I)	Hyperthyroidism: 5–10 mCi in Graves' disease, 15–29 mCi in toxic adenoma and toxic multinodular goitre	Hypothyroidism. Usually none; new patients may suffer some thyroiditis, occasionally with mild pain. Nausea may occur.		A single dose usually cures patients with Graves' disease.	$$$$ per dose
propylthiouracil ‡ Propyl-Thyracil	Hyperthyroidism: 50–100 mg PO BID–QID Thyrotoxic crisis: 200 mg PO QID	GI upset, rash, elevated liver function tests (not common), neutropenia (rare, but most serious of side effects; usually reversible with discontinuation of the drug, but may present with serious bacterial sepsis).	Oral anticoagulants – altered hypothrombinemic response; monitor prothrombin time.	Patients started on either drug should be counseled regarding side effects.	$
methimazole ‡ Tapazole	Hyperthyroidism: 5–10 mg PO BID–QID Thyrotoxic crisis: 20 mg PO QID			Methimazole should not be used in pregnancy or lactation.	$
iodine Lugol's solution (Strong Iodine Solution)	Before thyroidectomy: 2–6 drops Lugol's sol'n TID for 10 days before surgery Thyrotoxic crisis: 2 drops of Lugol's sol'n QID for 2–3 days or 1 dose IV contrast dye, given after PTU or MMI has been started	Hypersensitivity reactions: skin rashes, mucous membrane ulcers, anaphylaxis, metallic taste, rhinorrhea, parotid and submaxillary swelling.		Must not be used before PTU or MMI for thyrotoxic crisis. If used, ^{131}I therapy cannot be used for at least 3 mos.	$†

Drug	Dosage	Adverse Effects	Drug Interactions	Comments	Cost*
propranolol Inderal, Inderal-LA, generics	Hyperthyroidism: 20–40 mg PO BID Painless (silent) thyroiditis: 10–20 mg PO BID Thyrotoxic crisis: 20–40 mg PO BID. Titrate dose cautiously based on cardiac status	Bradycardia, hypotension, dyspnea, fatigue, depression.	With digoxin, Ca++ channel blockers, amiodarone, additive bradycardia. ↑ hypoglycemic effect when added to hypoglycemic agents.	Contraindicated in patients with asthma or congestive heart failure.	$ LA: $$
dexamethasone Decadron, generics *hydrocortisone* A-Hydrocort, Solu-Cortef, generics	Thyrotoxic crisis: 2 mg dexamethasone Q6H or 100 mg hydrocortisone Q6H (for 2–3 days or until stable) Myxedema coma: hydrocortisone 100 mg IV Q8–12H until patient is stable	Glucose intolerance, weight gain, mood alteration, hypertension, osteoporosis, adrenal suppression, cataracts, myopathy.	With barbiturates, phenytoin, and rifampin (may ↓ steroid effect).		$π $$$$π
levothyroxine (L-T4) Eltroxin, Synthroid, generics	Hypothyroidism: Initially, 50–100 µg PO once daily, titrated with serum TSH Q6–12 wks until TSH normalizes. Older patients – initially 12.5–25 µg daily, titrated upwards more slowly Myxedema coma: Initially, 500 µg IV, followed by 50–100 µg daily, given IV or PO	Due to overdosage and induced hyperthyroidism (e.g., heat intolerance, weakness, fatigue, nervousness, insomnia, tachycardia).	Cholestyramine, colestipol, ferrous sulfate and sucralfate decrease thyroxine absorption. Anticonvulsants and rifampin accelerate thyroxine metabolism. Effects of oral anticoagulants are ↑ by T4; monitor for excessive hypoprothrombinemia. Dose of antidiabetic agent may need to be ↑; monitor blood glucose.	Sensitive TSH assays allow dosing to be individualized. When stable, TSH levels should only be performed at intervals of 6–12 mos.	$

† Extemporaneously compounded.
‡ Initial doses are arbitrary. Patients with larger goitres and more active disease may require larger initial doses.
π Cost of 3 days of therapy.
*Cost of 30-day supply – includes drug cost only.
Legend: $ <$10 $$ $10–20 $$$ $20–30 $$$$ $30–60 $$$$$ >$60

- Secondary to hypopituitarism
- External radiation

Most causes of hypothyroidism are primary in nature (i.e., due to disease in the thyroid itself). Therefore, as free T_4 falls, serum TSH rises (loss of negative feedback). By contrast, secondary hypothyroidism is due to pituitary or hypothalamic damage (hypopituitarism), where both thyroid hormone and TSH are low.

Investigations

- A thorough history with attention to symptoms (weakness, tiredness, lethargy, fatigue, cold intolerance)
- Physical examination. Clinical manifestations include cold intolerance, weight gain, dry skin, constipation, delayed relaxation of the deep tendon reflexes and bradycardia. When manifestations are severe, particularly in skin and soft tissues, the condition is called *myxedema* and the effects seen are due to the accumulation of hydrophilic substances, such as hyaluronic acid in subcutaneous tissues
- Laboratory tests (primary hypothyroidism):
  – elevated TSH, normal free T_4 and T_3 (very mild, e.g., compensated hypothyroidism)
  – elevated TSH, reduced free T_4 and T_3 (overt hypothyroidism)

Therapeutic Choices

Pharmacologic Choices

Oral **levothyroxine** (T_4) is used to treat hypothyroidism. Different brands of levothyroxine are not interchangeable as bioavailability differs between preparations. Since T_4 is converted to T_3 in peripheral tissues, the administration of T_3 is not needed.

There is individual variability in dosing, but in otherwise healthy adults the usual starting dose is 50 to 100 µg once daily, titrated with serum TSH every 6 to 12 weeks until the TSH normalizes (if caused by hypopituitarism free T_4, not TSH, is followed). Since thyroxine has a half-life of 8 days, it is important to wait at least 6 to 8 weeks after a dosage adjustment to retest TSH.

Older individuals, or those with heart disease, should start at a lower dosage (i.e., 12.5 to 25 µg daily) and be titrated upwards more slowly. Thyroxine increases myocardial oxygen consumption which may potentially worsen cardiac ischemia.

Lifelong treatment is required for most causes of hypothyroidism, with yearly thyroid function tests and dosage adjustments as needed. The exception is the hypothyroid phase of transient thyroiditis (subacute or painless), when therapy can be stopped after approximately 12 months, and thyroid function tests repeated 6 to 8 weeks later to determine if recovery has occurred.

Hypothyroidism in Special Circumstances

Papillary or Follicular Thyroid Cancer

Most patients with papillary or follicular cancer have had near-total thyroidectomy plus ^{131}I ablation of any residual thyroid tissue, followed by lifelong thyroid replacement. Because TSH may be a growth factor for thyroid tumors, higher doses of levothyroxine are given to suppress TSH below the lower limit of normal. Thyroxine is stopped periodically (every 1 to 5 years) for 4 to 6 weeks to prepare the patient for ^{131}I total body scan to check for residual or metastatic disease. Discontinuing thyroxine enables TSH to rise, thereby ensuring any remaining thyroid tissue will avidly take up ^{131}I. **Oral T$_3$** (Cytomel), in an average dose of 25 μg TID, can be given for the first 2 weeks after levothyroxine is stopped, to help ameliorate symptoms of hypothyroidism. Because the half-life of T$_3$ is short (about 1 day), it can then be discontinued 2 to 3 weeks prior to the ^{131}I scan. This is the only "routine" use for T$_3$.

Myxedema Coma

A rare endocrine emergency, with profound hypothyroidism manifested by hypothermia, bradycardia, hypotension, hypoventilation and coma. Even when treated, the mortality rate is high. Death typically occurs in an older patient, with undiagnosed or undertreated primary hypothyroidism, in which another illness (e.g., sepsis, myocardial infarction, pneumonia) worsens the clinical status. Myxedema coma is a clinical diagnosis, since a decision to treat with thyroxine must be made quickly prior to the availability of thyroid function test results.

Myxedema coma is treated with a single 500 μg IV dose of **levothyroxine** followed by 50 to 100 μg of levothyroxine daily, given IV or orally. In case there is coexisting primary adrenal insufficiency, **hydrocortisone** (100 mg IV Q8–12H) must also be given until the patient is stable.

Thyroid Enlargement (Goitre)

Thyroid enlargement may be classified as diffuse or nodular.

Diffuse Goitre

The most common causes of diffuse goitre are: any form of thyroiditis, Graves' disease, congenital enzyme defects or iodine deficiency.

Hashimoto's thyroiditis is the most common cause in areas where iodine deficiency does not occur (i.e., Canada – where all table salt is iodized). Patients with thyroiditis can be euthyroid, hypothyroid, or hyperthyroid, depending on the nature and phase of their condition (see previous section). Therapy, therefore, depends on these factors.

Therapy of congenital enzyme defects involves levothyroxine (T_4) replacement. Therapy of iodine-deficiency goitres consists of iodine repletion.

Nodular Thyroid Enlargement

Nodular thyroid enlargement can consist of either a solitary nodule or be multinodular. Therapy of toxic nodules has previously been discussed.

The pathogenesis of thyroid nodules is poorly understood. Nodules are more common in women, in the older age group, following radiation exposure to the head and neck, and in areas of iodine deficiency.

Approximately 1 in 20 nontoxic (cold) thyroid nodules is malignant.

Investigations

- Review of risk factors for malignancy (i.e., male gender, presentation in childhood, and previous ionizing radiation)
- Evaluation of clinical features of concern for malignancy (i.e., rapid growth of the nodule, regional lymphadenopathy, and evidence of extrathyroidal invasion [i.e., hoarse voice])
- Fine needle aspiration, as well as thyroid isotope scanning, may be helpful in deciding which nodules require surgical excision. Fine needle biopsy cytologic results are classified as:
  – benign (follow unless other significant clinical risk factors for malignancy are present)
  – malignant (require surgical removal)
  – suspicious (require surgical removal) or
  – as nondiagnostic (warrant repeat biopsy) – 2 or more non-diagnostic results generally necessitate surgical excision
- Isotope scanning may be helpful. Hot nodules are much less likely to be malignant
- Ultrasound cannot distinguish benign from malignant nodules, but may be valuable in follow-up to determine if a nodule has increased in size (necessitating surgical removal)

Therapeutic Choices

For many years, therapy with levothyroxine (T_4) to suppress TSH was used in an attempt to shrink nodules. The belief was that nodules that shrink were less likely to be malignant. This practice is now controversial, since the success rate in shrinking nodules is variable, the required dosages of T_4 are high (not safe in elderly patients), and the differentiation of benign from malignant lesions is unreliable. As a result, when action is required, surgical excision appears to be the treatment of choice.

Suggested Reading List

Braverman LE, Utiger RD, eds. *Werner and Ingbar's the thyroid: a fundamental and clinical text.* 6th ed. Philadelphia: JB Lippincott, 1991.

Franklyn J. The management of hyperthyroidism. *N Engl J Med* 1994;330:1731–1738.

Larson PR, Ingbar SH. The thyroid gland. In: Wilson JD, Foster DW, eds. *Williams textbook of endocrinology.* 8th ed. Philadelphia: WB Saunders, 1992:357–487.

Mazzaferri EL. Management of a solitary thyroid nodule. *N Engl J Med* 1993;328:553-559.

CHAPTER 72

Common Anemias

N. Blair Whittemore, MD, FRCPC

The treatments of **iron deficiency anemia** and **megaloblastic anemia** are discussed in this chapter.

Definition

- In general, patients with hemoglobin (Hgb) values 2 standard deviations below the mean should be considered anemic and require investigation.
- Normal mean Hgb for men is 155 ± 20 g/L; for women, 140 ± 20 g/L

NB: Occasionally patients may be "normal" with Hgb values below 2 standard deviations of the mean, but one must exclude occult disease. Previous hemogram values are valuable in determining the significance of the current result.

Goals of Therapy

- To determine the etiology of the anemia and replace any identified deficiencies

Investigations

- History and physical examination including:
  - medication intake: antineoplastic and zidovudine therapy will usually cause macrocytosis; several drugs are associated with altered folate metabolism and macrocytosis including anticonvulsants (phenytoin, primidone), triamterene, trimethoprim and oral contraceptives
  - alcohol intake
  - dietary history (strict vegetarians are at risk of vitamin B_{12} deficiency)
  - gastric or small bowel surgery (terminal ileal resection) may predispose to B_{12} deficiency
  - chronic blood loss and other potential causes of iron deficiency (Table 3)
  - chronic inflammatory or malignant disease
  - diminished hepatic, renal or thyroid function
- Laboratory tests:
  - RBC indices, Hgb, hematocrit, white blood cell (WBC) count with differential, peripheral blood smear

- serum iron, total iron-binding capacity (TIBC), serum ferritin
- stool for occult blood
- other tests may include liver function tests, **red cell** folate rather than serum folate (the former is a better reflection of folate stores), serum B_{12}; with low serum B_{12} levels, a Schilling test with and without intrinsic factor, plus serum antibody to intrinsic factor should be done to clarify etiology
- urine for RBC, hemoglobinuria

Morphologic Classification of Anemia

- **microcytic:** low mean corpuscular volume (MCV) (Table 1)
- **normocytic:** normal MCV
- **macrocytic:** high MCV (Table 2). A falsely elevated MCV may be caused by cold agglutinins or marked leukocytosis, readily seen on a peripheral blood smear

Table 1: **Laboratory Evaluation of Microcytosis**

Cause	Serum Fe	TIBC	% saturation	Ferritin	Bone marrow Fe stores	Hgb A₂ and Hgb F
Iron deficiency (Table 2)	↓	↑	↓	↓	0	N
Anemia of chronic disease	↓	N or ↓	N or ↓	N or ↑	N or ↑	N
Thalassemia trait	N	N	N	N or ↑	N	↑ β thal, N α thal
Sideroblastic anemia	N or ↑	N or ↑	N or ↑	N or ↑	↑	N

Abbreviations: ↑ = increased; ↓ = decreased; N = normal; 0 = none; TIBC = total iron-binding capacity; Hgb A₂ = A₂ hemoglobin; Hgb F = fetal hemoglobin; β thal = β thalassemia; α thal = α thalassemia

Table 2: **Appearance on Peripheral Smear of Some Causes of Macrocytosis**

Appearance on Smear	Causes
Round macrocytes with target cells	Alcoholism or liver disease
Oval macrocytes with hypersegmented neutrophils	B₁₂ or folate deficiency (megaloblastic anemia)
Dimorphic red cell picture with or without hyposegmented neutrophils	Myelodysplasia

Iron Deficiency Anemia

Table 3: Potential Causes of Iron Deficiency Anemia

Inadequate ingestion (dietary deficiency/increased requirements)
  Growth spurts in infants, young children, adolescents
  Pregnancy
  Elderly "tea and toaster" (investigate other causes first)
Impaired absorption
  Partial gastrectomy
  Malabsorption syndromes
Blood loss (most important cause)
  Genitourinary
    Menstruation (most likely in women 15–45 yrs)
  Gastrointestinal (most likely in men and postmenopausal women)
    Peptic ulcer
    Hiatus hernia
    Cancer
    Telangiectasia
    Jogger's anemia
  Phlebotomy
    Polycythemia
    Blood donor
    Diagnostic phlebotomy
Trauma/surgery

Therapeutic Choices

Pharmacologic Choices (Table 4)
Iron Supplements

Various oral iron salts are available; they differ in their elemental iron content (see below).

Salt	mg/tablet	Elemental Fe/tablet
Ferrous sulfate	300 mg	60
Ferrous gluconate	300 mg	35
Ferrous fumarate	200 mg	66
Ferrous ascorbate	275 mg	33

With the diagnosis of iron deficiency anemia established, **oral iron replacement therapy** may be started immediately while the underlying cause is sought. Approximately 30 mg of elemental iron is absorbed from a dose of 180 mg of elemental iron per day. The Hgb should rise 10 g/L every 7 to 10 days if there are no complicating features (e.g., continued blood loss or impaired marrow production).

Upon restoration of the Hgb, iron stores begin to be replenished. This may take a further 6 to 9 months and can be monitored by measuring serum ferritin. Replenishing iron stores may be very difficult or only transient if menstruation causes the deficiency. In such cases it may be necessary to continue iron therapy (30 to 60 mg elemental iron per day) until menopause.

If there is a benign cause of recurrent bleeding for which surgery is not indicated, oral iron therapy may be continued indefinitely.

Parenteral iron therapy is required infrequently. Indications for its use are malabsorption/intolerance to oral iron preparations and iron losses exceeding maximal oral replacement. **NB:** Response to oral and parenteral iron occurs at same rate in normal circumstances.

Therapeutic Tips

- The cause of anemia should be established; iron deficiency is only a sign.
- Failure to respond to therapy may reflect:
  – continued bleeding, but there should be a good reticulocyte response indicating active red cell production
  – inadequate dose or duration of therapy
  – poor compliance
  – associated disease (e.g., inflammatory states, neoplastic disease) or concomitant deficiency (vitamin B_{12}, folic acid, thyroid)
  – incorrect diagnosis, for which a bone marrow aspirate is probably required
- Oral iron therapy is preferred.
- If GI side effects occur with oral iron, stopping therapy for 3 to 4 days and resuming at a lower dose may be helpful as this effect appears to be related to the amount of elemental iron. Switching to a liquid preparation to regulate dosage more precisely may also help.
- Nonenteric-coated iron salt should be used. Enteric-coated and time-released iron preparations are intended to reduce side effects but may be ineffective because of failure to release iron in the gastric environment.
- There is little evidence to support the therapeutic advantage of preparations of iron combined with substances to enhance iron absorption (e.g., ascorbic acid) and they are considerably more expensive.
- Treatment should continue long enough to replenish iron stores.

Megaloblastic Anemia

Megaloblastic anemia (MCV > 100 fL) occurs due to a deficiency of vitamin B_{12} or folate. Paresthesias with or without ataxia are the most common neurologic manifestations and may be present before anemia or macrocytosis.

Evaluation of macrocytosis should include serum folate, red cell folate and serum B_{12} to differentiate single deficiency of B_{12} or folate from combined deficiency.

Major causes of macrocytic anemia include alcoholism, vitamin B_{12}/folate deficiency and chemotherapy.

Therapeutic Choices

Nonpharmacologic Choices

For those with alcoholism, **abstinence** is necessary to reverse the macrocytosis.

Pharmacologic Choices (Table 4)

Vitamin B_{12}

Vitamin B_{12} (cyanocobalamin or hydroxocobalamin) is given in amounts sufficient to meet the daily needs of 2 to 3 μg and replenish tissue stores of 1 to 2 mg.

Parenteral therapy is necessary in B_{12} deficiency secondary to *lack of intrinsic factor or malabsorption*. Hydroxocobalamin has some advantage theoretically, but from a practical point of view cyanocobalamin is satisfactory and more readily available. Doses greater than 100 μg per day exceed available binding sites; the excess is renally excreted. Oral therapy with large daily doses (1 000 μg) of vitamin B_{12} has been used, but unpredictable absorption, cost and compliance make it of questionable value.

In those with *dietary* deficiency, oral therapy with 200 to 500 μg per day is satisfactory; parenteral administration to replenish B_{12} stores may be considered to ensure compliance and correction of the deficiency. Lower doses prevent dietary deficiency. This may be provided via a multivitamin tablet containing at least 15 μg of vitamin B_{12}.

Folic Acid

Inadvertent administration of pharmacologic doses of folic acid may aggravate the neurologic deficit seen in patients with neurologic manifestations secondary to vitamin B_{12} deficiency. Thus, folic acid should be administered **only** for folic acid deficiency or prophylactically where there is increased demand (e.g., pregnancy[1] or hemolysis).

Although a parenteral preparation is available, folic acid deficiency is generally treated orally; even in patients with malabsorption, the relatively large doses (usually 1 mg per day with the daily requirement being 100 to 400 μg) permit sufficient absorption to correct the deficiency.

---

[1] For recommended intake in pregnant women at high risk of having a pregnancy affected with a neural tube defect, see Chapter 99.

Table 4: Drugs Used to Treat Anemia

Drug	Dosage	Adverse Effects	Comments	Cost*
Iron Deficiency Anemia				
Oral Ferrous Salts†	100–195 mg elemental Fe/d	GI (nausea, epigastric distress, constipation and/or diarrhea).	Preferred replacement therapy (safe, inexpensive, generally well-tolerated). Optimal absorption occurs on an empty stomach, but frequency of GI side effects may ↑ (dose-related). Starting treatment with 1 tablet daily after a meal × 7–10 d and ↑ step-wise to 1 tablet after each meal often prevents side effects.	
ferrous sulfate many				$
ferrous gluconate many	Usual: 180 mg elemental Fe/d divided TID			$
ferrous fumarate Palafer, generics				$
ferrous ascorbate Ascofer	150 mg elemental Fe/d	Well-absorbed, excellent GI tolerance (indicated for patients who cannot tolerate other oral iron salts).	No iron salt has a particular advantage over another. Iron ↓ absorption of etidronate, tetracycline, levodopa, penicillamine, fluoroquinolones, methyldopa, levothyroxine (separate administration by 2 h).	$$$$
polysaccharide-iron complex Niferex-150			↓ hematological response to iron with concomitant vitamin E, chloramphenicol. ↓ absorption of iron with concomitant use of cholestyramine, antacids containing aluminum/magnesium salts, sodium bicarbonate, calcium carbonate.	$$$$
Parenteral Iron	Total dose = Hgb iron deficit + amount needed to replenish iron stores (refer to manufacturers' information for details)	IM: Discomfort and temporary discoloration at injection site, localized/generalized urticaria, transient metallic taste (common) rarely accompanied by loss of taste, nausea, vomiting, headache, dizziness, flushing of face, palpitations and sensations of pressure in the chest (occasional).	Iron sorbitol: given deep IM into upper outer quadrant of buttock by Z-track technique (↓ or prevents tracking to SC tissues and resultant discoloration, which may persist for years).	
iron sorbitol Jectofer (IM)				$2.70/100 mg
iron dextran Dexiron (IV) Infufer (IV)				$18.25/100 mg‡ $25.00/100 mg

(cont'd)

Table 4: Drugs Used to Treat Anemia *(cont'd)*

Drug	Dosage	Adverse Effects	Comments	Cost*
Parenteral iron *(cont'd)*			Systemic adverse effects occur more commonly with larger than normal doses, especially in underweight people.	
			IV: Anaphylaxis (< 1%), arthralgia, fever, myalgia, headache, GI distress, urticaria, exacerbation of arthritic symptoms in those with rheumatoid arthritis (may be managed with acetaminophen).	
Megaloblastic Anemia				
Parenteral Vitamin B$_{12}$ *cyanocobalamin* Rubramin, generics *hydroxocobalamin* generics	Suggested approach: 100 µg cyanocobalamin SC/IM daily × 1 wk, then 200 µg SC/IM weekly × 8–10 wks, then 200 µg SC/IM monthly for life	Usually nontoxic. However, mild transient diarrhea, peripheral vascular thrombosis, itching, transitory exanthema, feeling of swelling of entire body, pulmonary edema and congestive heart failure early in treatment and anaphylactic shock have been reported.		$ $
Folic Acid Folvite (oral and parenteral), generics	1 mg/d	Allergic reactions including erythema, pruritus and/or urticaria.		$

† *Liquid preparations are more expensive.*
‡ *Available from Luitpold Pharmaceuticals, USA (1–800–645–1706).*

* *Cost of 30-day supply – includes drug cost only.*
Legend: $ < $10 $$ $10–20 $$$ $20–30 $$$$ > $30

Therapeutic Tips

- Serum potassium should be monitored carefully in patients with severe pernicious anemia complicated by heart failure. Administration of diuretics and the intracellular shift of potassium associated with rapid reticulocytosis may cause hypokalemia and its complications unless supplementary potassium is given. Serum K^+ should be monitored daily for the first 3 to 5 days of diuretic treatment.

- As Hgb rises in response to vitamin B_{12}, the MCV gradually decreases and the patient may become microcytic, with Hgb plateauing below normal. If this occurs, oral iron should be added to therapy to achieve the maximum Hgb response.

Suggested Reading List

Brown RG. Determining the cause of anemia. *Postgrad Med* 1991;89:161–170.

Massey AC. Microcytic anemia. Differential diagnosis and management of iron deficiency anemia. *Med Clin North Am* 1992;76:549–566.

Schilling RF. Anemia of chronic disease: a misnomer. *Ann Intern Med* 1991;115:572–573.

Wymer A, Becker DM. Recognition and evaluation of red blood cell macrocytosis in the primary care setting. *J Gen Intern Med* 1990;5:192–197.

CHAPTER 73

Chemotherapy-induced Nausea and Vomiting

Lynne Nakashima, PharmD

Goals of Therapy

- To prevent acute (starting within 24 hours of chemotherapy), delayed (starting > 24 hours after chemotherapy) and anticipatory (starting before chemotherapy as a conditioned response) nausea and vomiting to ensure patient compliance with active treatment and to maintain quality of life
- To decrease incidence of nausea and vomiting (once it has occurred) and maintain patient comfort
- To prevent complications (esophageal tears, dehydration, anorexia, malnutrition, weight loss, pathological bone fractures, metabolic alkalosis, chloride and potassium depletion)

Investigations

- A thorough history including:
  - onset and duration of symptoms
  - timing of nausea and/or retching and/or vomiting
  - description of the vomiting episodes
  - medications the patient is taking
- Physical examination with particular attention to:
  - orthostatic hypotension
  - abdominal pain, distention, constipation, hemorrhage
  - neurologic assessment including cranial nerves, vestibular and pupillary function, extrapyramidal signs
- Laboratory tests:
  - BUN, creatinine, sodium, potassium, chloride (to assess hydration status), calcium, albumin (to assess for hypercalcemia)
  - drug screening, such as for digoxin if suspected as a cause of nausea and vomiting

Although medication is the most likely cause of nausea and vomiting in a patient receiving chemotherapy, other potential causes (e.g., fluid/electrolyte abnormalities, bowel obstruction, central nervous system or hepatic metastases, infections and radiation therapy) should be ruled out. Other drugs (e.g., narcotics, digoxin, antibiotics) may cause or exacerbate nausea and vomiting so a thorough medication history is essential. Some chemotherapeutic agents are more likely to cause nausea and

Figure 1: **Management of Nausea and Vomiting Due to Chemotherapy**

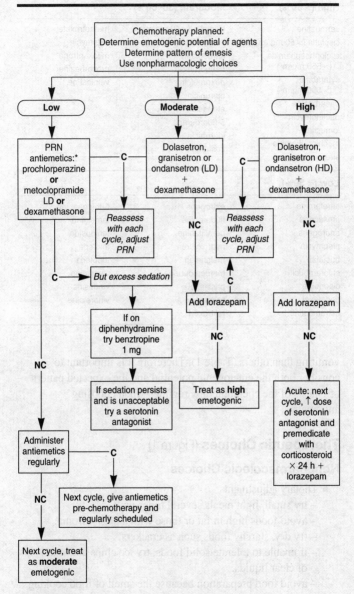

Add diphenhydramine 25–50 mg PO with metoclopramide dose.
Abbreviations: C = controlled; NC = not controlled; CT = chemotherapy.
Doses:
Dexamethasone 10 mg PO/IV pre and 4–8 mg Q12H.
Lorazepam 1 mg S/L pre and Q4H PRN.
Ondansetron: LD (low dose) 8 mg PO/IV pre CT;
HD (high dose) 16–32 mg PO/IV pre CT.
Metoclopramide: LD (low dose) 10–20 mg Q6H.

Table 1: **Emetogenic Potential of Chemotherapy Agents**

High (> 60%)	Moderate (30–60%)	
carmustine	cisplatin (< 50 mg/m^2)	methotrexate
cisplatin (> 50 mg/m^2)	L-asparaginase	mitomycin
cyclophosphamide (> 550 mg/m^2)	carboplatin	mitoxantrone
cytarabine (> 500 mg/m^2)	daunorubicin	procarbazine
	doxorubicin	vinblastine
dacarbazine	epirubicin	
dactinomycin	etoposide	
lomustine	5-fluorouracil	
mechlorethamine	idarubicin	
streptozocin	ifosfamide	

Low (< 30%)		
altretamine	estrogens	6-thioguanine
amsacrine	fludarabine	tamoxifen
androgens	gemcitabine	teniposide
bleomycin	hydroxyurea	thiotepa
busulfan	melphalan	topotecan
chlorambucil	mercaptopurine	vincristine
cladribine	paclitaxel	vindesine
docetaxel	progestins	vinorelbine
estramustine	ralitrexed	

vomiting than others (Table 1). Therefore it is important to consider both the emetogenic potential and the expected pattern of emesis of the chemotherapy regimen when choosing antiemetics.

Therapeutic Choices (Figure 1)

Nonpharmacologic Choices

- Dietary adjustments
  - try small, light meals several times daily.
  - avoid foods high in fat or those with a heavy aroma.
  - try dry, starchy foods such as crackers.
  - if unable to tolerate solid foods, try ice chips and small sips of clear liquids.
  - avoid food preparation because the smell of food cooking often worsens nausea.
- Behavioral methods
  - relaxation techniques may help decrease physiologic arousal and anxiety.
  - individualized exercise programs may help decrease anxiety and depression.

– systemic desensitization may be helpful for anticipatory nausea and vomiting.
- Other
  – keep movement to a minimum; rest in bed or a chair to avoid vestibular stimulation.
  – acupuncture and acupressure have been shown to have some effect on chemotherapy-induced emesis.
  – sleep has been shown to protect against chemotherapy-induced nausea and vomiting.

Pharmacologic Choices (Table 2)

Benzodiazepines

Benzodiazepines provide useful antianxiety, amnesic and sedating effects. Lorazepam is the most commonly used, usually in combination with other antiemetics.

Butyrophenones

Haloperidol and droperidol have reported efficacy and are generally used as alternatives to high-dose metoclopramide or ondansetron in refractory nausea and vomiting.

Cannabinoids

Nabilone and dronabinol are of limited use because they are available only as oral formulations and are associated with several side effects including mood alterations, hallucinations, delusions and increases in heart rate and blood pressure. They are generally used in refractory nausea and vomiting or in combination with other antiemetics.

Corticosteroids

Dexamethasone is the most commonly used, although several others including prednisone and methylprednisolone have been studied. The actual mechanism of action is unknown, but the efficacy of corticosteroids is documented. They appear to be effective as single agents, in combination with other antiemetics and for delayed nausea and vomiting. Dexamethasone in combination with a serotonin antagonist is the most effective antiemetic regimen for acute nausea and vomiting. Dexamethasone alone or in combination with metoclopramide appears to be the most effective regimen for delayed nausea and vomiting. The optimal dose has not been identified; the usual range is from 6 to 60 mg daily.

Dimenhydrinate

An antihistamine useful for treating vomiting due to motion sickness, it is considered no more effective than placebo against chemotherapy-induced nausea and vomiting.

Table 2: Drugs Used to Treat Chemotherapy-induced Nausea and Vomiting

Drug	Dosage	Adverse Effects	Drug Interactions	Cost*
Benzodiazepines *lorazepam* Ativan, generics	1 mg PO/SL pre CT, then 1–4 mg Q4H PRN	Sedation (up to 80%).	Sedating medications.†	$
Butyrophenones *haloperidol* Haldol, generics *droperidol* Inapsine	Haloperidol:1–2 mg PO/IM pre CT and Q8H Droperidol: 0.5–1 mg IV pre CT and Q4H	Sedation, extrapyramidal effects.†	Sedating medications.†	$ $$$
Cannabinoids *nabilone* Cesamet *dronabinol* Marinol	1 mg PO BID 5 mg/m² PO Q2–4H Max: 6 doses/d. May ↑ by 2.5 mg/m² to max 10 mg /m²/dose	Sedation (4–89%), dizziness, ataxia (12–65%), psychotropic effects ("high") (27%), tachycardia (7%), orthostatic hypotension (10%), dry mouth (6–62%).	Sedating medications.†	$ $$$–$$$$$
Corticosteroids *dexamethasone* Decadron, Dexasone	4–10 mg PO pre CT and Q6–12H 8–20 mg IV pre CT and Q6–12H	Mood changes, increased appetite, GI irritation, ulceration, fluid retention, weight gain, may mask signs of infection.	Warfarin – ↓ or ↑ response.	$ oral $–$$$ IV
metoclopramide 🔴 Maxeran, Reglan, generics	Low: 10–20 mg PO Q6H High: 1–3 mg/kg PO/IV Q3H	Sedation (up to 80%), dose-related diarrhea (up to 45%), extrapyramidal effects (3%).		$ low dose High dose varies

Phenothiazines

prochlorperazine
Stemetil, generics

perphenazine
Trilafon, generics

Prochlorperazine: 10 mg Q6H

Perphenazine: 2–4 mg Q8H

Sedation, anticholinergic effects (dry mouth, blurred vision, constipation, nasal congestion, urinary retention), extrapyramidal effects, hypotension, hypersensitivity (1.4%), rare pancytopenia.

Sedating medications.[†]

$

Serotonin Antagonists

dolasetron
Anzemet

granisetron
Kytril

ondansetron
Zofran

1.8 mg/kg IV pre CT or 100 mg PO pre CT

10 µg/kg IV or 2 mg PO pre CT or 1 mg pre CT and 12 h post

low: 8 mg PO/IV pre CT

high: 16–32 mg PO/IV pre CT

Headache (6–43%) constipation (4–19%), diarrhea (1–16%), sedation (4–10%), transient ↑ in LFTs (<1–19%), bradycardia (4%), dizziness (3%).

$$ PO
$ IV
$$$ PO
$$$$$ IV
$$–$$$$$ IV and PO

[†] Additive sedation occurs with, for example, narcotic analgesics, hypnotics, alcohol; avoid or minimize use if possible.

Abbreviations: LFTs = liver function tests; CT = chemotherapy.

⚑ Dosage adjustment may be required in renal impairment – see Appendix I.
* Cost per day – includes drug cost only.
Legend: $ < $15 $$ $15–30 $$$ $30–45 $$$$ $45–60 $$$$$ > $60

Metoclopramide

Metoclopramide blocks the dopaminergic receptors in the chemoreceptor trigger zone and has serotonin antagonistic activity at higher doses. Low doses (10 to 20 mg) are generally as effective as prochlorperazine; however, in high doses (1 to 3 mg/kg), metoclopramide shows significantly greater antiemetic activity. When compared to serotonin antagonists for acute antiemetic efficacy against highly emetogenic chemotherapy, serotonin antagonists are superior and have fewer side effects. For delayed nausea and vomiting, metoclopramide plus a corticosteroid are as effective as a serotonin antagonist plus a corticosteroid and more cost-effective. One limitation is the development of extrapyramidal side effects; diphenhydramine, 25 to 50 mg, should be administered prophylactically to all patients receiving high-dose metoclopramide.

Phenothiazines

The most commonly used are prochlorperazine and perphenazine. Considered moderately effective, they are usually used in low emetogenic regimens or as rescue medication. The availability of a wide variety of dosage forms (tablet, suppository, injectable) facilitates prochlorperazine use, especially for outpatients.

Propofol

Propofol is an anesthetic agent with antiemetic properties. Studies suggest that a continuous infusion at low doses (1 mg/kg/ hour) is effective in patients with cisplatin-induced nausea and vomiting that is refractory to serotonin antagonists combined with cortico-steroids.[1–3] Its use is still considered investigational, however, propofol use may be considered in severe, refractory vomiting.

Serotonin Antagonists

The various serotonin antagonists are equivalent in efficacy and toxicity. Dolasetron, granisetron and ondansetron are currently available. Single agent efficacy is reported, but in combination with corticosteroids, efficacy is improved and the 2-drug regimen is recommended unless the patient has a contraindication to corticosteroids.[4,5] Serotonin antagonists plus corticosteroids are reported to be no more effective for delayed nausea and vomiting than metoclopramide plus corticosteroids or corticosteroids

[1] *Can J Anaesth 1992;39:170–172.*

[2] *Oncology 1993;50:456–459.*

[3] *Anaesth Analg 1992;74:539–541.*

[4] *J Clin Oncol 1991;9:675–678.*

[5] *Eur J Cancer 1993;29A (Suppl).*

alone.[6,7] These drugs are well tolerated. The major drawback to their use is cost. However, because of their superior efficacy, serotonin antagonists should be used for the prophylaxis of acute nausea and vomiting for moderate and highly emetogenic regimens. The choice of serotonin antagonist can be based on cost.

Therapeutic Tips

- Use antiemetic therapy to prevent anticipatory nausea and vomiting, which usually worsens with each cycle; up to 30% of patients refuse further chemotherapy because of intolerable nausea and vomiting.

- Regularly scheduled and administered antiemetics (i.e., not PRN) are more effective at preventing nausea and vomiting.

- If the patient can tolerate oral antiemetics, this is the recommended route of administration. However, rectally administered antiemetics such as prochlorperazine are especially useful in patients who are vomiting or unable to take oral medications and who are at home. For hospitalized patients, the IV route of administration is recommended in patients who are vomiting.

Suggested Reading List

Berard CM, Mahoney CD. Cost-reducing treatment algorithms for antineoplastic drug-induced nausea and vomiting. *Am J Health-Syst Pharm* 1995;52:1879–1885.

Cooke CE, Mehra IV. Oral ondansetron for preventing nausea and vomiting. *Am J Hosp Pharm* 1994;51:762–771.

Grunberg SM, Hesketh PJ. Control of chemotherapy-induced emesis. *N Engl J Med* 1993;329:1790–1796.

Hesketh P, Navari R, Grote T, et al. Double-blind, randomized comparison of the antiemetic efficacy of intravenous dolasetron mesylate and intravenous ondansetron in the prevention of acute cisplatin-induced emesis in patients with cancer. *J Clin Oncol* 1996;14:2242–2249.

Osoba D, Warr DG, Fitch MI, et al. Guidelines for the optimal management of chemotherapy-induced nausea and vomiting: a consensus. *Can J Oncol* 1995;5(3):381–400.

---

[6] *Cancer 1995;76:1821–1828.*
[7] *J Clin Oncol 1995;13:2417–2426.*

CHAPTER 74

Prevention and Treatment of Side Effects of Antineoplastics

Louis A. Fernandez, MD, FACP, FRCPC

Goals of Therapy

- To recognize and provide optimal management of chemotherapy-induced side effects in order to deliver 100% of the recommended dose with curative intent

Side Effects of Chemotherapy

Acute (Table 1)

- Extravasation
- Thrombophlebitis
- Hypersensitivity reactions
- Rapid tumor lysis syndrome
- Nausea and vomiting (Chapter 73)

Chronic, Organ-Specific (Table 2)

- Skin
- Bone marrow
- Heart
- Lungs
- Nervous system
- Gastrointestinal
- Liver
- Kidneys
- Gonads
- Eyes

Conclusions

The number of side effects that may occur in a patient is formidable, yet many can be prevented, others are spontaneously reversible and some are treatable. For example, amifostine is a cytoprotective agent which reduces hematologic (anemia, leukopenia, thrombocytopenia) and nonhematologic (mucositis, xerostomia, loss of taste) toxicity in patients treated with antineoplastic agents. In spite of the potential side effects, many patients are able to take most types of chemotherapy in the hope of "cure" or long-term disease-free survival. The ideal chemotherapeutic regimen would be effective if given orally and have no side effects; obviously, we are a long way from the ideal. Researchers have therefore moved their attention to developing biological response modifiers in the hope of controlling malignancies.

Table 1: Acute Side Effects of Antineoplastic Drugs

Acute Side Effect	Investigation(s)	Management	Prevention
Extravasation Vesicant drugs: Dactinomycin Daunorubicin Doxorubicin Epirubicin Idarubicin Mechlorethamine Mitomycin Plicamycin Streptozocin Vinblastine Vincristine Vindesine Vinorelbine	Diagnose clinically; burning at the site of infusion.	Stop infusion immediately. Measures such as application of ice, heat, local steroids, IV steroids may provide patient comfort.	Do not insert an IV needle or catheter in the dorsum of the hand or cubital fossa; extravasation in these areas may cause serious damage to tendons. Always try to insert IV lines distally; if unsuccessful move to a proximal site to ensure there is no puncture site proximal to where the IV is finally placed. Do not use force when giving vesicant drugs by IV push. It may be better to let them drop in by gravity. When accessing a Port-A-Cath, be sure that the Huber needle is in the Port-A-Cath receptacle.
Thrombophlebitis	None specific; diagnosed clinically.	Infuse offending drug slowly.	Peripheral veins may be protected by placing central lines.
Hypersensitivity Reactions Seen frequently with paclitaxel (10%), l-asparaginase (20%)	None helpful. Mechanism of hypersensitivity reactions is unpredictable.	Stop infusion. Intravascular volume expansion with saline. Administer steroids.	When the offending agent is used in future, premedication with steroids and antihistamines may prevent anaphylaxis. Erwinia-derived source of l-asparaginase may be substituted for E. coli-derived source (some cross reactivity) or use pegaspargase, a modified form of l-asparaginase which does not cross react. (Neither are commercially available as yet.)

(cont'd)

Table 1: **Acute Side Effects of Antineoplastic Drugs** *(cont'd)*

Acute Side Effect	Investigation(s)	Management	Prevention
Rapid Tumor Lysis Syndrome Occurs when large numbers of tumor cells are lysed rapidly by chemotherapy. Symptoms are malaise, tetany, oliguria, fluid overload, arrhythmia.	Biochemical profile shows ↓ calcium and ↑ serum phosphate, potassium and uric acid. ECG may show QT interval prolongation.	IV hydration to maintain urine output > 3 L/24 h. Alkalinize urine to pH 7. Allopurinol 600 mg/d beginning 24–48 h before chemotherapy for 2–3 d, then 300 mg/d until uric acid levels normal. If metabolic derangements occur, hemodialysis may be needed.	

Table 2: Organ-specific Side Effects

Organ/System	Goal(s)	Management	Prevention
Skin/Appendages Alopecia Nail changes Dry skin Pigmentation changes	Recognize changes in skin and its appendages secondary to chemotherapy.	Wig for alopecia. Most changes in skin and its appendages return to normal after chemotherapy ceases.	Scalp tourniquet is not recommended, particularly for hematological neoplasms due to concerns re: safety and efficacy.
Bone Marrow Suppression	To titrate dose to avoid prolonged neutropenia and life-threatening thrombocytopenia. To avoid anemia and/or development of myelodysplastic syndrome.	Absolute neutrophil count and platelet count (usually 10 d after chemotherapy) and CBC before next dose of chemotherapy. Macrocytosis is commonly seen due to interference with DNA synthesis. Observe carefully for changes in red cell morphology (poikilocytosis, anisocytosis) that may foretell development of myelodysplastic syndrome. For febrile neutropenia, use broad-spectrum antibiotics (Chapter 98). Platelet transfusions for a platelet count < 15 × 10⁹/L if patient not bleeding,[2,3] If bleeding, transfuse if platelets are 30–40 × 10⁹/L. Packed red blood cell transfusions or erythropoietin for anemia.	Dose intensity of chemotherapeutic agents causing myelosuppression can be ↑ approximately five-fold if supplemented by use of granulocyte colony stimulating factor (G-CSF) and approximately ten-fold if rescued by autologous bone marrow transplantation.[1] Neither survival nor mortality changes. Although therapy is costly, prolonged and dangerous neutropenia can be avoided by prophylactic use of G-CSF (usual dose 5 µg/kg SC daily starting 48 h after chemotherapy and continuing for 10 d).

(cont'd)

[1]*Demetri G. Presented at ASH Satellite Symposium, St. Louis, Mo. Dec 3–7, 1993.*
[2]*Wandt H, et al. (Abstract 1760). Presented at ASH, Orlando, Fl, 1996.*
[3]*GIMEMA group (Abstract 1761). Presented at ASH, Orlando, Fl, 1996.*

Table 2: Organ-specific Side Effects *(cont'd)*

Organ/System	Goal(s)	Management	Prevention
Cardiotoxicity	Recognize that risk of congestive heart failure (CHF) is dose-related; 0.1% to 1.2% when the cumulative dose of anthracyclines is 550 mg/m², increasing to 50% at 1 000 mg/m². Other cardiac risk factors (if present), combination with other chemotherapeutic agents or mediastinal radiation may ↑ the risk of developing CHF.	Look for cardiac risk factors (i.e., hypertension and ischemic heart disease). ECG, serial ejection fractions. If arrhythmias occur during anthracycline infusion, there is no need to discontinue or ↓ the dose of anthracyclines.	Dexrazoxane (500 mg/m²–30 min prior to administration of adriamycin) protects against cardiomyopathy. If serial ejection fraction ↓ by 25% from baseline, consider stopping anthracyclines.
Pulmonary Toxicity	Recognize toxicity and distinguish it from infection; pulmonary toxicity is commonly seen with bleomycin, carmustine, cyclophosphamide and mitomycin.	Sputum for Gram's stain, culture and sensitivity, bronchial washings; possibly gallium scan and lung biopsy. Rule out infections.	Steroids may be helpful if damage is due to hypersensitivity and should be given prophylactically when these drugs are used.
Neurotoxicity	Recognize that neurotoxicity will occur with vinca alkaloids and may present as peripheral neuropathy, ileitis, urinary retention, impotence and/or cranial neuropathy. Chemical meningitis, myelopathy with paraplegia and/or leukoencephalopathy are more common with intrathecal administration.	Rule out other causes (e.g., metastatic involvement of the nervous, GI or urinary system). With mild, stable level of toxicity, there is no need to discontinue the drug; however, increasing or severe toxicities mandate discontinuation.	

Gastrointestinal Toxicity Mucositis Nausea and vomiting (Chapter 73)	Recognize that mucositis occurs with drugs such as doxorubicin, methotrexate, 5-fluorouracil and bleomycin and distinguish it from an infective process.	Rule out infection: swab for Gram's stain; bacterial, fungal, viral cultures. For small ulcers apply benzocaine in Orabase. For generalized mucositis, topical rinses such as lidocaine viscous (maximum 120 mL/24 h) or Kaopectate mixed with diphenhydramine may help; in severe cases pain is relieved by IV morphine. Spicy, salty, acidic, hot, cold or rough foods should be avoided. Caloric intake should be supplemented with milk shakes. If unable to swallow, the patient may be fed by gastric tube or total parenteral nutrition.
Hepatotoxicity	Recognize that hepatotoxicity may occur with the nitrosoureas (e.g., carmustine, lomustine), cytarabine, methotrexate, 6-mercaptopurine, l-asparaginase, etoposide, plicamycin, streptozocin and azathioprine.	Rule out other causes of hepatic damage. No specific treatment; may have to discontinue drug depending upon the severity of liver damage. Liver function tests including bilirubin. Liver biopsy may be needed.
Nephrotoxicity Uric acid nephropathy	Prevention, particularly if large number of tumor cells will be lysed.	Serum uric acid, creatinine and BUN. ↑ hydration such that urine output is > 3 L/24 h. Alkalinize urine to pH > 7. Allopurinol 300–600 mg/d PO, 24–48 h before starting chemotherapy.

(cont'd)

Table 2: **Organ-specific Side Effects** *(cont'd)*

Organ/System	Goal(s)	Management	Prevention
Other nephrotoxicity	Recognize that drugs such as cisplatin and the nitrosoureas are nephrotoxic.	Urinalysis. Serum creatinine and BUN.	The key to prevention of cisplatin-induced nephrotoxicity is hydration: give 2–3 L of normal saline IV over 8–12 h.
	Methotrexate may precipitate in the kidney.		Prophylactic magnesium supplements. Methotrexate precipitation may be avoided by ↑ diuresis and alkalinizing urine to pH > 7.
	Ifosfamide and cyclophosphamide may cause hemorrhagic cystitis.		Mesna is used to prevent ifosfamide-induced hemorrhagic cystitis and may prevent cyclophosphamide-induced hemorrhagic cystitis; mesna should be given at 20% of the ifosfamide dose before and Q4H for 3–5 doses. Rigorous diuresis is also helpful.
	Mitomycin may cause a hemolytic–uremic syndrome.	Red cell morphology for presence of schistocytes and disseminated intravascular coagulation screen if mitomycin is the offending agent.	
Ocular Toxicity	Recognize effects: **Effect** Cataracts Optic neuritis Visual blurring ↑ lacrimation Oculomotor palsies, cortical blindness Conjunctivitis	Follow-up by ophthalmologist and may include CT scan of the brain to rule out cortical blindness. Cataract surgery.	Prophylactic steroid eye drops may prevent conjunctivitis.

Ocular Toxicity drug list:

Effect	Drug
Cataracts	Busulfan, corticosteroids
Optic neuritis	Cisplatin
Visual blurring	Cyclophosphamide
↑ lacrimation	Doxorubicin
Oculomotor palsies, cortical blindness	Vincristine
Conjunctivitis	Cytarabine, 5-fluorouracil, methotrexate, 2'-deoxycoformycin

Gonadal Toxicity	Prevent sexual dysfunction and infertility.	Baseline sperm count, motility and reproductive hormone levels in males and females (to rule out primary infertility). Assisted reproductive technology.	Sperm banking before chemotherapy and suppression of ovulation during chemotherapy. Counseling against conception while on chemotherapy.
Miscellaneous Myelodysplastic syndrome (MDS) Secondary malignancy Vascular complications vasospasm, Raynaud's, thromboembolism, cerebral ischemia		Specific for each (e.g., bone marrow cytology and chromosomal abnormality for MDS). Routine screening methods for diagnosing other malignancies, vascular problems. Successful treatment of secondary MDS and malignancies by standard protocols is disappointing. Standard guidelines for treatment of vascular complications.	

Suggested Reading List

Perry MC, ed. *The chemotherapy source book*. Baltimore: Williams & Wilkins, 1992.

Perry MC, Yarbro JW, eds. *Toxicity of chemotherapy*. Orlando: Gruenne & Stratton, 1984.

Principles of chemotherapy. In: DeVita VT, Hellman S, Rosenberg SA, eds. *Cancer: Principles and practice of oncology*. 5th ed. Philadelphia: J.B. Lippincott–Raven, 1997.

CHAPTER 75

Drug Exposure During Pregnancy and Lactation

Orna Diav-Citrin, MD, Shlomit Ben-David, MD and Gideon Koren, MD, FRCPC

Many pregnant women are exposed to a variety of medications that may exert therapeutic, toxic or teratogenic effects on the fetus. Since the thalidomide disaster, many physicians and pregnant women tend to withhold any medication during pregnancy, although the risk of teratogenic effect from most drugs in therapeutic doses is nonexistent. Major congenital defects occur in 1 to 3% of the general population at birth. Of the major defects, about 25% are of genetic origin (genetically inherited diseases, new mutations and chromosomal abnormalities) and 65% are of unknown etiology (multifactorial, polygenic, spontaneous errors of development and synergistic interactions of teratogens). Only 2 to 3% of malformations is thought to be associated with drug treatment. The remaining defects are related to other environmental exposures including infectious agents, maternal disease states, mechanical problems and irradiation.

Proper prescribing in pregnancy is a challenge and should provide maximal safety to the fetus as well as therapeutic benefit to the mother. To date, very few drugs are proven teratogens in humans. However, drug-induced malformations are important because they are potentially preventable.

Maternal physiologic changes during pregnancy may alter the pharmacokinetics of drugs. Clearance rates of many drugs increase during late pregnancy due to increases in both renal and hepatic elimination (e.g., digoxin, phenytoin), while in others the clearance rate decreases (e.g., theophylline). Generally, little is known about the relationship between maternal serum drug concentration and risk of teratogenicity.

The importance of **timing of drug exposure** is better understood; the effect produced by a teratogenic agent depends upon the developmental stage in which the fetus is exposed. Several important phases in human development are recognized:

- The **"all or none" period**, the time from conception until implantation. Insults to the embryo in this phase are likely to result in death and miscarriage or intact survival. The embryo is undifferentiated and repair and recovery are possible through multiplication of the still totipotential cells. Exposure to teratogens during the preimplantation stage usually does not cause congenital malformations unless the agent persists in the body beyond this period.

- The **embryonic period**, from 18 to 60 days after conception when the basic steps in organogenesis occur. This is the period of maximum sensitivity to teratogenicity since tissues are differentiating rapidly and damage becomes irreparable. Exposure to teratogenic agents during this period has the greatest likelihood of causing a structural anomaly. The pattern of anomalies produced depends on which systems are differentiating at the time of teratogenic exposure.

- The **fetal phase**, from the end of the embryonic stage to term, when growth and functional maturation of formed organs and systems occurs. Teratogen exposure in this period will affect fetal growth (e.g., intrauterine growth restriction) and the size or function of an organ, rather than cause gross structural anomalies. The term fetal toxicity is commonly used to describe such an effect. The potential effect of psychoactive agents (e.g., antidepressants, antiepileptics, alcohol and other drugs of abuse) on the developing central nervous system has lead to a new field of behavioral teratology.

Many organ systems continue structural and functional maturation long after birth. Most of the adenocarcinomas associated with first trimester exposure to diethylstilbestrol occurred many years later.

Teratogens must reach the developing conceptus in sufficient amounts to cause their effects. Large molecules with a molecular weight greater than 1 000 (e.g., heparin) do not easily cross the placenta into the embryonic-fetal bloodstream. Other factors influencing the rate and extent of placental transfer of xenobiotics include polarity, lipid solubility and the existence of a specific protein carrier.

In an attempt to provide the practitioner, who is considering treatment of the pregnant woman, with a better assessment of fetal risk, the FDA developed a classification of fetal risk in 1979. These categories initially appeared logical but were *not* found to be very *helpful* in counseling individual patients. Drug manufacturers may have legal rather than scientific reasons for assigning particular designations. The classification frequently resulted in ambiguity and even false alarm. For example, oral contraceptives are denoted as X (i.e., contraindicated in pregnancy), despite failure of two meta-analyses to show increased teratogenic risk. In 1994 the Teratology Society stated that the FDA ratings were inappropriate and should be replaced by narrative statements that summarize and interpret available data regarding hazards of developmental toxicity and provide estimates of teratogenic risk.

Teratogenic Counseling

- Ascertain the clinical facts regarding the nature of the exposure: the length, dosage, and timing during pregnancy, as well as other exposures of concern (e.g., alcohol, cigarette smoking).

- All available current data regarding the agent are collected, and conclusions regarding the risk of exposure are drawn.

- Counseling should include background human baseline risk for major malformations, whether the fetus is at increased risk, which anomaly has been associated with the agent in question, a risk assessment, methods of prenatal detection when available, limitations in our knowledge, and limitations of prenatal diagnostic capabilities.

- Additional aspects include the potential risk of the medical condition for which a drug is prescribed, known interactions (in both directions) between the disease state and the pregnancy, and preventive measures when applicable (e.g., folic acid supplementation in carbamazepine exposure).

- Because more than 50% of pregnancies are unplanned, teratogenic risk assessment should be started prior to pregnancy.

Table 1 lists drugs with sufficient evidence to prove their teratogenic effect in humans. They should be avoided, when possible, in pregnancy. Table 2 lists possible teratogenic drugs with yet insufficient evidence for teratogenicity in humans. Table 3 presents drugs of choice during gestation for common maternal conditions.

Drug Use During Lactation

The extent of drug exposure in the infant depends on several factors: the pharmacokinetic properties of the drug in the infant and mother; milk composition; the amount of milk consumed; the physiology of the breast and the infant's suckling pattern. The susceptibility of an infant to adverse effects from drugs depends on the extent of exposure and the infant's sensitivity. Adverse drug reactions can be dose-related and reflect the pharmacologic effect of the drug or idiosyncratic (rarely).

To be excreted in the breast milk, a drug must be absorbed into the maternal circulation then pass into the breast milk. This process involves crossing of several membrane barriers by passive diffusion or active transport. This movement of drug is influenced by protein binding, lipid solubility, degree of ionization, concentration gradient and molecular weight. These factors influence the ratio of drug concentration in milk to drug concentration in maternal plasma—the M/P ratio.

Table 1: **Proven Teratogenic Drugs in Humans**

Drug	Adverse Effects
Alcohol	Fetal alcohol syndrome: intrauterine growth restriction (which commonly continues postnatally), microcephaly, developmental delay, and dysmorphic facies (low nasal bridge, midface hypoplasia, long featureless philtrum, small palpebral fissures and thin upper lip). Cleft palate and cardiac anomalies may occur. Full expression of the syndrome occurs with chronic daily ingestion of 2 g alcohol per kg (8 drinks per day). The full syndrome is present in about $1/3$ and partial effects in ¾ of offspring.
Angiotensin converting enzyme inhibitors (ACEI)	Adverse effects related to hemodynamic effects of ACEI on the fetus, teratogenic risk with first trimester exposure appears to be low. In late pregnancy: intrauterine renal insufficiency, neonatal hypotension, oliguria with renal failure, hyperkalemia, complications of oligohydramnios (i.e., fetal limb contractures, lung hypoplasia, and craniofacial anomalies), prematurity, intrauterine growth restriction and fetal death.
Carbamazepine	First trimester exposure: 1% risk of neural tube defects (10 times baseline risk). A pattern of malformations similar to the fetal hydantoin syndrome has also been associated.
Cocaine	Abruptio placenta, prematurity, fetal loss, decreased birth weight, microcephaly, limb defects, urinary tract malformations, and poor neurodevelopmental performance. Methodological problems make the findings difficult to interpret. Cocaine abuse is often associated with poly-drug abuse, alcohol consumption, smoking, malnutrition and poor prenatal care. Human epidemiology indicates the risk of major malformation from cocaine is probably low, but the anomalies may be severe.
Coumarin anticoagulants	First trimester exposure (6–9 wks gestation): fetal warfarin syndrome (nasal hypoplasia and calcific stippling of the epiphyses). Intrauterine growth retardation and developmental delay (CNS damage), eye defects and hearing loss. Warfarin embryopathy is found in $1/3$ of the cases where a coumarin derivative was given throughout pregnancy. Associated with high rate of miscarriage. After the first trimester: risk of CNS damage due to hemorrhage.
Diethylstilbestrol	Vaginal clear cell adenocarcinoma in offspring exposed in utero before 18th wk (> 90% of the cancers occurred after 14 years of age). High incidence of benign vaginal adenosis. Exposure starting at 4 wks associated with adenosis in 56% of the offspring, decreasing to 30% at 16 wks and 10% at 20 wks. Increased miscarriage rate and preterm delivery. In 134 males exposed in utero there were no signs of malignancy, but 27% had genital lesions (epididymal cysts, hypotrophic testes, or capsular induration of the testes). In 29%, pathologic changes were found in spermatozoa.
Folic acid antagonists: aminopterin and methotrexate	Fetal aminopterin syndrome: CNS defects (hydrocephalus, meningomyelocele), facial anomalies (cleft palate, high arched palate, micrognathia, ocular hypertelorism, external ear anomalies), abnormal cranial ossification, abnormalities in first branchial arch derivatives, intrauterine growth restriction and mental retardation. Maternal dose of methotrexate needed to induce defects is probably above 10 mg per wk with a critical period of 6–8 wks postconception.

(cont'd)

Table 1: **Proven Teratogenic Drugs in Humans** *(cont'd)*

Drug	Adverse Effects
Hydantoins (phenytoin)	Fetal hydantoin syndrome: craniofacial dysmorphology (wide anterior fontanelle, ocular hypertelorism, metopic ridge, broad depressed nasal bridge, short anteverted nose, bowed upper lip, cleft lip, cleft palate), anomalies and hypoplasia of distal phalanges and nails, growth restriction, mental deficiency and cardiac defects.
Lithium	Small increase in risk for major anomalies and a specific risk for cardiac teratogenesis in early gestation. The risk of Ebstein's anomaly exceeds spontaneous rate of occurrence. Fetal echocardiography if exposed in first trimester.
Misoprostol	First trimester exposure: limb defects and Moebius sequence. The teratogenic risk of misoprostol seems real, although not very high.
Retinoids (acitretin, isotretinoin) and megadoses of vitamin A	Systemic exposure: potent human and behavioral teratogen. Retinoic acid embryopathy: craniofacial anomalies (microtia or anotia, accessory parietal sutures, narrow sloping forehead, micrognathia, flat nasal bridge, cleft lip and palate and ocular hypertelorism), cardiac defects (primarily conotruncal malformations), abnormalities in thymic development and alterations in CNS development. Risk for associated miscarriage 40%.
Tetracyclines	Discoloration of the teeth after 17 wks gestation when deciduous teeth begin to calcify. Close to term: crowns of permanent teeth may be stained. Oxytetracycline and doxycycline associated with a lower incidence of enamel staining.
Thalidomide	Malformations limited to tissues of mesodermal origin, primarily limbs, ears, cardiovascular system, and gut musculature. Critical period: 27th–40th day of gestation. A single dose of < 1 mg per kg has produced the syndrome. Phocomelia, polydactyly, syndactyly, oligodactyly were all reported. Defects of external ears (20%), facial capillary hemangiomas, palsies of cranial nerves VI or VII, cardiovascular defects (10%). Visceral anomalies: agenesis of kidneys, spleen, gallbladder and appendix and atresias or stenoses of the esophagus, duodenum and anus. Embryopathy found in about 20% of the pregnancies exposed in the critical period.
Valproic acid	First trimester exposure: neural tube defects with 1–2% risk of meningomyelocele, primarily lumbar or lumbosacral. Fetal valproate syndrome: narrow bifrontal diameter, high forehead, epicanthal folds, infraorbital creases, telecanthus, low nasal bridge, short nose with anteverted nares, midfacial hypoplasia, long philtrum, thin vermillion border, small mouth, cardiovascular defects, long fingers and toes, hyperconvex fingernails and cleft lip, has been delineated by some investigations.

Table 2: **Possible Teratogenic Drugs in Humans**

Drug	Adverse Effects
D-penicillamine	High dose treatment: connective tissue disorders (cutis laxa) [case reports].
Methimazole	Scalp defects (aplasia cutis congenita) [case reports and an epidemiological study in which methimazole had been added to animal feeds as a weight enhancer and in those areas a higher incidence of aplasia cutis congenita was found].
Diazepam	A small increase in the incidence of cleft lip and palate [small studies]. Larger studies did not confirm the association.

Infants and adults differ in drug absorption, distribution, metabolism and excretion. In neonates, gastric acid secretion is decreased, gastric emptying time is variable and unpredictable, total body water is higher, fat content is lower and protein binding is decreased. The neonate's capacity for oxidative metabolism, and drug conjugation and glucuronidation is lower. The kidney's ability to eliminate drugs is also reduced.

Drugs Usually Contraindicated During Breast-feeding

- **Antineoplastic drugs** — potential risk for toxicity.
- **Ergot alkaloids** (ergotamine, bromocriptine) — potential risk of suppression of lactation and adverse effects in infant.
- **Lithium** — drug reaches one-third to one-half therapeutic blood concentration in infant.
- **Drugs of abuse** — potential hazard to nursing infant and concern that a mother using these substances may not be capable of proper infant care.
- **Gold** — potential adverse effects and long half-life in infant.
- **Oral contraceptives** — not recommended in early lactation, may change milk composition and decrease yield.
- **Radioactive compounds** — potential exposure of the nursing infant to excessive radioactivity.
- **Iodine-containing compounds** — iodine is transported into breast milk and may induce goitre and hypothyroidism.

In summary, most drugs taken by the breast-feeding mother are excreted into the milk. The amount of drug consumed by the infant is usually less than 5% of the maternal dose (weight adjusted). When maternal drug therapy is indicated, the agent with minimal risk to the infant should be chosen. The infant should be monitored for potential adverse effects. When toxicity is likely, drug concentration in the milk and infant's plasma may sometimes be measured.

Table 1: **Proven Teratogenic Drugs in Humans** (cont'd)

Drug	Adverse Effects
Hydantoins (phenytoin)	Fetal hydantoin syndrome: craniofacial dysmorphology (wide anterior fontanelle, ocular hypertelorism, metopic ridge, broad depressed nasal bridge, short anteverted nose, bowed upper lip, cleft lip, cleft palate), anomalies and hypoplasia of distal phalanges and nails, growth restriction, mental deficiency and cardiac defects.
Lithium	Small increase in risk for major anomalies and a specific risk for cardiac teratogenesis in early gestation. The risk of Ebstein's anomaly exceeds spontaneous rate of occurrence. Fetal echocardiography if exposed in first trimester.
Misoprostol	First trimester exposure: limb defects and Moebius sequence. The teratogenic risk of misoprostol seems real, although not very high.
Retinoids (acitretin, isotretinoin) and megadoses of vitamin A	Systemic exposure: potent human and behavioral teratogen. Retinoic acid embryopathy: craniofacial anomalies (microtia or anotia, accessory parietal sutures, narrow sloping forehead, micrognathia, flat nasal bridge, cleft lip and palate and ocular hypertelorism), cardiac defects (primarily conotruncal malformations), abnormalities in thymic development and alterations in CNS development. Risk for associated miscarriage 40%.
Tetracyclines	Discoloration of the teeth after 17 wks gestation when deciduous teeth begin to calcify. Close to term: crowns of permanent teeth may be stained. Oxytetracycline and doxycycline associated with a lower incidence of enamel staining.
Thalidomide	Malformations limited to tissues of mesodermal origin, primarily limbs, ears, cardiovascular system, and gut musculature. Critical period: 27th–40th day of gestation. A single dose of < 1 mg per kg has produced the syndrome. Phocomelia, polydactyly, syndactyly, oligodactyly were all reported. Defects of external ears (20%), facial capillary hemangiomas, palsies of cranial nerves VI or VII, cardiovascular defects (10%). Visceral anomalies: agenesis of kidneys, spleen, gallbladder and appendix and atresias or stenoses of the esophagus, duodenum and anus. Embryopathy found in about 20% of the pregnancies exposed in the critical period.
Valproic acid	First trimester exposure: neural tube defects with 1–2% risk of meningomyelocele, primarily lumbar or lumbosacral. Fetal valproate syndrome: narrow bifrontal diameter, high forehead, epicanthal folds, infraorbital creases, telecanthus, low nasal bridge, short nose with anteverted nares, midfacial hypoplasia, long philtrum, thin vermillion border, small mouth, cardiovascular defects, long fingers and toes, hyperconvex fingernails and cleft lip, has been delineated by some investigations.

Table 2: **Possible Teratogenic Drugs in Humans**

Drug	Adverse Effects
D-penicillamine	High dose treatment: connective tissue disorders (cutis laxa) [case reports].
Methimazole	Scalp defects (aplasia cutis congenita) [case reports and an epidemiological study in which methimazole had been added to animal feeds as a weight enhancer and in those areas a higher incidence of aplasia cutis congenita was found].
Diazepam	A small increase in the incidence of cleft lip and palate [small studies]. Larger studies did not confirm the association.

Infants and adults differ in drug absorption, distribution, metabolism and excretion. In neonates, gastric acid secretion is decreased, gastric emptying time is variable and unpredictable, total body water is higher, fat content is lower and protein binding is decreased. The neonate's capacity for oxidative metabolism, and drug conjugation and glucuronidation is lower. The kidney's ability to eliminate drugs is also reduced.

Drugs Usually Contraindicated During Breast-feeding

- **Antineoplastic drugs** — potential risk for toxicity.

- **Ergot alkaloids** (ergotamine, bromocriptine) — potential risk of suppression of lactation and adverse effects in infant.

- **Lithium** — drug reaches one-third to one-half therapeutic blood concentration in infant.

- **Drugs of abuse** — potential hazard to nursing infant and concern that a mother using these substances may not be capable of proper infant care.

- **Gold** — potential adverse effects and long half-life in infant.

- **Oral contraceptives** — not recommended in early lactation, may change milk composition and decrease yield.

- **Radioactive compounds** — potential exposure of the nursing infant to excessive radioactivity.

- **Iodine-containing compounds** — iodine is transported into breast milk and may induce goitre and hypothyroidism.

In summary, most drugs taken by the breast-feeding mother are excreted into the milk. The amount of drug consumed by the infant is usually less than 5% of the maternal dose (weight adjusted). When maternal drug therapy is indicated, the agent with minimal risk to the infant should be chosen. The infant should be monitored for potential adverse effects. When toxicity is likely, drug concentration in the milk and infant's plasma may sometimes be measured.

Table 3: **Drugs of Choice for Selected Conditions During Pregnancy**

Condition	Drugs of Choice	Alternative	Comments
Fever and Pain	acetaminophen	ASA, NSAIDs	Avoid full anti-inflammatory dose of NSAIDs in 3rd trimester.
Dyspepsia	alginic acid compound – Gaviscon antacids – numerous aluminum hydroxide–magnesium hydroxide combinations	H_2-antagonists, cisapride, omeprazole	
Nausea/ Vomiting	doxylamine/pyridoxine – Diclectin	dimenhydrinate, metoclopramide	
Hypertension	methyldopa, hydralazine	calcium channel blockers, beta-blockers	With beta-blockers, reduced birth weight and persistent beta-blockade in newborn possible.
Epilepsy	carbamazepine	valproic acid, benzodiazepines	With carbamazepine and valproic acid, periconceptual folate supplementation and level II ultrasound for NTD prevention.
Depression	tricyclic antidepressants, fluoxetine	newer selective serotonin reuptake inhibitors	
Hyperthyroidism	propylthiouracil	methimazole	Fetal ultrasound near term for goitre detection.

Suggested Reading List

Bennett PN. *Drugs and human lactation: A comprehensive guide to the content and consequences of drugs, micronutrients, radiopharmaceuticals, and environmental and occupational chemicals in human milk.* 2nd ed. Amsterdam: Elsevier, 1996.

Briggs GG, Freeman RK, Yaffe SJ. *Drugs in pregnancy and lactation: A reference guide to fetal and neonatal risk.* 4th ed. Baltimore: Williams and Wilkins, 1994.

Committee on drugs. The transfer of drugs and other chemicals into human milk. *Pediatrics* 1994;93:137–150.

Hale TW. *Medications and mother's milk.* 5th ed. Amarillo: Pharmasoft Medical Publishing, 1996.

Koren G, ed. *Maternal fetal toxicology: A clinician's guide.* 2nd ed. New York: Marcel Dekker, 1994.

CHAPTER 76

Dehydration in Children

Gary I. Joubert, MD, FRCPC

Goals of Therapy

- To treat shock/impending shock
- To treat dehydration using an appropriate fluid and route
- To treat electrolyte imbalances
- To prevent complications (seizures or edema)

Fluids in Infants and Children

Newborn and young children have a much higher water content than adolescents and adults (Table 1) and are thus more prone to both water and salt (sodium [Na^+], potassium [K^+]) loss during illness.

Table 1: Age vs Percentage of Body Water

Age	% Body Water
Newborn	75–80
Child ≤ 1 yr	70–75
Child 1–12 yrs	60-70
Adolescent/adult	55–60

Investigations

- Thorough history with attention to:
  - underlying cause(s): vomiting and/or diarrhea or other excessive fluid loss
  - frequency and amount of loss
  - frequency and amount of urinary output
- Physical examination to assess clinical manifestations and degree of dehydration
- Laboratory tests: electrolytes, BUN, creatinine, glucose, urinalysis as indicated clinically

The **assessment of dehydration** in infants and children is challenging (Table 2). This difficulty is related to a child's ability to maintain adequate blood pressure in the face of moderate to severe dehydration.

Table 2: **Estimation of Dehydration**

Extent of Dehydration	Mild	Moderate	Severe
Weight loss – Infants (under 1 yr)	5%	10%	15%
Weight loss – Children (over 1 yr)	3–4%	6–8%	10%
History	decreased intake duration of illness decreased urine output activity frequency of vomiting diarrhea	decreased intake duration frequency of vomiting and diarrhea marked decreased urine listless, weight loss	very decreased intake longer duration frequency of vomiting and diarrhea anuria obtunded
Pulse	normal	slightly increased	rapid
Blood pressure	normal	normal to orthostatic, > 10 mm Hg change	orthostatic to shock
Behavior	normal	irritable	hyperirritable to lethargic
Thirst	slight	moderate	intense
Mucous membranes*	normal	dry	parched
Tears	present	decreased	absent, sunken eyes
Anterior fontanelle	normal	normal to sunken	sunken
External jugular vein	visible when supine	not visible except with supraclavicular pressure	not visible even with supraclavicular pressure
Skin* (less useful in children > 2 yrs)	capillary refill < 2 sec	slowed capillary refill (2–4 sec), decreased turgor	significant delayed capillary refill (> 4 sec) and tenting; skin cool, acrocyanotic, or mottled*
Urine specific gravity (SG)	> 1.020	> 1.020, oliguria	oliguria or anuria
Lab values	normal BUN/creatinine	increased BUN/creatinine	increased+++ BUN/creatinine increased Hgb low glucose

These signs are less prominent in patients who have hypernatremia.

Figure 1: **Management of Isonatremic Dehydration**

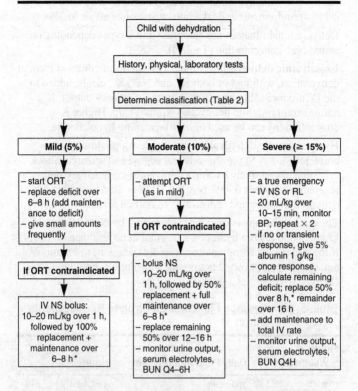

* *Replacement therapy after bolus should contain 50–60 mmol/L Na⁺ plus a source of glucose (e.g., D5W) plus appropriate K⁺. An ideal solution is 0.33% NaCl (Na⁺ 51.3 mmol/L) + D3.3W (3.3 g glucose/100 mL) + appropriate K⁺. K⁺ should not exceed 4 mmol/kg/d and replenishment should be done gradually over 2 d. **No urine output, no K⁺.***
Abbreviations: NS = 0.9% NaCl; ORT = oral replacement therapy; RL = Ringer's lactate.

Therapeutic Choices

Treatment of dehydration involves replacing fluid deficits, then maintaining normal hydration.

The calculation of the **fluid deficit** for a given degree of dehydration can be based on historical or objective information (e.g., predehydrational and present dehydrated weight). When the predehydrational weight is known:

Deficit liters (L) = predehydrational weight (kg) – present weight (kg).

Predehydrational body weight can be estimated by:

Body weight (kg) = (age × 2) + 10. This gives an estimated weight at or about the 50th percentile for age and can be used for children up to 10 years of age.

Maintenance fluid (Table 3) is the amount of fluid required to maintain normal hydration. Maintenance fluids are linked to caloric requirements and take into account insensible losses.

Dehydrational illnesses are classified into 3 types depending on serum Na^+ concentration (Table 4).

Isonatremic dehydration (Figure 1) is the most common form of dehydration, with loss of both K^+ and Na^+. K^+ can be added to the IV mixture following establishment of urinary output. K^+ administration should not exceed 4 mmol/kg/d. Higher K^+ concentrations can be used in life-threatening hypokalemia.

Hypernatremic dehydration usually develops slowly and is corrected slowly to prevent cerebral edema and seizures. Shock is treated aggressively by using 0.9% NaCl until urinary output is re-established, then 0.45% NaCl + D5W is used to correct dehydration states and restore Na^+ to normal levels.

The goal of therapy is to reduce serum Na^+ by 10 to 15 mmol/L/day and to restore hydration to normal in no less than 48 hours. If the serum concentration drops rapidly (i.e., > 10 to 15 mmol/day or > 1 mmol every 2 hours), the IV solution should be changed to 0.9% NaCl + D5W.

Table 3: **Maintenance Fluid and Electrolyte Requirements in Children**

Fluids

Weight (kg)	Daily Fluid Requirement	Hourly Rate
0–10	100 mL/kg	4 mL/kg
11–20	1 000 mL + (50 mL/kg × each kg > 10)	40 mL/h + (2 mL/kg × each kg > 10)
> 20	1 500 mL + (20 mL/kg × each kg > 20)	60 mL/h + (1 mL/kg × each kg > 20)

Daily Electrolytes	Na^+	2.5–3 mmol/kg
	K^+	2–2.5 mmol/kg

Calculation of Maintenance Fluid Requirements (using information from Table 3)

Example: For a 15-kg child use information for 11–20 kg

Fluids:	Daily fluid	Hourly fluid rate (quick calculation)
For the first 10 kg	10 kg × 100 mL/kg = 1 000 mL	10 kg × 4 mL/kg = 40 mL
For the next 5 kg	5 kg × 50 mL/kg = 250 mL	5 kg × 2 mL/kg = 10 mL
	Total 1 250 mL or 52 mL/h	**Total 50 mL/h**

Electrolytes:

Na^+ 15 kg × 3 mmol/kg/d = 45 mmol/d
(45 mmol/1 250 mL or 36 mmol/L)

K^+ 15 kg × 2 mmol/kg/d = 30 mmol/d
(30 mmol/1 250 mL or 24 mmol/L)

Suggested commercially available solution best meeting the needs would be 0.2% NaCl/D5W + 20 mmol KCl/L.

Table 4: **Types of Dehydration**

Type of Dehydration (frequency)	Serum Na$^+$ (mmol/L)	Serum Osmolality (mOsm/kg)
Isonatremic (80%)	130–150	Normal: 280–295 mOsm/kg Equal water and salt loss
Hypernatremic (15%)	> 150	Elevated: 295 mOsm/kg Water loss > salt loss
Hyponatremic (5%)	< 130	↓ or normal or ↑ Must determine subgroup

Hyponatremic dehydration is classified into 3 subgroups:
- excessive water.
- Na$^+$ depletion.
- fictitious lowering of serum Na$^+$ concentration due to increased glucose, electrolytes, lipids and proteins.

Shock must be treated aggressively using isotonic saline (0.9% NaCl).

Symptomatic hyponatremia is usually related to the degree of serum Na$^+$ depletion. Children with serum Na$^+$ > 120 mmol/L rarely demonstrate any clinical manifestations; when serum Na$^+$ drops below 120 mmol/L, neurologic manifestations (e.g., seizures) are common. Children who are symptomatic require aggressive replacement using hypertonic saline (3% NaCl) to achieve a serum Na$^+$ > 125 mmol/L.

Serum Na$^+$ deficit can be calculated as follows:

[Na$^+$] deficit = ([Na$^+$] desired − [Na$^+$] actual) × body weight (kg) × total body water (L/kg).

After initial elevation of Na$^+$ to > 125 mmol/L, the remaining deficit can be replaced over 24 to 48 hours.

Calculation of Fluid Deficit and Replacement for Isonatremic Dehydration

Example: For a 15-kg child who is 10% isonatremic dehydrated
Fluids: Total fluid replacement equals *deficit* replacement plus *maintenance*. Fluid deficit in 10% dehydration is 100 mL/kg; in 5% dehydration 50 mL/kg
(i)   Deficit replacement calculation = 15 kg × 10% (100 mL/kg)
                                         = 1.5 L or 1 500 mL
      Need to replace 50% or 750 mL over first 8 h at a rate of 94 mL/h
(ii) Maintenance = 52 mL/h (from Table 3 calculation)
(iii) Total = 146 mL/h (94 mL/h + 52 mL/h) for first 8 h, then reduce to 100 mL/h for next 16 h (replacing remaining 750 mL over 16 h + maintenance [47 mL/h + 52 mL/h ≈ 100 mL/h])
Electrolytes:
      Na$^+$ loss would be approximately 120 mmol (8–10 mmol/kg/d) and K$^+$ loss would be approximately 120 mmol (8–10 mmol/kg/d).

Using a rehydration solution of 0.45% NaCl + D5W at the above rate will replace 115 mmol of Na$^+$. K$^+$ 40 mmol/L (not to exceed 4 mmol/kg/d) will replace 60 mmol of total loss. Replacement of K$^+$ will make up losses over the next 2 d.

Oral Rehydration Therapy (ORT)

ORT is the treatment of choice in children with mild to moderate dehydration. It can be used in all types of dehydration provided that hypo- and hypernatremic dehydration are not at the extreme of the spectrum.

The fluid deficit is calculated and replaced over 6 to 8 hours using frequent small amounts of fluids. The fluid should be a balanced electrolyte solution that will be acceptable to the GI tract and will help facilitate Na^+ transport. Solutions ideal for ORT contain Na^+ 45 to 75 mmol/L, K^+ 20 mmol/L and glucose 20 to 24 g/L; 100 to 150 mL/kg/day is given to the child.

Commercially available preparations (Table 5) may be used to rehydrate the child with observation in an ambulatory/emergency room setting or at home.

Children who have been started on IV replacement therapy can be switched to ORT at any point. It is important to ensure that no contraindications (shock or impending shock, high diarrheal purge rates, intractable vomiting, altered sensorium) are present.

Table 5: **Oral Replacement Solutions**

Product	Composition				Cost*
	Dextrose g/L	K^+ mmol/L	Na^+ mmol/L	Cl^- mmol/L	
Enfalac Lytren	20	25	50	45	$$$$
Gastrolyte	17.8	20	60	60	$$
Pedialyte	25	20	45	35	$$
Pediatric Electrolyte	20	20	45	35	$$

* Cost per liter – includes drug cost only (retail mark-up not included).
Legend: $ < $5 $$ $5–10 $$$ $10–15 $$$$ $15–20

Suggested Reading List

Boineau FG, Lewy JE. Estimation of parenteral fluid requirements. *Pediatr Clin North Am* 1990;37:257.

Castell HB, Fidorick SC. Oral rehydration therapy, fluid and electrolyte therapy. *Pediatr Clin North Am* 1990;37:295.

Jospe N, Gorbes G. Fluids and electrolytes – clinical aspects. *Pediatr Rev* 1996;17(11):395–403.

Kallen RJ. The management of diarrheal dehydration in infants using parenteral fluids. *Pediatr Clin North Am* 1990;37:265.

CHAPTER 77

Edema

David J. Hirsch, MD, FRCPC

Edema is a sign, not a specific illness. Therapy is inappropriate until the underlying cause is defined.

Unilateral dependent edema should prompt an assessment of local venous and lymphatic drainage and a search for local infection. **Bilateral dependent edema** or anasarca is usually seen in patients with pregnancy, nephrotic syndrome, renal insufficiency, liver disease, heart failure or pericardial disease. Because of the wide range of serious illnesses causing edema, the approach outlined here must be general, and should be individualized for every patient.

Goals of Therapy

- To define the cause
- To reduce swelling if it causes reduced mobility, skin breakdown or infection, or discomfort
- To avoid elimination of all edema
- To avoid electrolyte disturbances

Investigations

- History with attention to:
  - salt intake
  - location of edema (peripheral, facial, ascites)
  - evidence of pregnancy, heart disease, renal disease, liver disease
  - previous diuretic use
- Physical examination:
  - weight, postural BP and pulse
  - severity of edema and its location (unilateral vs. bilateral)
  - evidence of cardiac failure, pleural effusion, ascites, hepatic enlargement or stigmata of hepatic failure
- Laboratory tests:
  - urinalysis
  - serum electrolytes and creatinine
  - liver function tests
  - chest radiograph

Figure 1: **Management of Edema**

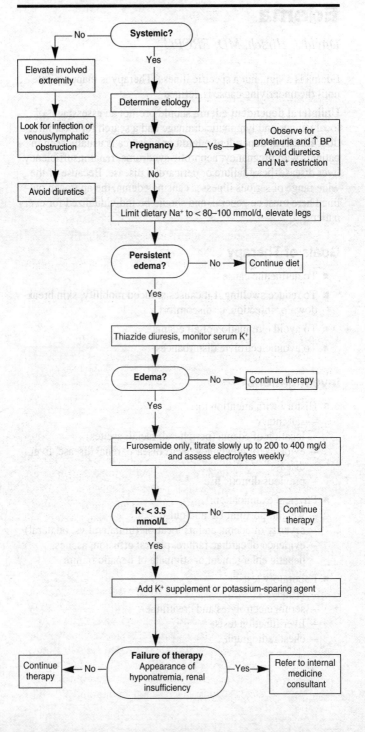

Therapeutic Choices (Figure 1)

Nonpharmacologic Choices

- Restriction of dietary sodium intake to < 80 mmol/day.
- Rest and elevation of the legs.
- Addition of supportive hose (if possible).

Pharmacologic Choices

Medications should only be used if nonpharmacologic measures have failed to control edema after attempted treatment of any underlying specific disease process.

Diuretic Therapy (Table 1)

- Indications:
  - if edema cannot be reduced to the point where shoes can be worn.
  - presence of skin breakdown in the lower limbs.
  - scrotal or vulvar edema.
  - pitting edema extending to the thighs or anterior abdominal wall.
- Pregnant women should **not** receive diuretics for edema without advice from a consultant.

Thiazides

Mild edema in the absence of renal insufficiency can be treated with a thiazide diuretic, using up to 100 mg of **hydrochlorothiazide** per day if nonpharmacologic measures fail. Serum potassium should be monitored.

Loop Diuretics

Failure of a thiazide response usually indicates a need for a loop diuretic, e.g., **furosemide**. Dosage starts at 20 to 40 mg per day as a single dose, and is doubled every 2 days until the patient notes the onset of diuresis. The effective dose should then be used as a single daily dose until sufficient edema reduction improves the patient's symptoms. The patient should monitor daily weight and avoid a reduction of more than 1 kg per day. Serum electrolytes and creatinine should be carefully followed.

Potassium-sparing Therapy

Hypokalemia (< 3.5 mmol/L) indicates a probable need for potassium supplements or the use of K^+-sparing agents, e.g., **spironolactone, triamterene** or **amiloride**. Although all are effective, amiloride has the least number of long-term side effects. Triamterene can occasionally result in decreased renal function and spironolactone can cause gynecomastia, if taken for long periods of time. All K^+-sparing agents may increase diuresis, so that volume depletion must be constantly monitored.

Table 1: Diuretic Agents

Drug	Daily Dose	Adverse Effects	Drug Interactions	Comments	Cost*
Thiazide Diuretics					
hydrochlorothiazide HydroDiuril, generics	25–100 mg	Hypokalemia, hyponatremia, hypovolemia, hyperuricemia, hyperglycemia, impotence, rash.	For all thiazides: Lithium: lithium toxicity (monitor Li+ levels).	Good initial agent, often ineffective if renal insufficiency present.	$
Others:					
metolazone Zaroxolyn	2.5–10 mg		Digoxin: digoxin toxicity if ↓ K+ (monitor K+).	No advantage over hydrochlorothiazide, generally more expensive.	$
chlorthalidone Hygroton, generics	25–100 mg		Antidiabetic agents: ↑ blood glucose (monitor).		$
indapamide Lozide, generics	1.25–2.5 mg		Corticosteroids: hypokalemia. NSAIDs: ↓ diuretic effect, ↑ renal toxicity.		$–$$
Loop Diuretics					
furosemide Lasix, generics	20–500 mg	As for thiazides; ototoxicity if rapidly injected.	As for thiazides.	Effective in refractory edema, useful in renal insufficiency.	$
ethacrynic acid Edecrin	25–200 mg	As for furosemide.		No advantage over furosemide clinically, more ototoxic.	$–$$
bumetanide Burinex	0.5–10 mg	As for furosemide.		No advantage over furosemide.	$–$$
torsemide Demadex	5–100 mg	As for furosemide.		No advantage over furosemide.	$–$$

Potassium-sparing Agents			
spironolactone Aldactone, generics	25–300 mg	Hyperkalemia, gynecomastia, GI upset, headache.	Gynecomastia is common.
triamterene Dyrenium	100–300 mg	Hyperkalemia, acute renal failure (esp. with NSAIDs).	Occasional reports of renal stones or acute renal failure.
amiloride Midamor	5–20 mg	Hyperkalemia.	Probably fewest side effects clinically.
		Avoid NSAIDs, ACE inhibitors, potassium supplements: may cause severe hyperkalemia.	All: $–$$

⊗ *Dosage adjustments may be required in renal failure – see Appendix I.*

* Cost of 30-day supply – includes drug cost only.
Legend: $ < $20 $$ $20–40

Hyperkalemia in diabetics or those patients taking NSAIDs or ACE inhibitors is common.

Combination Diuretic Therapy

If furosemide alone fails to induce a diuresis after doses of up to 400 mg per day, combination diuretic therapy may be required; the combination of **furosemide with a potassium-sparing agent** may be effective. However, on many occasions the use of a combination of **thiazide and furosemide** is required to cause diuresis in refractory patients. There is no evidence that metolazone is preferable to other thiazide diuretics. This type of therapy should be monitored closely, preferably in a hospital, because of the risk of complications including sudden massive diuresis, hypokalemia, hypomagnesemia, hyponatremia and acute hypotension with volume depletion. A combination of 25 mg hydrochlorothiazide with 80 to 200 mg of furosemide is often effective, but diuresis may be delayed for a few days following initiation of treatment.

Idiopathic Edema

Commonly seen in young to middle-aged females, particularly those very concerned with their appearance or weight. In some patients, there will be considerable complaint about edema not apparent to physicians. In other cases, patients have been able to document sudden shifts in weight of 3 or 4 kg from one day to another, often with the appearance of mild ankle edema. Thorough investigation in these cases fails to identify the usual causes of edema listed above, and the pathophysiology of this syndrome is not clear. The use of diuretics in these patients is best avoided: many do not respond to thiazide diuretics and require slow tapering of the dosage to avoid rebound edema on discontinuation of the diuretic. This group of patients reinforces the point that edema should not be treated pharmacologically unless there are clear indications to do so. **Diuretics should not be used for cosmetic purposes alone.**

Therapeutic Tips

- The goal of therapy is to reduce edema to the point of comfort, not to abolish it: pre-renal azotemia and volume depletion can result if edema is completely removed.

- The appearance of refractory hypokalemia, elevated serum creatinine, or hyponatremia usually indicates overdiuresis and/or progression of the underlying problem to a more complicated state; consultation and reduction of medication is appropriate.

- K^+-sparing agents should be avoided in patients with diabetes or reduced renal function. Dosage reductions of diuretics are not generally needed in liver or renal disease.

- Combination diuretic preparations (e.g., thiazide plus K⁺-sparing agent) should be avoided due to inflexibility in dosage adjustment.

- For all classes of diuretic agents, there is no reason to use more than one daily dose except in emergencies such as pulmonary edema.

- In patients where a target weight can be set, thiazides or loop diuretics can be given intermittently. Once an effective dose has been found by titration, that dose can be given only on days when the target weight is exceeded. This will reduce the risks of volume depletion, hyperuricemia, and electrolyte disturbance.

Suggested Reading List

Rose BD. Diuretics. *Kidney Inter* 1991;39:336–352.

Schrier RW. Pathogenesis of sodium and water retention in high-output and low-output cardiac failure, nephrotic syndrome, cirrhosis, and pregnancy. *N Engl J Med* 1988;319:1065–1072,1127–1134.

de Wardener H. Idiopathic edema: role of diuretic abuse. *Kidney Inter* 1981;19:881–892.

CHAPTER 78

Hypovolemia

Glen R. Brown, Pharm D, FCSHP, BCPS

Dehydration in children is discussed in Chapter 76.

Goals of Therapy

- To restore normal state of hydration
- To replace associated electrolyte deficiencies
- To identify and rectify the cause of the dehydration

Investigations

- Physical examination with attention to:
  - cardiac and respiratory system (a search for orthostatic hypotension may identify dehydration when supine BP appears appropriate)
  - estimate of volume deficit (often greater than anticipated) (Table 1)
- Identify factors limiting route and rate of rehydration
  - search for physical signs or symptoms which would prevent use of oral rehydration (e.g., upper GI pathology, severe vomiting, decreased alertness)
  - physical examination and history to determine if cardiac, renal, or pulmonary function will limit rate or volume of rehydration
- Identify associated electrolyte disturbances
  - if dehydration is moderate or severe (Table 1), measure serum sodium, potassium, phosphate, and creatinine concentration to identify associated deficiencies and renal function
- Identify cause of dehydration – look for:
  - excessive urine production – including use of diuretics (for diuresis or weight loss), unexplained polyuria and associated polydipsia
  - excessive GI losses – including vomiting (cause, frequency, quantity, and quality) or diarrhea (frequency, consistency, cause). The potential for "third spacing" of fluid in the abdomen, as a result of development of ascites or pancreatitis, should be excluded
  - excessive losses through the skin – burns, exfoliative dermatitis, fever
  - inadequate intake – history of lack of access to fluids, immobility, crush injury, loss of consciousness, mental changes, excessive perspiration through exercise without

fluid replacement, medications (e.g., antipsychotic therapy) which may blunt the thirst response

Therapeutic Choices (Figure 1)

Therapy should provide prompt rehydration, replace electrolyte deficiencies, utilize the least invasive route and avoid toxicities related to excessive or too rapid rehydration. Oral rehydration should be considered as the initial method unless volume of deficit (and resulting severity of symptoms) or lack of feasibility of oral intake suggest parenteral therapy is necessary.

Pharmacologic Choices

Oral Rehydration Therapy (ORT) (Table 2)

- should be attempted in patients with adequate blood pressure and those able to consume oral fluids. For patients with very low or undetectable blood pressure, IV administration of initial fluid is recommended.
- ORT solution should contain both sodium and glucose to maximize absorption of sodium and water.
- water, commercial soft drinks and fruit juices are not adequate for treating fluid and electrolyte deficiencies of moderate to severe dehydration.
- in hypernatremic dehydrated patients, use low sodium rehydration solutions (20 to 30 mmol Na+/L).
- when using oral hydration solutions with > 60 mmol/L of sodium, have water readily available to allow the patient to respond to changes in serum sodium concentrations and avoid hypernatremia.
- for hypokalemic patients, a minimum 20 mmol KCl/L of ORT is recommended.
- the addition of a base (bicarbonate or citrate) to ORT has not been demonstrated to be of value regardless of the presence or absence of systemic acidosis.
- for mild dehydration (Table 1) administer ORT–50 mL/kg; for moderate dehydration administer 100 mL/kg, over initial 2 to 4 hours of treatment given in frequent small volumes. The patient should then be re-evaluated for maintenance fluid requirements.
- if ongoing GI losses occur, replacement with 10 mL/kg for each diarrheal stool and 2 mL/kg for each episode of vomiting will approximate losses.

Intravenous Rehydration Therapy (Table 3)

- **normal saline** is the fluid of choice for replenishing intravascular volume.
- required for patients with severe dehydration or where use of oral hydration is not possible (e.g., unconciousness, noncompliance, upper GI pathology).

Figure 1: **Management of Hypovolemia**

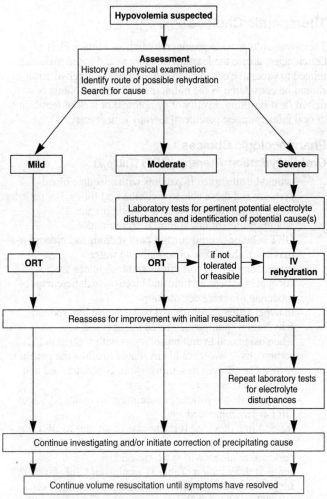

- correction of extracellular fluid deficit will resolve cardiovascular abnormalities (Table 3).
- colloid solutions (5% albumin, pentastarch) have not been demonstrated to produce more rapid rehydration or improve clinical outcome over crystalloid solutions. Albumin solutions may contribute to pulmonary edema if an intrinsic albumin leak is present in the lungs.
- consider blood administration if low hemoglobin.
- for severe dehydration, administer a liter of normal saline over 30 minutes followed by a second liter over the next hour. Repeat physical examination and serum electrolyte

measurement to determine subsequent rate of administration and electrolyte requirements.
– once hemodynamics are stabilized, the serum sodium
concentration will determine the rate of administration of
rehydration fluids (see below).

Electrolyte Replacement

Sodium

If the patient is hypernatremic, use hypotonic sodium solutions; if
hyponatremic, use isotonic sodium solutions (normal saline). To
avoid neurologic toxicities the rate of sodium administration
should not exceed 12 mmol/L/24 hours.

Potassium (See also Chapter 80.)

For mild dehydration, potassium replacement may not be
required. With moderate to severe dehydration caused by
gastrointestinal or renal losses, addition of potassium is usually
required.

If the serum potassium concentration is less than 3.5 mmol/L,
administer at least 20 mmol KCl/L of replacement solution. If
renal function is impaired, a repeat measurement after the initial
20 mmol will guide the need for further KCl.

KCl is unpalatable but can be administered as tablets or flavored
elixirs. Parenteral administration of KCl in concentrations
> 40 mmol/L is very irritating to veins.

Magnesium

When serum potassium concentration is low, consider magnesium
supplementation. If the serum creatinine is normal, magnesium
can be administered without measuring serum concentration
(of questionable value in determining total body stores). If renal
impairment is evident, measuring serum magnesium prior to
initiating replacement is prudent. If the concentration is elevated,
no supplementation is necessary. If it is normal, a single IV
dosage of 8 mmol can be given if clinical symptoms of deficiency
exist.

Oral magnesium supplementation is difficult since adequate
doses cause diarrhea. Parenteral administration is preferred.
Determining the required amount is difficult; however, 20 mmol
(5 g) of magnesium sulfate administered IV over 24 hours is an
appropriate initial dose in patients with normal renal function.

Phosphate

If the patient has a condition which could result in prolonged
phosphate loss (e.g., prolonged, sustained ethanol consumption)
or inadequate phosphate intake (prolonged starvation), measuring
serum phosphate concentration and supplementing if low is

Table 1: **Physical Findings in Association with Degree of Dehydration**

Clinical Signs	Mild	Moderate	Severe
Fluid loss*	< 6%	6–10%	> 10%
Mentation	alert	restless	drowsy to comatose
Radial pulse			
rate	normal	rapid	very rapid
pulse	normal	weak	feeble to impalpable
Respirations	normal	deep	deep and rapid
Systolic BP	normal	low	very low or undetectable
Skin elasticity	retracts rapidly	retracts slowly	retracts very slowly
Eyes	normal	sunken	very sunken
Voice	normal	hoarse	inaudible
Urine production	normal	scant	oliguria

Given as percentage of body weight.

Table 2: **Oral Replacement Therapy Fluids**

Fluid	Na⁺ (mmol/L)	K⁺ (mmol/L)	Comments
Water	0	0	Intake of solutions with low sodium will not replace sodium losses and does not maximize the absorption of water. Risk of precipitating hyponatremia.
Soft drinks	3	1	
Fruit juices	2	28	
Gatorade	20	3	
Commercial products			
Gastrolyte	60	20	Palatable. Useful for replacing losses of diarrhea.
Pedialyte	45	20	
World Health Organization	90	20	Not commercially available. Also contains glucose 111 mmol/L, chloride 80 mmol/L, citrate 10 mmol/L.
Broths	110–250	2–120	Easily available through commercial soup broths. Do not contain glucose.
Homemade	60	0	Half teaspoon salt (Na⁺ 60 mmol), 8 teaspoons sugar (sucrose 110 mmol) per liter water. Does not contain potassium.

Adapted from: Schreiber M, Halperin ML. Hypovolemia (Adults). In: Gray J, ed. Therapeutic Choices. Ottawa: Canadian Pharmaceutical Association, 1995: 561.

Table 3: **Intravenous Rehydration Solutions**

Solution	Concentration (mmol/L)		Volume (mL) expanded by 1 L of solution	
	Na$^+$	Glucose	ICV	ECV
Normal Saline (0.9% NaCl)	154	0	0	1 000
Half-normal saline (0.45% NaCl)	77	0	333	667
5% Dextrose	0	278	667	333
2/3–1/3	51	186	445	555

Abbreviations: ICV = intracellular volume; ECV = extracellular volume.
Adapted from: Schreiber M, Halperin ML. Hypovolemia (Adults). In: Gray J, ed.
Therapeutic Choices. Ottawa: Canadian Pharmaceutical Association, 1995:562.

appropriate. A serum concentration < 0.4 mmol/L warrants
therapy with potassium phosphate 15 mmol/L (in 250 mL IV
fluid over 6 hours), repeated if hypophosphatemia persists.
Patients at risk for phosphate deficiency may require phosphate
supplementation as the serum phosphate level may decrease with
reinitiation of caloric intake (re-feeding syndrome).

Reversal of Cause of Dehydration

The search for the underlying cause of the dehydration should
be concurrent with the rehydration therapy to prevent the
re-emergence of dehydration from ongoing fluid losses.

Therapeutic Tips

- ORT will allow rehydration of many patients without the
  need for initiation of IV therapy.
- Parenteral fluid administration by SC route (clysis) may be
  an alternative for hydration of adults who are unable to take
  fluids orally and for whom IV therapy is undesirable. A
  maximum of 3 L of fluid may be administered by clysis.

Suggested Reading List

Avery ME, Snyder JD. Oral therapy for acute diarrhea. The
    underused simple solution. *N Engl J Med* 1990;323:891–894.

Farthing MJG. Oral hydration therapy. *Pharmac Ther*
    1994;64:477–492.

Hussain NA, Warshaw G. Utility of clysis for hydration in
    nursing home residents. *J Am Geriatr Soc* 1996;44:969–973.

Rivin B, Santosham M. Rehydration and nutritional management.
    Bailliere's Clin Gastroenterol 1993;7:451–476.

CHAPTER 79

Hypercalcemia

Donna M.M. Woloschuk, Pharm D

Goals of Therapy

- To correct dehydration
- To enhance renal excretion of calcium
- To inhibit accelerated bone resorption
- To treat the underlying disorder

Investigations

- Initiating treatment (general measures) immediately will not interfere with diagnostic tests
- History and physical examination, with special attention to:
  - duration of symptoms if symptomatic (anorexia, nausea, vomiting, constipation, malaise, drowsiness, polydipsia, polyuria), or of hypercalcemia if asymptomatic
  - history of, or physical findings consistent with, familial hypocalciuric hypercalcemia, primary hyperparathyroidism, granulomatous diseases, malignancy, nonparathyroid endocrine disorders, immobilization, acute/chronic renal insufficiency or milk-alkali syndrome
  - medications that cause or aggravate hypercalcemia (thiazide diuretics, lithium, excess vitamin A or D, estrogens, antiestrogens, progestins, androgens, parenteral nutrition, ingestion of > 3 g elemental calcium per day)
- Laboratory evaluation:
  - serum calcium and albumin (see Table 1 to calculate correction) *or* ionized calcium
  - serum phosphate, serum creatinine, BUN, 24-hour urine creatinine and calcium
  - alkaline phosphatase (fractionated for bony source, if available)
  - serum parathyroid hormone
  - other tests based on history or physical findings of hypercalcemia-associated conditions, as required

Therapeutic Choices (Figure 1)

- Aggressiveness of initial interventions depends on the magnitude of the hypercalcemia.
- Definitive therapy for long-term control of hypercalcemia requires diagnosis of the underlying condition.

Figure 1: **Management of Hypercalcemia**

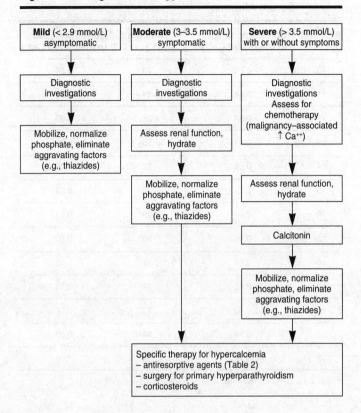

Nonpharmacologic Choices
Mobilize

Hypercalcemia is exacerbated by immobilization. Ambulation helps to reduce bone resorption and normalize serum calcium.

Diet

Dietary changes rarely correct hypercalcemia. Patients with vitamin D-mediated hypercalcemia may benefit from dietary calcium restriction. Excessive use of calcium supplements or calcium-containing antacids should be curtailed in all patients.

Pharmacologic Choices
General Measures
Stop Offending Agents

If possible, offending agents should be discontinued and replaced with agents that do not exacerbate hypercalcemia.

Table 1: Serum Calcium Correction (mmol/L) for Low Serum Albumin*

Albumin (g/L)	Correction (add to measured Ca++)	Albumin (g/L)	Correction (add to measured Ca++)
10	0.60	23	0.34
11	0.58	24	0.32
12	0.56	25	0.30
13	0.54	26	0.28
14	0.52	27	0.26
15	0.50	28	0.24
16	0.48	29	0.22
17	0.46	30	0.20
18	0.44	31	0.18
19	0.42	32	0.16
20	0.40	33	0.14
21	0.38	34	0.12
22	0.36	35	0.10

* $(40 - measured\ albumin)(0.02) + measured\ Ca^{++} = corrected\ Ca^{++}\ value.$

Hydrate

Expansion of intravascular volume enhances renal calcium clearance. Hydration alone usually reduces serum calcium by ≤ 0.6 mmol/L. This effect is present only while hydration is administered. Serum magnesium and potassium may also decrease. They should be monitored and replaced as needed.

Patients with mild to moderate asymptomatic hypercalcemia should drink 3 L per day of noncaffeinated beverages to achieve and maintain euvolemia. Patients with moderate to severe symptomatic hypercalcemia should receive 0.9% NaCl injection until euvolemic, then the infusion rate should be reduced to maintain normal hydration. Volume correction may require 2 to 3 L of fluid within the first 8 hours. Patients with a significant volume deficit may need 3 to 5 L of fluid therapy in the first 24 hours. Renal dysfunction, a result of volume loss or permanent renal damage, is common among hypercalcemic patients. Careful monitoring of hydration is essential, especially in elderly patients and those with permanent renal damage.

A loop diuretic (e.g., furosemide) should be used to prevent fluid overload and heart failure, as needed, but only after dehydration is corrected. Thiazide diuretics are contraindicated because they impair calcium excretion.

Normalize Serum Phosphate

Hypophosphatemia (seen mostly in primary hypoparathyroidism and malignancy-associated hypercalcemia) exacerbates hypercalcemia by increasing renal synthesis of 1,25–dihydroxy-vitamin D, reducing bone formation and increasing bone resorption. Oral phosphates (1 to 2 g elemental phosphate per day) can be safely given in all patients except those with renal insufficiency, to increase serum phosphate into the low normal range (0.8 to 1 mmol/L). Calcium phosphate can precipitate and cause serious organ damage (heart, kidney, lungs, blood vessels) if phosphate levels are increased to > 1 mmol/L or if IV phosphate is administered.

Specific Measures (Table 2)
Primary Hyperparathyroidism

Surgery is the first-line measure for control of primary hyperparathyroidism. In the < 10% of patients for whom surgery is not an option, pharmacologic therapy may be required. **Estrogen** therapy (conjugated estrogens 0.625 to 2.5 mg per day) lowers serum calcium concentrations (0.25 to 0.5 mmol/L) without affecting parathyroid hormone levels in postmenopausal women. This may be useful for women with mild to moderate hyperparathyroidism. Oral **phosphate** therapy can also be used if the dose is titrated to normalize serum calcium, and appropriate monitoring is provided.

Granulomatous Diseases

Excess production of 1,25–dihydroxyvitamin D is characteristic of granulomatous diseases. Specific therapy includes restriction of vitamin D and calcium intake, and avoiding excessive exposure to sunlight. **Corticosteroids** counteract the effects of vitamin D. Hydrocortisone 200 to 300 mg IV is given every 3 to 5 days in acutely ill patients. Ambulatory patients may benefit from oral prednisone (or equivalent) 25 mg per day. The dose should be tapered when calcium control is achieved.

Malignancy

Antineoplastic therapy aimed at the underlying malignancy is the key to long-term calcium control. Not all patients, however, are candidates for this therapy. **Bisphosphonates** are first-line drugs if effective antineoplastic therapy is not available

Table 2: Antiresorptive Agents for Treatment of Hypercalcemia

Drug	Dosage	Adverse Effects	Comments	Cost*
calcitonin salmon Calcimar, Caltine	3–8 IU/kg Q12H SC max. 8 IU/kg Q6H	Nausea, vomiting (dose dependent), hypersensitivity reactions.	Inhibits release of Ca^{++} from bone and stimulates urinary Ca^{++} excretion. Used for rapid early effect (within 6 h). Tachyphylaxis develops in 2–7 d; combining with glucocorticoids may ↑ efficacy and ↓ tachyphylaxis. Use with bisphosphonate for long-term control. Extent of Ca^{++} lowering ≤ 0.2 mmol/L. Skin test before therapy if suspected sensitivity.	$$–$$$$$/5 d
clodronate disodium ⬥ Bonefos, Ostac	300 mg/d IV over 2 h (usually × 5 d) or 600–1 500 mg IV single dose over 2 h 800–1 600 mg PO BID (2 h AC or 2 h PC)	Uncommon. GI upset, diarrhea, muscle cramps.	**Dilute in 0.5–1 L saline or dextrose before infusion;** fatal acute renal failure reported from infusion < 2 h. Onset – 2 d; maximal effect – 6 d; duration – variable (2–3 wks in hypercalcemia of malignancy). Significant drug interactions with PO iron, calcium, magnesium, aluminum (e.g., antacids).	$$$/5 d $–$$/single dose $$–$$$$/30 d
etidronate disodium ⬥ Didronel IV	7.5 mg/kg/d IV over 2 h × 3 d	Febrile reaction within 24–48 h, interferes with normal bone mineralization and increases risk of fractures with long-term exposure.	**Dilute in ≥ 250 mL saline or dextrose before infusion;** acute renal failure reported with infusions ≤ 2 h. Onset – 24 h; maximal effect – 72 h after first dose.	$$$/3 d
pamidronate disodium ⬥ Aredia	30–90 mg IV over 2 h single dose	Febrile reaction within 24–48 h of infusion.	Same as clodronate.	$–$$$$/ single dose

| plicamycin †● (mithramycin) Mithracin | 12.5–25 µg/kg IV over 4–12 h | Nausea, vomiting (worse with rapid infusion), renal tubular necrosis, thrombocytopenia, hepatotoxicity. | Very effective, potent agent. Onset 6–12 h; maximal effect – 10 d; duration up to 6 wks. Risk of bone marrow toxicity ↑ if dose is repeated. Rarely used – safer alternatives available. May be given in smaller fluid volume; therefore, an alternative agent in heart failure or fluid overload. | † |

● Dosage adjustment may be required in renal impairment — see Appendix I.
† Available through the Special Access Program (formerly the Emergency Drug Release Program), Therapeutic Products Directorate, Health Canada.

* Cost of supply for specified treatment period – drug cost only.
Legend: $ < $200 $$ $200–300 $$$ $300–400 $$$$ $400–500 $$$$$ > $500

or appropriate, or if the patient has severe hypercalcemia (> 3.5 mmol/L, with or without symptoms). For acute management, parenteral **pamidronate** or **clodronate** are drugs of choice. **Etidronate** is also effective but requires repeated daily doses, has a higher risk of renal toxicity, and is more likely to interfere with normal bone mineralization. In patients who respond, prolonged therapy with clodronate or pamidronate can maintain calcium at acceptable levels. Patients with multiple myeloma or selected solid tumors also benefit from reduced bone pain, slower progression of bony disease and prevention of hypercalcemia recurrence if prolonged therapy is used. Recent information about the safety of rapid infusion techniques makes outpatient IV bisphosphonate therapy more convenient. Although other bisphosphonates (e.g., alendronate) might also be effective, there are insufficient data to recommend their use in hypercalcemic states.

Therapeutic Tips

- Overly aggressive use of loop diuretics can aggravate hypercalcemia by depleting extracellular fluid volume. Routine prescription of a loop diuretic with hydration therapy is discouraged.

- To reduce serum calcium rapidly (within 6 to 12 hours) in severe hypercalcemia of malignancy, use calcitonin plus hydration. Serum calcium usually declines ≤ 0.8 mmol/L at 12 to 24 hours following combined therapy. To augment and prolong serum calcium control, give definitive therapy (e.g., chemotherapy) for the underlying cause. If chemotherapy is not an option, give a bisphosphonate when dehydration is corrected and adequate urine output is achieved (preferably within 24 hours of hypercalcemia diagnosis).

- Premedication with acetaminophen 650 mg can prevent bisphosphonate-induced fever in patients with hypercalcemia of malignancy.

- Adjunctive glucocorticoid therapy (e.g., prednisone 40 to 100 mg per day for up to 1 week) is particularly useful in patients with lymphoma, myeloma, lymphoid leukemia and breast cancer (if hypercalcemic flare is caused by hormonal treatment).

Suggested Reading List

Bilezikian JP. Management of acute hypercalcemia. *N Engl J Med* 1992;30:1196–1203.

Chisolm MA, Mulloy AL, Taylor AT. Acute management of cancer-related hypercalcemia. *Ann Pharmacother* 1996;30:507–513.

Consensus Development Conference Panel. Diagnosis and management of asymptomatic primary hyperparathyroidism: consensus development conference statement. *Ann Intern Med* 1991;114:593–597.

Kaye TB. Hypercalcemia: how to pinpoint the cause and customize treatment. *Postgrad Med J* 1995;97:153–156, 159–160.

CHAPTER 80

Potassium Disturbances

Jean Ethier, MD, FRCPC

Goals of Therapy

- To restore the ratio of intracellular to extracellular potassium to prevent life-threatening cardiac arrhythmias and improve neuromuscular conductivity
- To re-establish normal body stores of potassium (K^+) and prevent undue losses or accumulations

Investigations

- History with attention to possible etiology (Table 1)
- Physical examination to assess cardiac rhythm, paresis, muscle weakness, paresthesias, blood pressure (in suspected hypokalemia)
- Laboratory tests:
  - urea, creatinine, Na^+, K^+, Cl^-, glucose
  - arterial or venous gases or total CO_2
  - spot urine for Na^+, K^+, Cl^- and osmolality to calculate the transtubular K^+ concentration gradient (TTKG); 24-hour urine collection for Na^+, K^+ and creatinine
  - renin, aldosterone, cortisol in selected cases
  - magnesium in refractory hypokalemia, especially when patient is at risk for hypomagnesemia (e.g., taking diuretics, cisplatinum)

Table 1: Common Causes of Potassium Disturbances

Hyperkalemia	Hypokalemia
Drug-induced: K^+ supplements, NSAIDs, ACE inhibitors, K^+-sparing diuretics, digoxin overdose, cyclosporine, trimethoprim or co-trimoxazole (high-dose or in susceptible patients i.e., elderly, renal failure), heparin, beta-blockers, pentamidine	Diarrhea, vomiting
	Inadequate dietary intake
	Drug-induced: diuretics, laxatives, amphotericin, aminoglycosides, long-term corticosteroid therapy, antipseudomonal penicillins
Digoxin use (potentiates risk of arrhythmia)	Digoxin use (potentiates risk of arrhythmia)
Renal failure, diabetes, adrenal insufficiency	Familial history (Bartter's syndrome)
Familial history of hyperkalemia	Mineralocorticoid excess (hypertension)
Acidosis	Metabolic alkalosis
Crush injury, trauma, hemolysis, tumor lysis	Osmotic diuresis (diabetes)

Figure 1: **Management of Hyperkalemia**

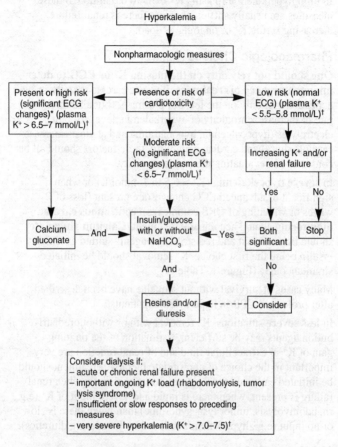

* Loss of P waves or widening of QRS complexes or more severe changes are considered significant but not isolated peaked T waves.

† Plasma potassium level is given only as indicative; **therapy should not rely only on the plasma level.**

- rule out pseudohyperkalemia (possible with thrombocytosis, severe leukocytosis, in vitro hemolysis or forearm contraction)
- ECG

Hyperkalemia

Therapeutic Choices (Figure 1)

Nonpharmacologic Choices

- K⁺ supplements and drugs inducing hyperkalemia should be stopped.

- Dietary K^+ intake should be reduced to ≤ 60 mmol/d.

In mild hyperkalemia (plasma $K^+ < 5.5$ to 6.0 mmol/L) these measures are usually sufficient unless there is renal failure, increasing serum K^+ or ongoing K^+ load.

Pharmacologic Choices (Table 2)

One should not rely only on the plasma K^+ or ECG to determine the urgency of treatment. Because cardiac toxicity is dependent not only on the level of plasma K^+ but also on the rate of increase, chronicity of hyperkalemia, levels of other electrolytes (hypocalcemia, hyponatremia and acidosis increase cardiotoxicity) and cardiac irritability, these factors should all be considered in evaluating the cardiac toxicity.

In **severe hyperkalemia** ($K^+ > 6.5$ to 7 mmol/L) or when significant or advanced ECG changes are present (loss of P waves or widening of QRS complexes), **continuous cardiac monitoring** should accompany treatment. **Calcium gluconate** should be used first and redistribution agents started quickly, insulin being the first choice. K^+ removal should be initiated simultaneously (Figure 1, Table 2).

Many cases of survival without sequelae have been described after prolonged CPR in hyperkalemic patients.

In **less severe** situations, K^+ removal with or without redistribution agents may be sufficient. Estimation of the ongoing gain of K^+ in extracellular fluid and of renal function are very important in the choice of appropriate therapy. Treatment should be initiated early and more aggressively, especially when renal failure is present, when there is rapid and severe input of K^+ (e.g., rhabdomyolysis, tumor lysis syndrome) than when there is slow or no input (e.g., hyperkalemia induced by K^+-sparing diuretics).

Membrane Antagonists

Hyperkalemia reduces the magnitude of the resting potential (RP) (less negative) that approaches the threshold potential (TP), leading to an increased risk of arrhythmia and conduction defects. Membrane antagonists correct the difference between RP and TP in excitable tissues. They have a rapid onset but a relatively short duration of action.

IV infusion of **calcium gluconate** raises the TP, restoring the difference between the TP and the RP. **NB:** Calcium should be infused more slowly in patients receiving digoxin because of the risk of hypercalcemia-induced digoxin toxicity.

Redistribution Agents

Redistribution agents promote an intracellular shift of K^+ and increase [$K_{intracellular}$]/[$K_{extracellular}$] (RP). These agents act quickly and for a longer period than membrane antagonists.

Table 2: Treatment of Hyperkalemia

Therapy	Dose	Onset (O), Duration (D) of Action	Comments
calcium gluconate 10%	10–20 mL IV over 2–5 min; may repeat once after 5 min (depending on ECG)	O: 1–3 min D: 30–60 min	Continuous ECG monitoring required; ↑ digoxin toxicity; incompatible with NaHCO₃-containing solutions (precipitation).
hypertonic saline (NaCl 3%)	50–100 mmol IV	O: 5–10 min D: 2 h	Risk of hypertonicity.
sodium bicarbonate (NaHCO₃)	50–100 mmol IV over 5 min; repeat Q10–15 min (depending on ECG)	O: variable, within 1 h D: 2 h	Variable response; risk of tetany if hypocalcemia present (give calcium first); watch for Na⁺ overload.
insulin with glucose	Bolus: 5–10 units IV with 25–50 g of glucose over 5 min. If less urgent, infuse 10 units insulin in 500 mL of 10% dextrose	O: 30 min D: 4–6 h	Risk of hypoglycemia.
salbutamol Ventolin, generics	10–20 mg by nebulizer	O: 30 min D: 2–4 h	Reserved for life-threatening cases when other treatments have failed; risk of arrhythmia or angina; variable response.
sodium polystyrene sulfonate resin Kayexalate, generics	PO: 20–30 g in 50–100 mL of 20% sorbitol Q4–6H PRN PR: 30–50 g in 100–200 mL of water or 10% dextrose Q4–6H PRN; retain at least 30–60 min	O: 1–2 h PO 30–60 min PR D: 4–6 h	Constipating; watch for Na⁺ overload; risk of colonic ulceration or necrosis with hypertonic enema. Cleansing enema before PR use recommended. Cleansing enema after PR use is to be given after evacuation of the resins or after retention for 1–6 h.
furosemide ● Lasix, generics	40–250 mg PO/IV depending on renal function	O: 30–60 min D: to end of increased diuresis (about 4–6 h)	Risk of volume depletion; transient ototoxicity with high-dose furosemide.

● *Dosage adjustment may be required in renal impairment – see Appendix I.*

Insulin increases the cellular uptake of K^+ independent of glucose uptake. This effect is proportional to insulinemia; to achieve the expected result, insulin must be administered IV. **Glucose** (40 to 50 g per 10 units insulin) is given to avoid hypoglycemia. Bolus administration of glucose should be avoided because the acute increase in plasma tonicity can induce a rise in plasma K^+.

The correction of metabolic acidosis with **sodium bicarbonate (NaHCO$_3$)** induces an intracellular shift of K^+. $NaHCO_3$ administration in the absence of a low serum bicarbonate concentration or pH has a similar effect but to a much smaller degree. $NaHCO_3$ administration also can induce bicarbonaturia with an increase in renal K^+ excretion. The increased Na^+ concentration has a membrane antagonist effect. To avoid an acute increase in K^+, hypertonic $NaHCO_3$ solutions should not be used.

Insulin administration may be faster, more reliable and more effective than $NaHCO_3$. $NaHCO_3$ may not be useful as the sole initial treatment of hyperkalemia, especially if there is no, or only mild, acidosis present. It has, however, a synergistic effect with insulin in the presence of mild metabolic acidosis. $NaHCO_3$ is still recommended when severe acidosis is present. **NB:** The correction of acidosis in hypocalcemic patients may induce tetany.

The beta$_2$-agonist, **salbutamol**, is effective in lowering plasma K^+. Its effect is similar to insulin, but the mechanism is different; concurrent administration of insulin and salbutamol has a synergistic effect. High doses of nebulized salbutamol have a similar effect to IV salbutamol; however, up to 50% of renal failure patients are resistant to this therapy. Salbutamol should be reserved for young patients or life-threatening situations when other therapies have failed, because it is arrhythmogenic and has the potential to exacerbate angina.

Potassium Removal

Cation-exchange resins (e.g., sodium polystyrene sulfonate) promote the exchange of Na^+ for K^+ in the bowel; they also bind calcium and magnesium. **NB:** The Na^+ released in exchange for K^+ (2 mmol of Na^+ per mmol of K^+) may lead to volume overload. Because they are constipating, they must be given with a laxative, usually sorbitol. Sorbitol-induced diarrhea can enhance K^+ loss. Oral administration is more effective but is much slower than the rectal route.

Rectal ulceration or colonic necrosis has been described when sodium polystyrene sulfonate mixed in sorbitol is given orally or by enema postoperatively. Necrosis may be caused by sorbitol rather than by resins. The duration of drug contact with the mucosa may be a risk factor. A cleansing enema (sodium-free) is recommended to reduce the risk. Use of sorbitol should be

avoided when the resin is administered by enema, especially in postoperative patients.

The administration of **loop diuretics** in patients with sufficient renal function can significantly increase renal K^+ excretion.

Dialysis

If large amounts of K^+ need to be removed rapidly, **hemodialysis** is the technique of choice. Because time is required to prepare the equipment and to insert a catheter, other treatments must be initiated while preparing for dialysis. Continuous hemodialysis may also be useful. Peritoneal dialysis is far less efficient in acutely reducing plasma K^+.

Therapeutic Tips

- The treatment of chronic hyperkalemia should focus on the cause or pathophysiological mechanism (Table 1). The modalities are similar to the ones used in acute hyperkalemia ($NaHCO_3$, diuretics, resins).
- Mineralocorticoids (9-alpha-fludrocortisone) may be used in patients with hypoaldosteronism.

Hypokalemia

Therapeutic Choices

Nonpharmacologic Choices

- Reduce or stop medication leading to K^+ loss if clinically appropriate.
- Determine and treat the etiology (Table 1).
- If the deficit is slight (plasma K^+ = 3.0 to 3.5 mmol/L) and there are no ongoing losses or clinical conditions warranting prompt treatment, dietary intake of potassium-rich foods should be adequate. If there are still unusual losses, K^+ supplements will be needed.

Pharmacologic Choices

The appropriate pharmacologic approach is determined by:

- **Relative urgency for treatment** (Table 3).
- The **estimated deficit** for an adult with plasma K^+ = 3.0 mmol/L is approximately 200 to 400 mmol and for plasma K^+ = 2.0 mmol/L, approximately 500 to 700 mmol. **NB:** The true deficit will be *smaller* with an intracellular shift of potassium (e.g., periodic paralysis or hyperadrenergic state) and *larger* with an extracellular shift of potassium (e.g., acidosis or insulin deficit).

Fluid and Electrolyte Disorders

Table 3: **Management of Hypokalemia**

Urgency to Treat	Clinical Status	Rate of K^+ Administration
Urgent (immediate treatment required)	Severe hypokalemia (plasma K^+ < 2.5 mmol/L) Symptomatic hypokalemia (respiratory muscle weakness or paresis, paralysis) Cardiac arrhythmia or conduction disturbances	20–40 mmol* in the first hour with continuous ECG monitoring and frequent serum K^+ measurements to adjust further rate of administration. When plasma K^+ = 3.0 mmol/L, remaining deficit should be corrected more slowly.
Less urgent (prompt treatment required)	Plasma K^+ = 2.5–3.0 mmol/L Hypokalemia with digitalis toxicity, myocardial infarction or ischemia Hypokalemia with diabetic ketoacidosis (risk of insulin-induced life-threatening hypokalemia) Hypokalemia with hepatic insufficiency (risk of hepatic encephalopathy)	10–20 mmol over one hour (↑ serum K^+ by 0.25–0.5 mmol/L) with ECG monitoring if > 10 mmol/h. Should be repeated according to control value of serum K^+. The remaining deficit should be corrected more slowly.
Not urgent	Plasma K^+ > 3.0–3.5 mmol/L	Initially, 40–60 mmol/d (divided doses), preferably PO (or IV), is usually sufficient.

* *Larger quantities have been given in extreme life-threatening hypokalemia.*

- **Ongoing losses** must be added to the deficit when replacement therapy is planned. Renal losses can be estimated based on urine K^+ levels and the volume excreted per hour.

- In the presence of renal failure the treatment should be more cautious.

Potassium Salts (Table 4)

In most cases **potassium chloride** (KCl) is the salt of choice, and **oral administration** is the preferred route. If there is no paralytic ileus or suspected absorption problem, oral administration of KCl can rapidly increase plasma K^+ (40 to 60 mmol of a liquid preparation will increase plasma K^+ by 1.0 to 1.5 mmol/L).

Potassium bicarbonate or **potassium citrate** should be reserved for hypokalemic patients with metabolic acidosis (e.g., renal tubular acidosis, diarrhea). **Potassium phosphate** is used when severe hypophosphatemia is present.

IV administration of potassium should be reserved for patients requiring urgent treatment or those unable to take oral supplements (e.g., postsurgery, paralytic ileus). IV potassium should be administered via a large peripheral vein at a maximum concentration of 40 to 60 mmol/L to avoid sclerosis. Higher

Table 4: Oral Potassium Salts†

Salt	Dosage Form	Adverse Effects	Comments	Cost*
potassium chloride	Liquid or powder:‡ K-10, Kaochlor, Kay Ciel, K-Lyte/Cl, K-Lor, Roychlor, generics	Unpleasant taste, aftertaste, nausea, heartburn.	Rapid absorption, good bioavailability. Salt of choice, especially in alkalotic patients. Inconvenient for transport.	$-$$
	Wax matrix: Slow-K, Kalium Durules, generics	GI symptoms (less frequent than with liquid), GI ulceration (rare).	Avoid in patients with delayed GI transit or impaired esophageal or intestinal motility. Empty wax matrix may appear in stool.	$
	Micro-encapsulated: K-Dur, Micro-K	May be less ulceration than with wax matrix.		$
potassium citrate (bicarbonate/citric acid)	Effervescent tablets: K-Lyte	Same as potassium chloride.	Useful for patients with metabolic acidosis. More convenient for transport.	$$
	Crystals or liquid: Polycitra-K		Useful for hypokalemia secondary to thiazides given for kidney stones. ↑ urinary citrate excretion.	$$
potassium gluconate	Liquid: Kaon		Useful in patients with acidosis.	$$
potassium chloride and potassium bicarbonate	Effervescent tablets: Potassium-Sandoz		Convenient for transport.	$

† Potassium chloride and potassium phosphate are available in parenteral form.
‡ Salt substitutes also contain potassium chloride.

* Cost of 30-day supply of a 20 mmol/d dose – includes drug cost only.
Legend: $ <$10 $$ $10–20

concentrations should be administered via a central line with the catheter positioned away from the right atrium or ventricle. In patients with severe hypokalemia, K^+ should be administered in a dextrose-free solution to avoid stimulating insulin secretion and subsequent intracellular K^+ shift.

The **rate of administration** depends on the urgency to treat (Table 3).

Potassium-sparing Diuretics (Table 5)

If renal K^+ losses are involved in the pathogenesis of hypokalemia (e.g., hyperaldosteronism, concomitant use of other diuretics), K^+-sparing diuretics may be used to decrease these losses; they also prevent or decrease magnesium losses. **Triamterene, amiloride and spironolactone** are equally effective but differ in side effects. The most frequent and serious side effect is hyperkalemia.

K^+-sparing diuretics should be avoided in patients with renal or adrenal insufficiency, the elderly, patients with diabetes, and patients taking other drugs that may increase plasma K^+ (Table 1).

Therapeutic Tips

- Using K^+ supplements and K^+-sparing diuretics together greatly increases the risk of hyperkalemia and should be avoided. Combined use may be required temporarily at the beginning of replacement therapy if renal K^+ losses are very high; however, frequent monitoring of plasma K^+ is mandatory, and one of the drugs should be stopped when plasma K^+ reaches 3.0 to 3.5 mmol/L.

Table 5: **Potassium-sparing Diuretics***

Drug	Dosage	Adverse Effects
spironolactone ❥ Aldactone, generics	25–200 mg/d (in single or divided doses); up to 400 mg/d in patients with hyperaldosteronism	Hyperkalemia, gynecomastia, androgen-like side effects, GI symptoms
triamterene ❥ Dyrenium	50–300 mg/d (in single or divided doses)	Hyperkalemia, muscle cramps, GI symptoms, triamterene renal stones (1 in 1 500), acute renal failure (especially with NSAIDs)
amiloride ❥ Midamor	5–20 mg/d	Hyperkalemia, muscle cramps, headaches, GI symptoms (rare)

* *For information on drug interactions and costs, see Chapter 77.*

❥ *Dosage adjustment may be required in renal impairment – see Appendix I.*

Suggested Reading List

Allon M. Treatment and prevention of hyperkalemia in end-stage renal disease. *Kidney Int* 1993;43:1197–1209.

DeFronzo RA, Smith JD. Clinical disorders of hyperkalemia. In: Narins RG, ed. *Clinical disorders of fluid and electrolyte metabolism*. 5th ed. New York: McGraw-Hill, 1994:697–754.

Halperin ML, Goldstein MB. Hyperkalemia. In: Dyson J, ed. *Fluid, electrolyte and acid-base emergencies*. Philadelphia: W.B. Saunders, 1988:252–273.

Halperin ML, Goldstein MB. Hypokalemia. In: Dyson J, ed. *Fluid, electrolyte and acid-base emergencies*. Philadelphia: W.B. Saunders, 1988:228–251.

Krishna GG, Steigerwalt SP, Pikus R, et al. Hypokalemic states. In: Narins RG, ed. *Clinical disorders of fluid and electrolyte metabolism*. 5th ed. New York: McGraw-Hill, 1994:659–696.

Rose BD. *Clinical physiology of acid-base and electrolyte disorders*. 4th ed. New York: McGraw-Hill, 1994:776–799.

CHAPTER 81

Acute Otitis Media in Childhood

Ross A. Pennie, MD, FRCPC

Definition

Acute otitis media (AOM) is a suppurative infection of the middle ear cavity. It occurs most commonly in preschool children. Affected children usually have earache and fever and may appear toxic. Two-thirds of cases are due to bacteria; the remaining third are probably due to viruses, *Mycoplasma* and *Chlamydia*. While most patients recover without antibiotics, it has been shown that antibiotic therapy hastens the resolution of symptoms and reduces the incidence of complications such as mastoiditis and meningitis.

Goals of Therapy

- To control pain
- To eradicate infection
- To prevent complications
- To avoid unnecessary antibiotics

Investigations

- Presenting signs of earache in children:
  - children will usually describe an earache
  - infants react by crying, sleeplessness, irritability
- Inspection of the eardrum (otoscopy):
  - wax and debris should be removed from the ear canal to obtain a clear view
  - the eardrum should be examined for opacity, bulging, loss of light reflex, loss of ossicular landmarks and redness

NB: The following also cause redness of the eardrum in children **without** AOM:

  - crying and agitation
  - the common cold
  - chronic otitis media with effusion
  - aggressive examination or manipulation of the external ear canal

- If the diagnosis of AOM is uncertain, the presence of fluid/pus behind the eardrum should be determined by looking for one of the following:
  - decreased drum mobility on pneumatic otoscopy
  - abnormal profile on tympanometry
  - abnormal reading with acoustic otoscope
- Examination for other causes of apparent earache:
  - pharyngitis, tonsillitis
  - tooth abscess
  - foreign body in the ear canal
- Examination for complications of AOM:
  - ruptured eardrum (perforation visible, pus oozing)
  - mastoiditis (tender, boggy, swollen mastoid region)
  - intracranial infection (lethargy, confusion, stiff neck, vomiting, focal neurologic signs)

Therapeutic Choices (Figure 1)

Nonpharmacologic Choices

- Heat applied to the painful ear may provide comfort to an older child.
- Aspiration of pus from the middle ear cavity (tympanocentesis or myringotomy) may relieve the infection when earache and fever do not resolve after 3 days of antibiotics.

Pharmacologic Choices

- Acetaminophen is indicated for pain relief.
- Oral antihistamines and decongestants have been shown **not** to improve outcome.
- Antibiotic therapy is the mainstay of treatment (Tables 1 and 2).

The choice of antibiotic rests mainly on which one of the following three scenarios best represents the episode of AOM:

New Infections (Table 1):
  - no episodes of AOM have occurred in previous 2 months
  - most bacterial causes are susceptible to amoxicillin
  - co-trimoxazole is an effective, low-cost alternative for patients allergic to penicillin

Failure of current treatment or recurrence within 2 months after an episode of AOM (Table 2). Such infections may be due to:
  - beta-lactamase-producing bacteria resistant to amoxicillin or pivampicillin
  - Pneumococci with reduced susceptibility to penicillins and cephalosporins (higher dose is needed). Such strains are often resistant to macrolides
  - organisms resistant to co-trimoxazole

Infection in a newborn less than 1 month of age:
  - gram-negative enteric bacteria frequently cause AOM in this age group
  - hospital admission to rule out bacterial sepsis and initial treatment with IV ampicillin and cefotaxime are recommended

Figure 1: **Management of Acute Otitis Media**

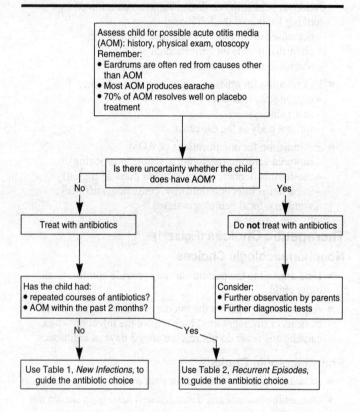

Therapeutic Tips

- Two weeks after the start of successful antibiotic therapy, 80% of children with AOM may have middle ear effusions (and thus abnormal-looking eardrums). Do not prescribe antibiotics for a child who looks and feels better but has abnormal-appearing eardrums on follow-up.

- Optimal duration of therapy has not been determined for most antibiotics (usually 7 to 10 days). A 5-day course of azithromycin is effective.

Prevention of Recurrent Acute Otitis Media

- Children with more than 3 episodes of AOM in a 6-month period should be considered for prophylaxis; unfortunately, even the most effective interventions are associated with only modest reductions in AOM episodes.

Table 1: Antibiotics for *New Episodes* of Acute Otitis Media*

Antibiotic	Pediatric Dosage	Advantages	Disadvantages	Cost†
amoxicillin 🍂 Amoxil, generics	40–60 mg/kg/d divided TID‡	Effective against 85–90% of bacteria that cause AOM. Excellent safety profile. Used orally instead of ampicillin because of better absorption.	Occasionally causes mild diarrhea. Maculopapular skin rash occurs uncommonly but is difficult to distinguish from a concomitant viral exanthem.	Chewable tabs $$–$$$ Liquid $ Caps $
co-trimoxazole 🍂 Bactrim, Septra, generics	8–10 mg/kg/d trimethoprim divided BID	BID dosing. Liquid formulation has a long shelf-life at room temperature, making the drug suitable for travelers.	Not active against group A *Streptococcus*. Resistance is increasing among strains of Pneumococci and *H. influenzae*. Probably causes rash more commonly than amoxicillin. May cause leukopenia if taken for several weeks.	$
pivampicillin 🍂 Pondocillin	60–80 mg/kg/d divided BID‡	Better absorbed than ampicillin; therefore, higher blood levels can be achieved, permitting BID dosing. Same excellent safety profile as amoxicillin.	No improvement in antibacterial spectrum or side effect profile compared to amoxicillin, despite ↑ cost.	$$–$$$

* The child has had no episodes of AOM within the preceding 2 mos.

🍂 Dosage adjustment may be required in renal impairment – see Appendix I. In acute otitis media the recommended dosages are moderate and thus adjustments are not usually necessary.

† Cost of 10-day supply – includes drug cost only.

Legend: $ < $10 $$ $10–20 $$$ $20–30

‡ Ontario Anti-infective Review Panel. Anti-infective Guidelines for Community-acquired infections. 2nd edition, 1997:85–87.

Table 2: Antibiotics for *Recurrent Episodes* of Acute Otitis Media*

Antibiotic	Pediatric Dosage	Advantages	Disadvantages	Cost†
amoxicillin/ clavulanic acid Clavulin	40–60 mg/kg/d amoxicillin divided TID‡	Excellent safety profile of amoxicillin. Active against most bacteria likely to cause AOM.	Diarrhea occurs in about 50% of patients but does not necessarily lead to discontinuing the drug.	$$$–$$$$
cefaclor Ceclor	40 mg/kg/d divided BID or TID	Active against most bacteria likely to cause AOM.	Antimicrobial activity in vitro not as great as with other similar drugs. Serum-sickness reaction in about 1% of children.	$$$
cefixime Suprax	8 mg/kg/d given once daily	Active against amoxicillin-resistant strains of *H. influenzae* and *M. catarrhalis*. Once daily dosing.	Not active against *S. aureus*. Poor in vitro activity vs Pneumococci exhibiting reduced susceptibility to penicillins and cephalosporins. Diarrhea occurs in about 10% of patients.	$$$
cefprozil Cefzil	30 mg/kg/d divided BID	Active against most bacteria likely to cause AOM. Good-tasting liquid formulation is well absorbed. Low incidence of diarrhea or gastro-intestinal upset.		$$$$

cefuroxime axetil 🔎 Ceftin	30–40 mg/kg/d divided BID	Active against most bacteria likely to cause AOM. Pediatric suspension is available as single-dose sachets suitable for travelers.	Diarrhea occurs more frequently when higher doses are used. Because of the potential to cause bitter after-taste, Ceftin suspension should be taken with food and/or juice.	$$$$
azithromycin Zithromax	First day: 10 mg/kg Days 2–5: 5 mg/kg Administer once daily at bedtime	Active against most bacteria likely to cause AOM. Good-tasting liquid formulation. Low incidence of diarrhea or gastrointestinal upset. Convenient once daily dosing and short 5-day course	Pneumococci exhibiting reduced susceptibility to penicillins and cephalosporins are often resistant to azithromycin.	$$$
clarithromycin 🔎 Biaxin	15 mg/kg/d divided BID	Active against most bacteria likely to cause AOM. Better tolerated than erythromycin.	Pneumococci exhibiting reduced susceptibility to penicillins and cephalosporins are often resistant to clarithromycin. Diarrhea or vomiting occur in 15% of patients. Because of the potential to cause bitter after-taste, Biaxin suspension should be taken with food and/or juice.	$$$$
erythromycin/sulfisoxazole 🔎 Pediazole	40 mg/kg/d erythromycin divided TID or QID	Active against most bacteria likely to cause AOM.	About 40% of patients experience abdominal pain, nausea or vomiting because of the erythromycin component. Rashes are probably more common with sulfonamides than other antibiotics.	$$

(cont'd)

Table 2: Antibiotics for Recurrent Episodes of Acute Otitis Media* (cont'd)

Antibiotic	Pediatric Dosage	Advantages	Disadvantages	Cost†
co-trimoxazole 🌑 Bactrim, Septra, generics	8–10 mg/kg/d of trimethoprim divided BID	BID dosing. Liquid formulation has a long shelf-life at room temperature, making the drug suitable for travelers.	Not active against group A *Streptococcus*. Resistance is increasing among strains of Pneumococci and *H. influenzae*. Probably causes rash more commonly than amoxicillin, cefixime and cefuroxime. May cause leukopenia if taken for several weeks.	$

* Failure of current treatment or recurrence within 2 mos after an episode of AOM.

🌑 Dosage adjustment may be required in renal impairment – see Appendix I. In acute otitis media the recommended dosages are moderate and thus adjustments are not usually necessary.

† Cost of 10-day supply except 5-day supply for azithromycin – includes drug cost only.

Legend: $ < $10 $$ $10–20 $$$ $20–30 $$$$ $30–40

‡ Ontario Anti-infective Review Panel. Anti-infective Guidelines for Community-acquired infections. 2nd edition, 1997:85–87.

Figure 2: **Management of Serous Otitis Media (SOM)**

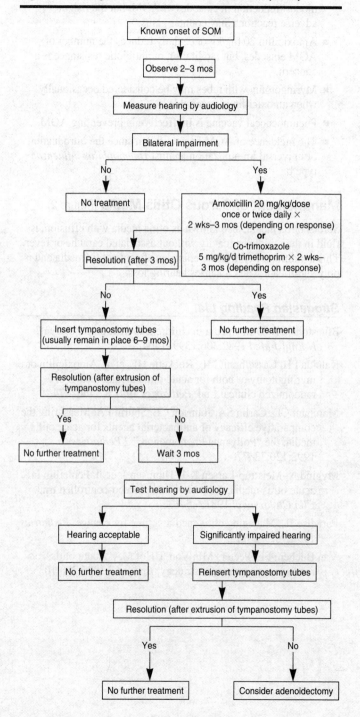

- Studies of prolonged courses of sulfonamides have shown modest reduction in episodes of AOM, but the risk of adverse reactions may counter gains.

- Amoxicillin 20 mg/kg once daily reduces the number of AOM episodes, but facilitation of antibiotic resistance is a concern.

- Myringotomy with tubes may be considered occasionally when amoxicillin is unsuitable.

- Pneumococcal vaccine is **ineffective** in preventing AOM.

- The incidence of AOM has not fallen since the introduction of universal immunization against *Haemophilus influenzae* type b.

Management of Serous Otitis Media (Figure 2)

Serous otitis media, also known as otitis media with effusion, is fluid in the middle ear cavity without associated earache or fever. This condition often follows episodes of acute otitis media and is only significant when it causes hearing loss.

Suggested Reading List

Bluestone CD. Otitis media in children: to treat or not to treat? *N Engl J Med* 1982;306:1399–1404.

Kaleida PH, Casselbrant ML, Rockette HE, et al. Amoxicillin or myringotomy or both for acute otitis media: results of a randomized clinical trial. *Pediatrics* 1991;87:466–474.

Marchant CD, Carlin SA, Johnson CE, Shurin PA. Measuring the comparative efficacy of antibacterial agents for acute otitis media: the "Pollyanna Phenomenon." *J Pediatrics* 1992;120:72–77.

Mygind N, Meistrup-Larsen K-I, Thomsen J, et al. Penicillin in acute otitis media: a double-blind placebo-controlled trial. *Clin Otolaryngol* 1981;6:5–13.

Paradise JL. Managing otitis media; a time for change. *Pediatrics* 1995;96:712–713.

Van Buchem FL, Peeters MF, Van'T Hof MA. Acute otitis media: a new treatment strategy. *Br Med J* 1985;290:1033.

CHAPTER 82

Streptococcal Sore Throat

David P. Speert, MD, FRCPC

Goals of Therapy

- To provide symptomatic relief
- To prevent suppurative complications
- To prevent nonsuppurative complications (acute rheumatic fever and poststreptococcal glomerulonephritis)
- To prevent spread of group A streptococci to contacts

Investigations

NB: Probability of culturing group A streptococci is greatest in a child with an acute sore throat who is > 3 years, lacks signs of a viral upper respiratory infection and has signs and symptoms as listed below. However, the diagnosis of streptococcal pharyngitis (strep throat) should be considered seriously in any child presenting with an acute sore throat, with or without "classical" signs and symptoms.

- Differential diagnosis: a partial list of etiologic agents for acute sore throat includes:

Streptococcus, group A

Streptococcus, groups C and G

Neisseria gonorrhoeae (if recovered from child's throat, sexual abuse should be considered)

Corynebacterium diphtheriae

Viruses (adenoviruses, enteroviruses, cytomegalovirus, Epstein-Barr, influenza and parainfluenza viruses)

*Mycoplasma pneumoniae**

*Chlamydia trachomatis**

*Arcanobacterium hemolyticum**

*Chlamydia pneumoniae**

*role in acute pharyngitis is controversial

- Clinical diagnosis of streptococcal infection: adenitis and positive throat cultures are the only predictive features. Although not diagnostic, signs and symptoms include:
  - signs: tender cervical adenopathy, erythematous pharynx and tonsils, pharyngeal exudate, excoriated nares, scarlatiniform rash
  - symptoms: sore throat, headache, abdominal pain, nausea, vomiting, fever (Chapter 105)

Figure 1: **Management of Acute Sore Throat**

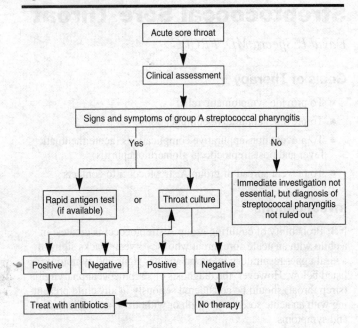

- Laboratory diagnosis:
  - throat culture is "gold standard" (results available in 24 to 48 hours). Viral throat culture rarely affects therapy (results available in days to weeks)
  - antigen screen of throat secretions (rapid test): results available in 7 to 70 minutes but only 50 to 70% sensitive
  - streptococcal serology (antistreptolysin O [ASO] and others): useful retrospectively in patients who have possible complications of streptococcal infection (e.g., rheumatic fever)

Therapeutic Choices (Figure 1)

Pharmacologic Choices (Table 1)

Antibiotic therapy for group A streptococcal pharyngitis can shorten the course of the acute illness and prevent both suppurative and nonsuppurative complications.

Penicillin is the drug of choice. **Erythromycin** is the preferred alternative in patients allergic to penicillin. Although **cephalo-sporins** are effective, they should **not** replace penicillin as the drug of choice.

Acetaminophen may be given for fever and pain. Lozenges and gargles may be indicated for symptomatic treatment of sore throat.

Table 1: Drugs for Treatment of Group A Streptococcal Pharyngitis

Drug	Dosage	Adverse Effects	Comments	Cost*
Penicillins				
penicillin V 🌸 PVF K, V-Cillin, generics	< 27 kg: 125 mg PO TID × 10 d ≥ 27 kg: 250 mg PO TID × 10 d	Hypersensitivity (mild to severe).	Drug of choice. Oral route for penicillin preferred. Should be given full 10 d for eradication of group A streptococci and prevention of rheumatic fever.	$ $$
benzathine penicillin G Bicillin L-A	< 27 kg: 600 000 units IM, single dose > 27 kg: 1 200 000 units IM, single dose	Hypersensitivity (mild to severe).	Highly efficacious. Advantage of administering entire dose. Pain of IM injection may be unacceptable to patient/parent.	$$†
Macrolides				
erythromycin estolate Ilosone, generics	20–30 mg/kg/d in 2 to 4 divided doses × 10 d Max.: 1 g/d	Nausea, vomiting, epigastric distress, diarrhea, elevated liver enzymes, cholestatic jaundice.	May ↑ blood levels of cisapride, digitalis, theophylline, warfarin, carbamazepine, astemizole, terfenadine, cyclosporine, methylprednisolone.	250 mg TID $$
erythromycin ethylsuccinate EES, generics	40–50 mg/kg/d in 2 to 4 divided doses × 10 d Max.: 1 g/d	As for erythromycin estolate.	As for erythromycin estolate.	400 mg TID $$$
clarithromycin 🌸 Biaxin	Adult: 250 mg PO BID × 10 d Children: 125 mg PO BID × 10 d	As for erythromycin estolate; lower frequency of GI effects.	Drug interactions as for erythromycin estolate. Can be taken BID.	$$$$$
azithromycin Zithromax	>16 yrs: 500 mg × 1 d, then 250 mg/d × 4 d		5-day course is effective. Less likely than other macrolides to interact with other drugs.	$$$$$

† Cost of single dose.
* Cost of 10-day supply of suspension (tablets may cost up to 50% less) except azithromycin 5-day supply of tablets – includes drug cost only.
Legend: $ < $5 $$ $5–10 $$$ $10–15 $$$$ $15–25 $$$$$ > $25

🌸 Dosage adjustment may be required in renal impairment – see Appendix I.

Therapeutic Tips

- If the antigen detection test is unavailable or is negative, a culture should be obtained and antibiotics may be withheld until the results are available in 24 to 48 hours. This approach does not increase the risk of acute rheumatic fever but avoids the unnecessary use of antibiotics. Patients with positive cultures for group A streptococci should be recalled and treated with antibiotics.

- Since there is no efficient way to differentiate between the acutely infected child and the carrier of group A streptococci, all symptomatic patients with positive cultures should receive antistreptococcal therapy. A large percentage of cases of acute rheumatic fever develop after mild or sub-clinical streptococcal infections.

- The early institution of antibiotic therapy shortens the duration of fever, cervical adenitis and pharyngeal injection and hastens the overall clinical improvement. Early treatment can hasten the return of children to school or to daycare and minimize work time lost by their parents.

- Repeat cultures are not necessary at the end of therapy, and cultures need not be obtained from asymptomatic family contacts.

- It is impossible to reliably differentiate between acute streptococcal infection and chronic carriage; a means of eradicating chronic carriage is therefore desirable. Unfortunately, penicillin, the drug of choice for treating acute streptococcal sore throat, often fails to eradicate pharyngeal streptococcal carriage. Some advocate the use of clindamycin (20 mg/kg/day divided TID for 10 days) or the addition of rifampin (20 mg/kg/day; maximum = 600 mg) for the final 4 days of penicillin therapy to attempt to interrupt chronic pharyngeal carriage of group A streptococci.

Suggested Reading List

Dajani A, Taubert K, Ferrieri P, Peter G, Shulman S. Treatment of acute streptococcal pharyngitis and prevention of rheumatic fever: a statement for health professionals. *Pediatrics* 1995;96:758–764.

Gerber MA. Treatment failures and carriers: perception or problems? *Pediatr Infect Dis J* 1994;13:576–579.

Markowitz M, Gerber MA, Kaplan EL, et al. Treatment of streptococcal pharygotonsillitis: Reports of penicillin's demise are premature. *J Pediatr* 1993;123:679–685.

Shulman ST. Evaluation of penicillins, cephalosporins and macrolides for therapy of streptococcal pharyngitis. *Pediatrics* 1996;97:955–959.

Tanz RR, Shulman ST, Barthel MJ, et al. Penicillin plus rifampin eradicates pharyngeal carriage of group A streptococci. *J Pediatr* 1985;106:876–880.

CHAPTER 83

Bacterial Meningitis

*Upton Allen, MBBS, MSc, FAAP, FRCPC and
Ronald Gold, MD, MPH, FRCPC*

Goals of Therapy

- To eradicate bacteria
- To manage acute complications (increased intracranial pressure, dehydration, seizures, subdural effusion)
- To minimize or prevent permanent neurologic damage

Investigations

Meningitis should be suspected in the following:

- **Infants less than 24 months of age:** any infant with fever and significant alteration in consciousness (irritability and/or lethargy); signs of meningeal irritation (neck stiffness, Brudzinski and Kernig signs) often lacking, especially in infants less than 6 months of age
- **Children and adults:** any person with sudden onset of fever, neck stiffness, severe headache, alteration in level of consciousness (occasionally agitation or combativeness rather than more usual lethargy or stupor)

In addition, pain on movement, vomiting and seizures may be present in all ages.

- Lumbar puncture (LP)
  - indicated in any person suspected of bacterial meningitis. The procedure is contraindicated only in the presence of **definite** signs of marked increase in intracranial pressure (coma, papilledema, decerebrate posture, hypertension, bradycardia, irregular respiration)
  - if performance of LP must be delayed, empiric antibiotic therapy should be started after blood culture obtained

- Examination of CSF
  - CSF in bacterial meningitis usually shows pleocytosis ($> 1 \times 10^9$/L WBC, mainly neutrophils), glucose ≤ 2 mmol/L and protein ≥ 0.4 g/L. However, initial CSF may have $< 1 \times 10^9$/L WBC in 33% of cases, normal glucose in 33% and normal protein in 20%
  - Gram's stain is positive in 80% of cases not previously treated with antibiotics
  - detection of bacterial antigens with latex agglutination correlates highly with Gram's stain and is most useful in cases treated with antibiotics before LP. Latex

Table 1: **Bacterial Meningitis – Risk Factors, Pathogens and Empiric Management**

Age Group/Risk Factor (Mechanism)	Pathogens	Initial Antibiotics*
Infants < 6 wks of age	E. coli Group B streptococcus Listeria monocytogenes S. pneumoniae N. meningitidis	Ampicillin + gentamicin or Ampicillin + cefotaxime
Infants 6 wks-3 mos of age (Lack of natural antibody; impaired host defenses in premature infants)	as above + H. influenzae (rare)	Ampicillin + cefotaxime
Otherwise normal infants ≥ 3 mos of age, children and adults (Lack of natural antibody up to 24 mos)	S. pneumoniae N. meningitidis H. influenzae (rare)	Ceftriaxone or Cefotaxime
Elderly (Impaired host defenses)	E. coli S. pneumoniae	Ampicillin + ceftriaxone
CNS malformation (Direct access of bacteria from skin)	S. epidermidis S. aureus S. pneumoniae	Vancomycin + cefotaxime
Head trauma (Direct access of bacteria from skin or nasal mucosa)	S. aureus S. pneumoniae	Cloxacillin
Neurosurgery (Foreign body impairs host defenses)	S. aureus S. epidermidis	Vancomycin
Chronic middle ear infection (Direct extension through petrous bone)	P. aeruginosa	Ceftazidime +/– tobramycin or amikacin
Asplenia, sickle cell disease (Impaired clearance of bacteremia; impaired IgM synthesis)	S. pneumoniae N. meningitidis H. influenzae (rare)	Ceftriaxone or Cefotaxime
Agammaglobulinemia (Lack of IgG)	S. pneumoniae N. meningitidis H. influenzae (rare)	Ceftriaxone or Cefotaxime
Terminal complement component deficiency (C5–8) (Lack of bactericidal activity against Neisseria)	N. meningitidis	Ceftriaxone or Cefotaxime
Cancer chemotherapy (Impaired cellular immunity)	S. pneumoniae N. meningitidis Listeria monocytogenes H. influenzae (rare)	Ampicillin + ceftriaxone or Ampicillin + cefotaxime

*Initial regimen should include vancomycin if S. pneumoniae is a likely possibility.

agglutination is reliable in detecting antigens in CSF of group A and C meningococci (*Neisseria meningitidis*), most pneumococci (*Streptococcus pneumoniae*), *Haemophilus influenzae* type b and group B streptococci. It is much less reliable in detecting group B meningococcal antigen

- Blood and CSF should be obtained for culture to maximize the probability of identifying the infective cause

- CT scan[1] or other imaging studies are indicated in the presence of definite signs of impending herniation due to increased intracranial pressure

Pharmacologic Choices

Antibiotic Therapy

Initial parenteral antibiotic choice should be based on age and risk factors so as to cover the most likely pathogens (Table 1). Meningitis due to *H. influenzae* type b has virtually disappeared in Canada. Because of the increasing prevalence of penicillin-resistant strains of meningococci and pneumococci, penicillin G should not be used until antibiotic susceptibilities have been determined. Once the pathogen and its antibiotic susceptibilities are known, therapy should be changed, if possible, to drug of first choice that is less expensive and/or less toxic (Tables 2 and 3).

It is currently recommended that **vancomycin** be used in addition to **ceftriaxone** or **cefotaxime** as empiric therapy for presumed pneumococcal meningitis in children older than 1 month of age, because of the problem of **penicillin- and cephalosporin-resistant pneumococci.**

Children with immediate hypersensitivity to β-lactam antibiotics may be treated empirically with vancomycin and **rifampin** if they are presumed to have pneumococcal meningitis. Treatment failures have occurred with **chloramphenicol**, which should not be used unless the organism is known to have a minimal bactericidal concentration (MBC) value of 4 μg/mL or less for this drug.[2] Since at least 3 days are required to obtain this information, the use of chloramphenicol in combination with vancomycin is not a practical option for the child with presumed pneumococcal meningitis.

Due to the fact that infants under 1 month of age may have pneumococcal meningitis, most experts recommend that vancomycin be added to the usual antibiotic combination for neonatal sepsis if: (1) the CSF shows characteristic gram-positive diplococci or (2) bacterial antigen testing suggests pneumococcal meningitis.

---

[1] *J Pediatr 1987;111:201–205.*
[2] *Pediatrics 1997;99:289–299.*

Table 2: **Antibiotic Therapy for Meningitis**

Pathogen	Drug of First Choice	Alternative	Days of Treatment*
S. pneumoniae	Penicillin G	Vancomycin, Cefotaxime, Ceftriaxone	7
N. meningitidis	Penicillin G	Ceftriaxone, Cefotaxime	5
H. influenzae type b	Ceftriaxone, Cefotaxime	Ampicillin (if β-lactamase negative)	7
Group B *Streptococcus*	Ampicillin	Penicillin	14
E. coli	Cefotaxime, Ceftriaxone	Gentamicin	21
Listeria monocytogenes	Ampicillin	Vancomycin	14

* Minimum duration of therapy.

Response Monitoring

The most important criterion for assessing response to therapy is improved brain function (i.e., improvement in level of consciousness and normalization of behavior and responsiveness). Approximately 10% of patients will have persistent or recurrent fever that is rarely caused by failure of eradication of bacteria from the CSF.

In cases of pneumococcal meningitis, a repeat lumbar puncture should be considered after 24 to 48 hours if the organism is penicillin- or cephalosporin-resistant and the patient's condition has not improved or has worsened.

Given the emergence of penicillin- and cephalosporin-resistant pneumococci, an infectious disease expert should be consulted if the patient with presumed pneumococcal meningitis does not appear to be responding to the appropriate empiric therapy (e.g., vancomycin and cefotaxime or ceftriaxone) after 24 to 48 hours.

Anti-inflammatory Therapy

The use of adjunctive dexamethasone in children over 1 month of age with bacterial meningitis is recommended to reduce the incidence of deafness and other neurologic sequelae (Table 4). Such therapy enhances the rate of resolution of inflammation. Studies have shown a reduction in the incidence of severe deafness due to *H. influenzae* type b meningitis. The effectiveness of dexamethasone in meningitis caused by other bacteria and its safety and efficacy in neonatal or adult meningitis are not known.

Table 3: Intravenous Antibiotics for Treatment of Bacterial Meningitis

Antibiotic	Dose (Maximum)	Frequency	Adverse Effects	Drug Interactions	Cost*
penicillin G 🍁 generics	70 000 units/kg/dose (2–4 million units/dose)	Q6H	Hypersensitivity, rash, drug fever, positive Coombs' test.	Tetracycline may ↓ effect.	$$
ampicillin 🍁 Ampicin, Penbritin, generics	75 mg/kg/dose (2.5 g/dose)	Q6H	Hypersensitivity, GI effects, rash, seizures with excessively rapid IV.	With allopurinol ↑ rashes.	$$
cloxacillin Orbenin, Tegopen, generics	50 mg/kg/dose (3 g/dose)	Q6H	Hypersensitivity, rash, eosinophilia.		$
ceftriaxone Rocephin	80 mg/kg/dose (2 g/dose, 4 g/d)	Q12H × 48 h, then once daily	Phlebitis, hypersensitivity, ↑ AST, superinfection.		$$$$$
cefotaxime 🍁 Claforan	50 mg/kg/dose (2 g/dose)	Q6H	Phlebitis, hypersensitivity, positive Coombs' test.		$$$$
ceftazidime 🍁 Ceptaz, Fortaz, Tazidime	50 mg/kg/dose (2 g/dose)	Q8H	Phlebitis, hypersensitivity, positive Coombs' test, ↑ AST.		$$$$$

| gentamicin ❦ Cidomycin, Garamycin | 2.5 mg/kg/dose | Q8H | Nephrotoxicity – usually reversible, ↑ risk with dose, duration; ototoxicity (often reversible). | ↑ ototoxicity with loop diuretics. ↑ nephrotoxicity with nephrotoxic drugs. Can be inactivated if mixed with some penicillins. | $$ |
| vancomycin ❦ Vancocin | 10–15 mg/kg/dose (1 g/dose) | Q6H | Phlebitis, hypotension, flushing with rapid IV. | ↑ toxicity with other ototoxic or nephrotoxic drugs. | $$$$$ |

❦ *Dosage adjustment may be required in renal impairment – see Appendix I.*
* *Cost per 70 kg per day – includes drug cost only.*
Legend: $ < $25 $$ $25–50 $$$ $50–75 $$$$ $75–100 $$$$$ > $100

Table 4: **Use of Dexamethasone in Children With Bacterial Meningitis**

Age	Use in children ≥ 3 mos of age. Consider in infants 1–3 mos of age. Do **not** use in infants < 1 mo of age.
Dose	0.6 mg/kg/d, IV divided Q6H for 4 d.
Timing	IV push before or concurrently with first dose of antibiotics. Do **not** start dexamethasone more than 4 h after first dose of antibiotics.
Viral meningitis	Discontinue if bacterial meningitis unlikely.
Precautions	Measure hemoglobin and stool for occult blood daily. Discontinue if gross blood in stool or melena occurs.

Significant bleeding from the gastrointestinal tract, such as perforated duodenal ulcer or hemorrhage requiring transfusion, has been observed in approximately 0.8% of dexamethasone-treated children.

Prevention of Meningitis

The virtual disappearance of meningitis due to *H. influenzae* type b (Hib) is due to the efficacy of the vaccine. Vaccines are available against the A, C, Y and W135 serogroups of *N. meningitidis* but not against serogroup B; these are recommended only for outbreak control.

Household and close contacts of patients with meningitis due to *H. influenzae* and *N. meningitidis* should be given antibiotic prophylaxis. **Rifampin** (10 mg/kg/dose, Q12H for 4 doses or 20 mg/kg/day × 4 days, maximum 600 mg/dose) effectively eradicates nasopharyngeal carriage of *N. meningitidis*. **Ceftriaxone** (125 mg for children < 12 years, 250 mg for persons > 12 years, single dose IM) or **ciprofloxacin** (500 mg PO single dose for adults and postpubertal children) is also effective. The index case should receive chemoprophylactic antibiotics (in addition to the antibiotics used to treat the meningitis) before discharge from hospital unless the infection was treated with ceftriaxone or cefotaxime.

Suggested Reading List

American Academy of Pediatrics. Committee on Infectious Diseases. Therapy for children with invasive pneumococcal infections. *Pediatrics* 1997;99:289-299.

American Academy of Pediatrics. Pneumococcal Infections. In: Peter G, ed. *1997 Red Book: Report of the Committee on Infectious Diseases*. 24th ed. Elk Grove Village, IL: American Academy of Pediatrics, 1997:410-419.

Bonadio WA. The cerebrospinal fluid: physiologic aspects and alterations associated with bacterial meningitis. *Pediatr Infect Dis J* 1992;11:423–432.

Feigin RD, McCracken GH, Klein JO. Diagnosis and management of meningitis. *Pediatr Infect Dis J* 1992;11: 785–814.

Powell KR, Sugarman LI, Eskenazi AE, et al. Normalization of plasma arginine vasopressin concentrations when children with meningitis are given maintenance plus replacement fluid therapy. *J Pediatr* 1990;117:515–522.

Townsend GC, Scheld WM. Adjunctive therapy for bacterial meningitis: rationale for use, current status, and prospects for the future. *Clin Infect Dis* 1993;17(suppl 2):S537–S549.

CHAPTER 84

Prevention of Bacterial Endocarditis

Hillar Vellend, MD, FRCPC

Principles

- Systemic antibiotics should be administered to patients with types of valvular heart disease or cardiac history known to be associated with significant risk of endocarditis at the time of procedures associated with a high probability of transient bacteremia (Table 1). Most cases of endocarditis cannot be attributed to such invasive procedures.

- The prophylaxis for dental, oral, respiratory tract or esophageal procedures is directed against α-hemolytic (viridans) streptococci (Table 2).

- The prophylaxis for genitourinary or GI (excluding esophageal) procedures is directed against *Enterococcus faecalis* (enterococci) (Table 2).

- The antibiotic(s) should be administered to provide effective serum concentrations at the time of the anticipated bacteremia and for a few hours thereafter. How antibiotics interfere with bacteria during development of endocarditis is unknown.

Table 1: Conditions and Procedures Recommended for Endocarditis Prophylaxis

Cardiac Conditions Associated with Risk of Endocarditis	Dental or Surgical Procedures for Which Endocarditis Prophylaxis is Recommended
High Risk	All dental procedures likely to induce bleeding, including professional cleaning
Prosthetic cardiac valves	Tonsillectomy and/or adenoidectomy
Previous bacterial endocarditis	All operations that involve oral, respiratory or intestinal mucosa
Complex cyanotic congenital heart disease	Sclerotherapy for esophageal varices
Surgically constructed systemic-pulmonary shunts or conduits	Esophageal dilatation
	ERCP with biliary obstruction
Moderate Risk	Biliary tract surgery
Most congenital cardiac malformations	Cystoscopy
Rheumatic valvular heart disease	Urethral dilatation
Hypertrophic cardiomyopathy	Prostatic surgery
Mitral valve prolapse with valvular regurgitation (murmur and/or ECHO/ Doppler demonstration)	Any surgery or drainage procedure involving an abscess, infected tissue or body fluid (urine, bile, amniotic fluid, peritoneal fluid, etc.) if patient is not already receiving appropriate antibiotics

Prophylaxis is **NOT** recommended for flexible bronchoscopy or GI endoscopy with or without biopsy, transesophageal echocardiography, vaginal delivery, cesarean section, vaginal hysterectomy, therapeutic abortion, cardiac catheterization, transvenous pacemaker insertion.

Table 2: Antibiotic Prophylaxis for Bacterial Endocarditis

Dental, Oral, Respiratory Tract or Esophageal Procedures

Drug	Adult Dosing	Pediatric Dosing
Standard Regimen		
amoxicillin	2 g PO 1 h before procedure	50 mg/kg PO 1 h before procedure
Unable to Take Oral Medications		
ampicillin	2 g IV 30 min before procedure	50 mg/kg IV 30 min before procedure
Allergic to Penicillin		
clindamycin	600 mg PO 1 h before procedure	20 mg/kg PO 1 h before procedure
or cephalexin*	2 g PO 1 h before procedure	50 mg/kg PO 1 h before procedure
or clarithromycin	500 mg PO 1 h before procedure	15 mg/kg PO 1 h before procedure
or azithromycin	500 mg PO 1 h before procedure	15 mg/kg PO 1 h before procedure
Allergic to Penicillin and Unable to Take Oral Medications		
clindamycin	600 mg IV 30 min before procedure	20 mg/kg IV 30 min before procedure
or cefazolin*	1 g IV 30 min before procedure	25 mg/kg IV 30 min before procedure

(cont'd)

Table 2: **Antibiotic Prophylaxis for Bacterial Endocarditis** (cont'd)

Genitourinary or Gastrointestinal (Excluding Esophageal) Procedures

Drug	Adult Dosing	Pediatric Dosing
High-risk patient		
Standard Regimen		
ampicillin plus	2 g IV plus	50 mg/kg IV plus
gentamicin	1.5 mg/kg (max: 120 mg) IV 30 min before procedure	1.5 mg/kg IV 30 min before procedure
then *amoxicillin*	1.5 g PO 6 h later	then 25 mg/kg PO 6 h later
or *ampicillin*	1 g IV 6 h later	25 mg/kg IV 6 h later
Allergic to Penicillin		
vancomycin plus	1 g IV infused over 1–2 h plus	20 mg/kg IV infused over 1–2 h plus
gentamicin	1.5 mg/kg (max: 120 mg) IV 30 min before procedure	1.5 mg/kg IV 30 min before procedure
Moderate-risk patient		
Standard Regimen		
amoxicillin	2 g PO 1 h before procedure	50 mg/kg PO 1 h before procedure
or *ampicillin*	2 g IV 30 min before procedure	50 mg/kg IV 30 min before procedure
Allergic to Penicillin		
vancomycin	1 g IV over 1–2 h 30 min before procedure	20 mg/kg IV over 1–2 h 30 min before procedure

Cephalosporins should not be used in individuals with immediate-type hypersensitivity reaction (urticaria, angioedema or anaphylaxis) to penicillins.

Therapeutic Tips

- It is important to recognize the limitations of evidence on which current recommendations are based. No adequate clinical trials have been done to establish the efficacy of the recommended drug regimens. Well-documented cases of infective endocarditis have occurred in spite of appropriate prophylaxis.

Suggested Reading List

Dajani AS, Taubert KA, Wilson W, et al. Prevention of bacterial endocarditis. Recommendations by the American Heart Association. *JAMA* 1997;277:1794–1801.

Durack DT. Prevention of infective endocarditis. *N Engl J Med* 1995;332:38–44.

Freedman LR. To prevent or not to prevent bacterial endocarditis – that is the question. *Clin Infect Dis* 1993;17:195–197.

Hall G, Nord CE, Heimdahl A. Elimination of bacteremia after dental extraction: comparison of erythromycin and clindamycin for prophylaxis of infective endocarditis. *J Antimicrob Chemother* 1996;37:783–795.

Simmons NA and the Endocarditis Working Party of the British Society for Antimicrobial Chemotherapy. Recommendations for endocarditis prophylaxis. *J Antimicrob Chemother* 1993;31:437–438.

CHAPTER 85

Community-acquired Pneumonia

Harvey R. Rabin, MD, FRCPC

Goals of Therapy

- To relieve symptoms (fever, cough, sputum production, chest pain)
- To improve (or prevent) associated respiratory distress (dyspnea, hypoxemia, cyanosis)
- To minimize complications (bacteremia, hemoptysis, cavitation, pneumothorax, empyema, effusions, death)

Table 1: Defining Lower Respiratory Tract Infections

Endobronchial, interstitial or alveolar clinical and radiologic presentations.
Suppurative (cough with sputum production) vs nonsuppurative.
Typical or atypical* characteristics.
Community-acquired, nursing-home-acquired or nosocomial.
With or without comorbidity.†
Immunocompromised or immunocompetent patients.

* *Usually defined as a patient with a cough that is nonproductive or productive of mucoid sputum only, a more protracted clinical course before presentation to a physician and physical findings that do not correlate with the extent of radiologic infiltrates.*

† *Chronic obstructive pulmonary disease, alcoholism, diabetes mellitus, congestive heart failure, renal insufficiency, immunosuppression.*

The approach for the initial management of community-acquired pneumonia is based on a Canadian consensus report.[1] For the management of community-acquired pneumonia in immuno-compromised patients, see Chapter 97. For empiric management of nosocomial pneumonias in adults the reader is referred to another Canadian consensus report.[2]

Investigations

- A detailed history and a physical examination with special reference to:
  - age and comorbidity
  - risk factors for severe pneumonia (Figure 1)
  - presence of complications
  - clinical indication(s) for admission to hospital (Figure 1)

[1] Can J Infect Dis 1993;4:25–28.
[2] Can J Infect Dis 1993;4:317–321.

Figure 1: **Initial Management of Community-acquired Pneumonia**

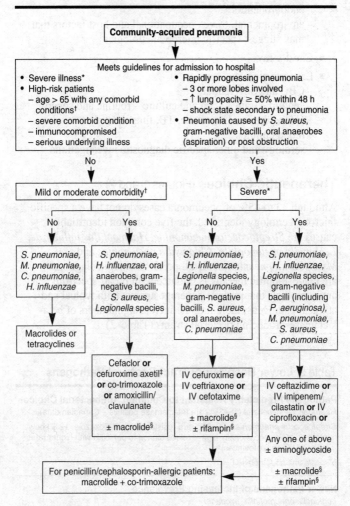

* **Severe Pneumonia** – Predictors of mortality
  Any one or more of:
  • Cavitation or involvement of more than one lobe on chest x-ray
  • Respiratory failure (PaO_2 < 60 mm Hg) on a FiO_2 > 35% except patients with
    chronic obstructive lung disease (COPD) who may be hypoxemic without
    pneumonia
  • Respiratory rate 30/min or greater
  • Sepsis with evidence of end organ dysfunction
  • Extrapulmonary septic complications

A prediction rule and point scoring system of severity for assignment of patients to risk
categories has been published (N Engl J Med 1997;336:243–250).
† Comorbid conditions: COPD, alcoholism, diabetes mellitus, congestive heart failure,
  renal insufficiency, immunosuppression.
‡ Cefixime or cefprozil may also be considered but are not approved for this indication in
  Canada.
§ If Legionella is a concern.

- To distinguish as much as is possible:
  - acute pneumonia from acute exacerbations of chronic endobronchitis
  - environmental, travel, occupational and host factors that may suggest specific microbial etiologies
- Chest x-ray
- Laboratory tests:
  - CBC and differential
  - sputum, Gram's stain and culture – routine and specific (*Mycoplasma, Legionella*, TB, fungal, viral)
  - blood cultures
  - serology and other specific diagnostic investigations

Therapeutic Choices (Figures 1 and 2)

Although 33 to 45% of pneumonia cases do not have a specific microbial etiology identified, the five common identifiable causes are *Streptococcus pneumoniae, Haemophilus influenzae, Legionella pneumophila, Chlamydia pneumoniae* and *Mycoplasma pneumoniae*. Until precise etiologic diagnoses are made, empiric therapy is initiated with broad-spectrum antimicrobials that provide coverage against both typical and atypical pathogens, including the increasing numbers of beta-lactamase-producing bacterial strains (Table 2).

Table 2: Lower Respiratory Tract Bacterial Pathogens

Pathogens Predictably Resistant to Common Antibacterial Choices

Haemophilus influenzae (15–35% are β lactamase positive – Canadian data).

Streptococcus pneumoniae (20–40% are resistant to co-trimoxazole; 12% show intermediate or occasionally high-level resistance to penicillin with higher rates reported in some provinces)*

Mycoplasma pneumoniae [†]

Newer Pathogens of Increasing Prevalence

Legionella pneumophila, micdadei

Moraxella (Branhamella) catarrhalis

*Chlamydia pneumoniae**

Pneumocystis carinii

Pathogens Requiring Very Specific Antimicrobial Choices

Staphylococcus aureus

Pneumocystis carinii

Klebsiella pneumoniae, Enterobacter species, *Escherichia coli, Pseudomonas aeruginosa, Proteus* species, *Serratia marcescens*

Mycobacterium tuberculosis, Mycobacteria other than *tuberculosis*

---

* *Antimicrob Ag Chemother 1996;40:2190–2193.*

[†] *Mycoplasma pneumoniae and Chlamydia pneumoniae account for approximately 25% of community-acquired pneumonia among outpatients.*

Figure 2: **Initial Management of Nursing-home-acquired Pneumonia**

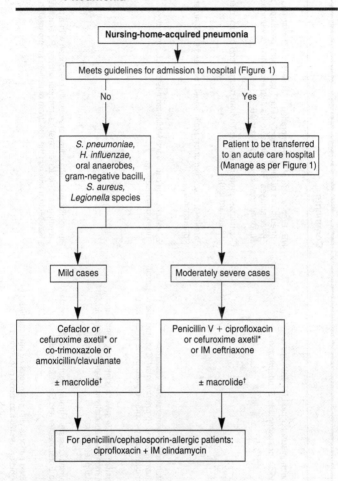

* *Cefixime or cefprozil may also be considered but are not approved for this indication in Canada.*
† *If Legionella is a concern.*

Therapeutic Tips

- Patients should have IV therapy stepped down to oral antibiotics as soon as:
  - they are afebrile (temperature < 38°C).
  - respiratory rate is < 24/minute.
  - oxygen saturation is > 92% breathing room air.
  - chest x-ray confirms that the pneumonia is stable or resolving.
  - oral medications can be tolerated.

Table 3: Pharmacologic Treatment of Community-acquired Pneumonia

Drug	Use (Spectrum)	Comments
Beta-lactams		
penicillin ampicillin amoxicillin	For culture **proven** common susceptible LRT pathogens. Penicillin is drug of choice for susceptible *S. pneumoniae*.	**NB:** Empiric use of first-generation β-lactams is not indicated in pneumonia because majority of LRT pathogens produce β-lactamases. They are also inactive against *M. pneumoniae, L. pneumophila, C. pneumoniae*.
amoxicillin/clavulanate cefaclor	*H. influenzae*.	Clavulanate protects amoxicillin from degradation by penicillinase (β-lactamase).
cloxacillin cefazolin	*S. aureus*.	Parenteral cloxacillin or cefazolin should be used for *S. aureus* pneumonia.
cefuroxime cefixime cefprozil	Pathogens often resistant to first-generation β-lactams – *H. influenzae, M. catarrhalis* and *K. pneumoniae*. Cefixime and cefprozil are not approved for community-acquired pneumonia in Canada.	*K. pneumoniae* can infect debilitated hosts in community or nosocomial setting.
ceftriaxone cefotaxime	Nosocomial gram-negative bacilli; in severe community- and nursing-home-acquired pneumonias, especially in hospitalized patients; first choice for nosocomial pneumonia.	
piperacillin piperacillin/tazobactam ceftazidime	Selectively for nosocomially resistant gram-negative bacilli, especially *P. aeruginosa*, some *Enterobacter* and *Serratia* species.	Piperacillin and ceftazidime are usually prescribed with an aminoglycoside for optimal bactericidal activity. Piperacillin/tazobactam extends the spectrum of activity for piperacillin.
imipenem/cilastatin meropenem	Reserved for hospitalized patients with polymicrobial pneumonias, including mixed aerobic/anaerobic aspiration pneumonia.	

Macrolides
erythromycin
azithromycin
clarithromycin

Erythromycin: most effective against *Mycoplasma*, *S. pneumoniae* and *S. pyogenes* and *S. aureus* (less). IV erythromycin is first choice for *C. pneumoniae* and *Legionella* species.

Azithromycin, clarithromycin: *H. influenzae*, *M. catarrhalis*.

No macrolides have a role in gram-negative bacillary pneumonia. 45% of *H. influenzae* resistant to erythromycin.
Legionella is best treated with erythromycin plus rifampin.
Data are not available on use of clarithromycin or azithromycin in severe pneumonia requiring hospitalization.

Fluoroquinolones
ciprofloxacin
levofloxacin
ofloxacin

All: *H. influenzae*, *M. catarrhalis* (including β-lactamase-producing strains), *E. coli* and *K. pneumoniae*.
Ciprofloxacin: *P. aeruginosa*.

Not first choice for *S. pneumoniae* or *S. aureus*.

Other
co-trimoxazole
tetracycline
doxycycline

Co-trimoxazole: in penicillin-allergic patients; alternative to β-lactams in uncomplicated LRTIs.

S. pneumoniae resistance to tetracycline and doxycycline restricts their use in LRTIs.
Are drugs of first choice for mild exacerbations of chronic endobronchitis.

Abbreviations: LRT = lower respiratory tract; LRTI = lower respiratory tract infection.

Table 4: Antibiotics Used in Pneumonia

Drug	Dosage	Adverse Effects/Comments	Cost*
Beta-lactams			
Penicillins		**Penicillins:** hypersensitivity reactions, rash, nausea, vomiting, pseudomembranous colitis, interstitial nephritis.	
penicillin V – Pen-Vee, PVF K, generics	300 mg TID PO		$
amoxicillin – Amoxil, generics	500 mg TID PO		$
amoxicillin/clavulanate – Clavulin	500 mg TID PO		$$
cloxacillin – Orbenin, Tegopen, generics	500 mg QID PO		$
piperacillin – Pipracil	3 g Q4H IV		$$$$
piperacillin/tazobactam – Tazocin	3.375 g Q6H IV		$$$$
First-generation Cephalosporins		**Cephalosporins:** hypersensitivity reactions, rash, nausea, vomiting, pseudomembranous colitis, renal and hepatic dysfunction, phlebitis and pain at site of IM injection.	
cefazolin – Ancef, Kefzol	2 g Q8H IV	Cefotaxime is safe in hepatobiliary disease.	$$$
Second-generation Cephalosporins			
cefaclor – Ceclor	250 mg TID PO		$$
cefprozil – Cefzil	500 mg Q24h		$$
cefuroxime axetil – Ceftin	500 mg BID–TID PO		$$
cefuroxime sodium – Kefurox, Zinacef	750 mg Q8H IV		$$$
Third-generation Cephalosporins			
cefixime – Suprax	400 mg daily PO		$$
ceftriaxone – Rocephin	1–2 g Q24H IV		$$$–$$$$
cefotaxime – Claforan	1–2 g Q6–8H IV		$$$–$$$$
ceftazidime – Ceptaz, Fortaz, Tazidime	1–2 g Q8H IV		$$$$
Penems			
imipenem/cilastatin – Primaxin	500 mg Q6H IV	**Imipenem:** hypotension, nausea with rapid infusion; seizure activity with high levels.	$$$$
meropenem – Merrem	0.5–1 g Q8H IV	**Meropenem:** less likely to cause seizures.	$$$$

Drug	Dosage	Comments	Cost*
Macrolides			
erythromycin ⬩ – E-Mycin, Erybid, Eryc, Erythromid, PCE, Ilosone, generics	1 g/d divided BID, TID or QID PO	Abdominal cramping, nausea, vomiting, diarrhea, rash, cholestatic hepatitis. (Fewer side effects with azithromycin and clarithromycin.)	$–$$
clarithromycin ⬩ – Biaxin	250–500 mg BID PO		$$
azithromycin ⬩ – Zithromax	500 mg 1st d, 250 mg × 4 d PO	Azithromycin given daily × 5 d is equivalent to erythromycin QID × 10 d.	$$
Fluoroquinolones			
ciprofloxacin ⬩ – Cipro	500–750 mg BID PO / 400 mg Q12H IV	Abdominal pain, photosensitivity, hepatitis, pseudomembranous colitis. Cartilage toxicity – avoid in children. *Drug interactions:* Ciprofloxacin may ↓ theophylline elimination; concomitant antacids, sucralfate ↓ absorption of quinolones; ciprofloxacin and ofloxacin may prolong INR if given with warfarin.	PO: $$ / IV: $$$
levofloxacin ⬩ – Levaquin	250–500 mg Q24H PO		$$
ofloxacin ⬩ – Floxin	400 mg BID PO		$$
Aminoglycosides			
gentamicin ⬩ – Garamycin, Cidomycin	2 mg/kg Q8H IV or 5–7 mg/kg once daily	Nephrotoxicity, ototoxicity.	$$$
tobramycin ⬩ – Nebcin			$$$
Other			
co-trimoxazole ⬩ – Bactrim, Septra, generics	160/800 mg BID PO	**Co-trimoxazole:** hypersensitivity reactions, nausea, vomiting, diarrhea, rash, false ↑ serum creatinine, renal impairment, neutropenia, thrombocytopenia, anemia, agranulocytosis. *Drug interactions:* ↑ phenytoin levels; ↑ INR with warfarin, hypoglycemia with sulfonylureas, ↑ nephrotoxicity with cyclosporine.	$
tetracycline ⬩ – Tetracyn, generics	500 mg QID PO		$
doxycycline – Vibramycin, Vibra-tabs, Doryx, generics	100 mg BID PO	**Tetracycline, doxycycline:** nausea, vomiting, photosensitivity, candidiasis, pseudotumor cerebri. *Drug interactions:* calcium, aluminum, magnesium, iron ↓ absorption.	$$
rifampin – Rifadin, Rimactane, Rofact	300 mg BID PO		$$

⬩ *Dosage adjustment may be required in renal impairment – see Appendix I.*
† *If appropriate for renal function.*

Cost of 1-day supply – includes drug costs only.
Legend: $ < $1 $$ $1–10 $$$ $10–50 $$$$ > $50

- In choosing any antimicrobial therapy, once issues of efficacy and toxicity have been addressed, costs should then be considered (Table 4).

- *Streptococcus pneumoniae* with reduced susceptibility to penicillin has now been reported in Canada.[3] Some intermediate- and high-level penicillin-resistant strains may also be resistant to cephalosporins, including third-generation agents (e.g., cefotaxime and ceftriaxone). Antimicrobial susceptibility testing of pneumococci, particularly if isolated from normally sterile body sites (blood and CSF), is now mandated by these results. When a high prevalence of penicillin-resistant pneumococci exists, vancomycin should be considered as empiric therapy of life-threatening pneumococcal infections (bacteremia, meningitis).

- Patients with COPD (Chapter 38) who present with increased sputum, increased sputum purulence and increased dyspnea but without radiologic evidence of pneumonia, respond to nonpharmacologic approaches to management (chest physiotherapy, oxygen, humidity and avoidance of respiratory irritants) and combined bronchodilators and either inhaled or oral corticosteroids. Empiric use of common antibiotics (erythromycin, doxycycline, tetracyclines, amoxicillin or co-trimoxazole) is reserved for more symptomatic patients and is often continued despite sputum culture confirmation of a resistant causative organism. Only if complicated with other risk factors or the patient fails to respond would one recommend a second- or third-generation cephalosporin, amoxicillin/clavulanate, a fluoroquinolone or a newer macrolide antibiotic.

- Recommendations of the National Advisory Committee on Immunization suggest that the polyvalent pneumococcal capsular polysaccharide vaccine is indicated for all persons ≥ 65 years of age and in all persons > 2 years of age in whom there is an increased risk of morbidity and mortality from pneumococcal infections.[4]

- A prediction rule that identifies patients with community-acquired pneumonia who are at low risk for death and other adverse outcomes may help physicians make more rational decisions about hospitalization for patients with pneumonia.[5] This should reduce the uncertainty in assessing the severity of illness and foster more appropriate use of hospital care in the management of patients with community-acquired

---

[3] *Antimicrob Agents Chemother 1996;40:2190–2193.*

[4] *Canadian Immunization Guide, 4th ed. Ottawa: Health and Welfare Canada, 1993.*

[5] *N Engl J Med 1997;336:243–250.*

pneumonia. The predictor variables and point scoring system are explicitly defined and can be readily assessed at the time of patient presentation.

Suggested Reading List

Balter ME, Hyland RH, Low DE, et al. Recommendations on the management of chronic bronchitis. *Can Med Assoc J* 1994;151(10)(suppl):1–23.

Jadavji T, Law B, Lebel MH, et al. A practical guide for the diagnosis and treatment of pediatric pneumonia. *Can Med Assoc J* 1997;156:S703–S711.

Mandell LA, Niederman M and The Canadian Community Acquired Pneumonia Consensus Conference Group. Antimicrobial treatment of community acquired pneumonia in adults: a conference report. *Can J Infect Dis* 1993;4: 25–28.

Mandell LA, Marrie TJ, Niederman MS and The Canadian Hospital Acquired Pneumonia Consensus Conference Group. Initial antimicrobial treatment of hospital acquired pneumonia in adults: A conference report. *Can J Infect Dis* 1993; 4:317–321.

Marrie TJ. Community-acquired pneumonia. *Clin Infect Dis* 1994; 18:501–515.

CHAPTER 86

Tuberculosis

Thomas J. Marrie, MD, FRCPC

Goals of Therapy

- To prevent latent infection from progressing to clinically active disease
- To treat active disease (by eradicating *Mycobacterium tuberculosis* from the affected organ) and relieve symptoms (fever, sweats, weight loss, cough)
- To prevent person-to-person spread

Investigations

- Thorough history with special attention to:
  - risk factors for acquisition of tuberculosis (TB) (e.g., exposure, travel, occupation)
  - history of TB and details of treatment
- Physical examination:
  - nutrition status, fever, choroid tubercles, rales, rhonchi, meningitis
  - concomitant diseases that may affect treatment (e.g., HIV)
- Laboratory tests:
  - chest x-ray
  - urinalysis
  - sputum smear and culture for acid-fast bacilli (AFB)
  - urine smear and culture for AFB if renal TB suspected
  - lumbar puncture with smear and culture of spinal fluid for AFB, plus sugar, protein and cell count if meningitis suspected
  - CBC, ESR
  - creatinine, ALT, AST, alkaline phosphatase, bilirubin
- Special procedures:
  - bronchoscopy with transbronchial biopsy in some cases. A rapid diagnosis is possible by demonstrating granulomata on biopsy
  - aspiration of pleural effusions with culture, chemical and cytological analysis, and pleural biopsy for culture and histology may be useful
- Polymerase chain reaction (PCR) for detection of mycobacterial antigens in body fluids is used in some laboratories
  - major advantage is rapid diagnosis, generally < 48 h
  - most useful in diagnosing meningeal or pleural TB

Figure 1: **Diagnosis and Management of Latent M. tuberculosis Infection**

Intradermal administration of 5 TU PPD (Mantoux test) to volar surface of forearm of:*

I	those with signs/symptoms or history suggestive of TB
II	recent contacts of known TB cases
III	those with a chest radiograph compatible with old (inactive) TB
IV	HIV-infected or immunosuppressed persons
V	those with medical conditions that ↑ the risk of TB
VI	groups at high risk of recent infection with M. tuberculosis

48–72 h later

< 5 mm induration	≥ 5 mm induration Groups II, III, IV	≥10 mm induration Groups V, VI	≥15 mm induration No risk factor
Negative: no TB infection; some of these (e.g., recent contacts) may need repeat testing in 12 wks	Tuberculosis infection	Tuberculosis infection	Tuberculosis infection

Chest radiograph → Normal → No disease / Old or active TB → See Figure 2

Chest radiograph → Normal → No disease

Chest radiograph → Normal → No disease / Old or active TB → See Figure 2

< 35 yrs old
Yes → INH
No → No INH

Consider INH

INH 300 mg/d × 6 mos; for children × 9 mos; for HIV-infected × 12 mos

Monitor LFTs monthly; discontinue INH if liver enzymes exceed 5 times normal

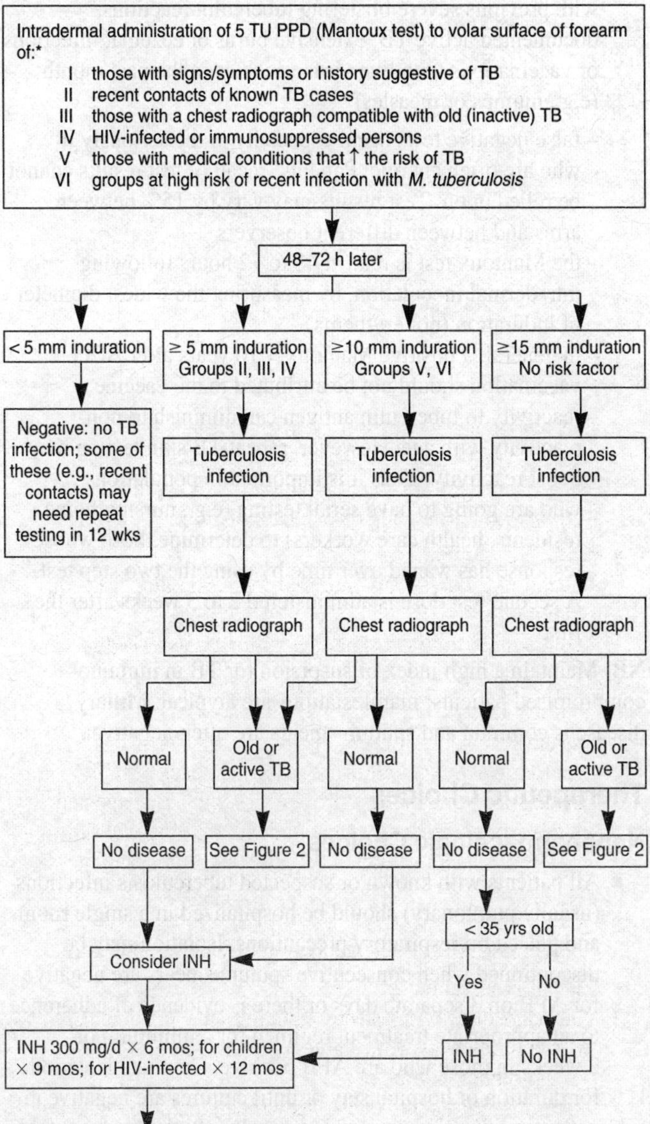

*Several other antigens (e.g., CMI Multitest) should be inoculated onto the other arm. If there is no reaction to these common antigens the patient is anergic, and a negative Mantoux is meaningless.
Abbreviations: LFTs = liver function tests; INH = isoniazid.

- Tuberculin skin (Mantoux) testing has 3 indications – diagnosis of infection, diagnosis of disease and as an epidemiologic tool. It should not be performed on persons with previous severe blistering tuberculin reactions, documented active TB, extensive burns or eczema, infections or vaccinations with live virus vaccines in the past month (e.g., mumps or measles)
  - false negative tests occur especially in the seriously ill who are often anergic. Patients' recall of test results cannot be relied upon. Test results may vary by 15% between arms and between different observers
  - the Mantoux test is read at 48 to 72 hours following intradermal inoculation, by measuring the widest diameter of induration (not erythema)
  - in general, a positive Mantoux > 10 years after BCG vaccination should not be attributed to the vaccine
  - reactivity to tuberculin antigen can diminish to non-reactivity with age. However, repeat TB skin testing may boost reactivity. Thus it is important in populations who are going to have serial testing (e.g., nursing home residents, health care workers) to determine those whose response has waned over time by using the two step test. A second test dose is administered 2 to 3 weeks after the first

NB: Maintain a high index of suspicion for TB in immuno-compromised patients; manifestations are atypical. Miliary disease is common and sputum smears are often negative.

Therapeutic Choices

Nonpharmacologic Choices

- All patients with known or suspected tuberculosis infections (usually pulmonary) should be hospitalized in a single room and placed on respiratory precautions. Isolation may be discontinued when consecutive sputum smears are negative for AFB on 3 separate days or there is evidence of adherence to an appropriate treatment regimen for a minimum of 2 weeks in those who are AFB positive. Continue isolation for duration of hospital stay or until cultures are negative in patients with pulmonary or laryngeal multiple drug resistant TB.
  - proper masks (which filter particles one micron in size, have a 95% filter efficiency when tested in the unloaded state and provide a tight facial seal), should be worn when caring for patients with known or suspected TB. Surgical masks do not prevent the inhalation of droplet nuclei.

- All patients with a chest x-ray consistent with TB should be isolated pending results of sputum smear for AFB. The radiographic appearance of TB is different in patients with HIV. In a group of patients with advanced AIDS and pulmonary TB, 60% had hilar or mediastinal adenopathy, 29% had localized middle or lower lung infiltrates and 12% had normal chest radiographs.

- The Department of Health must be notified for contact tracing.

- Close follow-up is mandatory (initially, monthly visits and monthly chest radiographs).

- If there is doubt about compliance with therapy, twice weekly directly observed therapy should be instituted. Failure to comply with therapy is the major reason for the marked increase in cases of multidrug-resistant TB.

- Adequate nutrition is necessary to enhance healing.

- BCG vaccine is not in general use in Canada.[1]

Pharmacologic Choices (Table 1)

Latent Infection (Figure 1)

Patients with latent infection have low numbers of tubercle bacilli in their bodies but do not have active disease. However, the risk of active disease in certain patient groups is high. Therapy with a single drug, isoniazid (INH), can greatly reduce this risk.

Anergic HIV infected patients are at high risk for development of TB. They should be offered preventive therapy with INH if they live in areas with a high prevalence of TB, at least when the CD_4 count decreases to 500 cells/mm^3.

For those who have a positive Mantoux test and are in a low-risk group (Figure 1), the risk of adverse effects from INH must be weighed against its benefit in reducing the risk of active disease. In patients with no risk factors, the risk of adverse effects from INH is low for those < 35 years of age. This group should be offered INH prophylaxis. For those who have a positive Mantoux test and either silicosis or chest x-ray demonstrating old fibrotic lesions and no evidence of active TB, acceptable regimens include INH plus rifampin for 4 months or INH for 12 months.

Active Tuberculosis (Figure 2)

Treatment should always be with multiple drugs. Knowledge of the local epidemiology of resistance is essential to appropriate treatment. A four-drug regimen (**INH, rifampin, pyrazinamide** and **streptomycin** or **ethambutol**) is preferred for initial empiric

[1] *JAMA 1994;172:698–702.*

Table 1: Drugs Used in the Treatment of *M. tuberculosis*

Drug	Dosage	Adverse Effects	Drug Interactions	Cost*
First-line Therapy – primary drug resistance unlikely (e.g., persons born in Canada, no previous exposure to drug-resistant *M. tuberculosis*)				
isoniazid[†] Isotamine, generics	5 mg/kg, up to 300 mg/d (↓ dose in severe liver disease) For directly observed therapy, 15 mg/kg twice/wk	Asymptomatic ↑ hepatic transaminases and bilirubin (10–20%), clinical hepatitis, peripheral neuropathy, gynecomastia, seizures, galactorrhea, drowsiness, drug-induced lupus, toxic encephalopathy, fever, skin rash, mood changes, lymphadenopathy, hematologic effects.[‡]	INH ↑ concentrations of phenytoin, theophylline, carbamazepine, warfarin, benzodiazepines. Corticosteroids, aluminum salts ↓ INH concentrations. ↑ hepatotoxicity of INH[π] with rifampin, ethanol, acetaminophen (INH may also ↑ acetaminophen hepatotoxicity). Alcohol ↑ risk of hepatotoxicity; intake should be minimized.	$
rifampin Rifadin, Rimactane, Rofact	10 mg/kg, up to 600 mg/d (↓ dose in severe liver disease) For directly observed therapy, 600 mg twice/wk	GI upset, hepatitis, discoloration of urine and tears (contact lenses can be stained), cholestatic jaundice, subclinical disseminated intravascular coagulation, skin rash, diarrhea, hematologic effects,[‡] urticaria, ataxia, confusion, visual disturbances, fever, flu-like symptoms (may occur with intermittent therapy), acute interstitial nephritis.	↓ serum concentration of many drugs due to hepatic enzyme induction (e.g., oral contraceptives – use **additional/alternative method of birth control**), protease inhibitors (which ↑ serum levels of rifampin), glucocorticoids, oral anticoagulants, hypoglycemics, barbiturates, theophylline, cyclosporine, ketoconazole, fluconazole, β-blockers, phenytoin, methadone, some Ca++ channel blockers, diazepam, some antiarrhythmics. May ↑ hepatotoxicity of acetaminophen, halothane.	$–$$$

pyrazinamide ✎ Tebrazid, generics	25 mg/kg, up to 2 g/d (divided doses). Reduce dose in patients with ↓ renal function	Hepatotoxicity (rare with 2-mo therapy), rash, arthralgia, ↑ uric acid (acute gout rarely seen), drug fever, hematologic effects,‡ GI upset.	↓ levels of INH.	$$$
ethambutol†✎ Myambutol, Etibi	15–25 mg/kg/d	Ocular toxicity (↓ visual acuity, central scotomata, red–green color blindness due to retrobulbar neuritis [rare at 15 mg/kg/d]). GI upset, rash, Stevens-Johnson syndrome (rare), toxic epidermal necrolysis, hematologic effects,‡ headache, dizziness, confusion, hallucinations.	↓ cyclosporine blood levels.	$–$$
streptomycin ✎	15 mg/kg/d, up to 1 g IM or 15–25 mg/kg IM twice/wk Not to exceed total of 120 g	Vestibular/cochlear toxicity, ataxia (may be permanent), nystagmus, proteinuria, hypersensitivity with fever, rash, hematologic effects.‡	Additive toxicity with other neurotoxic, ototoxic or nephrotoxic drugs.	$$$–$$$$$
Second-line Therapy				
ethionamide# Trecator#	15–30 mg/kg/d, up to 1 g/d given BID	Hepatitis, arthralgia, GI disturbances, altered taste, peripheral neuritis, possible antithyroid effects (has produced clinical hypothyroidism); fatigue, depression, frozen shoulder syndrome, galactorrhea, ↑ salivation.	May ↑ CNS toxicity of cycloserine.	#

(cont'd)

Table 1: Drugs Used in the Treatment of *M. tuberculosis* (cont'd)

Drug	Dosage	Adverse Effects	Drug Interactions	Cost*
cycloserine ❂ Seromycin#	15 mg/kg/d, up to 1 g/d	Headache, irritability, behavior abnormalities, psychosis, seizures, aggravation of pre-existing psychiatric condition; peripheral neuropathy (especially when used with INH); rarely, may cause megaloblastic or sideroblastic anemia.	Ethionamide and alcohol may potentiate CNS toxicity of cycloserine.	$$$$$
Aminoglycosides				
kanamycin ❂ – Kantrex#	15 mg/kg/d IM	Vestibular/cochlear toxicity, nephrotoxicity.	Other oto- or nephrotoxic drugs may potentiate aminoglycoside toxicities.	# $$$$$
amikacin ❂ – Amikin	15 mg/kg/d IM			$$$$$
capreomycin ❂ Capastat Sulfate#	15 mg/kg/d IM (max. 1 g/d)			

* Cost of 30-day supply – includes drug cost only.
Legend: $ < 25 $$ $25–50 $$$ $50–75 $$$$ $75–100 $$$$$ > $100
† See Therapeutic Tips.
‡ May include any of eosinophilia, thrombocytopenia, transient leukopenia, hemolytic anemia, agranulocytosis, or sideroblastic or aplastic anemia.

π Cross-hepatotoxicity may occur between drugs that are chemically related (e.g., INH, pyrazinamide and ethionamide). All of these agents should be avoided if a reaction to one of them occurs.
❂ Dosage adjustment may be required in renal impairment – see Appendix I.
Available through Special Access Program (formerly the Emergency Drug Release Program), Therapeutic Products Directorate, Health Canada.

Figure 2: **Management of Pulmonary *M. tuberculosis* Infection**

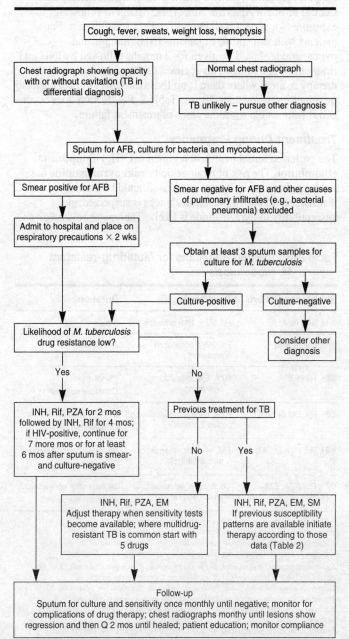

Abbreviations: INH = isoniazid; Rif = rifampin; SM = streptomycin; PZA = pyrazinamide; EM = ethambutol.

therapy. Adjust therapy when susceptibility results are available. Suspect resistance when disease is contracted in Africa, Asia, Central or South America, New York, Miami or following exposure to a patient with known drug resistant disease. For patients with susceptible organisms INH, rifampin and pyrazinamide should be given for 2 months followed by INH and rifampin for 4 months. This regimen can be used for empiric therapy in areas where there is no INH resistance. For regimens to treat multidrug-resistant TB, see Table 2. Reinfection does occur and is responsible for some cases of treatment failure.

Treatment During Pregnancy

The preferred initial treatment regimen is **INH, rifampin** and **ethambutol**. The risk of teratogenicity with **pyrazinamide** has not been determined; however, its use should be considered if resistance to one of the initial choices is suspected and susceptibility to pyrazinamide is likely. Therapy should be given

Table 2: **Suggested Regimens for Multidrug-resistant** *M. tuberculosis*

Resistance Pattern	Treatment	Duration
INH, SM, PZA	Rif, PZA, EM, amikacin*	9 mos
INH, EM (± SM)	Rif, PZA, oflox/cipro, amikacin*	6–12 mos
INH, Rif (± SM)	PZA, EM, oflox/cipro, amikacin*	18–24 mos Consider surgery†
INH, Rif, EM (± SM)	PZA, oflox/cipro, amikacin* plus 2 others‡	24 mos after conversion[π] Consider surgery†
INH, Rif, PZA (± SM)	EM, oflox/cipro, amikacin* plus 2 others‡	24 mos after conversion[π] Consider surgery†
INH, Rif, PZA, EM (± SM)	Oflox/cipro, amikacin* plus 3 others‡	24 mos after conversion[π] Consider surgery†

* *Capreomycin may be used if there is resistance to amikacin.*
† *Surgery may be required to resect nonhealing cavitary lesions.*
‡ *May choose from ethionamide, cycloserine, para-aminosalicylic acid.*
π *Refers to conversion from positive to negative sputum smear and culture.*

Abbreviations: INH = isoniazid; SM = streptomycin; PZA = pyrazinamide; EM = ethambutol; Rif = rifampin; Oflox = ofloxacin; Cipro = ciprofloxacin.
Data from a murine model indicate that ethionamide, sparfloxacin, ofloxacin, capreomycin, clarithromycin and clofazimine are active against a multidrug-resistant tuberculous isolate. In this system, despite in vitro resistance, INH had moderate activity.[1]
Sparfloxacin, ciprofloxacin and ofloxacin have activity against M. tuberculosis. Ciprofloxacin and ofloxacin are synergistic when combined with rifampin or INH. The role of these agents in the treatment of TB awaits further study.[2]

[1] *J Antimicrob Agent Chemother 1993;37:2344–2347.*
[2] *J Antimicrob Agent Chemother 1993;32:797–808.*

for a minimum of 9 months. Breast-feeding need not be discouraged since only small concentrations of anti-TB drugs appear in breast milk, and they do not produce toxicity in the newborn.

Therapeutic Tips

- All patients given INH should receive pyridoxine 25 to 50 mg per day to prevent peripheral neuropathy.
- Color vision should be monitored every 6 months in patients receiving ethambutol.

Suggested Reading List

Barnes PF, Barrows SA. Tuberculosis in the 1990's. *Ann Intern Med* 1993;119:400–410.

Barnes PF, Le HQ, Davidson PT. Tuberculosis in patients with HIV infection. *Med Clin North Am* 1993;77:1369–1390.

Bass JB, Farer LS, Hopewell PC, et al. Treatment of tuberculosis and tuberculosis infection in adults and children. *Am J Respir Crit Care Med* 1994;149:1359–1374.

Belusa MLF, Cocchiarella L, Conly J, et al. Guidelines for preventing the transmission of tuberculosis in Canadian health care facilities and other institutional settings. *Can Commun Dis Rep* 1996;2251:1–50.

Brausch LM, Bass JB Jr. The treatment of tuberculosis. *Med Clin North Am* 1993;77:1277–1288.

Canadian Thoracic Society, Standards Committee (Tuberculosis). *Canadian Tuberculosis Standards*. Fourth Edition. Ottawa: Canadian Lung Association, 1996.

Initial therapy for tuberculosis in the era of multidrug resistance. *MMWR* 1993;42(No. RR-7):1–8.

Miller B. Preventive therapy for tuberculosis. *Med Clin North Am* 1993;77:1263–1275.

Schluger NW, Rom WN. Current approaches to the diagnosis of active pulmonary tuberculosis. *Am J Respir Crit Care Med* 1994;149:264–267.

CHAPTER 87

Acute Osteomyelitis

Simon Dobson, MD, FRCPC

Goals of Therapy

- To cure the acute infection
- To minimize morbidity (e.g., loss of limb function)
- To prevent recurrence and progression to chronic osteomyelitis

Investigations

- History:
  - duration of symptoms: fever, pain, redness, swelling, limp or other loss of function or movement
  - any penetrating wound
  - vascular insufficiency
  - neuropathic ulcer of the diabetic foot
- Examination:
  - tenderness over affected bone (often exquisite). No pain is elicited if advanced neuropathy of diabetic foot
  - range of movement in affected limb (any suggestion of septic arthritis)
- Laboratory tests:
  - CBC and acute-phase reactants (erythrocyte sedimentation rate, C-reactive protein) as baseline
  - blood culture (positive in 30 to 60%)
  - culture of diabetic ulcer unreliable as colonizers will be present. Best to culture bone obtained surgically through intact skin
- Imaging:
  - x-ray – may be normal initially; changes (e.g., periosteal reaction) are not evident for at least 10 days after onset
  - rarefaction of bone visible only when 50% loss of bone density (early in neonates, later in older children)
  - x-ray does not rule out diagnosis in diabetic foot. Chronic osteopathy may be present
- Bone scan: imaging using technetium 99^m-labeled methylene diphosphonate has improved early diagnosis. Early "blood pool images" should be taken as well as later bone uptake images to help differentiate cellulitis from bone infection. A negative bone scan does not rule out osteomyelitis. In neonates an x-ray may be more reliable. Other causes of enhanced bone turnover (e.g., fracture or tumor) will also give a positive result

NB: If the clinical findings suggest osteomyelitis, management should not be delayed for lack of ready access to a bone scan.

- Probe diabetic ulcer with sterile instrument. If bone can be reached, this has high specificity and positive predictive value for osteomyelitis (89%) but low sensitivity. Best initial evaluation is x-ray plus a probe for bone. If both negative, treat for soft tissue infection but repeat x-ray in 2 weeks (Figure 2)

Table 1: **Initial Empiric Therapy of Acute Osteomyelitis***

Characteristics	Causative Organisms	Empiric IV Antibiotic
Hematogenous Osteomyelitis		
Most common type. Predominantly in children. Blood-borne bacteria lodge in bone as nidus of infection. Possible in any bone but usually in long bones: femur 36%, tibia 33%, humerus 10%. Vertebral osteomyelitis not uncommon in adults. Predisposing factors are IV drug abuse, trauma, other source of infection (e.g., urinary tract). In neonates, septic arthritis often coexists.	**Children:** *S. aureus*, group A streptococci Rare: *H. influenzae*,[†] *S. pneumoniae*, gram-negative enterics **Neonates:** group B streptococci, gram-negative enterics, *S. aureus* **Adults:** *S. aureus*, gram-negative enterics	**Children:** cloxacillin[‡] + cefotaxime (if *H. influenzae* suspected) **Neonates:** cloxacillin[‡] + cefotaxime (to cover gram-negative enterics) **Adults:** cloxacillin[‡]
Spread from Contiguous Sites		
Common in elderly. Predisposing factors include surgery, soft tissue infection. e.g., mandible, skull.	*S. aureus*, anaerobes, gram-negative organisms, mixed infection	Clindamycin ± gentamicin
Penetrating Trauma		
All ages. e.g., puncture wound of foot.	*P. aeruginosa*, *S. aureus*	Cloxacillin[‡] and ticarcillin + gentamicin (to cover *Pseudomonas*)
Vascular Insufficiency		
Diabetic foot.	*S. aureus*, streptococci, G-bacilli, anaerobes	Imipenem-cilastatin, ciprofloxacin + clindamycin

* The site and origin of infection and organism responsible are largely related to age.
† H. influenzae is of decreasing importance due to success of immunization.
‡ A semisynthetic, penicillinase-resistant penicillin (e.g., cloxacillin) provides coverage against S. aureus and streptococci.

■ Aspiration: A bacteriologic diagnosis of aspirate from the
subperiosteum or bone greatly aids further management.
An organism can be obtained in up to 80% of cases. Early
consultation with an orthopedic surgeon is recommended.

Figure 1: **Management of Acute Osteomyelitis**

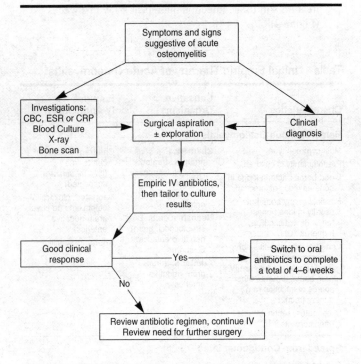

Abbreviations: ESR = erythrocyte sedimentation rate; CRP = C-reactive protein.

Therapeutic Choices (Figure 1)

Surgical Drainage

Antibiotics do not penetrate well into collections of pus or into
bone in which blood supply is compromised by infection.
Surgical decompression and exploration are necessary when there
has been a delay in presentation or diagnosis, when pus has been
found on aspiration or when there is x-ray evidence of bone
destruction. For early disease the role of immediate surgery has
been controversial. However, if swelling, pain, tenderness and
fever do not resolve within days after starting antibiotics, surgical
exploration should be considered. Suspicion of osteomyelitis
secondary to a penetrating injury (e.g., to the calcaneus) requires
bone exploration, débridement and culture. Osteomyelitis

Figure 2: **Management of Diabetic Foot Osteomyelitis**

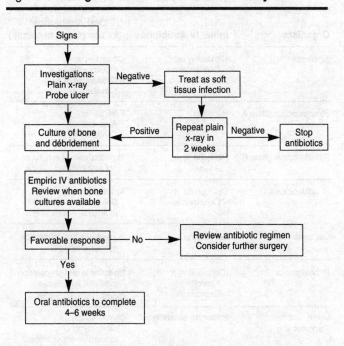

associated with diabetic foot requires surgical débridement. This should be aggressive and may involve amputation of the infected bone.

Pharmacologic Choices

Antibiotics

While cultures are pending, empiric IV antibiotic therapy, based on the most likely infecting organism, should be started (Table 1). A definitive choice can be made once the organism and sensitivities are identified (Table 2). The role of adjunctive antibiotics such as fusidic acid or rifampin has not been studied systematically. They cannot be used alone for staphylococcal infections because resistance develops rapidly.

Mild diabetic foot infection may be treated with an oral regimen of amoxicillin/clavulanic acid or ciprofloxacin plus clindamycin.

Duration of antibiotic therapy should be a minimum of 4 weeks; many authorities recommend 6 weeks. More severe initial presentation, extensive bone involvement, and slow resolution of systemic and local signs indicate a 6-week course. In osteomyelitis following penetrating injury, 10 to 14 days of treatment is sufficient if adequate débridement has been performed.

Table 2: **Choice of Antibiotics for Acute Osteomyelitis**

Organism	Initial IV Antibiotic	Oral Antibiotics (for completion of course)
S. aureus	Cloxacillin or Clindamycin	Cloxacillin or Flucloxacillin or Cephalexin or Clindamycin
Streptococcus group A	Penicillin	Penicillin or Amoxicillin or Clindamycin
Streptococcus group B	Penicillin	In neonates oral antibiotics not appropriate
H. influenzae	Cefotaxime or Cefuroxime	Amoxicillin or Cefixime (if ampicillin-resistant)
Coliforms	Cefotaxime	In neonates oral antibiotics not appropriate
P. aeruginosa	(Ceftazidime or Ticarcillin) + Gentamicin	No suitable oral preparation available for children. Ciprofloxacin for adults
Mixed aerobic/ anaerobic	Imipenem-cilastatin	Ciprofloxacin+ clindamycin or amoxicillin-clavulanate

In diabetic foot, 4 to 6 weeks of therapy is required. If no débridement of bone occurs, a 10- to 12-week course has been curative. If all infected bone has been completely removed, 2 to 3 weeks may be sufficient.

Sequential Intravenous–Oral Antibiotic Therapy

Since a long course is required, a switch from the IV to oral route has many advantages, particularly shortened hospital stay and reduced complications from IV cannulae. This has been the subject of a position paper by the Canadian Paediatric Society.[1] IV antibiotics should be continued until the patient is systemically better, the temperature is normal and local signs of inflammation and tenderness are improved. This may take several days. The same high concentrations of antibiotic can be achieved with the oral route but with certain provisos:

- Compliance is vital. For children, the taste of the oral antibiotic is the most important factor. Cloxacillin and flucloxacillin liquid preparations are particularly unpalatable; cephalexin has a more acceptable taste.

[1] Can J Infect Dis 1994;4:10–12.

Table 3: Antibiotics Used in Treatment of Acute Osteomyelitis*

Antibiotic	Dosage Pediatric (P)/Adult (A)	Adverse Effects	Comments	Cost†
amoxicillin 🍃 Amoxil, generics	(P) 100 mg/kg/d divided Q8H PO	GI effects, rash, eosinophilia.	Can be taken with food.	$
amoxicillin-clavulanate 🍃 Clavulin	(A) 2 g–0.2 g Q8H PO			$$
cefazolin 🍃 Ancef	(P) 100 mg/kg/d divided Q8H IV (A) 2 g Q8H IV			$ $$
cefixime 🍃 Suprax	(P) 8 mg/kg/d given Q24H PO	GI effects, especially diarrhea; hypersensitivity.	Can be taken with food.	$
cefotaxime 🍃 Claforan	(P) 150 mg/kg/d divided Q8H IV (A) 2 g Q8H IV	Phlebitis, hypersensitivity, positive Coombs' test.		$$ $$$
cefuroxime 🍃 Kefurox, Zinacef	(P) 150 mg/kg/d divided Q8H (A) 1.5 g Q8H IV	Phlebitis, eosinophilia, ↓ hematocrit, positive Coombs' test, neutropenia.		$$ $$
ceftazidime 🍃 Ceptaz, Fortaz, Tazidime	(P) 150 mg/kg/d divided Q8H (A) 2 g Q8H IV	Phlebitis, eosinophilia, positive Coombs' test, ↑ AST, superinfections.		$$ $$$$
cephalexin 🍃 Keflex, generics	(P) 100–150 mg/kg/d divided Q6H	GI effects, rash, eosinophilia, leukopenia, positive Coombs' test, ↑ AST.	Oral liquid preparations more palatable than cloxacillin and flucloxacillin.	$
ciprofloxacin 🍃 Cipro	(A) 400 mg Q12H IV or 750 mg Q12H PO			$$ $
clindamycin 🍃 Dalacin C	(P) 40 mg/kg/d divided Q6H IV or 30 mg/kg/d divided Q8H PO (A) 450–600 mg Q8H IV or PO	Rash, neutropenia, ↑ AST and alkaline phosphatase, pseudomembranous colitis.	May need to ↓ dosage in hepatic failure.	IV $$ PO $

(cont'd)

Table 3: Antibiotics Used in Treatment of Acute Osteomyelitis* *(cont'd)*

Antibiotic	Dosage Pediatric (P)/Adult (A)	Adverse Effects	Comments	Cost†
cloxacillin Orbenin, Tegopen, generics	(P) 200 mg/kg/d IV or 150–200 mg/kg/d PO divided Q6H (A) 2 g Q4H IV or 1 g Q6H PO	Rash, eosinophilia, GI effects.	May alter INR with warfarin. Oral liquid preparations unpalatable. Should be taken on empty stomach.	$ $ $$ $$
flucloxacillin Fluclox	(P) 150 mg/kg/d divided Q6H	Rash, eosinophilia, GI effects.	Oral liquid preparation unpalatable. Should be taken on empty stomach.	$$
gentamicin Cidomycin, Garamycin	(P) 6 mg/kg/d divided Q8H (A) 5–7 mg/kg/d Q8H or once daily if renal function permits	Nephrotoxicity usually reversible, ↑ risk with dose, duration. Ototoxicity often reversible.	↑ toxicity with other nephrotoxic or ototoxic drugs.	$
imipenem-cilastatin Primaxin	(A) 500 mg Q6H IV	Caution in beta-lactam sensitivity. Risk of seizures if dose exceeded in renal failure.		$$$$
penicillin G (IV) generics	(P) 200 000 units/kg/d divided Q4–6H (A) 4 million units Q6H	GI effects, hypersensitivity, rash, drug fever, positive Coombs' test. Monitor K+ and Na+ when using high-dose parenteral penicillin G.		$ $$
penicillin V (PO) Pen-Vee, PVF K, V-Cillin K, generics	(P) 100 mg/kg/d divided Q6H PO			$
ticarcillin Ticar	(P) 300 mg/kg/d divided Q6H IV (A) 3 g Q6H IV	Hypersensitivity, inhibition of platelet function, hypokalemia.	Contains 5.2 mmol of sodium/g. Can inactivate aminoglycosides if mixed.	$$ $$$

* *Therapy is initiated with IV antibiotics. When the patient is systemically better, a switch can be made to oral antibiotics under certain conditions – see Pharmacologic Choices.*
● *Dosage adjustment may be required in renal impairment – see Appendix I.*

† *Cost per day (pediatric dosage based on 20 kg) – includes drug cost only.*
Legend: $ < $10 $$ $10–50 $$$ $50–100 $$$$ $100–150

- No underlying immunocompromise is present.
- Patient is beyond neonatal age group.
- The dose of oral antibiotic is larger than that usually used for minor infections (Table 3).
- Patient will attend for regular review.
- Adequacy of antibiotic concentrations is measured. The most practical method is to measure the serum bactericidal titre (SBT) against the organism, using a blood sample drawn 45 to 90 minutes after an oral dose is given. The desired titre is ≥ 1:8. An inadequate dose of antibiotic, refusal to take all the dose or poor absorption may lead to failure in reaching the desired level. Inability to achieve this target or failure to improve clinically should lead to resumption of IV antibiotics. If no organism was isolated but the patient has recovered well on the empiric antibiotic regimen, a switch to a comparable oral antibiotic can still be made.

Follow-up

Success of treatment is judged by careful follow-up of systemic signs (i.e., fever and well-being, local signs of decreasing inflammation and tenderness and return of full function). ESR gradually returns to normal over several weeks. The C-reactive protein returns to normal in a matter of days.

Suggested Reading List

Canadian Paediatric Society, Infectious Diseases and Immunization Committee. The use of antibiotic therapy as an adjunct in treatment of bone and joint infections. *Can J Infect Dis* 1994;4:10–12.

Caputo GM, Cavanagh PR, Ulbrecht JS, et al. Assessment and management of foot disease in patients with diabetes. *N Engl J Med* 1994;331:854–860.

Eckman MH, Greenfield S, MacKey WC, et al. Foot infections in diabetic patients: decision and cost-effectiveness analyses. *JAMA* 1995;273:712–720.

Grayson MC, Gibbons GW, Balogh K, et al. Probing to bone in infected pedal ulcers. *JAMA* 1995;273:721–723.

Lew DP, Waldvogel FA. Osteomyelitis. *N Engl J Med* 1997;336: 999–1007.

Nade S. Acute haematogenous osteomyelitis in infancy and childhood. *J Bone Joint Surg Br* 1983;65:109–119.

Unkila-Kallio L, Kallio M, Eshola J, et al. Serum C-reactive protein, erythrocyte sedimentation rate and white blood cell count in acute haematogenous osteomyelitis of children. *Pediatrics* 1994;93:59–62.

CHAPTER 88

Cellulitis

Sandra A.N. Tailor, PharmD, Anita R. Rachlis, MD, MEd, FRCPC and Neil Shear, MD, FRCPC, FACP

Definitions

Cellulitis: a spreading infection of the skin that involves deeper subcutaneous tissues.

Erysipelas: a superficial cellulitis of the skin associated with extensive involvement of the lymphatics.

Necrotizing fasciitis: a spreading infection that involves the superficial layer of the deep fascia of muscle and may secondarily involve the surrounding muscle and subcutaneous tissues.

For **impetigo**, see Chapter 60.

Goals of Therapy

- To cure infection and prevent dissemination
- To minimize tissue damage

Causative Organisms/Presentation (Table 1)

Therapeutic Choices

Nonpharmacologic Choices

- **Surgical treatment:** Incision and drainage are **rarely** indicated to treat cellulitis. However, they are essential in necrotizing fasciitis.
- **Supportive therapy:** Elevation and immobilization of the affected area may decrease swelling.

Pharmacologic Choices (Tables 1 and 2)

Table 1: Presentation and Treatment of Cellulitis

Infection	Common Causative Organisms	Antibiotic Choice(s)	Comments
Uncomplicated streptococcal or staphylococcal cellulitis	Group A streptococci, *Staphylococcus aureus*	(1) Cloxacillin PO or IV*† Cephalexin PO‡π Cefazolin IV‡π (2) Clindamycin IV (if severe)π# Clindamycin POπ# (3) Erythromycin PO or IV†π# Clarithromycin POπ# Azithromycin POπ#	Lesions are red, hot and edematous with borders that are not sharply demarcated. Since streptococcal and staphylococcal cellulitis cannot be distinguished from each other clinically, the treatment of choice for both is **cloxacillin**.
Cellulitis in children	Group A streptococci, *S. aureus*, *Haemophilus influenzae* (usually < 2 yrs of age)	(1) Cefuroxime IV (2) Amoxicillin/clavulanate PO (if less severe) (3) Co-trimoxazole PO (4) Chloramphenicol IV	*H. influenzae* cellulitis may present with the child being very ill with upper respiratory tract symptoms, bacteremia or septicemia. **Cefuroxime** is the drug of choice (ensures coverage of *H. influenzae*).
Diabetic foot infections (mild)	Group A streptococci, *S. aureus*; commonly polymicrobic (*P. aeruginosa* and anaerobes)	(1) Co-trimoxazole PO + metronidazole PO (2) Amoxicillin/clavulanic acid PO Co-trimoxazole PO + clindamycin PO (3) Cephalexin PO + metronidazole PO (4) Clindamycin PO + ciprofloxacin PO**	Antimicrobial regimen should have broad-spectrum activity (gram-positive, gram-negative and anaerobes). **Metronidazole + co-trimoxazole** is effective and inexpensive. **NB:** Patients with severe diabetic foot infections should be referred to an infectious diseases specialist.

(cont'd)

Table 1: Presentation and Treatment of Cellulitis *(cont'd)*

Infection	Common Causative Organisms	Antibiotic Choice(s)	Comments
Erysipelas	Group A streptococci (*S. pyogenes*) most common. Others: group C streptococci, group G streptococci, group B streptococci, *S. aureus* (rare)	(1) Cloxacillin PO or IV*† Cefazolin IV or Cephalexin PO*π Penicillin V PO or Penicillin G IV*†‡ (2) Clindamycin PO or IV*π# (3) Erythromycin PO or IV†π# Clarithromycin PO*π# Azithromycin PO*π#	Skin lesion is initially small and may go unnoticed. However, fever and rigors may occur early and abruptly in the process. Lesions are edematous, brawny, hot, indurated, shiny and erythematous, with a sharply demarcated margin. Microbiological culture of the involved skin is often not helpful; diagnosis is clinical. **Penicillin, cloxacillin or cefazolin** is the treatment of choice. Facial involvement requires antimicrobials that penetrate into the CNS (e.g., **penicillin, cloxacillin** or **vancomycin**).
Necrotizing fasciitis	Group A streptococci (*S. pyogenes*)	Clindamycin 600 mg IV Q8H + penicillin G (3 million units IV Q6H) + in patients with streptococcal toxic-shock syndrome (STSS), intravenous immunoglobulin (IVIG) (0.4 g/kg/d × 5 d as single infusion over 6–9 h)	Surgical management and supportive care as required. Invasive group A streptococcal infection is a reportable disease in some provinces in Canada. Recent data indicate that close contacts of patients with necrotizing fasciitis may have a higher risk than the general population of developing necrotizing fasciitis. The Ontario provincial health policies indicate that close contacts of patients with STSS or necrotizing fasciitis should receive chemoprophylaxis. However, consensus has not been reached on either the use of chemoprophylaxis or specific drug therapy for chemoprophylaxis. **NB:** Patients with necrotizing fasciitis and chemoprophylaxis of close contacts should be referred to an infectious diseases specialist.

Abbreviations: (1) = *First line;* (2) = *Second line;* (3) = *Third line;*

* *In patients having questionable/minor allergic reactions with penicillin, cephalosporins are an alternative, but they should be avoided in patients describing an anaphylactic reaction to penicillin. Vancomycin, clindamycin, erythromycin, clarithromycin and azithromycin are good alternatives.*

† *IV route is recommended in severe cases.*

‡ *Vancomycin IV is recommended in patients not tolerating or not responding to therapy and in β-lactam-allergic patients (including those with facial involvement of cellulitis/erysipelas).*

π *Avoid in facial cellulitis, since assurance of meningeal penetration is required (in the clinical opinion of the authors).*

\# *Organisms resistant to erythromycin will also be resistant to clindamycin, clarithromycin and azithromycin.*

** *Although this regimen is third line for mild diabetic foot infections, it may be considered first line in patients with severe diabetic foot infections when oral therapy is the selected route.*

Table 2: Antibiotics Used to Treat Cellulitis

Antibiotic	Dosage	Adverse Effects	Drug Interactions	Cost*
amoxicillin/clavulanic acid 🍂 Clavulin	**Cellulitis in children** 40 mg/kg/d of amoxicillin PO divided Q8H (suspension) **Diabetic foot cellulitis** 500 mg PO Q8H	Nausea, vomiting, diarrhea, rash, eosinophilia.		$$
azithromycin 🍂 Zithromax	500 mg PO on day 1 followed by 250 mg on days 2–5 (total 1.5 g) (for mild cellulitis in patients not tolerating erythromycin)	Nausea, vomiting, diarrhea, abdominal cramps, rash (rare), hepatotoxicity (rare).	Inhibits cytochrome P-450 enzyme system.†	$$
cefazolin 🍂 Ancef, Kefzol	1g IV Q8H	Rash, ↑ AST and ALP, phlebitis, positive Coombs' test (rare).		$$
cefuroxime 🍂 Kefurox, Zinacef	100–150 mg/kg/d IV divided Q8H to maximum of 750 mg IV Q8H	Phlebitis (2%), eosinophilia (7%), anemia (10%), positive Coombs' test (< 1%), neutropenia (< 1%), rash (< 1%), ↑ LFTs (4%).		$$$$
cephalexin 🍂 Keflex, generics	500 mg PO QID	Nausea, vomiting, diarrhea (2%), rash (1%), eosinophilia (9%), leukopenia (3%), positive Coombs' test (rare), ↑ AST.		$
chloramphenicol 🍂 Chloromycetin	50–75 mg/kg/d IV divided Q6H	Eosinopenia, aplastic anemia, gray syndrome, fever, rash.	↑ toxicity of phenytoin. ↑ INR with warfarin. Hypoglycemia with sulfonylureas.	$$$$

(cont'd)

Table 2: Antibiotics Used to Treat Cellulitis *(cont'd)*

Antibiotic	Dosage	Adverse Effects	Drug Interactions	Cost*
ciprofloxacin Cipro	500–750 mg PO BID	Nausea, vomiting, diarrhea, abdominal pain.	Cimetidine ↑ levels of ciprofloxacin. Multivalent metallic cations, antacids and sucralfate ↓ absorption of ciprofloxacin. Inhibits cytochrome P-450 enzyme system.†	$$
clarithromycin Biaxin	500 mg PO BID (for mild cellulitis in patients not tolerating erythromycin)	Nausea, vomiting, diarrhea, abdominal cramps, dyspepsia, headache, ↑ BUN and serum creatinine.	Inhibits cytochrome P-450 enyzme system.†	$$
clindamycin Dalacin-C	PO: 300–450 mg QID (alone or with other antibiotics) IV: 450–600 mg Q8H ↓ dose in hepatic impairment	Diarrhea, rash (4%), neutropenia, eosinophilia, ↑ AST and ALP, pseudomembranous colitis.		PO: $-$$ IV: $$$$$
cloxacillin Orbenin, Tegopen, generics	**Uncomplicated cellulitis** PO: 500 mg QID IV: 1–2 g Q4–6H **Erysipelas** PO: 500 mg PO QID IV: 2 g IV Q4–6H	Nausea, vomiting, diarrhea, rash (1–5%), drug fever, eosinophilia, positive Coombs' test (rare), hemolytic anemia, neutropenia, interstitial nephritis,↑ AST.	Warfarin (may alter INR).	PO: $ IV: $$$-$$$$

Drug	Dosage	Adverse Effects	Drug Interactions	Cost*
co-trimoxazole ● Bactrim, Septra, generics	10 mg/kg/d of TMP component PO divided Q12H	Nausea, vomiting, diarrhea, rash, false ↑ serum creatinine, renal impairment, neutropenia, thrombocytopenia, anemia, agranulocytosis.	↑ phenytoin levels. ↑ INR with warfarin. Hypoglycemia with sulfonylureas. Cyclosporine (↑ nephrotoxicity). Bone marrow suppressing agents (↑ hematologic toxicity).	$
erythromycin Ilotycin, Eryc, PCE, EES, E-Mycin, Erythromid, Ilosone, generics	PO: 1 g/d PO divided BID, TID or QID IV: 500 mg Q6H	Nausea, vomiting, diarrhea, abdominal cramps, rash (rare), hepatotoxicity (rare).	Inhibits cytochrome P-450 enzyme system.[†]	PO: $ IV: $$$$$
metronidazole Flagyl, generics	500 mg PO BID	Nausea, vomiting, diarrhea, metallic taste, headache, dark urine, neutropenia.	Disulfiram reaction with alcohol. Acute toxic psychosis with disulfiram. ↑ INR with warfarin. Phenobarbital, phenytoin (↑ metabolism of metronidazole ↓ effectiveness). ↓ phenytoin clearance.	$
penicillin V (PO) ● Pen-Vee, PVF K, generics	PO: 300 mg QID × 7–10 d	Rash (1–5%), drug fever, positive Coombs' test.		$
penicillin G (IV) ● Crystapen, generics	IV: 2 million units Q4–6H	Electrolyte imbalance possible with high-dose IV penicillin G sodium or potassium (> 10 million IU/d).		

[†] Potential ↑ effect/toxicity of carbamazepine, corticosteroids, cyclosporine, digoxin, terfenadine, astemizole, theophylline and warfarin.

● Dosage adjustment may be required in renal impairment – see Appendix I.

* Cost per day – includes drug cost only.

Legend: $ < $2 $$ $2–10 $$$ $10–20 $$$$ $20–30 $$$$$ > $30

Infectious Diseases

Suggested Reading List

Danzinger LH, Fish D, Hassan E. Skin and soft tissue infections. In: *Pharmacotherapy, a pathophysiologic approach.* 3rd ed. Connecticut: Appleton and Lange, 1996:2059–2080.

Ontario Anti-infective Review Panel. *Anti-infective guidelines for community-acquired infections.* 2nd ed. Toronto: Queen's Printer for Ontario, 1997:32–35.

Sanford JP, Gilbert DN, Gerberding JL, et al. *Guide to antimicrobial therapy 1997.* Vienna, Virginia: Antimicrobial Therapy Inc., 1997.

Swartz MN, Weinberg AN. Infections due to gram-positive bacteria. In: Fitzpatrick TB, Eisen AZ, Wolff K, et al, eds. *Dermatology in general medicine.* 4th ed. New York: McGraw-Hill Inc., 1993:2309–2334.

CHAPTER 89

Septic Shock

Anthony W. Chow, MD, FRCPC, FACP

Goals of Therapy

- To restore fluid volume
- To improve tissue perfusion and oxygen delivery
- To correct metabolic acidosis and coagulation defects
- To reduce oxygen demand
- To eradicate causative pathogens
- To neutralize the biologic effects of exotoxins and/or endotoxins
- To manage complications (e.g., acute renal failure, acute respiratory distress syndrome [ARDS], disseminated intravascular coagulation [DIC], multiple organ dysfunction syndrome [MODS])
- To prevent nosocomial infections
- To prevent progression from sepsis syndrome to full septic shock

Classification of Sepsis and Septic Shock

Patients should be categorized into 1 of 3 syndromes (Table 1).

Table 1: **Classification of Sepsis and Septic Shock**

Clinical Staging	Diagnostic Criteria
Sepsis syndrome without shock (incipient septic shock)	Clinical evidence suggestive of infection plus: Signs of a systemic inflammatory response to infection (all of the following): Tachypnea: > 20 breaths/min or > 10 L/min if mechanically ventilated. Tachycardia: > 90 beats/min. Hyperthermia or hypothermia > 38.4°C or < 35.6°C. Evidence of altered organ perfusion (one or more of the following): Hypoxia: $PaO_2/FIO_2 < 280$ (in the absence of other pulmonary or cardiovascular disease). Oliguria: < 0.5 mL/kg for at least 1 h in patients with urinary catheters. ↑ plasma lactate (> normal upper limit). Altered mental status.
Septic shock Early Refractory	Clinical diagnosis of sepsis syndrome as outlined above plus: Early: Hypotension* lasting < 2 h, responsive to conventional therapy. Refractory: Hypotension* lasting > 2 h despite conventional therapy.

* < 90 mm Hg or a 40 mm Hg decrease below baseline.

Figure 1: **Early Management of Septic Shock (First 4 Hours)**

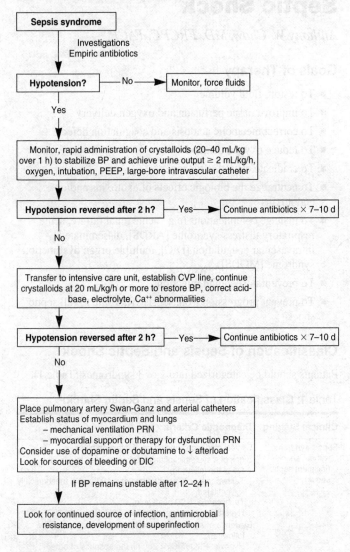

Abbreviations: PEEP = positive end-expiratory pressure; CVP = central venous pressure; DIC = disseminated intravascular coagulation.

Investigations

- Thorough history with special attention to underlying disease, precipitating event and possible sites of infection
- Physical examination to localize the site and extent of infection, assess end organ dysfunction and ascertain

- evidence of DIC or disseminated infection (e.g., skin rash, purpura, ecthyma gangrenosum, subcutaneous nodules)
- Clinical monitoring of vital signs, urine output, weight, level of consciousness
- Laboratory monitoring:
  - arterial blood gases
  - electrolytes, plasma lactate, acid-base status
  - BUN or serum creatinine
  - liver function tests
  - serum calcium and phosphate
  - chest x-ray, ECG
  - coagulation status
  - stool for occult blood
  - Gram's stain and cultures from blood, urine, sputum, other body sites
  - imaging studies to search for loculated infection
- Additional investigations may be necessary to monitor cardiopulmonary status and to localize the site of infection

Therapeutic Choices (Figure 1)

Nonpharmacologic Choices

Resuscitation and Monitoring

Meticulous monitoring of the patient's circulating volume and ventilatory status and immediate resuscitation if required, is essential. If simple measures do not quickly restore hemodynamic stability, intensive care should be considered with invasive hemodynamic monitoring and aggressive cardiovascular support.

Early institution of **mechanical ventilation** and **sedation** and the judicious use of muscle **relaxants** or **neuromuscular blockade** may help to reduce oxygen demand and improve oxygen delivery and extraction at the tissue level. **Adequate caloric intake** with trace element and vitamin supplements is important to retard intense catabolism in patients with significant protein–calorie malnutrition.

Localization and Evacuation of Loculated Infections

In addition to plain radiographs and tomograms, ultrasonography and computed tomography are invaluable for localizing nidus of infection in the thorax, abdomen, pelvis or the central nervous system. Loculated abscesses should be drained, and necrotic tissues must be adequately débrided. Infected foreign bodies should be removed.

Anticipation and Prevention of Complications

Acute respiratory distress syndrome (ARDS): Anticipate and treat supportively (the value of corticosteroids, ibuprofen, prostaglandin E_1, pentoxifylline or antioxidants is unproven).

Electrolyte and acid-base status: Correct initial hyponatremia and acidosis; anticipate and correct hypocalcemia and tetany.

Edema, pericardial and pleural effusions: Maintain adequate intravascular volume before using diuretic to mobilize extravascular fluid.

Acute renal failure: Avoid nephrotoxic drugs; monitor and dialyze PRN.

Thrombocytopenia and DIC: Administer fresh frozen plasma and platelets PRN. Heparin sulfate (50 to 100 units/kg Q4H) reduces thrombin generation, interrupts formation of fibrin microthrombi and reduces fibrinolysis but has not been shown to affect survival.

Impaired gastrointestinal motility and stress ulcers: Impaired motility may manifest as abnormal gastric emptying or as adynamic ileus. Stress ulceration is another common complication in the acutely ill. The judicious use of a gastrointestinal prokinetic agent (e.g., cisapride 10 mg Q6H) and agents to prevent stress ulcers (e.g., antacids, cytoprotectives or histamine H_2-receptor antagonists) may be beneficial.

Hepatic dysfunction: Avoid drugs requiring biotransformation in the liver.

Central nervous system dysfunction: Anticipate irrational behavior; manage seizures with anticonvulsants.

Nosocomial infections: Strict adherence to aseptic technique and infection control principles are required to minimize the development of nosocomial infections. Every effort should be made to reduce the number of invasive intravascular catheters. Peripheral venous catheters should be changed routinely every 48 to 72 hours; when such catheters are inserted emergently, they should be replaced within 24 hours. Nasogastric and nasotracheal intubation should be avoided to prevent nosocomial sinusitis. The value of selected digestive tract decontamination in reducing the incidence of nosocomial pneumonia remains controversial.

Pharmacologic Choices
Empiric Antimicrobial Therapy

Antimicrobial therapy remains the cornerstone of treatment for sepsis syndrome and septic shock. However, the underlying disease, comorbid conditions and development of complications (e.g., ARDS, MODS) often dictate the eventual outcome of therapy.

Table 2: **Common Pathogens in Patients with Sepsis Syndrome or Septic Shock**

Source of Infection	Common Pathogens	Initial Antibiotic Regimen
Oral cavity, lower respiratory tract	*Streptococcus viridans, Streptococcus pyogenes, Streptococcus pneumoniae, Haemophilus influenzae, Klebsiella pneumoniae, Peptostreptococcus* spp., *Bacteroides* spp., *Fusobacterium* spp., *Legionella pneumophila*.	Third-generation cephalosporin or Extended spectrum penicillin
Gastrointestinal tract, female pelvis	Enteric gram-negative bacilli, *Bacteroides fragilis, Peptostreptococcus* spp., *Clostridia* spp., *Enterococcus* spp.	Extended spectrum penicillin +/– aminoglycoside or Ciprofloxacin + metronidazole
Urinary tract	*Escherichia coli, Pseudomonas aeruginosa*, other enteric gram-negative bacilli, *Staphylococcus saprophyticus, Enterococcus* spp.	Ciprofloxacin or Aminoglycoside
Cardiac valves	*Staphylococcus aureus, Streptococcus viridans, Enterococcus* spp., *Corynebacterium* spp., *Coxiella burnetii*, HACEK group (*Haemophilus aphrophilus, Actinobacillus actinomycetemcomitans, Cardiobacterium hominis, Eikenella corrodens, Kingella* spp.).	Penicillin +/– vancomycin
Central nervous system	*Neisseria meningitidis, H. influenzae, S. pneumoniae, S. aureus*, enteric gram-negative bacilli, *Bacteroides* spp., *Nocardia asteroides, Peptostreptococcus* spp.	Extended spectrum penicillin
Necrotizing skin and soft tissues	*S. aureus*, enteric gram-negative bacilli, *B. fragilis, Clostridia* spp., *Peptostreptococcus* spp., *Enterococcus* spp.	Extended spectrum penicillin +/– aminoglycoside
Intravascular devices-associated	*S. aureus, Staphylococcus epidermidis, Staphylococcus haemolyticus*, enteric gram-negative bacilli, *Candida* spp.	Vancomycin

Initial antimicrobial therapy is empiric because gram-positive and gram-negative infections as well as mycobacterial, fungal and viral infections can present as sepsis syndrome or septic shock, which are clinically indistinguishable. Antibiotic selection is based on the most likely source/site of infection and hence the most likely causative microorganisms and their anticipated susceptibility profiles (Tables 2 and 3). The choice of anti-microbial agents (Table 4) may also be influenced by the presence of acute renal or hepatic failure, hypersensitivity

Table 3: **Spectrum of Antibiotics Used in Sepsis Syndrome and Septic Shock**

Pathogen	β-lactams	Aminogly-cosides	Fluoro-quinolones	Glyco-peptides
Staphylococci	++ I/C, P/T + others	±	++	+++ (incl. MRSA)
Streptococci	++ ctaz +++ others	−	+	+++
Enterococci	++ I/C +++ P/T ± others	++	+	+++
Haemophilus	+++	−	++	−
Enteric gram-negative bacilli	++ ctrx, cfax, ctiz +++ others	+++	+++	−
Pseudomonas, resistant gram-negative bacilli	++ ctrx, cfax, ctiz +++ others	++	+++	−
Anaerobes	+++ I/C, P/T (incl. *B. fragilis*) + ctaz, ctrx ++ ctiz	−	−	−

MRSA = methicillin-resistant S. aureus.
Activity: *− none; ± negligible; + some; ++ moderate; +++ excellent.*
β-lactams: *imipenem/cilastatin (I/C), piperacillin/tazobactam (P/T), ceftazidime (ctaz), ceftriaxone (ctrx), ceftizoxime (ctiz), cefotaxime (cfax).*
Aminoglycosides: *gentamicin, tobramycin, amikacin.* **Fluoroquinolones:** *ciprofloxacin.*
Glycopeptides: *vancomycin, teicoplanin.*

reactions, need for fluid restriction, local antimicrobial susceptibility patterns, emergence of resistance and drug interactions.

Antibiotics should be administered IV in critically ill patients and be reassessed within 3 to 5 days. Adjustments are guided by culture results, in vitro susceptibility patterns and clinical response.

Vasoactive Agents for Cardiovascular Support

Although rapid fluid administration alone may be sufficient to restore hemodynamic stability, vasopressors are often necessary to restore minimal tissue perfusion pressure and enhance myocardial contractility.

Dopamine (2 to 25 μg/kg/min) is usually selected first because it more effectively maintains organ blood flow. The dose is titrated until systolic BP is maintained at > 90 mm Hg and urine output at > 30 mL/h. Renal and mesenteric circulations may be selectively

Table 4: Intravenous Antimicrobial Drugs Used in Sepsis Syndrome and Septic Shock

Drug	IV Dosage	Adverse Effects	Comments	Cost*
Extended Spectrum β-lactams 🎔		Hypersensitivity, hepatitis, interstitial nephritis, neutropenia, hypoprothrombinemia, eosinophilia, positive Coombs' test, pseudomembranous colitis, seizures.	Have become mainstay of treatment due to lack of nephrotoxicity and broad-spectrum activity vs gram-negative organisms.	
imipenem/cilastatin Primaxin	1 g Q6H		No drug interactions; serum concentration monitoring not required.	$$$$$
piperacillin/tazobactam Tazocin	2 g Q4H		Imipenem, ceftazidime may be used with caution in patients allergic to penicillin.	$$
ticarcillin/clavulanate Timentin	3 g Q4H			$$
ceftazidime Ceptaz, Tazidime	2 g Q6H		Ceftizoxime is often chosen to cover anaerobes in head/neck, intra-abdominal, female pelvic or necrotizing skin infections.	$$$$$
ceftriaxone Rocephin	1–2 g Q24H			$$
ceftizoxime Cefizox	1–2 g Q8H			$$
cefotaxime Claforan	2 g Q6-8H			$$–$$$

Aminoglycosides 🎔

Drug	IV Dosage	Adverse Effects	Comments	Cost*
gentamicin Garamycin, generics	1.5 mg/kg Q8H or 4–7 mg once daily†	Nephrotoxicity, ototoxicity, neuromuscular blockade.	May be required as combination therapy with β-lactams for *Pseudomonas* or multiresistant gram-negative bacilli.	$
tobramycin Nebcin	1.5 mg/kg Q8H or 4–7 mg/kg once daily†		Often avoided in septic shock due to nephrotoxicity and ototoxicity; serum drug levels monitored to guide dosing and avoid toxicity.	$
amikacin Amikin	7.5 mg/kg Q12H or 15–20 mg/kg once daily†		Desired levels (µg/mL):	$$

	Gentamicin	*Tobramycin*	*Amikacin*
Peak	10	10	40
Trough	<2	<2	<10

↑ nephrotoxicity when used with vancomycin.

(cont'd)

Table 4: Intravenous Antimicrobial Drugs Used in Sepsis Syndrome and Septic Shock *(cont'd)*

Drug	IV Dosage	Adverse Effects	Comments	Cost*
Fluoroquinolones ❦ *ciprofloxacin* Cipro	400 mg Q8–12H	GI upset, insomnia, headache, rash, cartilage damage, seizures (rare).	Oral formulations available for step-down therapy. Serum levels not monitored. Ciprofloxacin:↑ theophylline (toxicity), ↑ caffeine levels; may cause nephrotoxicity with cyclosporine; may ↑ INR with warfarin.	$$$
Glycopeptides ❦ *vancomycin* Vancocin	1 g Q12H	Nephrotoxicity, ototoxicity, phlebitis; "red man syndrome" (flushing/rash, hypotension) if vancomycin infused too rapidly (< 1 h).	Enhanced nephrotoxicity when vancomycin used with aminoglycosides.	$$$
teicoplanin ‡	10 mg/kg/d		Teicoplanin has longer half-life. Desired serum levels: *peak* 40 µg/mL, *trough* < 10 µg/mL. Useful if serious infection with coagulase-negative staphylococci or enterococci or if methicillin-resistant *S. aureus* present.	‡
Others *clindamycin* Dalacin C	600 mg Q6H	Rash, thrombophlebitis, GI effects, pseudomembranous colitis, blood dyscrasias, ↑ liver function tests (clindamycin), metallic taste (metronidazole).	Often chosen to cover anaerobes in head/neck, intra-abdominal, female pelvic or necrotizing skin infections, but lack coverage against facultative gram-negative organisms (most often used with aminoglycosides or fluoroquinolones).	$$
metronidazole Flagyl, generic	500 mg Q8H		Clindamycin: may ↑ neuromuscular blocking action of other agents; may require dosage adjustment in hepatic failure. Metronidazole: ↑ lithium levels; ↑ INR with warfarin; disulfiram-like reaction with alcohol; acute psychosis and confusion with disulfiram.	$$

| *erythromycin* Ilotycin, Erythrocin | 15–20 mg/kg/d, divided Q6H | Venous irritation/ thrombophlebitis; rarely pro- longation of QT interval, ventricular arrhythmias, ototoxicity. Administer with caution if hepatic dysfunction. | Often included in initial empiric therapy if *Legionella* is suspected. Erythromycin: ↑ theophylline, carbamazepine, cyclosporine levels; ↑ INR with warfarin; ↑ risk of ventricular arrhythmias with astemizole and terfenadine. | $ |

‡ *Available through Special Access Program (formerly the Emergency Drug Release Program), Therapeutic Products Directorate, Health Canada.*
† *If appropriate for renal function.*
● *Dosage adjustment required in renal impairment – see Appendix I.*
* *Cost of 7-day supply – includes drug cost only:*
Legend: $ < $200 $$ $200–500 $$$ $500–750 $$$$ $750–1000 $$$$$ > $1000

preserved. **Dobutamine** (2 to 25 μg/kg/min, titrated as with dopamine) is similar to dopamine but has little chronotropic activity. **Isoproterenol** (5 μg/mL/min) increases the cardiac index but has little effect on mean arterial pressure. Its marked effect on increasing heart rate in some patients may limit its usefulness. **Norepinephrine** (0.1 to 0.2 μg/kg test dose, then 0.5 μg/kg/min) has intense peripheral vasoconstricting activity but can be used effectively to restore arterial pressure in patients with severe cardiovascular collapse. It may be administered as an adjunct to dopamine if hypotension persists but should be tapered down and discontinued in favor of dopamine infusion as soon as the clinical situation has improved.

Other Therapies

The routine use of **corticosteroids** as adjunctive therapy in septic shock cannot be recommended because benefits have not been demonstrated in controlled clinical trials.

Immunotherapy to neutralize or remove specific exotoxins may be worthwhile if etiologic agents are identified (e.g., diphtheria, botulism, anthrax, clostridial septicotoxemia, toxic shock syndrome); however, specific antisera are seldom available, and thus **immunoglobulins** pooled from healthy donors are often used empirically.

IV immune globulins (IVIG) (0.4 g/kg/day for 5 to 7 days) have been used as empiric adjunctive therapy for fulminant *Haemophilus*, pneumococcal, group A and group B streptococcal and *Pseudomonas* sepsis, and sepsis associated with staphylococcal toxic shock syndrome and streptococcal superantigens. Their efficacy in sepsis syndrome remains unproven except in hereditary or acquired immunodeficiency. Recent evidence suggests that IVIG can at least neutralize staphylococcal and streptococcal superantigen activity in vitro.

Naloxone, ibuprofen, indomethacin and **pentoxifylline** have been or are being investigated as adjunctive therapies in septic shock. Additional studies are needed before these agents can be recommended for routine clinical use. **Antitumor necrosis factor antibody** and **interleukin-1 receptor antagonists** were investigated but not found to be effective as adjunctive therapies in septic shock.

Therapeutic Tips

- Empiric broad-spectrum antibiotic therapy primarily directed at enteric gram-negative bacilli must be initiated early in **neutropenic** patients (Chapter 98). The classic symptoms and signs of infection, other than fever, are often absent, making it much more difficult to localize the primary source of infection. Infections (especially gram-negative) in these patients tend to disseminate rapidly and widely and are associated with a high mortality rate. The clinical response and eventual outcome is often dictated by the speed of bone marrow recovery and successful avoidance of complications (e.g., superinfections).

- **Persistent bacteremia,** despite appropriate antimicrobial therapy, suggests a valvular or endovascular infection, a loculated abscess with dissemination or the emergence of resistant microorganisms.

- **Culture-negative infections** are particularly common among patients who have received partial antimicrobial therapy before cultures are obtained and in immunocompromised patients undergoing bone marrow or solid organ transplants. The possibility of fastidious or culture-negative organisms, particularly *Legionella* spp., rickettsia, invasive fungi and viruses, should be seriously considered and appropriate investigations implemented.

Suggested Reading List

Bone RC. Managing sepsis: what treatments can we use today? *J Crit Illness* 1997;12:15–24.

Bone RC. Diagnosing sepsis: what do we need to consider today? *J Crit Illness* 1996;11:658–665.

Bone RC. Immunologic dissonance: a continuing evolution in our understanding of the systemic inflammatory response syndrome (SIRS) and the multiple organ dysfunction (MODS). *Ann Intern Med* 1996;125:680–687.

Crow S, Penn R. Controlling nosocomial infection in the intensive care unit. *J Crit Illness* 1996;11:380–391.

Lamothe F, D'Amico P, Ghosn P, Tremblay C, Braidy J, Patenaude JV. Clinical usefulness of intravenous human immunoglobulins in invasive group A streptococcal infections: case report and review. *Clin Infect Dis* 1995;21:1469–1470.

Lynn WA, Cohen J. Adjunctive therapy for septic shock: a review of experimental approaches. *Clin Infect Dis* 1995;20: 143–158.

CHAPTER 90

Sexually Transmitted Diseases

John W. Sellors, BSc, MSc, MD, CCFP, FCFP

Goals of Therapy

- To abolish symptoms of the infection, if any
- To prevent recurrence
- To prevent the spread of infection to sexual partners
- To decrease the probability of complications (which may be life-threatening or disabling) or permanent damage to reproductive and other systems
- To eliminate genital warts with as little pain and residual damage as possible, for cosmetic or psychosexual reasons or symptoms
- To reduce the frequency and severity of outbreaks and the associated symptoms of genital herpes (Chapter 95)

Investigations

- History for:
  - duration of symptoms, if any
  - duration of specific risk factors
  - specific complaints of sexual partner (e.g., anogenital sores, discharge)
  - previous therapy and response
  - recent childbirth, urinary tract surgery or intrauterine contraceptive device (IUCD) insertion (for pelvic inflammatory disease)
- Physical examination:
  - inspection of affected areas for lesions; genital herpes lesions/crusts are usually on an erythematous base
  - anoscopy (if perianal warts are present)
  - in women: speculum examination for signs of infection, using water as a lubricant
  - in men: signs of urethral discharge; palpation for inguinal lymphadenopathy or abnormalities of the testes/epididymides
  - systemic signs of syphilis
- Laboratory tests and other investigations:
  - swabs from affected areas and smears for Gram's stain
  - urine specimen microscopic examination and culture

 – scrotal ultrasound if available and epididymo-orchitis
   suspected
 – CBC, ESR, C-reactive protein, urine and serum
   β-HCG, VDRL, transvaginal pelvic ultrasonography
   (preferable to transabdominal) if PID suspected[1]
 – darkfield microscopy examination of specimen, VDRL

Table 1: **Differential Diagnosis of Vaginitis/Vaginosis**

	Candidiasis	Trichomoniasis	Bacterial Vaginosis
Signs/symptoms			
Pruritus	+	+	–
Odor	–	+	+
Discharge	cheesy	purulent	grey/milky
Inflammation	+	+	–
Simple tests			
pH	≤ 4.5	> 4.5	> 4.5
"Whiff" test	–	±	+
Microscopic findings			
Specific	mycelia	trichomonads	clue cells
PMNs	+ +	+ + +	–
Lactobacilli	+	–	–

Therapeutic Choices

Vaginitis (Table 1)

For management see Figure 1; for treatment see Table 2.

Patients should be instructed to complete the full, continuous
course of therapy, even during menstruation.

Recurrent vulvovaginal candidiasis (at least 4 proven episodes
per year) requires investigation and possibly referral. Predisposing causes, if present, should be addressed (e.g., use of
systemic antibiotics, poorly controlled diabetes, consideration
of HIV testing and counseling).

Nonsexually transmitted causes of vaginitis are numerous
(e.g., tampons/other foreign bodies, douches, deodorant sprays,
lubricants, perfumes, contraceptive chemicals, dyes in colored
toilet tissue, scented napkins, bubble bath, detergents, seasonal
allergy, allergy to latex condoms/semen).

Cervicitis and Urethritis due to Chlamydia Trachomatis or Neisseria Gonorrhoeae

For management see Figure 1 (cervicitis) and Figure 2
(urethritis); for treatment see Table 3.

---

[1] *Because the accuracy of clinical and laboratory diagnosis for PID is not good,
clinicians must follow women carefully and judge when to refer them for more definitive
tests (e.g., laparoscopy).*

Selective screening of high-risk women (shaded box, below) is important for detection of sexually transmitted (chlamydial) cervicitis because symptoms are often minor and unlikely to result in health-care-seeking behavior.

> **Indications for Chlamydial Screening[2]**
> Intermenstrual bleeding
> Frequent urination (on enquiry, not a presenting complaint)
> New sexual partner in previous year
> Mucopurulent (opaque or yellow) endocervical discharge
> Cervical friability with swabbing

Test of cure is usually not obtained for chlamydial infection but is recommended for gonococcal infection (1 to 2 months after treatment).

Epididymo-orchitis

Epididymo-orchitis is treated the same way as urethritis (Table 3, Figure 2), but the antichlamydial regimen should be given for at least 10 days and until resolution occurs. Scrotal elevation and bed rest are advisable.

In men over 35 years of age, urethral cultures may be negative but urine cultures suggestive of infection; in this case, treat for urinary tract infection (Chapter 91).

Pelvic Inflammatory Disease (PID)

For management algorithm, see Figure 3; for drugs used in outpatient treatment, see Table 4.

Syphilis

For management algorithm, see Figure 4; for drugs used to treat syphilis, see Table 5.

Individuals with HIV infection and syphilis and those with suspected or proven tertiary syphilis should be referred.

Genital Herpes (Chapter 95)

Genital Warts (Human Papillomavirus [HPV]) (Figure 5)

There is no specific laboratory test commonly available to detect HPV. Examination (3 minutes after applying 3 to 5% acetic acid)

[2] *Arch Intern Med 1992;152:1837–1844.*

Figure 1: **Management of Vaginitis and Cervicitis**

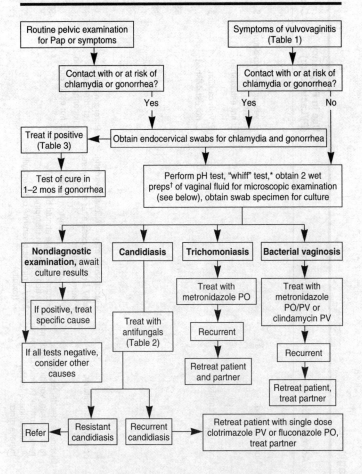

* Malodor often intensified after addition of 10% potassium hydroxide (KOH).
† One sample mixed in a few drops of normal saline; second sample mixed with 10% KOH.
Abbreviations: PV = vaginally

using a magnification device may detect subclinical exophytic and flat lesions, but the clinical utility of this is not proven, and it therefore is not recommended.

There is a frustratingly high recurrence rate (approximately 33%) of genital warts 1 year after apparent cure.

Hepatitis B (Chapter 94)

Table 2: Drugs Used for Vaginitis and Vaginosis

Drug	Dosage	Adverse Effects	Drug Interactions	Use in Pregnancy (P)/Lactation(L)	Cost*
Vulvovaginal Candidiasis					
Polyene Macrolides					
nystatin Mycostatin, Nilstat, generics	100 000 units PV daily × 14 d	None reported.		P: yes, until 6 wks before term. L: not established.	$
Imidazoles†					
clotrimazole Canesten, Myclo, generics	200 mg ovule PV QHS × 3 or 500 mg tab PV (1 dose)	Local hypersensitivity.		P: with caution. L: not established.	$
econazole Ecostatin	150 mg ovule PV QHS × 3				$$
miconazole Monistat, Micatin	400 mg PV QHS × 3				$$
tioconazole Gynecure	300 mg ovule or 6.5% oint (1 applicatorful) PV QHS × 1				$$
Triazoles					
terconazole Terazol	80 mg ovule or 0.8% cream (1 applicatorful) PV × 3	Local hypersensitivity.	Fluconazole: may ↑ INR with warfarin. May ↓ blood glucose after sulfonylurea administration.	P: terconazole – not in 1st trimester; fluconazole – no. L: not established.	$$
fluconazole† Diflucan, Diflucan-150	150 mg PO (1 dose)	Dizziness, headache, pruritus, rash, nausea, vomiting, abdominal pain, diarrhea, thrombocytopenia, ↑ transaminase levels, hypokalemia.	May markedly ↑ phenytoin levels. Fluconazole dose should be ↑ 25% when used with rifampin. May ↓ plasma clearance of theophylline (toxicity).		$$

Bacterial Vaginosis

clindamycin Dalacin Vaginal Cream, Dalacin-C	Topical: 5 g/d PV × 7 d Oral: 300 mg PO BID × 7 d	Nausea/vomiting, diarrhea, abdominal pain, constipation, heartburn, dizziness, headache, vertigo (< 1% with topical). Oral: pseudomembranous colitis. Topical: candidal vaginitis (10%).	**Topical:** P: yes. **Oral:** P: yes. L: with caution. $ $$
metronidazole Flagyl, NidaGel	Topical: 5 g (1 applicatorful) PV BID × 5 d Oral: see below	Candidal vaginitis.	See below. $$

Trichomoniasis or Bacterial Vaginosis

metronidazole Flagyl, generics	Oral: 2 g single dose[1] or 500 mg PO BID × 7 d Recurrences: same as above If not effective, 2 g PO daily × 3–5 d	Vertigo, headache, ataxia, abdomi- nal cramps, diarrhea, nausea, vomiting, pseudomembranous colitis, transient leukopenia, candidal vaginitis, taste altera- tions, gynecomastia.	Disulfiram-like reaction with alcohol. ↑ INR with oral anticoagulants. Psychosis/confusion with disulfiram. Barbiturates, phenytoin may ↑ metronidazole metabolism.	P: Safe use in 1st trimester uncertain; may use with caution during 2nd and 3rd trimesters.‡ L: no. $ $$ $$

[1] JAMA 1992;268:92–95.
† Use with caution in liver dysfunction.
‡ For symptomatic relief of trichomonal vaginitis during the 1st trimester; clotrimazole PV may suppress symptoms until definitive oral treatment can be given simultaneously to woman and partner(s) after 1st trimester.

* Cost of indicated course of therapy – includes drug cost only.
Legend: $ < $10 $$ $10–25

Figure 2: **Management of Urethritis and Epididymo-orchitis**

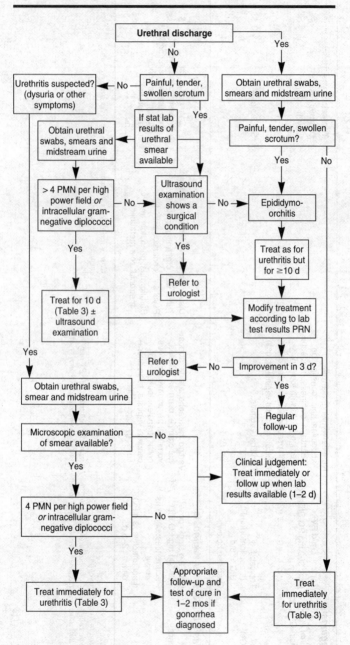

Abbreviations: PMN = polymorphonuclear leukocytes.

Table 3: Drugs Used in Gonococcal or Chlamydial Cervicitis and Urethritis *

Drug	Dosage	Comments	Use in Pregnancy (P)/Lactation (L)	Cost†
Gonococcal Cervicitis and Urethritis (should **ALWAYS** be followed by a regimen effective against *Chlamydia*)				
Cephalosporins				
ceftriaxone Rocephin	125 mg IM (1 dose)		P and L: caution.	$$
cefixime Suprax	400 mg PO (1 dose)		P and L: unknown.	$
Quinolones				
ciprofloxacin Cipro	500 mg PO (1 dose)		P and L: unknown.	$
ofloxacin Floxin	400 mg PO (1 dose)		P and L: unknown.	$
Spectinomycin Trobicin	2 g IM (1 dose)	Second-line therapy. Not effective in pharyngeal gonococcal infection. Alternative in pregnant patients allergic to cephalosporins.	P and L: caution.	‡
Chlamydial Cervicitis and Urethritis (should **ALWAYS** accompany gonococcal treatment)				
Tetracyclines				
doxycycline Vibra-Tabs, Vibramycin, Doryx, generics	100 mg BID × 7 d		P: 1st half. L: no.	7 d = $ 10–14 d = $$
tetracycline Tetracyn, generics	500 mg QID × 7 d			$

(cont'd)

Table 3: Drugs Used in Gonococcal or Chlamydial Cervicitis and Urethritis** *(cont'd)*

Drug	Dosage	Comments	Use in Pregnancy (P)/Lactation (L)	Cost†
Chlamydial Cervicitis and Urethritis *(cont'd)*				
Macrolides				
erythromycin base Eryc, Erybid, E-Mycin, PCE, Erythromid, generics	500 mg QID × 7 d; if not tolerated, 250 mg QID × 14 d may be used	May be substituted for doxycycline if tetracycline allergy, intolerance or pregnancy.	P: yes. L: with caution.	$
azithromycin Zithromax	1 g stat PO × 1 dose			$$
Ofloxacin 🟡 Floxin	300 mg BID × 7 d		P: unknown. L: unknown.	$$$
Sulfamethoxazole 🟡 generics	1 g BID × 10 d	Alternative to erythromycin for men or for pregnant women (1st, 2nd trimesters only).	P: 1st, 2nd trimester. L: with caution.	$
Amoxicillin 🟡 Amoxil, generics	500 mg TID × 10 d	Alternative to erythromycin for pregnant women in 3rd trimester.	P and L: with caution.	$

🟡 *Dosage adjustment may be required in renal impairment – see Appendix I.*
* *Epididymo-orchitis is treated similarly but for at least 10 d. For PID, see Table 5.*
‡ *Available through the Special Access Program (formerly the Emergency Drug Release Program), Therapeutic Products Directorate, Health Canada.*

† *Cost of one course of therapy – includes drug cost only.*
Legend: $ < $10 $$ $10–25 $$$ $25–50

Figure 3: **Management of Pelvic Inflammatory Disease**

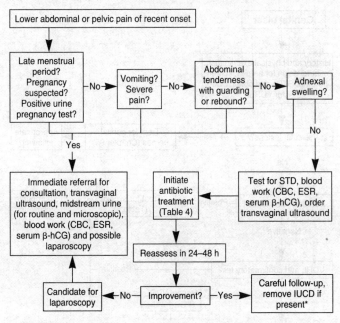

NB: If the patient has an IUCD in place, it should not be removed until after at least 2 d of antimicrobial therapy has been given.

Table 4: **Drugs Used for Outpatient Treatment of PID**

Drug Regimen		Cost*
Ceftriaxone 250 mg IM (single dose)	**plus** doxycycline† 100 mg PO BID	$$$
Cefoxitin‡ 2 g IM + probenecid†† 1 g PO (single dose)	**plus** doxycycline† 100 mg PO BID	$$
Cefixime ● 400 mg PO BID	**plus** doxycycline† 100 mg PO BID	$$$$$
Ciprofloxacin ● 500 mg PO BID	**plus** doxycycline† 100 mg PO BID	$$$$$
Ofloxacin ● 400 mg PO BID	π	$$$$$

NB: Duration of therapy for all oral agents is 14 d unless otherwise noted.

† *Erythromycin 500 mg PO QID × 14 d may be used instead of doxycycline if tetracycline allergy, intolerance or pregnancy.*

‡ *Safety in pregnancy is unknown.*

†† *Not needed if renal impairment is present. Use with caution in pregnancy and lactation.*

π *Ofloxacin covers both C. trachomatis and N. gonorrhoeae. Some experts would also add metronidazole 500 mg PO BID for anaerobes.*

● *Dosage adjustment may be required in renal impairment – see Appendix I.*

* *Cost of one course of therapy – includes drug cost only.*

Legend: $ < $10 $$ $10–25 $$$ $25–50 $$$$ $50–75 $$$$$ > $75

Figure 4: **Management of Genital Ulcers (Herpes, Syphilis)**

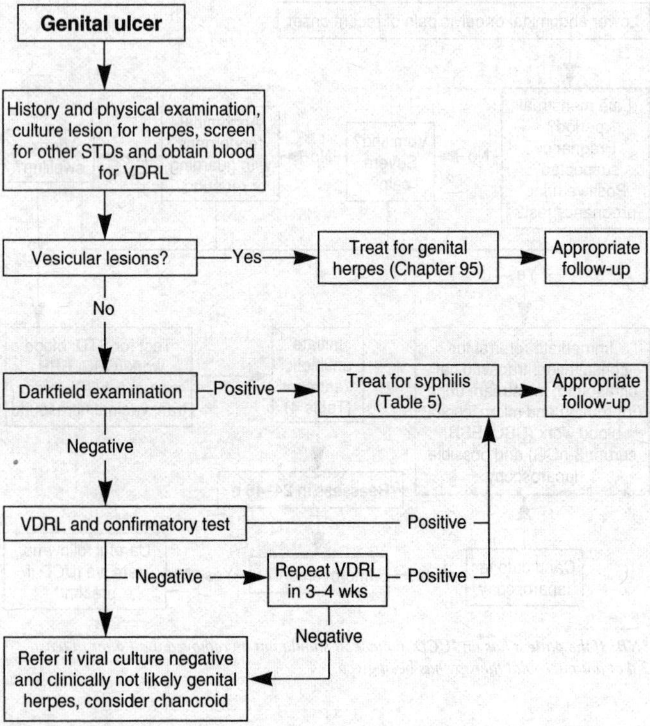

Therapeutic Tips

■ Treatment of sexual partner(s):

Infection	Treatment Required for Partner(s)?
Vulvovaginal candidiasis	Not unless symptomatic, or vaginitis is recurrent
Bacterial vaginosis	No
Trichomoniasis	Partner(s) always treated
Chlamydial or gonorrheal cervicitis, urethritis, epididymo-orchitis, PID	Refer all recent (< 6 wks) partners for testing and empirical treatment
Primary syphilis	Partners in previous 3 mos
Secondary syphilis	Partners in previous 6 mos
Early latent syphilis	Partners in previous yr
Late latent syphilis	Consider long-term partners and children
Genital herpes	No (condoms advised)
HPV	No (sexual contact should be avoided until warts have resolved)

- Testing and counseling for HIV and STD should be offered, when appropriate, to all patients.
  - patients testing positive for gonorrhea or chlamydia should be screened for syphilis
  - patients with genital herpes should be counseled on how to reduce the risk of transmission
  - the need for regular Pap smears should be emphasized to women with HPV infection

Table 5: Drugs Used to Treat Syphilis

Drug	Dosage	Comments	Cost*
benzathine penicillin G Bicillin 1200-LA	**Primary, secondary, early latent (< 1 yr):** 2.4 million units IM once (half in each buttock) **Late latent (> 1 yr):** 2.4 million units IM weekly × 3	Safe in pregnancy and lactation. May cause Jarisch-Herxheimer reaction in secondary syphilis (chills, fever, headache, myalgia, tachycardia, malaise, sweating, sore throat, hypotension).	$$ $$$
tetracycline 🍗 Tetracyn, generics	**Primary, secondary, early latent (< 1 yr):** Tetracycline: 500 mg PO QID × 14 d	Tetracyclines are alternatives in penicillin-allergic patients. Do not use in pregnancy and lactation.	$
doxycycline Vibramycin, Vibra-Tabs, Doryx, generics	Doxycycline: 100 mg PO BID × 14 d **Late latent (> 1 yr):** Same dosages × 28 d		14 d = $$ 28 d = $$$
erythromycin Eryc, Erybid, Erythromid, PCE, generics	**Primary, secondary, early latent (< 1 yr):** 500 mg PO QID × 14 d **Late latent (> 1 yr):** Same dosage × 28 d	Use only if penicillin desensitization is unsuccessful in pregnant, penicillin-allergic patients.	14 d = $ 28 d = $$

🍗 *Dosage adjustment may be required in renal impairment – see Appendix I.*
* *Cost of indicated duration – includes drug cost only.*
Legend: *$ < $10*   *$$ $10–25*   *$$$ $25–50*

Figure 5: **Management of Anogenital Warts**

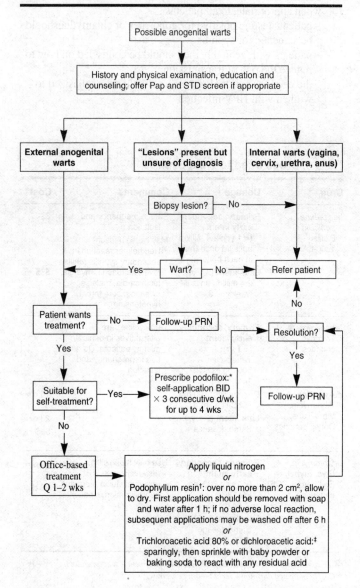

Adverse effects of:

* **Podofilox** (Condyline, Wartec): *inflammation, burning, erosion, pain, bleeding, pruritus, dizziness, insomnia. Do not use in pregnancy; safety in lactation unknown.*

† **Podophyllum resin** (Podofilm): *Systemic: urticaria, fever, paresthesia, polyneuritis, paralytic ileus, blood dyscrasias, coma, death. Local: severe necrosis, scarring, paraphimosis, pseudoepitheliomatous hyperplasia. Do not use in pregnancy; safety in lactation unknown.*

‡ **Dichloroacetic acid:** *Inflammation, erosion, pain, burning, ulceration. Safe for use in pregnancy and lactation.*

Suggested Reading List

Holmes KK, Mardh P-A, Sparling PF, et al, eds. *Sexually transmitted diseases*. 2nd ed. New York: McGraw-Hill, 1990.

MacDonald NE, Bowie WR, eds. 1995 Update. Canadian guidelines for the prevention, diagnosis, management and treatment of sexually transmitted diseases in neonates, children, adolescents and adults. *Can Commun Dis Rep* 1995;21 Suppl 4.

MacPherson DW, Sellors JW. Testing for HIV antibodies in family practice. A guide for obtaining informed consent. *Can Fam Physician* 1993;39:803–807.

Schlict JR. Treatment of bacterial vaginosis. *Ann Pharmacother* 1994;28:483–487.

Sellors JW, Pickard L, Gafni A, et al. Effectiveness and efficiency of selective vs universal screening for chlamydial infection in sexually active young women. *Arch Intern Med* 1992;152:1837–1844.

CHAPTER 91

Urinary Tract Infection

Lindsay E. Nicolle, MD

Goals of Therapy

- To ameliorate symptoms in acute infection
- To prevent recurrent infection
- To prevent pyelonephritis in pregnancy

Investigations (Table 1)

NB: Relapse is recurrence of UTI with the same organism, due to persistence of the organism within the urinary tract, usually in the prostate or kidneys. **Reinfection** is recurrent UTI with a new organism; it generally follows ascension of microorganisms from the periurethral area into the bladder.

Therapeutic Choices (Figure 1)

Pharmacologic Choices (Tables 2 and 3)

Co-trimoxazole and Trimethoprim

These are the drugs of choice for most UTIs. They are less useful for empiric therapy in individuals with complicated UTI due to increased antimicrobial resistance. Co-trimoxazole may be used as single dose (2 double-strength tablets) or 3-day therapy for acute uncomplicated UTI. Use of co-trimoxazole is limited by sulfa allergy (trimethoprim alone may be used in sulfa-allergic patients).

Nitrofurantoin

Nitrofurantoin, a urinary antiseptic, has been widely used to treat UTIs. It may not be as effective as co-trimoxazole for *short-course* therapy in the treatment of acute uncomplicated UTI. It is not recommended for treatment of pyelonephritis and is contra-indicated in renal failure. Pulmonary and hepatic toxicity may occur, usually with long-term use at full therapeutic doses. Nitrofurantoin macrocrystals may be better tolerated than the standard formulation.

Ampicillin and Amoxicillin

Resistance of *E. coli* to **ampicillin** limits its current use. It should be reserved for UTIs with streptococci or enterococci or in selected instances where other agents are not tolerated.

Empiric therapy of uncomplicated UTI with **amoxicillin** will be about 20% less effective than with co-trimoxazole. **Amoxicillin**

Figure 1: **Management of Recurrent Acute, Uncomplicated UTI**

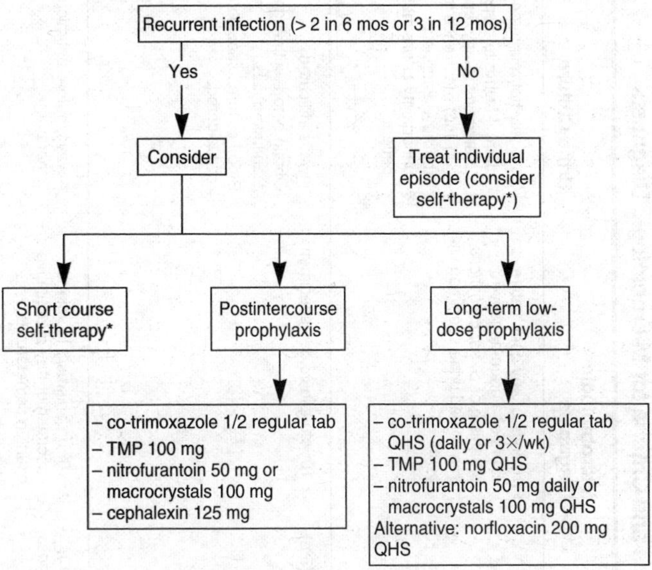

* 3-day course of treatment, self-administered on appearance of symptoms.
Abbreviations: TMP = trimethoprim.

with clavulanic acid is an effective alternative for resistant organisms, but it is more expensive and is associated with substantial gastrointestinal side effects (10 to 25% incidence).

Quinolones

Use of **nalidixic acid** is limited by development of resistance. The fluoroquinolones (**norfloxacin, ciprofloxacin** and **ofloxacin**) are as effective as co-trimoxazole for treatment of acute uncomplicated UTI due to susceptible organisms but are generally second-line therapy due to cost. Fluoroquinolones are important for treating complicated UTI and for patients infected with resistant organisms. They are **contraindicated** in children and pregnant women because of potential adverse effects on developing cartilage.

Cephalosporins

All the cephalosporins including **cephalexin, cefaclor, cefuroxime axetil** and **cefixime** are effective for the treatment of UTI. They are not as well studied as co-trimoxazole or quinolones and may be somewhat less effective, especially with short courses of therapy. Their use is limited by cost. Cephalosporins may be associated with a greater likelihood of vulvovaginal candidiasis.

Table 1: Clinical Syndromes of UTI, Most Frequent Infecting Organisms and Criteria for Microbiologic Diagnosis

Syndrome	Most Common Infecting Organisms*	Microbiologic Diagnosis	Urine Culture
Acute Uncomplicated UTI (Cystitis) Occurs in females with normal genitourinary tracts. These women have a genetic predisposition for recurrent UTI. Behavioral factors promoting infection include sexual intercourse and use of spermicides or diaphragm. Usual presenting symptoms include internal dysuria, frequency, suprapubic discomfort and urgency. Recurrences are common but of variable frequency.	*E. coli* (80–90%), *S. saprophyticus* (5–10%), *K. pneumoniae*, *P. mirabilis*, group B streptococcus.	Presence of any quantitative count of a gram-negative organism or *S. saprophyticus* in a voided urine specimen with pyuria.	Generally not recommended. Culture if failure to respond to empiric therapy, early (< 1 mo) recurrence following therapy, diagnostic uncertainty or pregnant patient.
Acute Nonobstructive Pyelonephritis Occurs in women with recurrent uncomplicated UTI but at lower frequency than cystitis. Classic presentation includes fever and flank pain with or without associated irritative urinary symptoms. Patients who present with UTIs with only lower tract symptoms or asymptomatic bacteriuria occasionally have associated "occult" renal infection. Bacteremic infection occurs most frequently in diabetic women or women > 65 yrs.	*E. coli* (80–90%), *P. mirabilis* (5%), *K. pneumoniae* (5%), *S. saprophyticus*.	$\geq 10^4$ cfu/L in voided specimen.	Always indicated. Obtain before initiating antimicrobials. Blood cultures should be considered.
Complicated UTI Occurs in individuals with an abnormal genitourinary tract due to structural or functional abnormalities or those with an indwelling catheter.	*E. coli* (50%), *P. mirabilis* (20%), *E. faecalis* (10%), *P. aeruginosa*, *P. stuartii*, *Citrobacter* spp.,	$\geq 10^5$ organisms/L in voided specimen or any quantitative count in catheterized specimen.	Always, before antimicrobial therapy.

Patients may present with cystitis (lower tract) symptoms or fever/pyelonephritis.

Management includes search for correctable anomalies; with persistent abnormalities, recurrent infection is common (50% by 6 wks post therapy).

Enterobacter spp., *Serratia* spp., group B streptococci (coagulase-negative), staphylococci.

Bacterial Prostatitis[†]

Acute: infection usually due to *E. coli* or *S. aureus*. Symptoms include sudden chills, fever, perineal and low back pain, irritative and obstructive voiding. The prostate is tender, swollen, indurated and warm. Prostatic massage is not recommended because it may cause bacteremia.

Enterobacteriaceae, *P. aeruginosa*, *S. aureus*, others.

Relapsing UTI > 10^5 cfu/L.

Triple glass test with potential pathogens isolated and pyuria in prostatic massage specimen or postprostatic massage urine specimen.

Voided urine specimen before empiric therapy.

Triple glass test.

Chronic: common, ↑ with age. Symptoms are variable, not diagnostic and may include mild to moderate urgency, frequency, nocturia, dysuria and discomfort in the perineal, suprapubic or genital area. Prostate examination is usually normal. It frequently presents as relapsing UTI in older men.

Asymptomatic Bacteriuria

Microbiologic evidence (≥ 10^5 cfu/L on 2 specimens) for UTI in the absence of associated symptoms.

Asymptomatic bacteriuria is more common in women, ↑ with age.

In pregnancy, screening should be performed for asymptomatic bacteriuria at 12–16 wks.

E. coli (60-70%), *P. mirabilis* (coagulase-negative) (10%), group B *streptococcus*, staphylococci (10–20%), others.

≥ 10^5 cfu/L in 2 consecutive specimens.

Screening of asymptomatic populations recommended only in pregnancy or before invasive genitourinary procedures.

---

† *Nonbacterial prostatitis is an inflammatory condition of unknown cause, diagnosed on the basis of prostatic fluid leukocytosis with negative culture. If there is no evidence for inflammation or infection of the prostate (triple glass test) the diagnosis is prostatodynia, which should not be treated with antibiotics.*

* *E. coli is the single most frequent organism causing UTI. Individuals with complicated UTI or recent exposure to antimicrobials are more likely to have organisms other than E. coli or organisms of increased antimicrobial resistance.*

Aminoglycosides

Aminoglycosides (**gentamicin, tobramycin, netilmicin and amikacin**) remain the therapy of choice for the treatment of acute pyelonephritis requiring parenteral therapy. Most gram-negative organisms, especially in patients with community-acquired infections, will remain susceptible to these agents. Initial parenteral therapy is switched to oral therapy as soon as symptoms and signs have settled (72 to 96 hours); with such short duration of therapy, ototoxicity and nephrotoxicity are unlikely. The aminoglycosides are usually interchangeable for the treatment of UTI; antimicrobial susceptibility and cost determine selection of an individual agent.

Table 2: **Antimicrobials for the Treatment of UTI**

Antimicrobial	Dose (Adult) ◗	Cost*
Oral Agents		
Amoxicillin/clavulanic acid	500 mg TID	$$$
Amoxicillin	500 mg TID	$
Cefaclor	250 mg TID	$$
Cefixime	400 mg/d	$$$
Cefuroxime axetil	250 mg BID	$$
Cephalexin	500 mg QID	$$
Ciprofloxacin	250–500 mg BID	$$$–$$$$
Co-trimoxazole†	160/800 mg BID	$
Nitrofurantoin	50 mg QID	$
Nitrofurantoin macrocrystals†	100 mg QID	$$
Norfloxacin	400 mg BID	$$$
Ofloxacin	400 mg BID	$$
Trimethoprim†	100 mg BID	$
Parenteral Agents		
Gentamicin‡	3–5 mg/kg/d	$$
Tobramycin	3–5 mg/kg/d	$$–$$$
Netilmicin	3–5 mg/kg/d	$
Amikacin	15 mg/kg/d	$$$
Ampicillin	1 g Q6H	$$
Piperacillin	3 g Q6H	$$$$
Cefazolin	1 g Q8H	$
Cefuroxime	750 mg Q8H	$$
Cefotaxime	1 g Q8H	$$$
Ceftazidime	1 g Q8H	$$$
Ticarcillin/clavulanate	1 g Q8H	$$$

† *First-line agents for acute uncomplicated UTI.*
‡ *First-line parenteral therapy for acute pyelonephritis.*
◗ *Dosage adjustment may be required in renal failure – see Appendix I.*
* *Cost per day – includes drug cost only.*
Legend: ***Oral Agents:***   *$ < $1*   *$$ $1–3*   *$$$ $3–5*   *$$$$ > $5*
       Parenteral Agents: *$ < $10*   *$$ $10–25*   *$$$ $25–50*   *$$$$ > $50–75*

Table 3: **Duration of Therapy**

Condition	Duration	Comments
Acute uncomplicated UTI	3 d	Generally sufficient unless amoxicillin or nitrofurantoin is used.
Use of nitrofurantoin or amoxicillin	7 d	
Therapy in postmenopausal women	7 d	Longer duration preferred in this population.
Pyelonephritis	14 d	
Complicated UTI	10–14 d	
Prostatitis	6 wks	Initial therapy; longer courses may be necessary following recurrence.*

Treatment is frequently unsuccessful; long-term suppressive therapy may be needed to prevent recurrences.

Therapeutic Tips

- Where possible, selection of antimicrobial therapy should be based on urine culture results.
- Antimicrobial susceptibility in populations is dynamic.
- Selection of empiric therapy in symptomatic patients should be based upon anticipated local antimicrobial susceptibilities and an individual patient's recent antimicrobial exposure and tolerance.
- Parenteral therapy should be used for patients who are septic, unable to tolerate oral medications, pregnant with pyelonephritis, or with resistant organisms requiring parenteral therapy.
- Prophylaxis should be considered for women with frequent recurrent uncomplicated UTI.

Suggested Reading List

Meares EM Jr. Acute and chronic prostatitis: Diagnosis and treatment. *Infect Dis Clin North Am* 1987;1:855–873.

Nicolle LE, Ronald AR. Recurrent urinary tract infection in adult women: diagnosis and treatment. *Infect Dis Clin North Am* 1987;1:793–806.

Nicolle LE. A practical guide to the management of complicated urinary tract infection. *Drugs* 1997;53:583–592.

Stamm WE, Hooton TM. Management of urinary tract infections in adults. *N Engl J Med* 1993;329:1329–1334.

CHAPTER 92

Malaria Prophylaxis

*W.L. Wobeser, MD, FRCPC and
J.S. Keystone, MD, FRCPC*

Goals of Therapy

- To assess risk of acquisition of malaria
- To provide safe and effective chemoprophylaxis

Considerations

- Malaria results in 5 million deaths worldwide each year.
- Determinants of acquisition risk include malaria endemicity, season, altitude, degree of rural travel and preventive measures for mosquito bites.
- Additional considerations in choosing prophylaxis include age, pregnancy, allergies and concurrent medications and illnesses.
- The risk of malaria for travelers is **greatest** in sub-Saharan Africa, Papua New Guinea and the Solomon Islands; **intermediate** on the Indian subcontinent and Haiti; and **low** in Southeast Asia and Latin America. There is regional variation of risk within these areas.
- All travelers to an endemic area require prophylaxis.
- When counseling a patient about malaria chemoprophylaxis, check an up-to-date source about the location and extent of drug-resistant *Plasmodium* species. Detailed recommendations for malaria prevention can be obtained on a 24-hour basis by calling the Centers for Disease Control (CDC) at (404) 332-4559. The Canadian Society for International Health provides a listing of local travelers' clinics at (613) 230-2654.

Therapeutic Choices (Figure 1)

Nonpharmacologic Choices

Malaria transmission by the anopheline mosquito mainly occurs between dusk and dawn; the following measures optimize protection during this time:

- **Insect repellents** containing N,N-diethyl-m-toluamide (DEET) should be used before outdoor activity during the main hours of malarial transmission (evening and nighttime). DEET has been associated (rarely) with neurologic side effects in children exposed to high concentrations (> 35%)

Figure 1: **Malaria Prophylaxis**

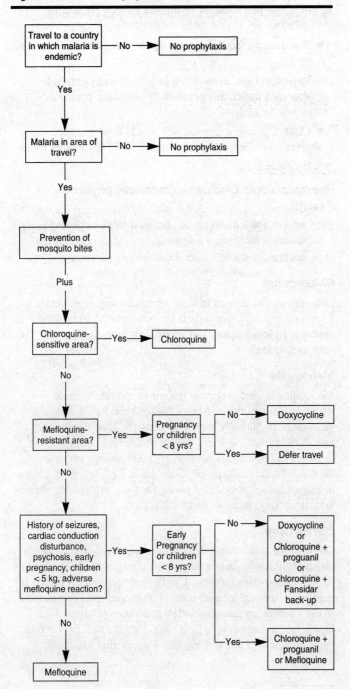

and prolonged use. Hourguard[1] (31.5% DEET) is formulated to reduce percutaneous absorption, thereby prolonging efficacy.

- **Bed nets**, preferably impregnated with permethrin, should be used.

- **Mosquito coils, aerosolized insecticides** or **electrically operated insecticide generators** containing pyrethroids should be used.

- **Clothes** covering exposed skin should be worn, weather permitting. Sleeping in an air-conditioned or screened room is preferable.

Pharmacologic Choices – Chemoprophylaxis
(Table 1)

Except for doxycycline, malaria chemoprophylaxis should begin 1 to 2 weeks prior to entry into a malarious area, continue during exposure and for 4 weeks after departure from a risk area.

Chloroquine

Chloroquine can be used in areas where chloroquine-resistant *Plasmodium falciparum* malaria has not occurred. Side effects appear to be less frequent and severe than those associated with mefloquine.

Mefloquine

Mefloquine is used to prevent malaria in travelers to areas reporting chloroquine-resistant *P. falciparum*. Resistance to mefloquine is clinically important along the Thai–Cambodian and Thai–Myanmar borders. Severe neuropsychiatric reactions (seizures and psychosis) occur in 1:13 000 patients who use the drug at appropriate prophylactic doses. Less severe, disabling, neuropsychological side effects (e.g., anxiety, nightmares, depression, irritability) occur in about 1:200 users.

Doxycycline

Doxycycline is recommended for those traveling to chloroquine-resistant areas who cannot take mefloquine and for those traveling to mefloquine-resistant areas. Unlike mefloquine, daily dosing is required. Users are advised to avoid prolonged sun exposure and to use a sunscreen that absorbs UVA radiation (Chapter 57). Doxycycline chemoprophylaxis should begin 1 to 2 days before entry into the area and continue for 4 weeks after departure.

---

[1] *Distributed by Amway.*

Table 1: Drugs Used for Malaria Chemoprophylaxis

Drug	Geographic Indication*	Dose Adult (A)	Dose Pediatric (P)	Adverse Effects	Comments	Cost†
chloroquine phosphate ‡ Aralen, generics	Central America (north of Panama), Haiti, parts of Middle East (e.g., Iraq, Turkey), Egypt, Dominican Republic, N. Africa, Asia	A: 500 mg (300 mg base) once/wk	P: 8.3 mg/kg (5 mg/kg base) once/wk (max: 500 mg)	GI disturbance, headache, visual disturbances, nonallergic pruritus (esp. in dark-skinned persons).	Hydroxychloroquine may also be used.	$
mefloquine ‡ Lariam	Africa, Asia, South America, SE Asia	A: 250 mg once/wk	P: 15–19 kg: 62.5 mg/wk; 20–30 kg: 125 mg/wk; 31–45 kg: 187.5 mg/wk; > 45 kg: adult dose	GI disturbance (nausea, diarrhea, abdominal pain), dizziness, headache, sleep disturbance, nightmares, skin rash, mood changes, vertigo, palpitations, seizures (rare), psychosis (rare).	Not recommended for those with known seizure disorder, history of severe neuropsychiatric problems, in the first half of pregnancy. Should be taken with caution in those with cardiac conductive disturbances or using chloroquine or quinine-like drugs.	$$
doxycycline ‡ Doryx, Vibra-Tabs, Vibramycin, generics	Thai borders	A: 100 mg once/d	P: > 8 yrs: 2 mg/kg/d (max.: 100 mg/d)	Photosensitivity, GI disturbance, vaginal candidiasis.	Contraindicated in pregnancy and in children < 8 yrs.	$$

(cont'd)

Table 1: Drugs Used for Malaria Chemoprophylaxis *(cont'd)*

Drug	Geographic Indication*	Dose Adult (A) Pediatric (P)	Adverse Effects	Comments	Cost†
proguanil ‡ *(chloroguanide hydrochloride)* Paludrine	Sub-Saharan Africa	A: 200 mg once/d in combination with chloroquine P: < 2 yrs: 50 mg/d 2–6 yrs: 100 mg/d 7–10 yrs: 150 mg/d > 10 yrs: 200 mg/d	Mouth ulcers (common), hair loss (rare).		$$
primaquine phosphate	Papua New Guinea, SE Asia, Central America	A: 26.3 mg (15 mg base) once/d × 14 d$^{\pi}$ P: 0.5 mg/kg (0.3 mg base/kg)$^{\pi}$ once/d × 14 d	GI disturbance, hemolytic anemia, methemoglobinemia.	Should not be given to patients with glucose-6-phosphate dehydrogenase deficiency. Used for terminal prophylaxis.	$
pyrimethamine/ sulfadoxine Fansidar		A: 3 tabs as a single dose P: < 1 yr: 1/4 tab 1–3 yrs: 1/2 tab 4–8 yrs: 1 tab 9–14 yrs: 2 tabs > 14 yrs: 3 tabs as a single dose	Skin rash, agranulocytosis (rare), hemolytic anemia (rare).	Contraindicated in persons allergic to sulfonamides. For self-treatment of a febrile illness when medical care is not immediately available. Travelers should seek medical attention as soon as possible after administering.	$

‡ Begin drugs 1 wk before (except doxycycline, which is started 1 to 2 d before) and continue until 4 wks after leaving malarious area.

* Check up-to-date resource for current areas of sensitivity and resistance.

$^{\pi}$ Double the daily dose for Papua New Guinea.

† Cost of 4-wk supply (primaquine: 2 wks only; Fansidar: 3 tabs only) – includes drug cost only.

Legend: $ < $10 $$ $10–20

Proguanil (Chloroguanide Hydrochloride)

Proguanil (administered daily) is used as an adjunct to chloroquine for travelers to chloroquine-resistant areas and for those for whom mefloquine is contraindicated (e.g., seizures, psychosis). However, the chloroquine/proguanil combination is considerably less effective than mefloquine.

Primaquine

Primaquine is used for terminal prophylaxis ("radical cure") in long-term travelers returning from areas with *P. vivax* and *P. ovale*, both of which have dormant liver forms (hypnozoites). Hypnozoites are not affected by chloroquine or mefloquine. Although recent studies suggest that primaquine may be used as a prophylactic agent against *P. vivax* and chloroquine-resistant *P. falciparum* malaria, large scale trials of primaquine use for this purpose have not been undertaken. Primaquine is not recommended for **routine** prophylaxis.

Primaquine is a potent oxidizing agent which can induce severe hemolytic anemia in those with G6PD deficiency. In risk groups for this enzyme deficiency, a G6PD level is recommended before primaquine is used. The drug is contraindicated in pregnancy.

Pyrimethamine/Sulfadoxine (Fansidar)

Fansidar is carried for self-treatment of a febrile illness when medical care is not immediately available. A single dose is recommended for areas (e.g., Asia) where chloroquine resistance is low.

Pregnancy and Infancy

Chloroquine with or without proguanil can be recommended for pregnant women and young children. Doxycycline is contra-indicated for both groups. Mefloquine has been shown to be safe in the second half of pregnancy and is recommended for children weighing ≥ 5 kg. Safety data are not available for children < 5 kg; however, mefloquine is likely to be safe in this group since it is safe in the second half of pregnancy. Limited data suggest that mefloquine is also safe in the first trimester. The risks of *P. falciparum* malaria in pregnancy far outweigh the potential risks of mefloquine. If a decision is made to travel to areas with intense chloroquine-resistant malaria transmission (e.g., sub-Saharan Africa), women and young children in particular should be strongly encouraged to utilize personal protection measures against mosquito bites.

Therapeutic Tips

- Mefloquine is not favored as a prophylactic regimen by some physicians in the United Kingdom and developing countries. Travelers may be advised by physicians and travelers from these areas that they are on the wrong regimen. In general, such advice should be accepted politely and ignored.

- No currently available regimen of malaria chemoprophylaxis is ideal and completely effective. Drug-resistant malaria continues to spread.

- All travelers in whom fever develops within 1 year (particularly within 2 months) of return from a malaria-endemic area must be considered to have malaria, regardless of chemoprophylaxis. Thick and thin blood films should be requested from a health care provider to rule out malaria.

Suggested Reading List

Hoffman SL. Diagnosis, treatment, and prevention of malaria. In: Wolfe MS, ed. *Med Clin North Am: Travel Medicine* 1992;76:1327–1356.

McCarthy AE, Keystone JS. Malaria. In: Rakel RE, ed. *Conn's Current Therapy 1994*. Philadelphia: W.B. Saunders, 1994:94–100.

Schwartz IK. Prevention of malaria. In: Gardner P, ed. *Infect Dis Clin North Am: Health Issues of International Travellers* 1992;6:313–332.

Suh K, Keystone JS. Malaria prophylaxis in pregnancy and children. *Infect Dis Clin Pract* 1996;5:541–546.

Wyler DJ. Malaria chemoprophylaxis for the traveller. *N Engl J Med* 1993;329:31–37.

Zucker JR, Campbell CC. Malaria: principles of prevention and treatment. In: Maguire JH, Keystone JS, eds. *Infect Dis Clin North Am: Parasitic Diseases* 1993;7:547–567.

CHAPTER 93

Traveler's Diarrhea

John R. Wright, MD, MBA, FRCPC

Goals of Therapy

- To reduce risk of infection
- To limit duration and severity of symptoms
- To prevent long-term persistence of symptoms (post-dysentery irritable bowel syndrome)

Investigations

- Abdominal pain and diarrhea develop in 40% of those traveling in tropical and semitropical areas. Bacteriologic investigations are usually impractical
- Patients should be counseled to distinguish mild symptoms (abdominal cramps, malaise, nausea and frequent bowel movements) from the high fever or dysentery (bloody diarrhea) of more severe infection requiring urgent antibiotic therapy
- Patients developing symptoms after returning home or presenting with persistent symptoms should be evaluated by:
  – physical examination (abdominal tenderness/guarding)
  – CBC
  – stool for occult blood, cultures, ova and parasites
- Symptoms persisting 6 weeks after antibacterial therapy should be further investigated with barium studies and endoscopy to rule out concomitant disease (inflammatory bowel disease, celiac disease, tropical sprue)

Therapeutic Choices (Figure 1)

Prophylaxis

Nonpharmacologic Choices

- Drink only bottled, carbonated beverages, pasteurized milk or purified water.
- Avoid ice cubes unless made from safe water.
- Eat only fruit (tomatoes are fruit) that has been washed in safe water and peeled. Do not eat watermelon.
- Avoid salads and raw vegetables.
- Eat only thoroughly and recently cooked meats or fish.

Figure 1: **Treatment of Traveler's Diarrhea**

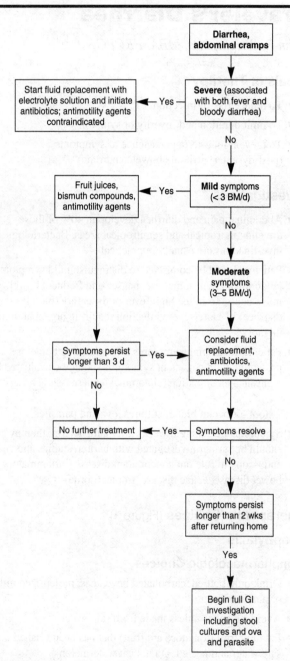

Abbreviations: BM = bowel movements.

- Avoid leftovers and condiments in open bottles.
- Choose food that is well cooked and served piping hot.

Pharmacologic Choices (Table 1)
Bismuth Subsalicylate (BSS)
Investigations suggest that BSS has a mild antibacterial effect and that it neutralizes bacterial toxins. Short-term attack rates of traveler's diarrhea have been reported as 14 to 24% with BSS and 40% with placebo. QID dosing may be advantageous. Those who are taking anticoagulants or salicylates or who are allergic to salicylates should not take BSS. Short-term side effects are minimal, and bismuth toxicity is uncommon with short-term use (i.e., less than 3 weeks) of recommended doses.

Antibiotics
Various antibiotics have been shown to significantly reduce the attack rate of traveler's diarrhea in endemic areas. **Norfloxacin** or **ciprofloxacin** effectively reduces attack rates of traveler's diarrhea and is relatively safe. **Co-trimoxazole** has also been shown effective in prophylaxis, reducing the incidence of traveler's diarrhea by as much as 86%. In spite of its effectiveness, side effects (including Stevens-Johnson syndrome rarely) limit its usefulness. **Doxycycline** has been effective for prophylaxis, but recent strains of bacteria have been shown to be resistant, reflecting overusage.

Treatment
Nonpharmacologic Choices
Maintenance of fluid balance is key to management:

- Patients with mild diarrhea will benefit from a clear fluid diet of carbonated beverages, fruit juices (for their potassium content), hot tea or safe water and salted crackers.
- Those with moderate diarrhea may benefit from electrolyte-containing solutions (e.g., Gatorade).
- Severe diarrhea, particularly in young children, requires careful fluid replacement with a solution of 3.5 g sodium chloride, 2.5 g sodium bicarbonate, 1.5 g potassium chloride and 20 g glucose in 1 L of water. Commercial preparations of Enfalac, Lytren, Gastrolyte, Pedialyte or Ricelyte[1] are available (Chapters 76, 78, 104).

---
[1] Not available in Canada.

Pharmacologic Choices (Table 1)
Antimotility Agents
Loperamide or **diphenoxylate with atropine** (Lomotil) provides
rapid relief for mild to moderate diarrhea (up to 3 to 5 loose stools
per day and mild cramping pain). Diphenoxylate has been shown
to prolong invasive infection with *Shigella, Salmonella* and
Campylobacter; thus, it should not be used in more severe
diarrhea associated with high fever or rectal bleeding (dysentery).
When given with antibiotics, loperamide may shorten the duration
of diarrhea. (See Therapeutic Tips.)

Antibiotics
Traveler's diarrhea is a mild, self-limiting disease that responds
promptly to appropriate therapy. Patients should be advised to
take a 2- to 5-day course of antibiotics with them on their travels
and initiate therapy with the onset of marked symptoms (severe
diarrhea, cramps or symptoms that extend beyond 3 days, bloody
diarrhea or high fever).

Although expensive, **ciprofloxacin** and **norfloxacin** are effective
and safe, reducing the duration of diarrhea by more than 50%
when compared to placebo. **Co-trimoxazole** should be given in
a single large dose followed by 1 tablet BID for 3 days (Table 1).
Doxycycline is a poor choice because several resistant enteric
pathogens have emerged. **Metronidazole** may be useful when
diarrhea persists and is associated with weight loss.

Therapeutic Tips

- Prophylaxis should only be used in patients at risk of the
  complications of diarrheal illness (e.g., prior gastrectomy,
  diabetes mellitus, ileostomy or immunocompromised) or
  those who cannot afford even a short interruption of their
  work. Prophylaxis should be infrequent and never continue
  for more than a few days.

- Several studies have suggested a role for loperamide **plus**
  antibiotics for moderately severe afebrile nondysenteric
  diarrhea, especially when the antibiotic is given in a high
  loading dose. Concurrent loperamide and co-trimoxazole
  resulted in 75% of subjects recovering from diarrhea within
  12 hours as compared with 34 hours for placebo.

- Mild traveler's diarrhea will usually resolve in 24 hours with
  antimotility agents and fluids.

- OTC agents should be discouraged as they are ineffective for
  prophylaxis. Foreign products may contain chloramphenicol,
  which may induce aplastic anemia, or iodochlorhydroxyquin
  (clioquinol), which can cause neurologic damage and optic
  atrophy.

Table 1: Drugs Used in Traveler's Diarrhea

Drug	Dosage Treatment	Dosage Prophylaxis*	Adverse Effects	Comments	Cost†
Quinolones					
norfloxacin Noroxin	400 mg BID × 1–3 d	400 mg once/d	Infrequently GI disturbance, CNS effects, skin rash.	Not recommended for children.	$$$
ciprofloxacin Cipro	500 mg BID × 1–3 d	500 mg once/d		Norfloxacin is less well-absorbed than other quinolones.	$$$
co-trimoxazole Septra, Bactrim, generics	160/800 mg BID × 6 doses or 320/1600 mg loading dose, then 160/800 mg × 5 doses	160/800 mg once/d	GI disturbance, blood dyscrasias, skin reactions (rarely, Stevens-Johnson syndrome).	For regions where co-trimoxazole resistance is uncommon (central Mexico in summer); not first choice in other geographic areas.	$
doxycycline Vibramycin, Vibra-Tabs, Doryx, generics	100 mg BID × 1–3 d	100 mg once/d	Photosensitivity, vaginal and esophageal candidiasis.	No longer recommended due to high incidence of resistance. Contraindicated in pregnancy, children < 8 yrs. Sunscreen recommended (Chapter 57). Antacids, bismuth may ↓ bioavailability.	$$
metronidazole Flagyl, generics	250 mg BID × 5–7 d		GI disturbance, metallic taste, CNS effects.	For symptoms suggestive of steatorrhea where *Giardia lamblia* infection is common. Avoid alcohol consumption (risk of disulfiram-like reaction).	$

(cont'd)

Table 1: Drugs Used in Traveler's Diarrhea *(cont'd)*

Drug	Dosage Treatment	Dosage Prophylaxis*	Adverse Effects	Comments	Cost†
bismuth subsalicylate Pepto-Bismol, generics	2 tabs (262 mg/tab) or 30 mL Q 30 min Max.: 8 doses/d	2 tabs (262 mg/tab) or 30 mL QID (with meals and QHS)	Darkening of tongue and stools, mild tinnitus.	Avoid in patients who cannot take salicylates or those already taking therapeutic doses of salicylates. May ↓ bioavailability of doxycycline if taken within 2 h.	$$
loperamide Imodium, generics	4 mg STAT, then 2 mg after each loose stool Max.: 16 mg/d	*Prophylactic anti-motility agents have no effect*	Abdominal cramping, rarely dizziness, dry mouth, skin rash.	Do not use if experiencing fever or bloody stools. Do not use longer than 48 h.	$$ (16 tabs)

* All drugs should be started on the first day in the area of risk and continued for 1 or 2 d after return home, to a maximum of 3 wks total.

† Cost of 3-day treatment – includes drug cost only.
Legend: $ < $2 $$ $2–10 $$$ $10–15 $$$$ > $15

- Symptoms persisting more than 2 weeks after the return home should be investigated thoroughly. Antibiotic-associated colitis, disaccharidase deficiency and inappropriate dietary alteration should be excluded. Inflammatory bowel disease or celiac disease may present while patients are traveling.

- Known cases of *Salmonella typhi* diarrhea should not be treated acutely with antibiotics.

Suggested Reading List

Chak A, Banwell JG. Traveller's diarrhea. In: Giannella RA, ed. *Gastroenterol Clin North Am*. Acute infection: Diarrhea. 1993;22:549–561.

Committee to Advise on Tropical Medicine and Travel. Statement on travellers' diarrhea. *Can Commun Dis Rep* 1994;20:149–155.

Dupont HL. Traveller's diarrhea: Which antimicrobial? Drugs 1993;45:910–917.

Ericson CD, Nicholls-Vasquez T, Dupont HI, et al. Optimal dosing of trimethoprim-sulfamethoxazole when used with loperamide to treat traveller's diarrhea. *Antimicrob Agents Chemother* 1992;36:2821–2824.

Mattila L, Peltola H, Siitonin A, et al. Short-term treatment of traveller's diarrhea with norfloxacin: a double-blind, placebo-controlled study during two seasons. *Clin Infect Dis* 1993;17:779–782.

Patrucelli BP, Murphy GS, Sanchez JL, et al. Treatment of traveller's diarrhea with ciprofloxacin and loperamide. *J Infect Dis* 1992;165:557–560.

Taylor DN, Sanchez JL, Candler W, et al. Treatment of traveller's diarrhea: Ciprofloxacin plus loperamide compared with ciprofloxacin alone. *Ann Intern Med* 1991;114:731–734.

CHAPTER 94

Viral Hepatitis

Jenny Heathcote, MB, BS, MD, FRCP, FRCPC

Goals of Therapy

- To prevent disease
- To minimize liver damage
- To reduce the spread of infection

Acute Viral Hepatitis

Acute viral hepatitis is a systemic viral infection that is present for less than 6 months and which causes inflammatory necrosis of the liver.

Important Features

- Most cases of acute viral hepatitis are asymptomatic.
- A fulminant course occurs in 0.1% (higher rate in pregnant women); immediate referral should be made to a liver transplantation centre because massive necrosis resulting in liver failure can occur.
- Diagnosis must be confirmed serologically.
- Hepatitis B becomes chronic in 1% of healthy adults.
- Hepatitis C becomes chronic in 70% of healthy adults.

Glossary of Abbreviations

HAV = Hepatitis A virus	HBeAg = Hepatitis Be antigen
HBV = Hepatitis B virus	Anti-HBe = Antibody to HBeAg
HCV = Hepatitis C virus	HDV = Hepatitis D (delta) virus
HBsAg = Hepatitis B surface antigen	Anti-HCV = Antibody to HCV
Anti-HBs = Antibody to HBsAg	HCV RNA = Hepatitis C RNA

Investigations

The clinical features are nonspecific, regardless of causative virus; viral type is identified by serologic markers.

- Check for parenteral/sexual exposure, medication list, travel/day care exposure, family history of hepatitis B
- Check for persistent nausea and vomiting, drowsiness, bruising (signs of severe disease)
- Check INR; if elevated refer patient to gastroenterologist

Figure 1: **Treatment of Acute Viral Hepatitis**

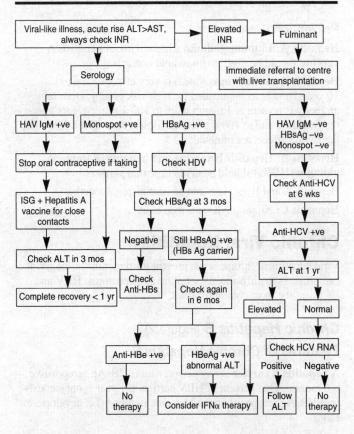

Abbreviations: HAV IgM = Hepatitis A IgM; HBsAg = Hepatitis B surface antigen;
HDV = Hepatitis D (delta) virus; ISG = Immune Serum Globulin; Anti-HCV = Antibody
to HCV; IFNα = Interferon alpha.

- Check serology
  – impossible to distinguish a flare-up of chronic hepatitis B
    or C from an acute case; only time will identify the carriers
    (i.e., all hepatitis B and C must be followed serologically)

Therapeutic Choices (Figure 1)

In most cases no specific therapy is indicated other than
supportive care. The majority of patients recover completely
without complications or chronic sequelae.

Nonpharmacologic Choices

- Avoid alcohol for at least 3 months.
- Stop oral contraceptives to avoid cholestatic symptoms.

- No particular diet is necessary.
- No restraint of physical activities is needed.

Prevention (Table 1)

Hepatitis A: Immune globulin with or without **hepatitis A vaccine** should be given to household contacts.

Hepatitis A vaccine (inactivated) is very effective (up to 10 years) and is recommended for high-risk groups. Detectable antibody is present at 1 month in 96 to 100% of recipients after the first dose and in 100% after the booster dose, given 6 months later. Side effects are minimal.

Hepatitis B: Hepatitis B vaccine and hepatitis B immune globulin (HBIG) should be given to sexual partners.

Hepatitis A and B vaccines can be administered together.

Hepatitis C: No prophylaxis is available.

Chronic Viral Hepatitis

Viral hepatitis is chronic when present for 6 months or longer. It can progress to cirrhosis, liver failure and hepatoma. HBV and HCV are the most common causes.

Chronic Hepatitis B (Figure 2)

Features of Chronic Hepatitis B

A hepatitis B carrier is any person who is HBsAg seropositive > 6 months. One percent of HBV carriers per year spontaneously lose HBsAg seropositivity and become immune (i.e, develop anti-HBs).

Investigations

- Check if patient is coinfected with hepatitis D virus
- Check "e" status (HBeAg and anti-HBe) and serum transaminase values

Therapeutic Choices

Nonpharmacologic Choices

- Advise against all but modest alcohol consumption (less than 4 drinks weekly).

Prevention (Table 1)

- All household members and sexual partners require hepatitis B vaccine.
- Hepatitis B vaccine and HBIG should be given at birth to infants of a carrier mother.

Figure 2: **Chronic Hepatitis B: Natural History**

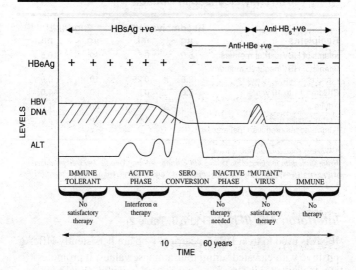

Figure 3: **Chronic Hepatitis B: Effect of Interferonα Therapy**
(ideal response: complete eradication HBsAg)

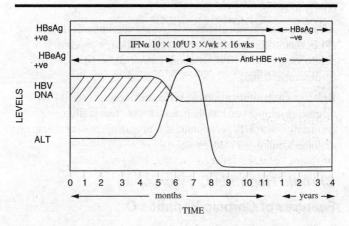

Pharmacologic Choices

Immunosuppressive drugs should be avoided (50% of hepatitis B carriers experience flare-up upon drug withdrawal).

Currently, no pharmacologic therapy is recommended for hepatitis B carriers with normal serum transaminase or for those who are anti-HBe positive.

Table 1: **Recommended Doses of Hepatitis B Vaccines Currently Licensed in Canada**

Recipients	Recombivax HB μg	Recombivax HB mL	Engerix-B μg	Engerix-B mL
Infants of HBV-carrier mothers	5.0	0.5	10	0.5
Infants of HBV-negative mothers and children ≤ 10 years	2.5	0.25	10	0.5
Children 11 to 19 years	5.0	0.5	20	1.0
Adults	10	1.0	20	1.0
Hemodialysis and immunocompromised patients	40	1.0*	40	2.0

* When special formulation is used.
From Canadian Immunization Guide, 4th Edition, Health Canada, 1993. Reproduced with permission of the Minister of Public Works and Government Services Canada, 1998.

Interferon Alfa (IFNα) (Figure 3, Table 2)

IFNα is used to treat HBsAg carriers who are persistently HBeAg positive with elevated serum transaminase values. It promotes HBeAg+ve to anti-HBe+ve seroconversion which is associated with a fall in serum transaminase to normal.

All patients with Hepatitis D coinfection relapse after IFNα therapy. HIV and other immunosuppressed patients respond poorly to IFNα.

Absolute contraindications to IFNα are autoimmune disease (SLE, rheumatoid arthritis), severe depression or psychosis, neutropenia ($< 1 \times 10^9$/L), thrombocytopenia ($< 50 \times 10^9$/L), cardiac arrhythmias.

Relative contraindications to IFNα are decompensated liver disease, insulin-dependent diabetes, chronic renal failure, coinfection with HIV, concomitant immunosuppressive therapy, ongoing alcohol or IV drug use.

Chronic Hepatitis C (Figure 4)

Features of Chronic Hepatitis C

- Anti-HCV is a marker of infection, not immunity.
- Measurement of RNA virus in serum is not routinely available.
- Most acute infections become chronic (in 70%) whether acquired parenterally or sporadically; up to 40% may later resolve spontaneously.
- 60 to 90% of persons who have ever been IV drug users have chronic hepatitis C.

- Immunosuppressed patients may lose anti-HCV but remain RNA positive.
- Sexual transmission (facilitated by HIV coinfection) rate is 0 to 5%; safe sex is recommended.
- Vertical transmission rate is 0 to 5%, depending on titre of RNA in mother (i.e., high titre if coinfected with HIV hence greater transmission rate).
- Risk factors for progressive fibrosis are male gender, age > 40 yrs at acquisition, alcohol consumption > 50 g daily and probably coinfection with HIV.

Figure 4: **Chronic Hepatitis C: Natural History**

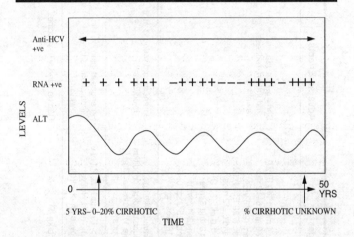

Figure 5: **Chronic Hepatitis C: Effect of Interferonα Therapy**

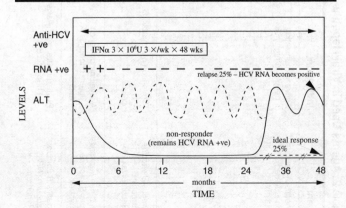

NB: 50% of treated patients do not respond to IFNα therapy.

Table 2: Agents Used in Viral Hepatitis

Agent	Indication	Dosage	Adverse Effects	Comments	Cost*
hepatitis A vaccine (inactivated) Havrix	Active immunization of people at high risk	Adults: 1 mL (1440 EL.U) IM at 0 and 6–12 mos Children: (2–18 yrs): 0.5 mL (720 EL.U) IM at 0 and 6–12 mos	Soreness at site, induration, redness, swelling.	Can be given with immune globulin if person at risk of contacting HAV before adequate anti-HAV antibody titres.	$$/2 doses $/2 doses
Vaqta		Adults: 1.0 mL (50 U) IM at 0 and 6 mos Children (2–17 yrs): 0.5 mL (25 U) at 0, 6 and 18 mos			$$/2 doses $$/2 doses
hepatitis B vaccine Engerix-B, Recombivax HB	Prevention of hepatitis B	Dose varies with age, product, medical condition (Table 1); 3 doses IM at 0, 1, 6 mos	Soreness and redness at injection site.	Booster not necessary in immunocompetent person. Can be used with HBIG.	$$/3 doses
combined hepatitis A and B vaccine Twinrex	Active immunization against hepatitis A and B	Adults > 19 yrs: 1 mL IM at 0, 1 and 6 mos. Not yet approved for children.	Soreness at injection site, induration, redness, swelling.	For high risk occupations and patients with cirrhosis.	$$$/3 doses
hepatitis B immune globulin (HBIG) Hyperhep	Postexposure prophylaxis of hepatitis B	0.06 mL/kg IM	Can be used with vaccine.	Used to prevent recurrence post liver transplant. It is of no value in treatment of fulminant acute or chronic active hepatitis B.	$$$$/dose

					$/dose
immune globulin Baygam	Prophylaxis of hepatitis A; postexposure prophylaxis of hepatitis A if within 2 wks of exposure	Adults: 0.08–0.12 mL/kg IM Children: 0.02–0.04 mL/kg IM If continued exposure, repeat dose in 5 mos	Soreness at injection site, anaphylaxis (rare).	Has no role in prophylaxis of hepatitis B.	
interferon alfa (IFNα) Intron A, Roferon-A, Wellferon	Treatment of chronic hepatitis B and C	**Hepatitis B:** 10×10^6 U $3\times$/wk $\times$ 16 wks, given SC **Hepatitis C** (ALT > 80 U/L): 3×10^6 U $3\times$/wk $\times$ 48 wks If ALT not normal in 8 wks, stop therapy	Common: fatigue, fever, muscle aches, asthenia, weight loss, headaches, irritability, hair loss, bone marrow suppression. Less common: pulmonary infiltrates, severe depression.	Intron A and Roferon-A are recombinant IFNαs, and Wellferon is a mixture of several IFNαs. No significant differences in efficacy have been shown among the 3 products.	HBV $5400/course HCV $6000/course

* *Cost of adult therapy, as indicated – includes drug cost only.*
Legend: $ < $50 $$ $50–100 $$$ $100–300 $$$$ > $300
Abbreviations: ELU = Elisa units.

Investigations

- Clinical signs of chronic liver disease are infrequent
- ALT > AST and wide fluctuations are observed; levels may be normal for long periods, although liver histology is rarely normal.

Therapeutic Choices

Nonpharmacologic Choices

- Any more than modest alcohol use should be avoided (less than 4 drinks weekly).

Prevention

- No vaccine is available.

Pharmacologic Choices

Interferon Alfa (Figure 5, Table 2)

IFNα is used in chronic hepatitis C with persistently elevated ALT (> 80 U/L). Fifty percent respond (ALT becomes normal); of these, 50% relapse when IFNα is stopped. If ALT increases during IFNα therapy, IFNα should be stopped.

Poor responders include those with established cirrhosis, long-term infection, coinfection with HIV, infection with genotypes 1 and 4.

Sustained remission, defined as loss of HCV RNA and normal transaminase levels at 1 year post cessation of IFN, is observed in 8% of cirrhotics and 15 to 25% of noncirrhotics when treatment is given for 12 months.

Contraindications to interferon therapy are the same as for Hepatitis B. As the doses are lower, side effects are similar but less severe.

Suggested Reading List

CASL Hepatitis Consensus Group. Treatment of chronic viral hepatitis with alpha-interferon: a consensus conference report. *Can J Gastroenterol* 1997;11:407–416.

Hoofnagle JH, Bisceglie AM. The treatment of chronic viral hepatitis. *N Engl J Med* 1997;336:347–356.

Lemon SM, Thomas DL. Vaccines to prevent viral hepatitis. *N Engl J Med* 1997;336:196–204.

CHAPTER 95

Herpesvirus Infections

Fred Y. Aoki, MD

The characteristics of some herpesvirus infections such as recurrent genital or orolabial herpes simplex virus (HSV) infection differ when caused by HSV type 1 or 2. However, knowledge of HSV type is not of practical value in guiding selection of drug therapy since both are similarly susceptible to available drugs. Therefore, drug choices can be based on the nature and severity of the disease.

In immunocompromised patients, HSV and varicella-zoster virus (VZV) infections may be more severe and resolve less rapidly than in immunocompetent hosts, but recommended drugs are not different in these two types of patients. The exception is that prolonged treatment of immunocompromised patients (most frequently HIV-infected individuals) with oral acyclovir can lead to drug resistance and therapeutic failure. Resistance is most commonly mediated by a mutation that causes cross-resistance between acyclovir, famciclovir, valacyclovir and ganciclovir. In such patients, foscarnet by injection is the preferred treatment and vidarabine is a less effective but better tolerated alternative.

Herpes Simplex Virus
Orolabial and Genital Infection
Goals of Therapy

- To ameliorate symptoms
- To prevent outbreaks

Primary HSV gingivostomatitis is primarily a disease of children. If the child can swallow, **acyclovir** oral suspension 600 mg/m^2 QID for 10 days is probably efficacious and safe.[1] If the severity of disease precludes ingestion of medication, IV acyclovir in pediatric doses analogous to those which are efficacious and safe in adults with primary genital herpes (Table 1) can be inferred to be appropriate treatment although no data have been published in support of this recommendation.

Recurrent orolabial herpes in immunocompetent adults should be treated with **penciclovir** 1% cream, the first treatment to clearly demonstrate an impact on the course of this infection. Patients

---

[1] Aoki FY, et al. *Acyclovir suspension for the treatment of acute HSV gingivostomatitis in children: a placebo-controlled, double blind trial (Abs). Interscience Conference on Antimicrobial Agents and Chemotherapy. New Orleans: October 1993.*

should be given a prescription and keep the drug close at hand. Treatment should be initiated at the earliest symptom of a recurrence (within 1 hour) and applied every 2 hours while awake for 4 consecutive days.[2] Oral **acyclovir** 400 mg 5 times per day for 5 days beginning within 1 hour of onset reduces pain duration by 0.9 days compared to placebo but no other disease parameter is altered. Topical acyclovir ointment is not effective. In immuno-compromised hosts, oral and IV acyclovir are effective.

For individuals in whom *recurrence of labial herpes* is *induced by exposure to sunlight*, oral **acyclovir** 400 mg BID begun 12 hours prior to sun exposure along with frequent sunscreen use prevents attacks by 76% compared to placebo. Prophylaxis is continued for the duration of sun exposure. In a strategy analogous to that which is effective in individuals with frequently recurring genital herpes *(vide infra)*, daily oral acyclovir 400 mg BID for up to 4 months prevents recurrent cold sores.

First episodes of genital herpes in otherwise healthy individuals may range from severe to inapparent. Therapy with IV **acyclovir** (5 mg/kg every 8 hours for 5 to 10 days) is optimal for severe cases. Oral acyclovir 200 mg 5 times daily for 5 to 10 days is licensed for this indication as well. Data suggest that, overall, IV treatment is approximately 25% better than PO, depending on the parameter (resolution of local symptoms 50%, systemic symptoms 0%, time to heal 33% and virus shedding 0%).

Recurrent genital herpes in immunocompetent and immuno-compromised patients can be treated for 5 to 7 days with oral **acyclovir** 200 mg 5 times daily, **famciclovir** 125 mg BID or **valacyclovir** 500 mg BID. Available data do not demonstrate clinically important differences between these drugs. For individuals with frequently recurring disease (6 or more episodes per year), it is important to recommend suppressive therapy because this is much more effective than episodic therapy of individual outbreaks. Suppression should be started with acyclovir 200 mg TID. If the response is favorable, the dose may be reduced to BID and if unfavorable, increased to 200 mg 5 times daily or 400 mg BID. Suppression should be interrupted periodically to evaluate the need for continued treatment. One strategy is to stop every 3 to 6 months and to await two recurrences. Only if these two recurrences are close together (maximum of 2 months apart) would another 3- to 6-month course be appropriate. This strategy can be continued almost indefinitely since safety of acyclovir during multiple years of use has been demonstrated. In immunocompromised patients, suppressive therapy will likely lead to resistance and clinical failure.

---

[2] *JAMA* 1997;227:1374–1379.

Table 1: **Antivirals for Treatment of Herpesvirus Infections**

Disease	Dose	Cost*
acyclovir – Zovirax, oral generics		
HSV gingivostomatitis (children)	600 mg/m² PO QID × 10 d	susp: $$$ tabs: $$
	250 mg/m² Q8H IV × 5–10 d	$420–840
HSV recurrent orolabial	400 mg 5 times daily × 5 d	$
Prophylaxis of recurrent orolabial HSV	400 mg BID 12 h prior to sun exposure × duration of exposure	$
Genital herpes – first episode	5 mg/kg Q8H IV × 5–10 d	$750–1 500
	200 mg PO 5 times daily × 5–10 d	$–$$
Genital herpes – recurrent	200 mg PO 5 times daily × 5–7 d	$
Genital herpes – suppression of recurrence	200 mg BID up to 5 times daily × 3–6 mos	$$$$$
Herpes simplex encephalitis	10 mg/kg IV Q8H × 10–14 d	$2 800–4 100
Chickenpox (children)	10–20 mg/kg PO QID × 5–7 d	$
(adults)	800 mg PO 5 times daily × 5 d	$$
	or 10 mg/kg IV Q8H × 5 d	$1 500
Acute herpes zoster	800 mg PO 5 times daily × 7 d	$$$
famciclovir – Famvir		
Recurrent genital herpes	125 mg PO BID × 5–7 d	$
Acute herpes zoster	500 mg PO TID × 7 d	$$$
valacyclovir – Valtrex		
Recurrent genital herpes	500 mg PO BID × 5–7 d	$
Acute herpes zoster	1 000 mg PO TID × 7 d	$
penciclovir 1% cream – Denavir		
Recurrent orolabial herpes	Apply Q2H while awake × 4 d	†
trifluridine ophthalmic drops – Viroptic		
HSV keratoconjunctivitis	1 drop Q2H while awake (max 9 drops) × 7 d, then 1 drop Q4H while awake (max 5 drops) × 7 d	$
idoxuridine ophthalmic drops – Herplex, Herplex D		
HSV keratoconjunctivitis	1 drop Q1H while awake and Q2H while sleeping × 5–7 d after healing, or 21 d	$

† *Expected to be available in 1998 from SmithKline Beecham Pharma.*

* *Cost per course of treatment – includes drug cost only. Cost of IV acyclovir assumes no wastage.*

$ <$50 $$ $50–100 $$$ $100–150 $$$$ $150–200 $$$$$ > $200

Encephalitis
Goals of Therapy

- To prevent death
- To prevent long-term neurologic sequelae

Herpes simplex encephalitis (HSE) is characterized by fever and confusion plus focal neurologic symptoms and signs (behavioral changes, speech disturbances and, less frequently, seizures). A brain abscess is the principal differential diagnostic possibility and antibiotic therapy should be included in the initial treatments prescribed, preferably with the help of an infectious diseases consultant. IV **acyclovir** should be initiated as soon as the diagnosis of HSE is considered. The dose is 10 mg/kg infused IV over not less than 60 minutes to prevent obstructive nephropathy caused by formation of acyclovir crystals in the renal tubular lumen. The dose should be repeated at 8-hour intervals in persons with normal renal function. Because acyclovir is eliminated exclusively by renal excretion by filtration and tubular secretion, dose intervals should be increased in those with renal dysfunction (Appendix I). Duration of treatment is usually 10 days. Rarely, relapse with virologically confirmed recrudescence occurs, necessitating prolonged therapy for 10 to 14 more days.

During therapy, diagnostic testing to demonstrate focal unilateral frontotemporal cerebritis (MRI, EEG, brain scan, CT) and HSV etiology (by detection of HSV in brain biopsy or, more commonly now, of HSV DNA in CSF) should be rapidly effected. Culture of CSF for HSV is uniformly negative. Acute phase serum will contain no HSV antibody in 2 out of 3 patients. A rise in titre will be demonstrated in a convalescent phase serum sample in these patients, indicating primary HSV infection.

Valacyclovir, penciclovir and famciclovir have not been evaluated as treatment for HSE.

Keratoconjunctivitis
Goals of Therapy

- To ameliorate symptoms
- To prevent corneal injury with vision impairment

HSV can cause keratitis and/or conjunctivitis. Because distinguishing HSV conjunctivitis from bacterial infection can be difficult, and because of the risk of visual impairment, consultation with an ophthalmologist is strongly advised if HSV infection is suspected. Topical **trifluridine** (Viroptic) applied every 2 hours during waking hours for 1 week and every 4 hours during waking hours for the second week is the treatment of choice. Topical **idoxuridine** (Herplex, Herplex-D) is the treatment of second choice. The role of oral acyclovir is controversial. Steroids may be recommended if concurrent uveitis is diagnosed.

Varicella-zoster Virus

Chickenpox

Goals of Therapy

- To accelerate healing of skin lesions
- To prevent complications

In healthy children and adults, the benefit of **acyclovir** therapy exceeds placebo effects only if initiated within 24 hours of rash onset. For children, the dose should be adjusted for age: 5 to 7 years of age, 20 mg/kg; 8 to 12 years, 15 mg/kg; 13 to 16 years, 10 mg/kg. This dose should be repeated QID for 5 to 7 days. Therapy may lessen the impact on parents by enabling children to return to day care or school earlier. Adults experience complications such as varicella pneumonia more commonly than children, albeit rarely. Oral acyclovir 800 mg 5 times daily for 5 days or IV acyclovir 10 mg/kg every 8 hours for 5 days accelerates healing and is well tolerated. No study of sufficient sample size to rigorously test the hypothesis that acyclovir prevents complications has been described. No data have been published on the utility of the oral prodrug famciclovir or its active moiety, penciclovir, or valacyclovir, for chickenpox therapy.

In immunocompromised hosts, it is intuitively sound to treat chickenpox even if more than 24 hours have elapsed since the rash began. However, available data do not document efficacy in this situation.

Acute Herpes Zoster (Shingles) (Figure 1)

Goals of Therapy

- To accelerate healing of skin lesions
- To prevent post-herpetic neuralgia (Chapter 15)

Glucocorticoids do not reduce the incidence of post-herpetic neuralgia compared to antiherpes drugs prescribed alone.

Figure 1: **Management of Acute Herpes Zoster**

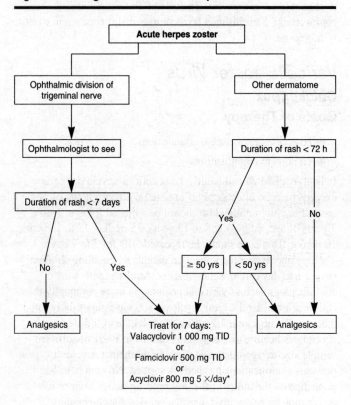

* Only acyclovir is approved for treatment of immunocompromised patients.

Suggested Reading List

Hirsch MS. Herpes simplex virus. In: Mandell GL, Bennett JE, Dolin R, eds. *Principles and practice of infectious diseases.* 4th ed. New York: Churchill Livingstone, 1995.

Hyndiuk RA, Tabbara KF, eds. *Infections of the eye.* Boston: Little, Brown, 1986.

Whitley, RJ. Varicella-zoster viruses. In: Mandell GL, Bennett JE, Dolin R, eds. *Principles and practice of infectious diseases.* 4th ed. New York: Churchill Livingstone, 1995.

CHAPTER 96

HIV Infection

*Valentina Montessori, MD, FRCPC and
Julio S.G. Montaner, MD, FRCPC, FCCP*

Goals of Therapy

- To prolong survival
- To slow disease progression
- To improve quality of life
- To decrease viral replication
- To prevent/reverse immunologic impairment
- To delay/prevent the emergence of HIV resistant strains

Investigations

- Clinical history:
  - risk behaviors, social support and need for counseling
  - establish date of infection based on review of past sexual contacts, period of needle sharing, availability of a previous negative test or a history of possible sero-conversion illness (i.e., mononucleosis or severe flu-like illness) shortly after a high risk exposure
  - general indicators: anorexia, weight loss, fatigue or malaise
  - symptoms of opportunistic infections (e.g., fever, night sweats, cough, dyspnea, diarrhea, headache or skin rashes)

- Past medical history:
  - sexually transmitted diseases (gonorrhea, syphilis, chlamydia, herpes simplex, genital warts)
  - past history or exposure to tuberculosis, hepatitis B or C
  - conditions that may compromise future drug therapy (i.e., kidney stones, peripheral neuropathy, liver disease, pancreatitis, gout)

- Physical examination:
  - focus on signs of immune dysfunction and indications of opportunistic disease
  - specific attention should be directed towards examination of the mental status, skin, visual fields, ocular fundi, oral cavity, lymph nodes, abdomen, rectal and genital exam (including PAP smear in women)

- Laboratory investigations:
  - plasma HIV RNA (also known as plasma viral load or pVL) is the best prognostic marker for progression to AIDS and survival. Plasma viral load ranges vary

according to the test employed. There is no "safe" level. The most sensitive plasma viral load assay currently available has a quantitation limit of 20 HIV-1 RNA copies/mL
- CD4 lymphocyte count and percentage is useful in determining where a patient is on the continuum of HIV disease and the need for specific intervention (Table 1). Knowledge of the CD4 count can also help to narrow the differential diagnosis in a symptomatic HIV infected patient. In adults, a CD4 count of 430 to 1 360 cells/mm^3 (0.43–1.36 Giga/Litre or G/L) is considered normal in most laboratories
- CBC, differential and platelet count
- liver (AST, ALT, alkaline phosphatase, bilirubin) and renal (BUN, creatinine) profiles
- hepatitis B, hepatitis C, syphilis, CMV and toxoplasmosis serologies
- cultures and smears for sexually transmitted diseases as indicated
- sputum cultures and smears for mycobacteria as indicated
- chest x-ray

Therapeutic Choices

Nonpharmacologic Choices (Table 1)
Pharmacologic Choices (Figure 1, Table 2)
Antiretroviral Therapy

Long-term nonprogression can be expected if plasma viral load is maintained below the level of detection of currently available assays on a long-term basis. When selecting the antiretroviral regimen, use agents with at least additive antiviral effect while minimizing additive toxicities. Also consider issues of cross-resistance, compliance, convenience and cost. Nonadherence to therapy promotes the emergence of drug-resistant strains, representing the single most important challenge remaining. Counseling and support are critical to ensure ongoing compliance.

Therapeutic Tips

- Develop a long-term treatment strategy ahead of time to deal with drug intolerance and treatment failure due to resistance.
- Compliance is the single most critical determinant of therapeutic failure: the simpler the regimen the better.

Table 1: **Management of Patients with HIV Infection**

CD4 count (cells/mm^3)

At all times	• Consider antiretroviral therapy (Figure 1) • General counseling (safer sex, nutrition, etc.) • History and physical examination every 3–6 months • Plasma viral load and CD4 count at least every 3–4 months • Herpes suppression if frequent recurrences (more than 4–6 outbreaks per year) (Chapter 95) • Syphilis serology • Pneumococcal vaccine • TB skin test and isoniazid prophylaxis if indicated (consider repeating yearly) • Update diphtheria, tetanus and inactivated polio vaccines • Hepatitis B vaccine if appropriate • Consider annual influenza vaccinations
< 500	• Plasma viral load and CD4 count every 3–4 months • Clinical evaluations and laboratory investigations at least bimonthly if symptomatic, diagnosed with AIDS, or on antiretroviral therapy
< 200	• Start PCP prophylaxis (Chapter 97)
< 100	• Start toxoplasmosis prophylaxis if seropositive and not on co-trimoxazole for PCP prophylaxis (Chapter 97)
< 75	• Consider MAC prophylaxis (Chapter 97)
< 50	• Screen by an ophthalmologist for early CMV retinitis; to be repeated at 3- to 6-month intervals or consider CMV prophylaxis (Chapter 97)

- Encourage initiation of therapy before immunodeficiency develops. Recognize, however, that antiretroviral therapy works at all stages of the disease and will be required on a long-term basis. Therefore, the best time to start therapy is when the patient is ready to commit to it.

- The current goal of therapy is to suppress plasma viral load below the level of quantitation of the assays (< 400 copies/mL).

- An alternative approach is to use partially suppressive therapy. This is often the only option available to patients who have failed previous courses of therapy. Even short-term decreases in plasma viral load in the order of 0.5 to 1.5 $\log_{10}$ have been associated with substantial (2- to 3-fold) reductions in disease progression and delayed mortality in clinical trials.

- Nonquantifiable levels in plasma do not imply cure, eradication or a reason for complacency with safer sex practices or similar safety measures.

Figure 1: **Approach to Antiretroviral Therapy**

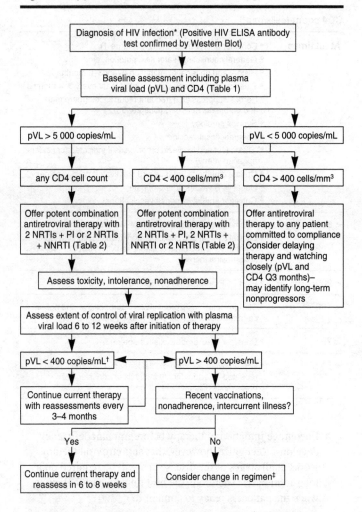

* If a patient presents with a history of possible exposure to HIV, with or without a history of a recent mononucleosis-like illness, consider HIV seroconversion. In this setting, the HIV antibody may be negative or "indeterminate", and a p24 antigen may be positive. These patients should be referred to specialists with experience in interpreting these results.
† The goal of therapy is to suppress viral replication to prevent the emergence of resistant strains and therefore, prolong the durability of the antiviral response. A goal of pVL < 400 copies/mL is recommended as this is the lower limit of quantitation common to all currently available clinical assays. As the newer, more sensitive assays become available, the goal will be revised to pVL < 20 copies/mL.
‡ Given the currently available therapeutic alternatives, it is reasonable to delay change in therapy until there is definitive evidence of rebound of viral replication. Full suppression of viral replication represents a very attractive therapeutic strategy. However, if this goal cannot be reached, the interim aim should become partial suppression of viral replication (i.e., pVL below baseline and below 10 000 to 20 000 copies/mL, as long as the CD4 count remains stable and there is no clinical evidence of disease progression).
Abbreviations: NRTI = nucleoside reverse transcriptase inhibitors; PI = protease inhibitors; NNRTI = non-nucleoside reverse transcriptase inhibitors.

- The variability of the plasma viral load assays is approximately 0.3 to 0.5 $\log_{10}$. Hence, changes in plasma viral load of < 50% are usually not regarded as clinically significant.

- Intercurrences (such as infections) or vaccinations can transiently but substantially increase plasma viral load.

- CD4 counts show diurnal variation, being lowest in the morning and highest in the evening. Fluctuations of up to 30% may occur which are not attributable to a change in disease status. Overall, it is important to monitor the trends in CD4 counts over time rather than placing too much emphasis on one specific reading.

- From a practical standpoint it is useful to consider the CD4 count as indicative of "the immunologic damage that has already occurred" and the plasma viral load as "the damage that is about to occur."

- If a patient experiences drug toxicity, brief cessation of all medications is recommended. Avoid decreasing dosage or stopping only one medication, as this will promote the development of resistance.

- If plasma viral load rebounds despite ongoing therapy, consider noncompliance and resistance as the most likely causes.

- Some antiretrovirals have variable pharmacokinetic profiles (i.e., delavirdine, saquinavir, indinavir) which may lead to subdosing even in a compliant patient.

- A confirmed rebound towards baseline in plasma viral load implies treatment failure. The regimen should then be changed to a new three-drug regimen, avoiding cross resistance with previous treatments.

- Treatment of HIV in pregnancy should be referred to specialists. While monotherapy with AZT in the second and third trimesters has resulted in a decrease in vertical transmission of HIV, study into the safety and efficacy of combination antiretroviral therapy in pregnancy is ongoing. Although prevention of HIV in the infant and avoidance of teratogenicity are important considerations in the treatment of HIV-infected pregnant women, at the present time, optimal therapy of the mother should be the primary treatment goal.[1] Furthermore, breast-feeding by HIV positive women is a recognized risk factor for HIV transmission to the infant and therefore is strongly discouraged.

---

[1] *JAMA 1997;277:1962–1969.*

Table 2: Antiretroviral Medications

Drug	Dosage	Comments	Cost*
Nucleoside Reverse Transcriptase Inhibitors (NRTI)			
zidovudine Retrovir (AZT)	400–600 mg/d divided 2–5 times/d	Most common adverse effects: nausea, headache, rash, anemia, leukopenia, elevated liver enzymes and elevated CPK. Should not be combined with d4T.	$
lamivudine (3TC) 3TC	150 mg BID	Most common adverse effect is neutropenia.	$$
didanosine (ddI) Videx	35–49 kg: 100 mg BID over 50 kg: 200 mg BID Full daily dose can be given once a day	Most common adverse effects: GI intolerance, pancreatitis, gout, reversible peripheral neuropathy. Should not be combined with ddC.	$
zalcitabine (ddC) Hivid	0.75 mg TID	Most common adverse effects: reversible peripheral neuropathy, mouth ulcers, pancreatitis. Should not be combined with d4T or ddI.	$
stavudine (d4T) Zerit	40–60 kg: 30 mg BID over 60 kg: 40 mg BID	Reversible peripheral neuropathy. Should not be combined with AZT.	$$

Non-nucleoside Reverse Transcriptase Inhibitors (NNRTI)

NNRTIs should be used within a highly suppressive regimen.

Drug	Dose	Adverse effects / Notes	Cost
nevirapine (NVP) Viramune	200 mg once daily for 2 weeks then increase to 200 mg BID. Full daily dose can be given once a day	Most common adverse effects: rash, elevated liver enzymes. Should not be combined with DLV.	†
delavirdine (DLV) Rescriptor	400 mg TID	Most common adverse effect is rash. Should not be combined with NVP.	‡

Protease Inhibitors (PI)

PIs have multiple drug interactions.

Drug	Dose	Adverse effects / Notes	Cost
saquinavir (SQV) Invirase	600 mg TID. If given with RTV use SQV 400 mg BID and RTV 400 mg BID	Most common adverse effect is elevated liver enzymes. Very poor bioavailability unless combined with RTV.	$$$$
ritonavir (RTV) Norvir	600 mg BID	Most common adverse effects: GI upset, diarrhea, circumoral paresthesia, elevated liver enzymes, hypertriglyceridemia. Should not be combined with IDV.	$$$$
indinavir (IDV) Crixivan	800 mg TID	Most common adverse effects: elevated liver enzymes, nephrolithiasis. Should not be combined with RTV.	$$$$
nelfinavir (NFV) Viracept	750 mg TID	Most common adverse effect is GI upset, mostly diarrhea.	π

Cost of 30-day supply – includes drug cost only.
Legend: $ $100–200 $$ $200–300 $$$ $300–400 $$$$ $400–500
† *Investigational (Boehringer-Ingelheim).*
‡ *Investigational (Upjohn).*
π *Investigational (Agouron).*

Suggested Reading List

Carpenter CCJ, Fischl MA, Hammer SM, Hirsch MS, Jacobsen DM, Katzenstein DA, et al. Antiretroviral therapy for HIV infection in 1996. Recommendations of an international panel. *JAMA* 1996;276:146–154.

Carpenter CCJ, Fischl MA, Hammer SM, Hirsch MS, Jacobsen DM, Katzenstein DA, et al. Antiretroviral therapy for HIV infection in 1996. An update. *JAMA* 1997;277:1962–1969.

Mellors JW, Rinaldo CR Jr, Gupta P, et al. Prognosis in HIV-1 infection predicted by the quantity of virus in plasma. *Science* 1996;272:1167.

Montaner JSG, Hogg RS, O'Shaughnessy MV. Emerging international consensus for use of antiretroviral therapy. *Lancet* 1997;349:1086.

Pantaleo G, Graziosi C, Demarest JM, et al. HIV infection is active and progressive in lymphoid tissue during the clinically latent stage of disease. *Nature* 1993;362:355–358.

Perelson AS, Neumann AU, Markowitz M, Leonard JM, Ho DD. HIV-1 dynamics in vivo: virion clearance rate, infected cell life-span, and viral generation time. *Science* 1996;271:1582–1586.

Wei X, Ghosh SK, Taylor ME, et al. Viral dynamics in human immunodeficiency virus type 1 infection. *Nature* 1995;373:117.

CHAPTER 97

Opportunistic Infections in HIV-positive Patients

Daniel B. Gregson, MD, FRCPC

In patients infected with the human immunodeficiency virus (HIV), the frequency of opportunistic infections increases as the CD4 count decreases. Most infections, other than *Mycobacterium tuberculosis* and *Pneumocystis carinii*, occur in patients with CD4 counts $< 0.1 \times 10^9$/L (100/mm^3). Management of common opportunistic infections is outlined; specialist support or other references should be sought for complicated problems.

Goals of Therapy

- To prevent opportunistic infection
- To prevent infectious complications
- To treat infections early to prevent permanent sequelae

Investigations

The initial evaluation of an HIV-positive patient determines the level of immune dysfunction both from a clinical and a laboratory standpoint and identifies specific risks for opportunistic infections.[1] Baseline tests include:

- HIV seropositivity (if documentation not available)
- CBC, electrolytes, creatinine, liver enzymes
- T-lymphocyte subsets (CD4)
- VDRL
- PPD skin test reactivity
- *Toxoplasma gondii* antibody
- Cytomegalovirus (CMV) antibody
- Hepatitis screening
- Chest x-ray
- HIV viral load determination

Therapeutic Choices

Preventive interventions are outlined in Table 1.

---

[1] *Antiretroviral therapy should be considered when CD4 $< 0.4 \times 10^9$/L (400/mm^3).*

Figure 1: **Management of Pulmonary Symptoms**

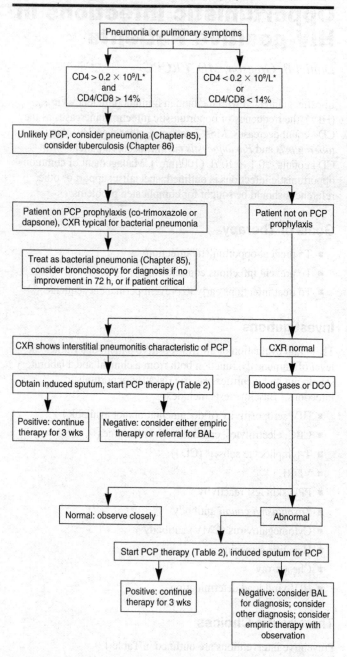

* These values apply to adults only. CD4 counts must be adjusted upwards in children.
Abbreviations: PCP = Pneumocystis carinii pneumonia; BAL = bronchoalveolar lavage;
DCO = diffusing capacity of carbon monoxide; CXR = chest x-ray.

Table 1: **Preventive Interventions for HIV-positive Patients**

Indications	Condition	Prophylactic Therapy
Independent of CD4 count	Immunization status	Update routine immunizations Pneumococcal vaccine *Haemophilus influenzae* b vaccine Hepatitis B vaccine (if nonimmune and ongoing risk behaviors)
Positive PPD (≥ 5mm), independent of CD4 count	*Mycobacterium tuberculosis*	Isoniazid 300 mg/d × 12 mos ± pyridoxine 50 mg/d
CD4 ≤ 0.2 × 10⁹/L or CD4/CD8 ≤ 0.2	*Pneumocystis carinii* pneumonia	Co-trimoxazole 160/800 mg/d or QM/W/F, or 80/400 mg/d, or dapsone 100 mg/d
CD4 < 0.1–0.2 ×10⁹/L and positive *T. gondii* serology	*Toxoplasma gondii* encephalitis	Co-trimoxazole (PCP dose) or dapsone (PCP dose) + pyrimethamine 50 mg/wk + folinic acid 25 mg/wk
CD4 < 0.05–0.1 × 10⁹/L	*Mycobacterium avium* complex	Azithromycin 1 250 mg PO once/wk Clarithromycin 500 mg PO BID Rifabutin 300 mg PO daily (in order of cost-effectiveness)
CD4 < 0.05 × 10⁹/L and positive CMV antibody	Cytomegalovirus	Ganciclovir 1 g PO TID (Does not prolong survival; newer assays, e.g., p65 antigenemia may identify patients most likely to benefit. Cost approx. $20 000/year)
CD4 < 0.05 × 10⁹/L	Fungal infections	Fluconazole 200 mg PO daily (reduces candidiasis and cryptococcosis but not mortality)

Abbreviations: PPD = purified protein derivative (of tuberculin).

Clinical Syndromes

Pneumonia

Although many opportunistic pathogens can cause pneumonia in HIV-infected patients, the majority of infections are caused by the agents commonly associated with community-acquired pneumonia or *P. carinii*. Figure 1 outlines an approach to the ambulatory patient.

Dysphagia

Esophageal candidiasis is the most common cause of dysphagia or odynophagia. This may occur without visible oral candidiasis. Herpes simplex, cytomegalovirus and malignancies are other causes of dysphagia. An empiric trial of oral imidazoles is

Figure 2: **Management of Fever and Neurologic Complaints**

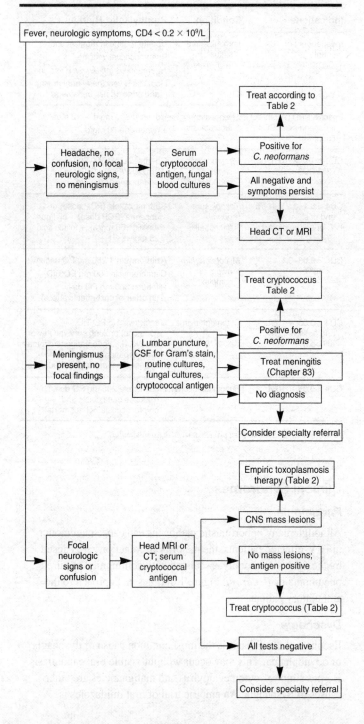

given initially. If the patient fails to respond after a week, esophagoscopy should be performed.

CNS Infections

Infectious CNS complications of chronic immunosuppression occur primarily in patients with late-stage HIV infection (CD4 $\leq 0.1 \times 10^9$/L). *Cryptococcus neoformans* and *Toxoplasma gondii* cause the majority of such infections (Figure 2).

Fever With No Focus of Infection

Patients often present with persistent fever without accompanying organ-specific symptoms. The HIV virus itself can produce fever, night sweats, malaise and weight loss. In patients in whom physical examination shows no focal source, *P. carinii* pneumonia should be considered (Figure 1). If the infection is not identified following routine work-up and blood cultures, do fungal and mycobacterial blood cultures and a serum cryptococcal antigen assay. If tests are still negative, consider specialty referral.

Diarrhea

Many pathogens have been associated with diarrhea in HIV-infected patients. Patients with acute symptoms (< 28 days) should have routine stool cultures and blood cultures ($\times$ 2 if febrile). Consider *Clostridium difficile* if the patient has taken antibiotics recently. Anti-infectives should be administered as per etiology, including salmonellosis.

Patients with chronic diarrhea (> 28 days) or undiagnosed acute diarrhea should have routine stool cultures, ova and parasite examinations ($\times$ 3), modified acid-fast (MAF) stain examination of stool and stool examination for microsporidia. Treat as per etiology. If tests are negative and diarrhea is associated with fever, abdominal pain or blood, do mycobacterial blood cultures and refer the patient for endoscopy with biopsy. Patients with watery nonbloody chronic diarrhea may be treated with loperamide. An empiric trial of metronidazole may be warranted.

Specific Infections

Management of selected infections is outlined in Table 2.

Table 2: **Management of Selected HIV-associated Infections**

Infection	Treatment (see also Table 3)
Candida Species Mucosal candidal infections: ↑ as CD4 count ↓; initially involve oral and vaginal mucosa; topical therapies used initially; systemic therapy may be required to maintain suppression. Esophageal candidiasis: usually a later manifestation; can occur without oral or vaginal disease. Severe discomfort or esophageal disease requires systemic therapy.	**Thrush, topical therapy:** nystatin suspension 500 000 U QID PO (swish and swallow) or vaginal tablet 100 000 U sucked QID, or clotrimazole vaginal tablet 100 mg sucked 5 ×/d or clotrimazole troche* 10 mg 5×/d. **Vaginal:** miconazole or clotrimazole vaginal cream or suppository. **Systemic oral therapy:** ketoconazole 200–400 mg/d or itraconazole 200 mg/d or fluconazole 100–200 mg/d × 2–3 wks. **Esophageal disease:** start with higher doses then taper when symptoms improved; if failure to respond to fluconazole, amphotericin B 0.3–0.5 mg/kg/d IV × 2–3 wks then weekly when symptoms resolved. Alternatives for patients with less advanced HIV disease are itraconazole 200 mg daily or amphotericin B suspension* 300–500 mg QID.
Cryptococcus neoformans Major cause of meningitis in later stages of HIV infection (in 10% of AIDS patients). Diagnosis includes positive serum or CSF cultures or detection of cryptococcal antigen in blood or CSF. Ongoing prophylactic therapy required after treatment of acute infection.	**Induction therapy:** amphotericin B 0.7 mg/kg/d IV × 2–6 wks ± flucytosine 100–150 mg/kg/d Q6H PO × 2 wks, then completion of 12-wk course with fluconazole 400 mg/d PO or IV (fluconazole may be used initially for patients who are well and followed closely). **Maintenance therapy:** fluconazole 200 mg/d PO or amphotericin B 1 mg/kg IV weekly.
Cytomegalovirus (CMV) Usually occurs with CD4 counts < 0.05 × 10⁹/L. Retinitis with visual disturbances most common manifestation. Enteritis, colitis, pneumonitis, encephalitis, myelitis and neuritis can also occur. Prognosis is poor without therapy. Life-long maintenance therapy required after initial therapy for CMV retinitis.	**Induction therapy:** ganciclovir 5 mg/kg/d IV Q12H × 14–21 d or foscarnet* 60 mg/kg IV Q8H × 14–21 d (prehydration with saline recommended) or ganciclovir implant* (lasts 30–40 wks with 15% risk of early retinal detachment, 50% develop disease in other eye and 25% other visceral disease within 6 mos) or cidofovir* 5 mg/kg IV Q weekly × 2 wks (prehydration and oral probenecid required). **Maintenance therapy:** ganciclovir 5 mg/kg/d IV daily or 6 mg/kg IV 5–7 × per wk or 1 g PO Q8H or 400 μg intravitreal implant (as above) or foscarnet 90–120 mg/kg/d (infused over 2 hours) or cidofovir 5 mg/kg IV Q2 wks.

Mycobacterium avium Complex (MAC)

Occurs with CD4 counts < 0.1×10^9/L.

Symptoms: fever, weight loss, fatigue, night sweats alone or with diarrhea, anemia, lymphadenopathy, hepatitis.

Diagnosis primarily by mycobacterial blood culture or biopsy and culture of involved tissue.

Prophylaxis with rifabutin 300 mg/d ↓ risk.

No standard therapy; consider specialty referral or entry into trials.

Multidrug regimens: usually include clarithromycin 500 mg BID PO or azithromycin 500 mg/d PO + ethambutol 15 mg/kg/d, ± 1–3 additional drugs (such as rifampin or rifabutin, ciprofloxacin, clofazimine and amikacin).

Initial therapy × 2–4 mos, followed by maintenance therapy.

Pneumocystis carinii

Primary cause of pneumonia (PCP) in HIV-positive patients with CD4 < 0.2×10^9/L.

All patients at risk of PCP should be receiving prophylaxis (Table 1).

Commonly presents as persistent fever with progressive shortness of breath and cough, often with normal chest x-ray.

Definitive diagnosis requires induced sputum, bronchoalveolar lavage or lung biopsy.

Addition of prednisone in severe PCP ↓ morbidity and side effects of co-trimoxazole.

Standard therapy: co-trimoxazole 15–20 mg/kg/d (trimethoprim) IV or PO (divided Q6–8H) × 21 d, or pentamidine 4 mg/kg/d IV × 21 d, or dapsone 100 mg/d PO + trimethoprim 15–20 mg/kg/d PO × 21 d (better tolerated than co-trimoxazole; no IV form), or

Other: atovaquone; clindamycin + primaquine; trimetrexate + folinic acid

Prednisone (adjunctive) 40 mg BID PO × 5 d, 20 mg BID × 5 d, 20 mg/d to completion of treatment.

(cont'd)

Table 2: Management of Selected HIV-associated Infections *(cont'd)*

Infection	Treatment (see also Table 3)
Toxoplasma gondii Up to 50% of HIV-positive patients with antibodies to this parasite will develop toxoplasma encephalitis as CD4 ↓ below 0.2 × 10⁹/L. Most commonly presents as fever with focal neurologic signs; usually a CT scan with contrast or MRI reveals multiple intracranial-enhancing lesions. Patients should be treated empirically; marked clinical response usually within 7 d; if no response, referral to a specialty centre should be considered. Patients with perilesional edema also require dexamethasone. Life-long prophylactic therapy required after acute therapy.	**Standard therapy:** pyrimethamine 100 mg Q12H × 2 doses, then 75 mg/d PO + folinic acid 10–20 mg/d PO + sulfadiazine 100–150 mg/kg Q6H (max. 6 g/d) × 4–8 wks or **Alternatives:** pyrimethamine + folinic acid (doses as above) + clindamycin 600 mg PO or 600–1 200 mg IV Q6H or azithromycin 1–1.5 g PO daily or clarithromycin 1 g PO Q12H or dapsone 100 mg daily or atovaquone 750 mg PO Q6H × 4–8 wks. **Maintenance therapy:** pyrimethamine 50 mg/d PO + sulfadiazine 1 g Q12H PO + folinic acid 10 mg/d; or pyrimethamine 50 mg/d PO + clindamycin 300 mg Q6H PO + folinic acid 10 mg/d.

* Available from Special Access Program (formerly the Emergency Drug Release Program), Therapeutic Products Directorate, Health Canada.

Table 3: Drugs Used in HIV-associated Infections

Drug	Major or Dose-limiting Toxicities	Comments	Cost*
amphotericin B 🝔 Fungizone	Nephrotoxicity, fever, chills, nausea during infusion, ↑ liver enzymes, bone marrow suppression.	↑ hemotoxicity of AZT, ↑ nephrotoxicity with nephrotoxic drugs. Should be used in all patients with *Cryptococcus neoformans* infections requiring hospitalization.	$$$
atovaquone Mepron	Generally well tolerated.	Should be taken with food (absorption ↑ with food, especially high fat). Less effective than co-trimoxazole for treatment of mild–moderate PCP.	$$
azithromycin Zithromax	GI disturbances.	Should be taken on empty stomach. Interchangeable with clarithromycin for MAC therapy.	$
cidofovir †‡ Vistide	Nephrotoxicity, ocular hypotony, neutropenia, metabolic acidosis.	Prehydration and probenecid ↓ risk of nephrotoxicity. Avoid other nephrotoxic drugs, e.g., NSAIDs.	†
clarithromycin 🝔 Biaxin	Generally well tolerated; diarrhea, vomiting, abdominal pain.	Terfenadine and astemizole should be avoided (↑ risk of arrhythmias). May ↑ carbamazepine and theophylline levels.	$
clofazimine ‡ Lamprene	Skin discoloration, peripheral neuropathy.		‡
co-trimoxazole 🝔 Bactrim, Septra, generics	Rash, nausea, vomiting and fever (common), leukopenia, thrombocytopenia, hypersensitivity reactions, ↑ liver function tests.	Adverse reactions common, often requiring alternate therapy. ↑ hemotoxicity with AZT, pyrimethamine. ↑ warfarin effect.	PO: $ IV: $$$$
dapsone Avlosulfon	Rash, nausea, hemolytic anemia, methemoglobine- mia (more common in G6PD deficiency).	Better tolerated than co-trimoxazole in PCP; ↑ hemotoxicity with AZT, pyrimethamine, primaquine, trimethoprim; absorption ↓ by ddl.	$

(cont'd)

Table 3: Drugs Used in HIV-associated Infections *(cont'd)*

Drug	Major or Dose-limiting Toxicities	Comments	Cost*
fluconazole 🍎 Diflucan	Generally well tolerated; nausea, vomiting, skin rash; ↑ liver function tests.	↓ levels with carbamazepine, phenytoin, rifampin; ↑ phenytoin levels; ↑ warfarin effect.	PO: $$-$$$$$ IV: $$$$$
flucytosine ‡ 🍎 Ancotil	Bone marrow toxicity, especially with high levels; GI disturbances.	↑ hemotoxicity with AZT, ganciclovir.	‡
foscarnet ‡ 🍎 Foscavir	Plasma electrolyte and mineral disturbances (may cause tetany, seizures), nephrotoxicity, anemia, nausea, vomiting, diarrhea, headache.	Prehydrate with normal saline to ↓ nephrotoxicity. Compared to ganciclovir, more difficult to administer. ↑ side effects, but may prolong survival.	‡
ganciclovir 🍎 Cytovene	Neutropenia, thrombocytopenia, nausea, vomiting, headache, confusion.	↑ hemotoxicity with AZT; G-CSF can be used to treat neutropenia; ganciclovir-resistant strains of CMV have emerged.	$$$
itraconazole Sporanox	Generally well tolerated; nausea, epigastric pain, rash, headache, edema, hypokalemia.	Terfenadine and astemizole should be avoided (risk of arrhythmias). ↓ levels with carbamazepine, H₂-blockers, isoniazid, phenytoin, rifampin. ↑ warfarin effect.	$
ketoconazole Nizoral	Anorexia, nausea, vomiting, hepatotoxicity.	Absorbed best in acidic environment; ↓ absorption with ddI, antacids, H₂-blockers. Terfenadine and astemizole should be avoided (↑ risk of arrhythmias). ↓ levels with carbamazepine, phenytoin, rifampin; ↑ warfarin effect; ↑ hepatotoxicity with AZT, co-trimoxazole.	$
pentamidine 🍎 Pentacarinat	Severe hypotension, hypo- and hyperglycemia, nephrotoxicity, cardiac arrhythmias, leukopenia, pancreatitis.	Aerosolized pentamidine well tolerated, but less effective for PCP treatment than IV. Should be injected over 1 h; monitor BP closely. ↑ nephrotoxicity with nephrotoxic drugs.	$$$

pyrimethamine Daraprim	Bone marrow suppression, blood dyscrasias, hematuria, anorexia, vomiting.	An antifolate agent, thus folinic acid (leucovorin) should be given concurrently to ↓ bone marrow toxicity; ↑ hemotoxicity with sulfonamides, AZT.	$
rifabutin Mycobutin	Hepatotoxicity, rash, pruritus, leukopenia, thrombocytopenia. Uveitis at doses > 300 mg/d.	May cause discoloration of urine/feces.	$
sulfadiazine ♥	Hypersensitivity reactions (e.g., rash, pruritus, fever, Stevens-Johnson syndrome); blood dyscrasias.	Used in combination with pyrimethamine.	$

* **Cost per day** – includes drug cost only. Cost based on dosages in Table 2 for 50 kg person.
Legend: $ < $10 $$ $10–20 $$$ $25–50 $$$$ $50–100 $$$$$ > $100
♥ Dosage adjustment may be required in renal impairment – see Appendix I.
† Investigational drug distributed by Upjohn in Canada.

‡ Available from Special Access Program (formerly the Emergency Drug Release Program), Therapeutic Products Directorate, Health Canada.
Abbreviations: AZT = zidovudine; ddI = didanosine; G-CSF = granulocyte colony-stimulating factor; G6PD = glucose-6-phosphate dehydrogenase.

Suggested Reading List

College of Family Physicians of Canada and Health Canada. *Comprehensive guide for the care of persons with HIV disease, Module 1: Adults – men, women, adolescents.* Ottawa: Health Canada, 1993.

Drugs for AIDS and associated infections. *Med Lett* 1995;37(959):87–94.

More new drugs for HIV and associated infections. *Med Lett* 1997;39(994):14–16.

Gallant JE, Moore RD, Chaisson RE. Prophylaxis for opportunistic infections in patients with HIV infection. *Ann Intern Med* 1994;120:932–944.

NIH Conference. Recent advances in the management of AIDS-related opportunistic infections. *Ann Intern Med* 1994;120:945–955.

USPHS/IDSA Prevention of Opportunistic Infections Working Group. 1997 USPHS/IDSA guidelines for the prevention of opportunistic infections in persons infected with human immunodeficiency virus. *MMWR* 1997;46(RR–12).

CHAPTER 98

Infections in the Cancer Patient

Lionel A. Mandell, MD, FRCPC

Goals of Therapy

- To diminish febrile morbidity associated with infection
- To minimize risk of death from infection

Investigations

- Thorough history with attention to:
  - nature of the malignancy and any associated defects in host defenses
  - use of cytotoxic, myelosuppressive or immunosuppressive therapy
  - neutropenia (severity and expected duration)
  - whether patient has had a splenectomy
  - whether nature of malignancy suggests obstruction of natural body passages (e.g., bronchus, bowel, ureter)
  - latent infections (e.g., tuberculosis)
  - travel and exposure to animals
- Complete physical examination (including perianal area) with attention to IV sites
- Laboratory tests:
  - CBC and differential to assess total granulocyte count
  - cultures of blood and any other suspected sites of infection (e.g., urine)
  - radiographic studies appropriate for suspected sites of infection (e.g., chest x-ray for pneumonia, CT scan of the head for cerebral abscess)

Therapeutic Choices

Nonpharmacologic Choices

- For neutropenic patients, avoid raw fruits and vegetables, and avoid flowers in the patient's room.

Pharmacologic Choices

Antibacterials

Bacteria are the most common pathogens causing infections in cancer patients. In non-neutropenic patients, the approach will depend on the clinical status of the patient and whether a focus of infection is present (Figure 1). The risk of death from infection is

Figure 1: **Management of Infection in Cancer Patients**

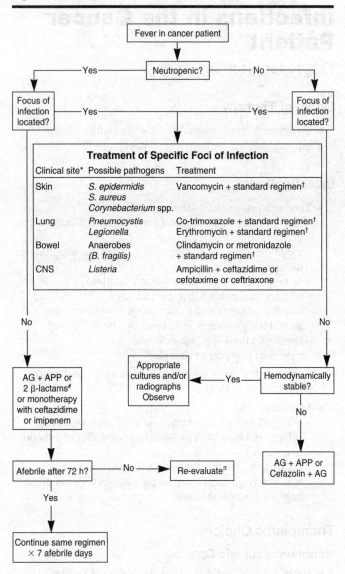

Fever in cancer patient

Neutropenic?

— Yes — / — No —

Focus of infection located? — Yes —

— Yes — Focus of infection located?

Treatment of Specific Foci of Infection

Clinical site*	Possible pathogens	Treatment
Skin	*S. epidermidis* *S. aureus* *Corynebacterium* spp.	Vancomycin + standard regimen†
Lung	*Pneumocystis* *Legionella*	Co-trimoxazole + standard regimen† Erythromycin + standard regimen†
Bowel	Anaerobes (*B. fragilis*)	Clindamycin or metronidazole + standard regimen†
CNS	*Listeria*	Ampicillin + ceftazidime or cefotaxime or ceftriaxone

No / No

AG + APP or 2 β-lactams# or monotherapy with ceftazidime or imipenem

Appropriate cultures and/or radiographs Observe

— Yes — Hemodynamically stable?

No

Afebrile after 72 h? — No → Re-evaluateπ

AG + APP or Cefazolin + AG

Yes

Continue same regimen × 7 afebrile days

---

* *Infection with aerobic gram-negative rods is possible in all of these sites; thus, the standard regimen should be used in addition to the specific agents that cover other possible pathogens from the specified site.*

† *Standard regimen: AG + APP or 2 β-lactams (e.g., piperacillin + ceftazidime) or monotherapy (ceftazidime or imipenem).*

‡ *Ceftazidime + piperacillin.*

π*Consider antifungal therapy if patient remains febrile after 7 days without obvious explanation.*

Abbreviations: AG = Aminoglycoside (e.g., gentamicin, tobramycin);
APP = Antipseudomonal penicillin (e.g., piperacillin, piperacillin-tazobactam).

greater in neutropenic patients, and antibacterials must be started regardless of whether a focus of infection has been found or a microbiologic diagnosis has been made. Single-agent therapy with ceftazidime or imipenem may be used if a patient is hemodynamically stable and there is no obvious site of infection (Table 1). For combination therapy, an antipseudomonal penicillin (e.g., **piperacillin** or **piperacillin-tazobactam**) plus an aminoglycoside or two beta-lactams is used. **Vancomycin** may be added if there is evidence of skin infection or infection with gram-positive organisms (e.g., coagulase-negative staphylococci, methicillin-resistant *S. aureus,* diphtheroids). These agents are generally well tolerated.

Antifungals

Amphotericin B is still the gold standard. It is given IV but is associated with some toxicity. Rigors, a common adverse effect, may be lessened by premedication with acetaminophen and IV meperidine and diphenhydramine. Amphotericin B may be used for resistant or persisting *Candida* infection, and should be given with oral **flucytosine** to treat cryptococcal infection.

Fluconazole may be given orally or IV; it is particularly useful for difficult cases of oral or esophageal candidiasis and cryptococcal infection. Data for treatment of disseminated *Candida* infections are not yet available. *Candida krusei* and *Candida glabrata* are usually resistant. Oral **itraconazole** has a similar spectrum to fluconazole but is also active against *Aspergillus.*

Antivirals

Acyclovir is used for treatment of herpes simplex and varicella zoster infections, whereas **ganciclovir** is the drug of choice for cytomegalovirus infection. Parenteral acyclovir should be used with caution in patients who have exhibited prior neurologic reactions to intrathecal methotrexate. Renal function should be monitored if acyclovir is used with other potentially nephrotoxic drugs (e.g., amphotericin B). If used with imipenem-cilastatin, the potential benefits should be weighed against the risk of seizures, which may occur when the two drugs are given together.

Antiparasitics

The most commonly used antiparasitic agent in cancer patients is **co-trimoxazole** for prevention and/or treatment of *Pneumocystis carinii* infection.

Adjunctive Measures

Hematopoietic growth factors such as granulocyte colony-stimulating factor (G-CSF) stimulate marrow recovery, thereby lessening the period of neutropenia.

Table 1: Drugs Used to Treat Infections in Cancer Patients

Drug	Dosage	Adverse Effects	Drug Interactions	Cost*
β-lactams				
piperacillin Pipracil	3–4 g IV Q4–6H	Hypersensitivity reactions; interstitial nephritis, neutropenia, hemolytic anemia; thrombocytopenia.	Some penicillins may inactivate aminoglycosides if mixed.	$$$$
piperacillin-tazobactam Tazocin	12–16 g/1.5–2 g/d IV divided Q6–8H			$$$–$$$$
ceftazidime Ceptaz, Tazidime	2 g IV Q8H			$$$$$
imipenem-cilastatin Primaxin	500 mg IV Q6H	Imipenem has been associated with seizures at doses of 1 g Q6H.		$$$$
ampicillin Ampicin, Penbritin, generics	2 g IV Q4H			$$
Aminoglycosides				
gentamicin Garamycin, generics	3–5 mg/kg/d IV divided Q8H or 5–7 mg/kg once daily†	Ototoxicity (auditory and/or vestibular), nephrotoxicity, neuromuscular paralysis (rare).	Synergistic or additive toxicity if used with vancomycin and/or platinum-derived antineoplastics or other nephrotoxic/ototoxic drugs.	$
tobramycin Nebcin	3–5 mg/kg/d IV divided Q8H or 5–7 mg/kg once daily†			$
amikacin Amikin	15 mg/kg/d IV divided Q8–12H or 15–20 mg/kg once daily†			$$
netilmicin Netromycin	4–6.5 mg/kg/d IV divided Q8H			$

vancomycin Vancocin	15 mg/kg IV Q12H	Shock after rapid IV infusion (over < 1 h), fever, chills, phlebitis, "red-neck" syndrome, tingling and flushing of head, neck, chest, rash (4–5%), transient leukopenia or eosinophilia, ototoxicity.	Nephrotoxicity may be enhanced if given with aminoglycosides or ethacrynic acid.	$$$$$
erythromycin Erythrocin, Ilotycin, generics	1 g IV Q6H	Abdominal pain, nausea, vomiting, diarrhea; thrombophlebitis, transient hearing loss with high doses.	May interfere with metabolism of theophylline, warfarin, carbamazepine, cyclosporine, methylprednisolone, terfenadine, astemizole, cisapride. May ↑ bioavailability of digoxin.	$$$$
Miscellaneous *clindamycin* Dalacin C	600 mg IV Q6H	Diarrhea, minor reversible ↑ liver transaminases, reversible neutropenia, thrombocytopenia, pseudomembranous colitis.	May enhance action of neuromuscular blocking agents.	$$$
metronidazole Flagyl, generic	500 mg IV Q12H	GI upset, reversible neutropenia, seizures, peripheral neuropathy (rare), rash, metallic taste.	Disulfiram reaction with alcohol. Potentiation of warfarin effects and other oral coumarin-type anticoagulants.	$

(cont'd)

Table 1: **Drugs Used to Treat Infections in Cancer Patients** *(cont'd)*

Drug	Dosage	Adverse Effects	Drug Interactions	Cost*
Antifungals				
amphotericin B Fungizone	0.3–1.5 mg/kg IV Q24H	Rigors, renal dysfunction (azotemia), headache, hypokalemia, phlebitis, thrombocytopenia, anemia, leukopenia (rare), hypotension.	↑ azotemia when used with other nephrotoxic drugs.	$$–$$$
fluconazole Diflucan	100–400 mg PO/IV Q24H	Nausea, headache, skin rash, abdominal pain, vomiting, diarrhea.	May cause hepatotoxicity if used with other potentially hepatotoxic drugs. Sulfonylureas, phenytoin, cyclosporine, coumarin-like drugs may require dosage adjustment (monitor). Avoid astemizole, terfenadine and cisapride (↑ risk of cardiac arrhythmias).	PO: $$–$$ IV: $$–$$$$$
flucytosine ‡ Ancotil	50–150 mg/kg/d PO divided Q6H	Nausea, vomiting, diarrhea, rash, leukopenia, thrombocytopenia, ↑ hepatic enzymes (reversible).		‡

Drug	Dosage	Adverse effects	Drug interactions	Cost
itraconazole Sporanox	100–200 mg PO daily–BID (PC)	Nausea, rash, headache, reversible ↑ hepatic enzymes.	Sulfonylureas, phenytoin, coumarin-like drugs, digoxin may require dosage adjustment (monitor). Didanosine, H$_2$-antagonists, rifampin, phenytoin, may ↓ itraconazole levels. Avoid astemizole and terfenadine (↑ risk of cardiac arrhythmias). Itraconazole ↑ levels of lovastatin.	$
Antiparasitics *co-trimoxazole* Septra, Bactrim	PO/IV: trimethoprim 20 mg/kg/d and sulfamethoxazole 100 mg/kg/d divided QID	Nausea, vomiting, diarrhea; hypersensitivity reactions, leukopenia, thrombocytopenia, hepatitis (rare).	INR may ↑ with warfarin.	PO: $ IV: $
Antivirals *acyclovir* Zovirax	5–12.4 mg/kg IV Q8H	Phlebitis, rash, hypotension, headache, nausea, tremors, confusion, seizures (1%), renal dysfunction.	Probenecid ↓ renal clearance.	$$$$$
ganciclovir Cytovene	Induction: 5 mg/kg IV Q12H Maintenance: 6 mg/kg IV Q24H	Leukopenia, nausea, headache, behavioral changes.	Avoid use with zidovudine (↑ hematological toxicity).	$$ (for maintenance)

† If appropriate for renal function.
‡ Available through Special Access Program (formerly the Emergency Drug Release Program), Therapeutic Products Directorate, Health Canada.
● Dosage adjustment may be required in renal impairment – see Appendix I.
* Cost per day – includes drug cost only. Where doses are expressed in mg/kg, costs were calculated for a 50 kg person.
Legend: $ < $25 $$ $25–50 $$$ $50–75 $$$$ $75–100 $$$$$ > $100

Prevention of Infection in Cancer Patients

Efforts at preventing infection are usually limited to patients with hematologic malignancy who are undergoing remission induction therapy. In these patients, fluoroquinolones (e.g., **ciprofloxacin**) have been shown to reduce febrile morbidity, but they do not prolong survival.[1]

Therapeutic Tips

- In neutropenic patients, consider adding an antifungal drug if fever does not subside without obvious explanation after 7 days of antibacterial therapy.
- Be aware of possible additive toxicity, particularly with drugs such as aminoglycosides, vancomycin and amphotericin B.

Suggested Reading List

Engervall P, Bjorkholm M. Infections in neutropenic patients II: management. *Med Oncol* 1996;13:63–69.

Hughes WT, Armstrong D, Bodey GP, et al. Infectious Diseases Society of America. Guidelines for the use of antimicrobial agents in neutropenic patients with unexplained fever. *J Infect Dis* 1990;161:381–396.

Pizzo PA. Management of fever in patients with cancer and treatment-induced neutropenia. *N Engl J Med* 1993;328:1323–1332.

The GIMEMA Infection Program. Prevention of bacterial infections in neutropenic patients with hematologic malignancies: a randomized multicenter trial comparing norfloxacin with ciprofloxacin. *Ann Intern Med* 1991;115:7–12.

Walsh TJ, Lee J, Lecciones J, et al. Empiric therapy with amphotericin B in febrile granulocytopenic patients. *Rev Infect Dis* 1991;13:496–503.

---

[1] *Ann Intern Med 1991;115:7–12.*

CHAPTER 99

Minerals and Vitamins

Stanley Zlotkin, MD, PhD, FRCPC

Goals of Therapy

- To ensure adequate intake of vitamins and minerals to maintain good health

Investigations

- History with special attention to:
  - dietary intake (particularly if there are diet restrictions)
  - surgical interventions, stool frequency and quality (if GI tract pathology)
  - medication intake
- Physical examination: unlikely to yield any findings
- Laboratory tests:
  - CBC with smear
  - individual vitamin (or metabolite) and mineral levels (rarely necessary in patients with dietary restrictions but useful for those with GI tract pathology)
  - if GI tract pathology, stool collection (for fat absorption) and breath hydrogen

Therapeutic Choices

Adults (including those over 65 years old) with no significant chronic health problems who are maintaining a stable weight and are eating a variety of foods from the 4 food groups (dairy, bread/pasta, meat and fruits/vegetables) **do not need** vitamin or mineral supplements.

Children who are free of chronic diseases who are growing and eating a variety of foods from the 4 food groups **do not need** vitamin and mineral supplements.

Anyone who is unable to meet the recommended nutrient intake (RNI) due to inadequate intake or increased requirements may need supplementation (Figure 1, Table 1).

Gastrointestinal Tract Pathology (Malabsorption)

Any condition leading to nutrient malabsorption (e.g., cystic fibrosis, sprue, radiation enteritis, Crohn's disease, surgical resections, short bowel, pancreatitis, cirrhosis, chronic cholestasis) may necessitate general or specific vitamin supplementation.

Figure 1: **Indications for Vitamin and Mineral Supplementation**

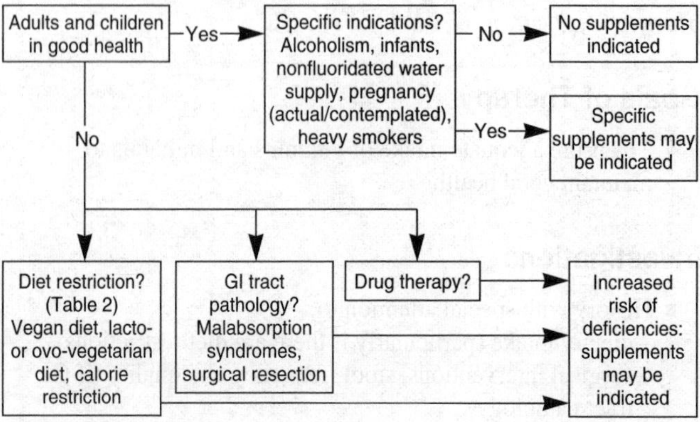

In patients with fat malabsorption, **water-miscible multivitamin preparations** that include the fat-soluble vitamins A, D, K and E should be used.

Surgical resection of specific sections of the GI tract will dictate the need for **mineral supplementation**. Iron, magnesium (200 to 250 mg per day) and calcium are the most common supplements required.

Malabsorption of **vitamin B$_{12}$** due to lack of intrinsic factor will lead to pernicious anemia (Chapter 72). Clinical manifestations may include glossitis, anorexia and diarrhea. Signs include paresthesias and decreased vibration and position sense. Lab evaluation will reveal increased MCV (usually 110 to 140 fL), low hematocrit and decreased serum levels of vitamin B$_{12}$ (< 73 pmol/L). Treatment is parenteral vitamin B$_{12}$ 100 μg daily for 1 week, followed by 200 μg weekly for 8 to 10 weeks, then monthly injections of 200 μg.

Drug Ingestion

Some drugs may decrease absorption, increase excretion or interfere with the utilization of vitamins and minerals. Often, **potassium losses** increase with diuretic and corticosteroid use. Dietary sources of potassium may not be adequate to replace losses in all cases (Chapter 80).

Vitamin supplements may be indicated during long-term therapy with certain drugs. Plasma **vitamin D** and **folate** concentrations should be monitored periodically in patients on phenytoin, carbamazepine and primidone and **fat-soluble vitamins** in patients on cholestyramine and colestipol. **Pyridoxine** supplements may be indicated in patients on isoniazid, penicillamine, cycloserine and hydralazine.

Table 1: Recommended Daily Nutrient Intake*

Age	Sex	Fat-soluble Vitamins			Vit. C (mg)	Water-soluble Vitamins					Minerals	
		Vit. A (RE†)	Vit. D (µg)	Vit. E (mg)		Folate (µg)	Thiamine (mg)	Riboflavin (mg)	Niacin (NE‡)	Vit. B₁₂ (µg)	Calcium (mg)	Iron (mg)
Months												
0–4	Both	400	10	3	20	25	0.3	0.3	4	0.3	250π	0.3#
5–12	Both	400	10	3	20	40	0.4	0.5	7	0.4	400	7
Years												
1	Both	400	10	3	20	40	0.5	0.6	8	0.5	500	6
2–3	Both	400	5	4	20	50	0.6	0.7	9	0.6	550	6
4–6	Both	500	5	5	25	70	0.7	0.9	13	0.8	600	8
7–9	M	700	2.5	7	25	90	0.9	1.1	16	1	700	8
	F	700	2.5	6	25	90	0.8	1	14	1	700	8
10–12	M	800	2.5	8	25	120	1	1.3	18	1	900	8
	F	800	2.5	7	25	130	0.9	1.1	16	1	1 100	8
13–15	M	900	2.5	9	30**	175	1.1	1.4	20	1	1 100	10
	F	800	2.5	7	30**	170	0.9	1.1	16	1	1 000	13
16–18	M	1 000	2.5	10	40**	220	1.3	1.6	23	1	900	10
	F	800	2.5	7	30**	190	0.8	1.1	15	1	700	12
19–24	M	1 000	2.5	10	40**	220	1.2	1.5	22	1	800	9
	F	800	2.5	7	30**	180	0.8	1.1	15	1	700	13

(cont'd)

Table 1: **Recommended Daily Nutrient Intake*** (cont'd)

| Age | Sex | Fat-soluble Vitamins | | | Water-soluble Vitamins | | | | | | Minerals | |
		Vit. A (RE†)	Vit. D (µg)	Vit. E (mg)	Vit. C (mg)	Folate (µg)	Thiamine (mg)	Riboflavin (mg)	Niacin (NE‡)	Vit. B₁₂ (µg)	Calcium (mg)	Iron (mg)
25–49	M	1 000	2.5	9	40**	230	1.1	1.4	19	1	800	9
	F	800	2.5	6	30**	185	0.8††	1††	14††	1	700	13
50–74	M	1 000	5	7	40**	230	0.9	1.2	16	1	800	9
	F	800	5	6	30**	195	0.8††	1	14††	1	800	8
75+	M	1 000	5	6	40**	215	0.8	1	14	1	800	9
	F	800	5	5	30**	200	0.8††	1	14††	1	800	8
Pregnancy (additional)												
1st Trimester		0	2.5	2	0	200	0.1	0.1	1	0.2	500	0
2nd Trimester		0	2.5	2	10	200	0.1	0.3	2	0.2	500	5
3rd Trimester		0	2.5	2	10	200	0.1	0.3	2	0.2	500	10
Lactation (additional)		400	2.5	3	25	100	0.2	0.4	3	0.2	500	0

* Recommended nutrient intake (RNI) is expressed on a daily basis but should be regarded as the average recommended intake over a period of time, such as a week.
† Retinol equivalents. 1 RE = 1 µg or 3.33 IU retinol. 1 RE = 6 µg or 10 IU beta-carotene.
‡ Niacin equivalents. 1 NE = 1 mg niacin or 60 mg tryptophan. About 3% of ingested tryptophan is oxidized to niacin.
π Infant formula with high phosphorus should contain 375 mg calcium per 750 mL of formula.
Breast milk is assumed to be the source of the mineral.
** Smokers should increase vitamin C by 50%.
†† Level below which intake should not fall.
Adapted with permission from Gillis MC, ed. Compendium of Pharmaceuticals and Specialties. Ottawa: Canadian Pharmaceutical Association, 1997.

Diet Restrictions (Table 2)

Table 2: **Supplements in Persons with Dietary Restrictions**

Dietary Restriction	Therapeutic Choices
Vegan Diets Contain no animal products, dairy products or eggs May not provide any vitamin B_{12} May be significantly low in iron, calcium, vitamin D May be low in vitamin A, some B vitamins, zinc	Include other foods from missing food groups; and Single daily multivitamin dose (must include vitamin B_{12}) with iron; and May need calcium supplement to meet RNI (especially women)
Ovovegetarian Diets Contain no animal or dairy products, but do contain eggs May be deficient in iron, calcium, vitamin D May be low in vitamin A, some B vitamins, zinc	Include other foods from missing food groups; and Single daily multivitamin dose with iron; and May need calcium supplement to meet RNI (especially women)
Lactovegetarian Diets Contain no animal products, no eggs, but do contain dairy products May be deficient in iron	Include other foods from missing food groups; and Iron supplement (Table 1)
Calorie-restricted Diets (< 1 200 kcal/d) Weight-reducing diets which are very calorie-restricted will not meet vitamin and mineral requirements	Increase food intake; and Single daily multivitamin plus mineral supplement (calcium and iron)

Specific Indications for Supplementation

Alcoholism

Chronic alcoholism is associated with poor dietary intake of **thiamine** and impaired thiamine absorption, metabolism and storage. Deficiencies of other water-soluble vitamins (including folic acid) may also be present.

Early clinical manifestations of thiamine deficiency are non-specific (anorexia, muscle cramps, paresthesias and irritability). Erythrocyte transketolase activity and urinary thiamine excretion are used to assess thiamine status. The clinical response to empiric therapy is used to support a diagnosis of thiamine deficiency.

For severe deficiency, thiamine 50 to 100 mg per day is given parenterally, followed by daily oral doses of 5 to 10 mg. Other water-soluble vitamins should be provided concurrently.

Patients Undergoing Dialysis

Dialysis removes some water-soluble vitamins; patients may also have dietary restrictions and anorexia. Clinical signs of early deficiencies are nonspecific, and biochemical evaluation is usually not worthwhile. An oral **multivitamin** preparation (including vitamin B_{12} and folic acid) should be recommended to dialysis patients.

Infants

Premature infants receiving breast milk as their primary source of nutrition will not receive an adequate intake of vitamin D or iron. These infants should receive **vitamin D** 10 μg per day (400 IU per day) and iron (2 to 2.5 mg/kg per day) supplements until breast-feeding has been discontinued and the diet supplies a mixture of iron-containing foods. Continuing the iron supplement until 12 months after birth is prudent.

Full-term infants receiving breast milk as their primary source of nutrition should receive a **vitamin D** supplement 10 μg per day (400 IU per day) until breast-feeding has stopped. This recommendation is particularly important for infants with dark skin who cannot endogenously synthesize vitamin D and for infants who will not be exposed to sunshine for prolonged periods.

Hemorrhagic Disease of the Newborn

A hemorrhagic disease of the newborn (HDNB), especially in breast-fed premature infants, has been well described. There is little vitamin K storage and limited synthesis in the newborn. In addition, human milk is low in vitamin K. For prevention of HDNB, the Canadian Paediatric Society recommends that all newborn infants should receive **vitamin K_1** as a single IM dose of 0.5 mg (birthweight ≤ 1 500 g) or 1 mg (birthweight > 1 500 g) within 6 hours after birth. For infants whose parents refuse an IM injection, recommend vitamin K_1 2 mg PO (no oral product available, use parenteral form) at the time of the first feeding, repeated at 2 to 4 weeks and 6 to 8 weeks of age. Advise parents that their infants remain at an increased risk of late HDNB using this regimen.[1]

Pregnancy and Women Contemplating Pregnancy

Folic acid has been demonstrated to protect against neural tube defects (NTD) if taken during the first trimester of pregnancy. Most women cannot achieve a high enough folic acid intake from diet alone. All pregnant women and **women contemplating pregnancy** should receive a folic acid supplement (0.4 mg/day). High-risk women (previous NTD) should take 4 mg/day for 3 months before and 3 months after conception under physician supervision.

[1] *Paediatr Child Health* 1997;2:429–431.

During the later stages of pregnancy, iron requirements are high. An iron supplement of 10 to 15 mg per day throughout pregnancy is often recommended.

Fluoride Supplements for Infants and Children

In Canada, dentists have observed an increased rate of dental fluorosis in communities with fluoridated and nonfluoridated water supplies. Excess fluoride intake from the ingestion of fluoridated toothpaste and other fluoridated products should be avoided to prevent dental fluorosis.

Infants (over age 6 months) and children living in communities or houses with nonfluoridated drinking water may require supplementation (Table 3).

Table 3: **Dosage Schedule for Dietary Fluoride Supplements (Canadian Paediatric Society)***

	Fluoride Concentration of Principal Drinking Water Source (parts per million)		
	< 0.3 ppm	0.3–0.6 ppm	> 0.6 ppm
Age	**Dosage of Supplement**		
6 mo – 3 yrs	0.25 mg/d	0	0
3–6 yrs	0.5 mg/d	0.25 mg/d	0
> 6–16 yrs	1.0 mg/d	0.5 mg/d	0

* Canadian Dental Association has different guidelines.

Heavy Smokers

Vitamin C (ascorbic acid) metabolism is about 50% greater in those smoking more than 20 cigarettes per day than in non-smokers. Recommended intake of vitamin C for heavy smokers is 60 mg daily (males) and 45 mg daily (females).

Vitamin Toxicity

Vitamins can be toxic if taken in large amounts. Because fat-soluble vitamins (vitamins A, D, E and K) are stored in adipose tissue and are not readily excreted, they are potentially more toxic than water-soluble vitamins. Nevertheless, water-soluble vitamins can also cause toxicity if taken in large amounts over long periods (Table 4).

Therapeutic Tips

- Large doses of Vitamin C cannot be recommended for the treatment of colds or other conditions, as clinical studies have not shown a significant benefit.

- Zinc lozenges may alleviate some symptoms of the common cold but can cause nausea and impart a bad taste. Caution is noted in that habitual or long-term ingestion of large doses of zinc (> 150 mg/day) may be hazardous by causing imbalances in copper levels and possibly other nutrients.[2]

Table 4: Vitamin Toxicities

Vitamin	Potential Toxic Effect
Fat-soluble:	
A	Toxic and teratogenic when consumed in large amounts (20 000–30 000 RE/d) for prolonged periods. (> 40 000 RE/d: ↑ CNS pressure – headache, irritability, pseudotumor cerebri; hepatosplenomegaly, hyperostosis, stomatitis, alopecia, anorexia, dry skin, hemorrhagic papilledema which may cause blindness.)
D	Excessive intake (> 1 000 IU/d [25 µg/d]) can lead to hypercalcemia. (75 000 IU/d [1875 µg/d]: osteoporosis associated with bone resorption, hypercalciuria with associated urinary stones, polyuria, weakness, nephrocalcinosis, nausea, diarrhea, anorexia.)
Water soluble:	
C	Adverse side effects can occur with the ingestion of large doses. (≥ 1 g/d: nausea, abdominal cramps, urinary stone formation due to oxaluria; > 4 g/d: ↑ uric acid clearance, rebound scurvy following sudden discontinuation, diarrhea.)
Pyridoxine (B_6)	Can cause ataxia and severe sensory neurotoxicity when taken in large amounts (gram quantities) for months or years as has been recommended for premenstrual syndrome. Can cause neurologic symptoms (usually reversible) at lower doses (≤ 500 mg/d) if taken for prolonged periods.
Niacin	Hepatotoxicity, hyperglycemia, peptic ulceration, diarrhea, facial flushing, pruritus, headache, abdominal cramps, skin effects – dryness, rash, pigmentation.

Suggested Reading List

Benzel RA, Lipman TO. Vitamin prescriptions on a hospital general medical ward: results of a drug utilization review. *J Parenter Enteral Nutr* 1989;13:262–264.

Durie PR. Vitamin K and the management of patients with cystic fibrosis. *Can Med Assoc J* 1994;151:933–936.

Health and Welfare Canada. *Nutrition recommendations. The report of the Scientific Review Committee.* Ottawa: Ministry of Supply and Services Canada, 1990.

---

[2] *Ann Intern Med 1996;125:81–88.*

McMillan DD. Administration of vitamin K to newborns: implications and recommendations. *Can Med Assoc J* 1996;154:347–349.

Russell RM, Suter PM. Vitamin requirements of elderly people: an update. *Am J Clin Nutr* 1993;58:4–14.

Swain R, Kaplan B. Vitamins as therapy in the 1990s. *J Am Board Fam Pract* 1995;8:206–216.

CHAPTER 100

Adverse Drug Reactions

Michael J. Rieder, MD, PhD, FRCPC

Adverse drug reactions (ADRs) are common and important problems. They complicate 5% of all courses of drug therapy and are responsible for 5% of hospital admissions.

Goals in Evaluation of ADRs

- To determine the role of medication in the etiology of untoward events
- To determine the most appropriate therapy for ADRs
- To determine if the goal of therapy has been reached and if dose adjustments or changes in therapy are needed
- To ensure patients, parents or guardians and other physicians understand the adverse event and how to proceed with therapy

Classification of ADRs (Table 1)

ADRs are classified as predictable or unpredictable. The majority of ADRs are related to the pharmacology of the drug and are often dose related and therefore **predictable**. Most of these are not severe in nature and do not require cessation of therapy but rather dose reduction. Many can be prevented by initiating therapy at 1/4 to 1/2 the usual recommended dose and then titrating upwards to the desired goal. This approach is best suited for nonurgent therapies.

Unpredictable ADRs are unrelated to the pharmacologic effects of the drug and include allergic and pseudoallergic reactions or "drug allergy." These ADRs are often more severe in nature and may require discontinuation of therapy.

Approach to Suspected ADRs (Figure 1)

- Careful **history and physical examination** should include associated symptoms and timing of the adverse event in relation to administration of the drug. Risk factors (Table 2) include factors intrinsic to therapy (multiple medications and high-dose therapy) and characteristics unique to the patient (previous drug reactions or organ failure). The very young and very old have increased risk, which may be related to developmental alterations in drug elimination and

Figure 1: **Management of Adverse Drug Reactions**

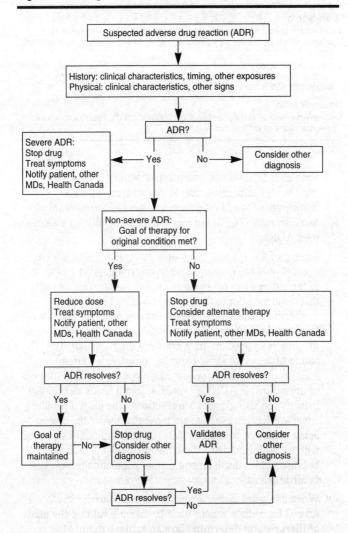

to polytherapy. Why women are at increased risk is not clear. Anthropologic differences (genetic and ethnic) in risk are only now beginning to be understood.

- Develop a **differential diagnosis** which includes details of the original diagnosis for which therapy was prescribed and considers if the events are related to therapy or are part of the disease pathophysiology. Patients often blame the drug while physicians tend to blame the disease. It may be necessary, especially for uncommon adverse events or drugs with which one is uncertain, to obtain additional information.

Table 1: **Classification of Adverse Drug Reactions**

Predictable

Overt – dose-related and due to known pharmacologic effects; occurs in all
patients with sufficient doses, may occur in patients with sensitivity to "standard"
doses

Covert – unsuspected pharmacologic effect; often similar to the underlying disease
(sudden death with antiarrhythmics) or seem unrelated to the drug's action
(cough with ACE inhibitors)

Unpredictable

Mechanism unrelated to the pharmacologic action of the drug (e.g., immune and
pseudoimmune or idiosyncratic reactions)

Specialized data bases, pharmacists or drug information
centres are useful resources. Manufacturers' product
monographs found in the *Compendium of Pharmaceuticals
and Specialties (CPS)* are less useful, especially for uncommon ADRs.

Timing of therapy and symptoms associated with the adverse
event should be considered when determining the probability
of the untoward event being related to therapy (e.g., a rash
that develops prior to therapy is unlikely to be related to
medication). Duration of symptoms can be important as well
(e.g., urticarial symptoms lasting more than 3 or 4 days after
the drug is stopped are frequently not drug-related). The
nature of the event should also be considered. Certain
reaction patterns (rash, urticaria) are common manifestations
of unpredictable ADRs, although selected foods and contact
irritants can also trigger such reactions. The most difficult
adverse effects to evaluate are those that mimic the disease
being treated or common events (e.g., arrhythmias associated
with the antihistamine terfenadine were not appreciated
because sudden death among certain population groups is a
familiar event).

- When untoward events appear to be related to therapy
several immediate actions must be taken. **Evaluate the goals
of therapy and determine how to achieve them.** Most
predictable ADRs are dose-related, mild and will decline or
even vanish over time. Many patients respond to lower
doses than originally prescribed, and dose reduction may
be a useful strategy. It is important not to make patients
"therapeutic orphans" because of mild adverse events which
may disappear with continued therapy. Elements of decision
making include the need for therapy and the availability of
suitable alternate therapy. As an illustration, in patients with
otitis media who develop a serum sickness-like reaction late
in therapy, it is likely that the infection has responded and no
further therapy is needed. However, if a patient with AIDS

Table 2: **Risk Factors for Adverse Drug Reactions**

History of adverse drug reactions to other agents
Use of multiple medications
Hepatic or renal compromise
Age (very young or very old)
Female gender

develops a rash to sulfonamides, the situation is more complex. In the absence of prophylaxis for *Pneumocystis carinii* pneumonia, AIDS patients have a demonstrably shorter life expectancy. The physician is compelled to consider suitable alternate therapy (e.g., pentamidine). As a general rule, examine the goals of treatment and determine if they have been achieved before discontinuing therapy.

- **Treat the adverse drug reaction.** Therapy is usually limited to supportive care and symptomatic relief (e.g., antihistamines used to relieve pruritus from a penicillin-related urticarial rash). When severe ADRs lead to organ failure (e.g., renal failure after accumulation of gentamicin), therapy includes support of the patient until organ function recovers (e.g., dialysis to enhance gentamicin clearance). In patients who develop severe delayed hypersensitivity type reactions, such as Stevens-Johnson syndrome, there is only anecdotal evidence that a brief course of high-dose adrenocorticosteroids may decrease severity. It is preferred not to treat side effects of drugs with other drugs on a chronic basis.

- It is critical that the patient and their family or guardian **understand** what drug caused **the adverse event**, the rationale for continuing or changing therapy and the risk further therapy or future exposure implies. Other physicians involved in the patient's care should also be notified, especially for those with chronic problems. The Adverse Drug Reaction Monitoring Program at Health Canada should be notified, especially if the reaction is severe or related to a newly introduced drug. (ADR reporting forms are included in the Clin-Info section of the *CPS* and intermittently in the *Canadian Medical Association Journal.*)

- Recent developments are promising, but presently the role of **testing for adverse drug reactions** is limited. The only widely available method is skin testing for urticarial or other IgE-mediated reactions to penicillins and local anesthetics. Oral challenge can be used if the drug is essential, but this should only be done under controlled circumstances.

- The best approach to ADRs is **prevention**; don't use a drug if at all possible and choose older, established drugs for which there is greater experience. Occasionally *adverse effects* can effectively be used as *desirable effects* (e.g., sedative antihistamines having better antipruritic and antimotion sickness effects).

Specific ADRs

Urticaria

Urticaria is a common clinical manifestation of ADRs and frequently seen with penicillins and sulfonamides. It is often caused by Type I or IgE-mediated hypersensitivity, although urticaria can occur via non-IgE-mediated mechanisms. Pruritus may be present; however, bronchospasm is not typical and, if present, may be an initial manifestation of anaphylaxis. The usual duration of drug-induced urticaria is 24 to 48 hours after drug exposure. If urticaria lasts longer than 3 to 4 days, nondrug etiologies should be considered.

Management is primarily symptomatic. Conventional antihistamines have been shown to be more effective for drug-related urticaria than newer nonsedating antihistamines. These agents should be used in conventional doses (e.g., diphenhydramine 25 to 50 mg Q4 to 6H or chlorpheniramine 8 mg once daily).

Anaphylaxis

Anaphylaxis is one of the most dreaded manifestations of an ADR, and unless treated promptly and aggressively, can lead to death or disability. Initial symptoms include urticaria, pruritus, cutaneous erythema, shortness of breath, vomiting, crampy abdominal pain, nausea and vomiting, lightheadedness, tight sensation in the throat and a feeling of doom. Symptoms develop within minutes to hours after exposure. Urticaria is the most common manifestation and can be accompanied by angioedema of the skin and upper airway. For angioedema of the upper airway, hoarseness and stridor are early signs; involvement of the larynx or epiglottis can lead to upper airway obstruction and death. Death may also result from vascular collapse, including myocardial ischemia and ventricular arrhythmias.

Prompt treatment is important in avoiding death or disability. Ensure the airway is not compromised. If the airway is involved, administer **epinephrine** in a dose of 0.1 mL (0.015 mg) SC (0.01 mL/kg [0.0015 mg/kg] in children). Oxygen is given concurrently. If bronchospasm occurs after epinephrine is administered, salbutamol can be given by aerosol. When bronchospasm is severe, assisted ventilation may be necessary. Cardiovascular instability is common, and circulatory support with IV fluids and inotropes may be needed. After an episode of anaphylaxis, antihistamines should be given every 4 to 6 hours for 48 hours.

Suggested Reading List

Avorn J. Putting adverse drug events in perspective. *JAMA* 1997;277:341–342.

Patterson R, DeSwarte RD, Greenberger PA, Grammer LC. Drug allergy and protocols for management of drug allergies. *N Engl Reg Allergy Proc* 1986;7:325–342.

Rieder MJ. *In vitro* and *in vivo* testing for adverse drug reactions. *Pediatr Clin North Am* 1997;44:93–111.

CHAPTER 101

Chronic Fatigue Syndrome

David B. Boyd, MD, FRCPC

Fatigue is a common symptom. Chronic fatigue syndrome (CFS) describes only a minority of the patients who present with chronic fatigue (Figure 1). CFS or myalgic encephalomyelitis has been described for many years with different names, e.g., post-infectious asthenia, neuromyasthenia.

The etiology of CFS is hotly debated but not certain; different patients may have different etiologies. Currently it is a trendy diagnosis and shares some features with fibromyalgia, depression, multiple somatic complaints and somatization disorder. The most widely accepted definition comes from the Centers for Disease Control (Table 1).

Goals of Therapy

- To exclude medical or psychiatric diagnoses that have specific and/or treatable causes
- To confirm the diagnosis based on the best data available
- To offer support and reassurance
- To offer therapies that may be helpful and safe

Investigations

No characteristic diagnostic tests have been validated for chronic fatigue syndrome. In general, any abnormalities of physical examination or laboratory testing should considerably amplify the prediagnosis likelihood that a medical diagnosis will be found (or should at least continue to be sought).

- A thorough *history* is essential. Questions should be asked to address "normal" causes of fatigue as well as standard review of symptoms. Habits of eating, sleeping, exercise, caffeine, nicotine and alcohol, as well as current life stresses, premorbid health and physiologic processes (e.g., pregnancy) should be queried.

- *Physical examination* is directed to both exclude other physical causes of fatigue and to include physical features of chronic fatigue syndrome (Figure 1).

- *Laboratory testing* (in the absence of directions suggested by the routine history and physical) should include CBC, electrolytes, urea, creatinine, glucose, alkaline phosphatase, AST, bilirubin, TSH and urinalysis. Further testing such as

Table 1: **Centers for Disease Control Case Definition of the Chronic Fatigue Syndrome**

Major Criteria

1. New onset of persistent or relapsing, debilitating fatigue in a person with no previous history of similar symptoms that does not resolve with bed rest and that decreases daily activity by > 50% for > 6 months.

2. Other clinical conditions that may produce chronic fatigue must be ruled out, based on history, physical examination and selected laboratory tests.

Minor Criteria

Symptom Criteria:

1. Mild fever (< 38.6°C) or chills.

2. Sore throat.

3. Painful cervical or axillary lymph nodes.

4. Unexplained generalized muscle weakness.

5. Muscle discomfort or myalgia.

6. > 24 hours of generalized fatigue after levels of exercise that were easily tolerated previously.

7. Generalized headaches.

8. Migratory arthralgias without arthritis.

9. Neuropsychologic complaints (photophobia, transient visual scotomata, forgetfulness, irritability, confusion, difficulty thinking, inability to concentrate, depression).

10. Hypersomnia or insomnia.

11. Onset of the symptom complex over a few hours to days.

Physical Criteria:

1. Low-grade fever (< 38.6°C orally or 38.8°C rectally).

2. Nonexudative pharyngitis.

3. Palpable or tender cervical or axillary lymphadenopathy ≤ 2 cm.

A case of chronic fatigue syndrome must fulfill major criteria 1 and 2, and 8 of the symptom criteria or 6 of the symptom criteria with 2 of the physical criteria.
As it appears in Epstein KR. The chronically fatigued patient. Med Clin North Am 1995;79(2):315–327 with permission. Adapted from Holmes GP, Kaplan JE, Gantz NM, et al: Chronic fatigue syndrome: A working definition. Ann Intern Med 1988;108: 387–389 with permission.

calcium, albumin, CK, ANA, ESR, HIV or Lyme serology and chest x-ray may be considered as a second tier of investigation.

- *Psychiatric evaluation*, psychometric testing or neuro-psychiatric assessment may be considered.

- A *medication history* to search for drugs that can cause fatigue (e.g., antihistamines, benzodiazepines, alpha-blockers, beta-blockers, antidepressants, antipsychotics, hypnotic-sedatives) can be invaluable.

Figure 1: **Assessment of Fatigue**

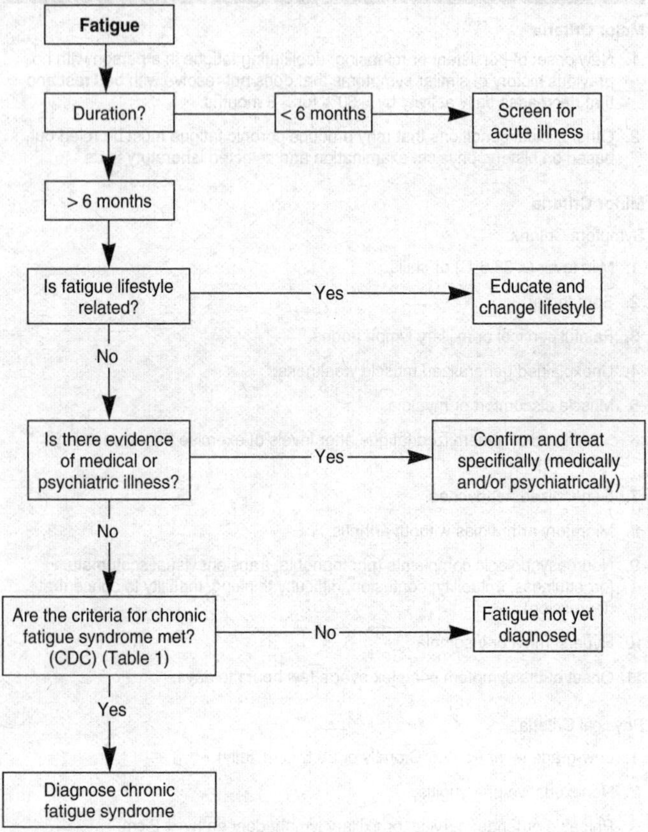

Therapeutic Choices

With the exception of cognitive behavioral therapy, evidence-based controlled trials do not support other therapies. No definitive treatments are known, but an individual may respond to sequential trials of the following.

Nonpharmacologic Choices

- Appropriate diet, sleep and exercise.
- Limit caffeine, nicotine, alcohol.
- Taper and discontinue unnecessary medications.
- Pace activities. Try graded aerobic exercise.[1]

---

[1] *BMJ 1997;314:1647–1652.*

Table 2: Drugs Used in the Treatment of Chronic Fatigue Syndrome

Drug	Initial Dose	Usual Dose	Comments	Cost*
Antidepressants†			Trial of 4 weeks.	
desipramine – Norpramin, Pertofrane, generics	50 mg/d	100–200 mg/d	Desipramine, nortriptyline: anticholinergic effects (dry mouth, constipation, blurred vision), sedation, weight gain, orthostatic hypotension, ↓ seizure threshold.	$$–$$$
nortriptyline – Aventyl	25 mg/d	75–150 mg/d		$$–$$$
fluoxetine – Prozac, generics	10 mg/d	20–40 mg/d	Fluoxetine, sertraline: nausea, nervousness, anorexia, insomnia, sexual dysfunction.	$$–$$$$
sertraline – Zoloft	25 mg/d	50–100 mg/d		$$$
venlafaxine – Effexor	37.5 mg/d	112.5–225 mg/d	Nausea, dry mouth, nervousness, dizziness.	$$$$–$$$$$
moclobemide – Manerix	200 mg/d	450–600 mg/d	Nausea, insomnia, dizziness.	$$$–$$$$$
Analgesics				
acetaminophen ● – Tylenol, generics	325 mg TID	1 g TID	Trial of 1 week.	$
ibuprofen ● – Motrin, Advil, generics	200 mg TID	600 mg TID		$
naproxen ● – Naprosyn, generics	250 mg BID	500 mg BID		$
Others				
evening primrose oil – Efamol	500 mg QID	1 g QID	Trial of 8 weeks.	$$

* Cost of 30-day supply – includes drug cost only.

Legend: $ < $20 $$ $20–40 $$$ $40–60 $$$$ $60–80 $$$$$ > 80

† See Chapter 5 for more information.
● Dosage adjustment may be required in renal impairment – see Appendix 1.

- Obtain psychological support and education. **Cognitive behavioral therapy** has been shown to be of benefit in a controlled trial.[2] Refer to a specialist psychologist or psychiatrist for this treatment.

Pharmacologic Choices (Table 2)

- Try **non-sedating antidepressants** (e.g., desipramine, nortriptyline, fluoxetine, sertraline, venlafaxine, moclobemide), starting with low dose and increasing slowly to therapeutic response. Antidepressants may be effective in the absence of depression but are particularly useful if depression coexists.

- Consider a trial of **acetaminophen** or **NSAIDs** (e.g., ibuprofen) for headache, myalgia or arthralgia. If there is no benefit after a week, stop the drug. If the patient perceives benefit, decrease the dose to find the minimal effective dosage.

- Consider a trial of **evening primrose oil** (Efamol) 1 g QID.

Therapeutic Tips

- Because an individual may respond to one of these therapies in spite of a lack of evidence-based trials, a short-term trial can be worthwhile.

- Keeping a log of therapies tried may maximize placebo effect (30 to 40%) and minimize toxicity, unique to the individual.

- Spontaneous resolution of chronic fatigue is not uncommon. Therefore, short courses of a therapy followed by tapering, discontinuation and re-evaluation over 2 weeks will prevent unnecessary long-term treatment.

Suggested Reading List

Epstein KR. The chronically fatigued patient. In: Merli GJ, Epstein KR, Reife CM, eds. *Med Clin North Am* 1995;79:315–327.

Holmes GP, Kaplan JE, Ganatz NM, et al. Chronic fatigue syndrome: A working definition. *Ann Intern Med* 1988;108:387–389.

Sharpe M. Cognitive behavior therapy for functional somatic complaints. The example of chronic fatigue syndrome. *Psychosomatics* 1997;38(4):356–362.

Straus SE. Chronic fatigue syndrome. In: Isselbacher KJ, Braunwald E, Wilson JD, et al, eds. *Harrison's Principles of Internal Medicine.* 14th ed. New York: McGraw-Hill:1998: 2483–2485.

---

[2] *Am J Psychiatry 1997;154:408–414.*

CHAPTER 102

Constipation

Hugh Chaun, MA, BM, FRCP, FRCP(Ed), FRCPC

Goals of Therapy

- To establish regular bowel function
- To abolish the need to strain and prevent the adverse effects of straining (e.g., hernia, coronary and cerebrovascular dysfunction in the elderly, gastroesophageal reflux)
- To prevent complications (e.g., hemorrhoids, anal fissure, rectal prolapse, stercoral ulcer, fecal impaction, fecal incontinence)
- To treat complications (e.g., fecal impaction, intestinal obstruction)
- To use laxatives wisely and prevent adverse effects of laxative dependence (e.g., cathartic colon)

Investigations

- Thorough history with special attention to:
  - duration of constipation
  - previous laxative use
  - dietary fibre and fluid
  - physical inactivity
  - drugs with constipating effects (e.g., anticholinergics such as antidepressants; narcotic analgesics such as codeine; antacids containing aluminum and calcium; sucralfate; iron supplements; calcium channel blockers; diuretics causing hypokalemia)
  - psychological factors (e.g., stressful events)
  - symptoms of obstructive disease (colonic neoplasm or stricture, anal stricture), painful hemorrhoid or fissure, pregnancy, neurological disease, endocrine disorder (hypothyroidism, diabetes mellitus), collagen vascular disease (progressive systemic sclerosis)
- Physical examination:
  - abdominal mass
- Laboratory tests:
  - CBC
  - stools for occult blood
- Sigmoidoscopy

Figure 1: **Management of Constipation**

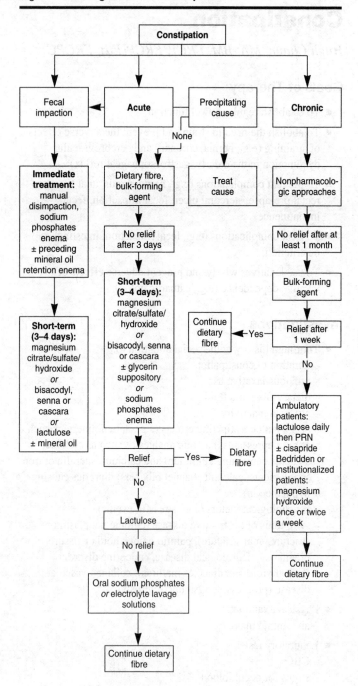

Table 1: **Drugs Used in Constipation**

Drug	Adult Daily Dosage (oral unless specified)	Approximate Time of Action	Adverse Effects	Comments	Cost*
Bulk-forming *psyllium hydrophilic mucilloid* Metamucil, Fibrepur, Prodiem plain, generics	4.5–20 g (psyllium)	All agents: 12–72 h	All agents: Bloating, abdominal pain, rare allergic reactions.	All agents: Increase stool weight; decrease GI transit time; enhance frequency of defecation. Should be taken with increased fluids.	$
sterculia gum Normacol	7–28 g			Can be used long term.	$
Hyperosmotic *glycerin* generics	Suppos: 2.6 g	15 min–1 h	Rectal discomfort or burning.	Stimulates peristalsis.	$
lactulose Lactulax, generics	15–60 mL (10–40 g)	24–48 h	Bloating, flatulence, cramps, diarrhea.	Induces bowel water retention.	$
Lubricant *mineral oil* generics	PO: 15–45 mL	6–8 h	Decreased absorption of fat-soluble vitamins (some drugs). Lipoid pneumonia if aspirated.	Oral dosage form: Avoid in bedridden patients because of risk of aspiration. Should not be used with stool softeners because ↑ absorption of mineral oil.	$
	Enema: 120 mL	2–15 min	Seepage from rectum causing pruritus and irritation.	Should be used for short period.	$$$$

(cont'd)

Table 1: **Drugs Used in Constipation** *(cont'd)*

Drug	Adult Daily Dosage (oral unless specified)	Approximate Time of Action	Adverse Effects	Comments	Cost*
Osmotic/Saline				All agents: Stimulate peristalsis. Useful for rapid response (e.g., preoperatively).	
magnesium citrate Citro-Mag (15 g/300 mL)	4–15 g	30 min–6 h	Hypermagnesemia in renal dysfunction (Mg++ salts).		$–$$$
magnesium hydroxide Milk of Magnesia, generics	2.4–4.8 g	30 min–6 h			$
magnesium sulfate Epsom Salts, generics	10–30 g	30 min–6 h			$
sodium phosphates Fleet Enema, generics Fleet Phospho-Soda, PMS Phosphates	Enema: 120 mL (22 g) Oral: 20 mL (laxative)– 45 mL (purgative)	2–15 min 30 min–6 h	Hyperphosphatemia.		$$ $$
Stimulant				All agents: Stimulate colonic peristalsis. Most potent purgatives. Usually used short term but may be long term in opioid users.	
bisacodyl Dulcolax, generics	PO: 5–15 mg Suppos: 10 mg Micro-enema: 10 mg	6–12 h 15 min–1 h 15 min–1 h	Abdominal pain, cramps, cathartic colon (all agents). Rectal microscopic mucosal changes (bisacodyl suppository, enema).		$ $ suppos $$ micro-enema
castor oil Neoloid, generics	15–60 mL	1–3 h			$–$$
senna Senokot, Glysennid	15–30 mg (sennosides)	6–12 h	Melanosis coli (anthraquinone derivatives). High sugar content in some senna preparations.		$

Stool Softeners			
docusate salts			
Colace, generics	100–200 mg	12–72 h	Act as surfactants. Used as $
Surfak, generics	240 mg		stool softeners following $
			rectal surgery and in long-term
			opioid users, but no
			documented beneficial effects.
Prokinetic Agents			
cisapride	15–40 mg	Gradual	Abdominal cramping, $–$$$
Prepulsid			flatulence. Seems beneficial. Releases
			acetylcholine from myenteric
			plexus and accelerates colonic
			transit.
Lavage Solutions			
electrolyte solutions	1 000–4 000 mL	30 min–1 h	Retching, nausea, abdominal $$$$
Golytely, Colyte,			fullness and bloating. Contain mainly sodium sulfate
Klean-Prep			and polyethylene glycol.
			Excellent cleansing for
			colonoscopy. Klean-Prep is
			available as 4×1 L sachets.

* Cost per day – includes drug cost only.
Legend: $ < $1 $$ $1–2 $$$ $2–3 $$$$ > $3

- Double contrast barium enema or colonoscopy if recent onset in older patients, severe symptoms, does not resolve with simple measures, cause of rectal bleeding not demonstrated on sigmoidoscopy, weight loss, anemia
- Psychological assessment when appropriate
- Transit study with radiopaque markers, anorectal manometry in selected patients, e.g., autonomic bowel paresis (diabetes).

Therapeutic Choices (Figure 1)

Nonpharmacologic Choices

- When possible, drugs with constipating effects (see Investigations) should be discontinued.
- Dietary fibre (20 to 30 g per day), flax seed, unprocessed bran, whole grains, fruits and vegetables should be encouraged. The daily amount should be increased slowly to minimize side effects.
- Fluid intake should be increased.
- Prune juice, stewed prunes, figs should be tried.
- Regular time for toilet use should be scheduled (e.g., after breakfast) to develop conditioned reflex for bowel action.
- Physical exercise should be encouraged.
- Relaxation exercises for pelvic floor and external anal sphincter muscles in conjunction with biofeedback can be tried.

Pharmacologic Choices (Table 1)

Therapeutic Tips

- Constipation is a symptom, not a disease. Establishing the cause, if any, and correcting it should be the primary objective of treatment.
- In general, drug therapy is used only when nonpharmacologic approaches have failed.
- Bulk-forming agents can be safely used for long-term therapy but should be taken with adequate fluids.
- Saline and stimulant laxatives should be used intermittently as needed and as sparingly as possible for short-term therapy, once or twice weekly at most.
- Patient's understanding and cooperation regarding general principles of therapy should be sought, and laxative tolerance should be monitored.
- Lactose-containing dairy products (milk, young cheese) may be the most cost-effective natural cathartic in patients with lactase deficiency.

- To discontinue chronic laxative use, gradually reduce frequency of laxative use over 3 to 4 weeks, while optimizing nonpharmacologic approaches; use an osmotic laxative (e.g., lactulose) intermittently PRN until bowel regularity is achieved.

Suggested Reading List

Smith MB, Chang EB. Antidiarrheals and cathartics. In: Wolfe MM, ed. *Gastrointestinal pharmacotherapy*. Philadelphia: W.B. Saunders, 1993:139–156.

Tedesco FJ. Laxative use in constipation. *Am J Gastroenterol* 1985;80:303–309.

Velio P, Bassotti G. Chronic idiopathic constipation: pathophysiology and treatment. *J Clin Gastroenterol* 1996;22:190–196.

CHAPTER 103

Cough

Tony R. Bai, MD, FRACP, FRCPC

Goals of Therapy

- To choose appropriate therapy based on cough etiology
- To decrease or abolish a nonproductive or distressing cough
- To resist nonspecific cough suppression therapy which may delay diagnosis of a curable cause

Investigations

- Clinical history including:
  - potential causes (Tables 1 and 2)
  - duration of cough – acute vs chronic (cough > 3 weeks)
  - presence and nature of sputum (blood-tinged, purulence)
  - timing and nature of cough (day or night)
  - associated diseases (sinusitis, esophageal reflux, asthma)
  - smoking habits
  - ACE inhibitor (ACEI) use; all ACEIs may cause cough (two-fold greater prevalence in women)
- Investigations of **acute cough** are guided by the presence and nature of sputum. In **chronic cough**, sequential investigation, including empiric therapy, is the most cost-effective approach (Figure 1)

Therapeutic Choices

Nonpharmacologic Choices

- Avoid stimuli causing cough: cigarette smoking, cold air, exercise, pungent chemicals.
- Stop or lower dose of drugs causing cough (e.g., ACEIs) if possible.
- In acute exacerbations of suppurative lung disease, postural drainage (physiotherapy referral) may be tried.

Table 1: **Causes of Acute Cough**

Infections: upper and lower respiratory tract
Asthma
Exacerbations of chronic bronchitis
Bronchogenic carcinoma
Foreign body inhalation
Esophageal reflux with aspiration
Left heart failure

Figure 1: **Management of Chronic Cough***

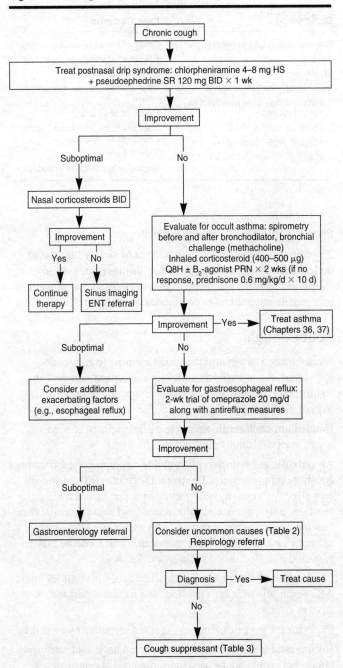

* *Algorithm assumes the chest x-ray is normal, and smoking has been discontinued for 4 weeks.*

Table 2: **Causes of Chronic Cough**

Common	Less Common
Postnasal drip syndrome/rhinitis	Carcinoma of upper respiratory tract
Asthma	Interstitial lung diseases
Chronic bronchitis	Chronic lung infections
Esophageal reflux with aspiration	Other disorders of upper respiratory tract
Sensitized cough reflex (postinfective and other causes)	Occult left heart failure
Lung tumors	Disorders of the diaphragm, pleura, pericardium, stomach
Drugs (e.g., ACE inhibitors)	Thyroid disorders
	Idiopathic ("psychogenic") cough

Pharmacologic Choices (Table 3)

A productive cough generally should not be simply suppressed (unless it interferes with sleep); rather, the underlying cause should be identified and treated. Nonproductive or harmful cough may require intermittent or continuous cough suppression.

Acute Cough

A combination of a **sympathomimetic amine** (e.g., pseudo-ephedrine) and an **antihistamine** (e.g., chlorpheniramine) can significantly decrease the severity of cough during the first few days of the common cold.

Inhaled anticholinergic agents (e.g., ipratropium) can reduce cough in exacerbations of bronchitis.

All **narcotic** and **non-narcotic opioids** can suppress a distressing cough and improve sleep. **Dextromethorphan** (DM), a proven cost-effective, centrally acting antitussive opioid, causes less sedation, constipation, histamine release and abuse potential than codeine. In a minority of patients who metabolize DM slowly, blurred vision and urinary hesitancy can occur. **Codeine** may be preferred if analgesia and sedation are desirable.

Combination of **antitussives with other drugs** in mixtures limits dose flexibility, adds little to effect, and increases cost and adverse effects.

Expectorant (e.g., guaifenesin) use is not supported by evidence.

Decongestants (e.g., pseudoephedrine) can have mild antitussive effects but should not be used indiscriminately because of side effects (e.g, increased blood pressure). They reduce nasal congestion when applied topically.

Table 3: Drugs Used in Cough Suppression

Drug	Dosage	Adverse Effects	Cost*
Antitussives *dextromethorphan* Benylin DM, Formula 44, Delsym (sustained release), generics	Adult: 15–30 mg Q6–8H 60 mg Q12H (sustained release) Pediatric: < 2 yrs: 1 mg/kg/d divided Q6–8H 2–5 yrs: 2.5–5 mg Q4H to 7.5 mg Q6–8H up to 30 mg/d 6–11 yrs: 5–10 mg Q4H to 15 mg Q6–8H up to 60 mg/d 12+ yrs: 10–20 mg Q4H to 30 mg Q6–8H up to 120 mg/d	Drowsiness, GI upset, blurred vision and urinary hesitancy in patients who metabolize DM slowly.	$†
codeine (if analgesia and sedation desired) generics	Adult: 5–20 mg Q4–8H Pediatric: < 2 yrs: 0.8–1.2 mg/kg/d divided Q4–6H 2–5 yrs: 0.25 mg/kg Q4–6H PRN up to 20 mg/d 6–11 yrs: 0.25 mg/kg Q4–6H PRN up to 60 mg/d ≥12 yrs: 0.25 mg/kg Q4–6H PRN up to 120 mg/d	Constipation, respiratory and CNS depression, dependence, nausea and vomiting.	$
Anticholinergics *ipratropium* Atrovent, generics	2–4 puffs QID	Dry mouth, metallic taste.	$$/inhaler
Antihistamines various agents, e.g., *chlorpheniramine* Chlortripolon, generics	Adult: 4–8 mg HS Pediatric: 1–2 mg HS	Mild sedation, decreases with tolerance.	$†

Legend: $ < $10 $$ $10–20

*Cost of 100 mL or 15 tablets – includes drug cost only.
† Available over the counter – retail mark-up may vary.

Antihistamines act indirectly as antitussives by reducing swelling, nasal discharge and itchiness.

Demulcent preparations (e.g., 5 to 10 mL simple syrup containing 125 mg citric acid monohydrate per 5 mL) or cough lozenges are soothing, largely because of their sugar content, which probably coats sensory endings in the hypopharynx. Their effect lasts only a few minutes.

Therapeutic Tips

- In most patients with chronic cough, treatment of the identifiable cause will resolve the symptom.

- Patients with a recurrence of cough within 3 months after treatment require chronic or episodic therapy.

- More than one cause of chronic cough may occur in the same individual.

- The cough reflex can become "sensitized", with a reduced threshold for sensory nerve activation following a variety of insults. This leads to a prolonged cough requiring prolonged antitussive therapy (e.g., DM) or nebulized lidocaine. Psychogenic cough is a diagnosis of exclusion; patients recognize emotional stress as a frequent trigger and nocturnal cough is absent. Psychiatrist/psychologist referral may be appropriate.

- If for medical reasons an ACEI that is inducing cough cannot be discontinued, inhaled sodium cromoglycate can be helpful.[1]

- Oral codeine and morphine remain the gold standard antitussives in cough associated with malignant or terminal respiratory disease. Oral DM is the nonaddictive gold standard for most other chronic coughs in which analgesia/sedation is not required.

- The increased cough and mucus production in acute exacerbations of asthma, COPD, cystic fibrosis and bronchiectasis should respond to appropriate treatment of the underlying cause; cough suppressants in such patients could lead to retention of mucus and deterioration in the underlying disease.

- Older antihistamines (e.g., chlorpheniramine) have been found to be more efficacious than the newer, relatively nonsedating group in treating postnasal drip syndrome. This may be attributed to their mild anticholinergic effect.

---

[1] *Lancet 1995;345:13–16.*

■ The antitussive effect of inhalations of warm water vapor with menthol and eucalyptus has not been adequately evaluated. Hypo-osmolar solutions can provoke cough.

Suggested Reading List

ACCP consensus conference: managing cough as a defense mechanism and as a symptom. *Chest* 1998: In press.

Carney IK, Gibson PG, Murree-Allen K et al. A systematic evaluation of mechanisms in chronic cough. *Am J Respir Crit Care* 1997;156:211–216.

Fuller RW, Jackson DM. Physiology and treatment of cough. *Thorax* 1990;45:425–430.

Pratter MR, Bartter T, Akers S, et al. An algorithmic approach to chronic cough. *Ann Intern Med* 1993;119:977–983.

CHAPTER 104

Diarrhea

Richard N. Fedorak, MD, FRCPC

Definition

Diarrhea is defined as the excretion of fecal matter at a rate greater than 200 g/24 h, with increased loss of fecal water and electrolytes. The increased fecal water content leads to a change in stooling frequency and consistency, symptoms the patient reports as diarrhea. Acute diarrhea occurs for less than 14 days, while diarrhea that persists for more than 14 days is considered chronic.

Goals of Therapy

- To reduce symptoms and re-establish normal fecal weight (volume)
- To prevent complications (dehydration, hemorrhoids, rectal prolapse)
- To identify and treat specific etiologies

Investigations

Prior to the initiation of therapy, 2 key questions must be addressed:

- Is this true diarrhea? Many people who complain of diarrhea actually have a motility disturbance (e.g., irritable bowel syndrome). They experience an increased frequency of very small bowel movements, but the 24-hour stool weight does not exceed normal amounts. Measuring fecal fat, osmolarity and bile acid levels can also help determine specific etiologies
- Is the diarrhea acute or chronic? In the absence of fever, dehydration or bloody stools, the management of acute diarrhea should alleviate symptoms rather than provide a specific diagnosis or therapy. **Acute diarrhea** is usually caused by viral agents, drugs or food toxins and irritants, for which there is no specific therapy, and usually remits spontaneously within 1 week. **Chronic diarrhea** is evaluated as in Figure 1

Therapeutic Choices

Nonpharmacologic Choices

- Discontinue drugs that cause diarrhea.

Figure 1: **Evaluation of Chronic Diarrhea**

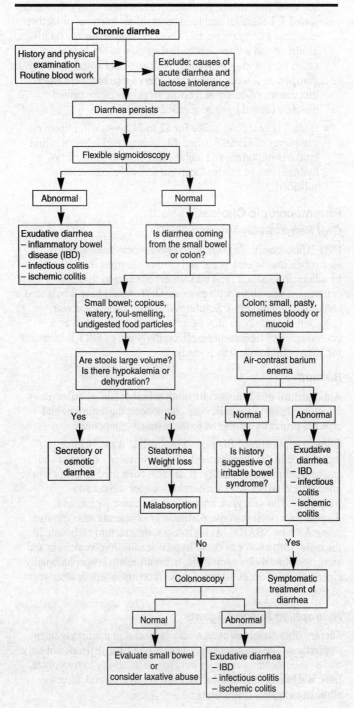

- Stop ingestion of carbohydrates that are poorly absorbed by the small intestine (e.g., dietetic candies and jams containing sorbitol; beverages and foods containing fructose; or lactose-containing dairy products). These carbohydrates are poorly absorbed and are fermented in the colon to produce short-chain fatty acids which cause both an osmotic and secretory diarrhea. A 2-week therapeutic trial of a lactose-restricted diet can avoid costly diagnostic work-ups of continued diarrhea caused by lactose malabsorption.
- Reducing oral food intake for 12 to 24 hours will improve symptoms of acute diarrhea. Maintenance of adequate fluid intake is important and a bland diet (low fat, low carbo-hydrate) can be reintroduced once bowel motions have subsided.

Pharmacologic Choices (Table 1)
Oral Rehydration Therapy (ORT)

ORT (Chapters 76, 78) is used to prevent dehydration and electrolyte loss in both acute and chronic diarrhea. It works by enhancing sodium (and thus water) absorption through cotransport of sodium with glucose. ORT should have a balanced sodium to glucose ratio. Solutions that have excess glucose (e.g., Jell-O, soda pop) may aggravate existing diarrhea as a consequence of their osmotic effect. Early use of ORT is essential for young children and the elderly.

Bismuth

Antidiarrheal mechanisms: Bismuth subsalicylate's antisecretory effect is related to the salicylate component; the antimicrobial effect is primarily attributed to the bismuth component.

Clinical applications: Bismuth subsalicylate is as effective as loperamide in the management of acute traveler's diarrhea and can be used prophylactically. It has also been used to treat chronic idiopathic diarrhea with a reduction in stool weight and frequency. The salicylate component can cause gastric and duodenal mucosal damage, particularly in patients who are also using ASA or NSAIDs. At high doses, the calcium carbonate in the tablet formation can cause hypercalcemia, hypercalciuria and associated metabolic symptoms. Bismuth-related encephalopathy can result from doses 10 times those recommended, or after years of use.

Hydrophilic Bulking Agents

Dietary fibre supplementation may be useful in the management of diarrhea. The ultimate effectiveness of a fibre depends not only on its water-holding capacity but also on its ability to hydrolyze fatty and bile acids which, if they are not hydrolyzed, directly stimulate intestinal secretion.

Table 1: Drugs Used to Treat Diarrhea

Drug	Dosage	Adverse Effects	Comments	Cost*
Bismuth				
bismuth subsalicylate Pepto-Bismol liquid	30 mL Q30 min to a max. of 8 doses/d	Salicylate toxicity, black tongue, black stool, bismuth-induced encephalopathy.	Solution: bismuth subsalicylate 17.6 mg/mL.	$†
bismuth subsalicylate with calcium carbonate Pepto-Bismol tablet	2 tablets Q30 min to a max. of 8 doses/d	Same as above. Hypercalcemia, hypercalciuria.	Tablet: bismuth subsalicylate 262 mg, calcium carbonate 350 mg.	$†
Hydrophilic Bulking Agents				
psyllium Fibrepur, Metamucil, generics	1 teaspoon (5–6 g) Q12H	Inhaled psyllium powder may cause allergic reactions.	Avoid products containing psyllium mixed with laxatives.	$†
cholestyramine resin Questran, generics	4 g Q12H	Nausea, fat soluble vitamin deficiency with long-term use.	1 packet contains 4 g and must be mixed with fluids. May bind other drugs in GI tract; do not take within 1 h before or 4 h after other medications.	$
Opiate Agonists				
loperamide Imodium, generics	2 mg after each loose bowel movement to a max. of 16 mg/d	Sedation, abdominal cramps.	Capsule: 2 mg. Solution: 2 mg/10 mL. After oral administration, absorption is poor (approx. 40% excreted unabsorbed in feces).	$†
diphenoxylate (with atropine sulfate) Lomotil, generics	5 mg initially then 2.5 mg after each loose bowel movement to a max. of 20 mg/d	Sedation, abdominal cramps, dry skin and mucous membranes (from atropine), some addiction potential.	Capsule: diphenoxylate 2.5 mg, atropine 0.025 mg.	$

(cont'd)

Table 1: Drugs Used to Treat Diarrhea *(cont'd)*

Drug	Dosage	Adverse Effects	Comments	Cost*
codeine generics	30–60 mg Q4H PRN	Sedation, nausea, tolerance, potentially addictive.	Tablet: 15 or 30 mg. Solution: 30 or 60 mg/mL.	$
opium and belladonna Opium & Belladonna, generics	1 suppository Q12H PRN	Sedation, nausea, dry mucous membranes, potentially addictive.	Suppository: opium 65 mg, belladonna 15 mg.	$
opium compound Diban	1 capsule Q4H PRN	Sedation, nausea, potentially addictive.	Capsule: opium 12 mg, hyoscyamine 52 µg, atropine 10 µg, scopolamine 3 µg, attapulgite 300 mg, pectin 71 mg.	$$
opium camphor *(paregoric)*	According to concentration of preparation	Sedation, nausea, potentially addictive.		$
Alpha₂-adrenergic Agonists				
clonidine Catapres, generics	0.1–0.6 mg Q12H	Centrally mediated sedation and hypotension.	Tablet: 0.1 and 0.2 mg.	$
Somatostatin				
octreotide Sandostatin	50–500 µg Q12H SC	Pain at injection site.	Ampul: 50, 100, 500 µg. Multidose vial: 200 µg/mL.	$$$

* Cost per day – includes drug cost only.
Legend: $ < $5 $$ $5–10 $$$ > $10
† Available without prescription; retail mark-up may vary.

Psyllium is a hydrophilic agent that increases fecal water-holding capacity and may reduce diarrheal symptoms. Many psyllium-containing products are mixed with laxatives; these products must be avoided in patients with diarrhea.

Cholestyramine resin, in addition to its hydrophilic action, has the ability to bind bile acids. Thus, it has a specific usefulness in treating bile acid-induced diarrhea (e.g., Crohn's disease). Cholestyramine's ability to bind luminal bacterial toxins has led to its adjunctive use in toxin-induced diarrhea (e.g., *C. difficile*).

Opioids

Antidiarrheal mechanisms: Opiates act to reduce diarrhea by decreasing intestinal secretion and/or promoting intestinal absorption, and reducing intestinal motility.

Clinical application: Available opioids include naturally occurring preparations (**paregoric** and **opium alkaloids**) and synthetic preparations (**codeine**, **diphenoxylate** and **loperamide**). These agents are very effective in both acute and chronic diarrhea; however, side effects limit their acute use but tolerance usually occurs with chronic use. Diphenoxylate and loperamide have fewer CNS side effects than the other opioids. Diphenoxylate has been combined with atropine to limit its potential for abuse. Loperamide, which has the least number of side effects or abuse potential, is available without prescription. Codeine may be considered if sedation or analgesia is also required.

Alpha$_2$-adrenergic Agonists

Antidiarrheal mechanisms: Alpha$_2$-adrenergic agonists are potent enhancers of net intestinal absorption, stimulating sodium and chloride absorption and inhibiting bicarbonate and chloride secretion, likely through stimulation of adrenergic receptors at the enterocyte level. In addition, they slow intestinal transit time.

Clinical application: **Clonidine** is effective against opioid-withdrawal diarrhea and diabetic diarrhea associated with autonomic neuropathy. Unfortunately, the dose required to achieve an antidiarrheal effect is often associated with sedation, dry mouth and symptomatic orthostatic hypotension.

Somatostatin

Antidiarrheal mechanisms: **Somatostatin** directly reduces intestinal motility, enteric hormone release and gastric and pancreatic secretion; it promotes large and small intestinal water and electrolyte absorption. Indirectly, somatostatin can inhibit the release of peptides that cause diarrhea from neuroendocrine tumors.

Clinical applications: Somatostatin has a short biological half-life and requires continuous IV infusion, thus limiting its role. **Octreotide**, a long-acting somatostatin analog, can be administered SC. It has been used to control diarrhea caused by neuroendocrine tumors (VIPoma, carcinoid, medullary carcinoma of the thyroid). Octreotide has also been shown to limit idiopathic and infant secretory diarrhea, as well as diarrhea associated with ileostomy, diabetic neuropathy, chemotherapy and HIV disease. In HIV disease, octreotide completely ameliorated diarrhea in 30% of patients, partially improved it in 30%, but had no effect in the remaining 40%.

Suggested Reading List

Barrett KE, Dharmsathaphorn K. Pharmacologic approaches to the therapy of diarrheal diseases. In: Field M, ed. *Diarrheal diseases.* New York: Elsevier, 1991:501–517.

DuPont HL. Nonfluid therapy and selected chemoprophylaxis of acute diarrhea. *Am J Med* 1985;78:81–94.

Fedorak RN. Anti-diarrheal therapy. In: Friedman E, Jacobson ED, McCallum RW, eds. *Gastrointestinal pharmacology and therapeutics.* Philadelphia: Lippincott-Raven, 1997:175–193.

Fedorak RN, Field M. Antidiarrheal therapy: prospects for new agents. *Dig Dis Sci* 1987;32:195–205.

Powell DW, Field M. Pharmacological approaches to treatment of secretory diarrhea. In: Field M, ed. *Secretory diarrhea.* Bethesda: American Physiological Society, 1980:187–198.

CHAPTER 105

Fever

R.G. Peterson, MD, PhD, MPH, FRCPC

Goals of Therapy

- To reduce body temperature to normal range
- To observe response to therapy as a possible diagnostic indicator of etiology
- To make the patient more comfortable

Investigations

NB: Persistent fever should be viewed as a pathological process whose etiology (frequently infectious) must be investigated.

- Careful history and physical examination to:
  - rule out serious or life-threatening infection
  - evaluate the patient's state of hydration
  - assess risk factors for febrile seizures[1] (in children < 7): previous febrile seizure or family history of febrile seizures; rapid change in body temperature (only in susceptible children)
- Measurement of core temperature when oral or axillary temperature > 37.5°C
- Laboratory tests (if indicated by history, physical examination or magnitude of temperature elevation):
  - CBC with differential, glucose (osmolality), electrolytes, BUN, chest x-ray, spinal fluid examination and culture
  - culture of other sources of infection (urine, blood, abscess)

Not all elevations in body temperature represent a fever. Noncentrally mediated responses include exercise, impaired heat loss, dehydration, anticholinergic drugs (commonly tricyclic antidepressants), elevated environmental temperature, toxins (e.g., ASA overdose, cocaine, amphetamines), hyperthyroidism, malignant hyperthermia and autoimmune tissue damage. *All* possible causes of elevated body temperature must be considered to make the correct therapeutic choice for temperature normalization.

---

[1] *Simple febrile seizures occur in 2–4% of all children and are not associated with morbidity or mortality.*

Figure 1: **Temperature Reduction**

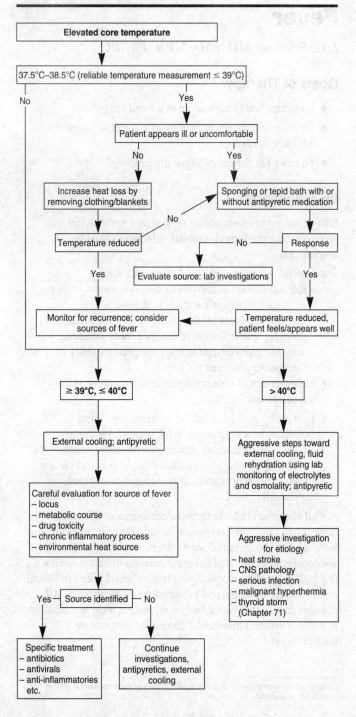

Table 1: Antipyretic Medications

Drug	Dosage	Adverse Effects	Comments
*acetaminophen** Abenol, Atasol, Tylenol, Tempra, generics	Pediatric: 10–15 mg/kg PO/PR Q4–6H Adult: 325–1 000 mg PO/PR Q4–6H	Rare: agranulocytosis, anemia, allergic dermatitis, hepatitis, renal colic, thrombocytopenia.	Risk of hepatotoxicity (with single toxic doses or prolonged use of excessive doses) may be ↑ in alcoholics or in patients regularly taking enzyme inducers.
*acetylsalicylic Acid (ASA)** 🏵 Aspirin, generics	Adult: 325–650 mg PO Q4–6H†	Not recommended for use in children (↑ risk of Reye's syndrome). Allergic reactions, anemia, GI toxicity, rectal irritation (with suppository).	Avoid ASA in patients on methotrexate (high dose), oral anticoagulants. May affect clearance of many other drugs. ↑ risk of bleeding when used concurrently with other medications that may inhibit blood clotting or cause GI bleeding/ulceration.
*ibuprofen** 🏵 Advil, Actiprofen, Motrin IB, generics	Pediatric: 4–8 mg/kg PO Q4–6H Adult: 200–400 mg PO Q4–6H	Allergic reactions, tinnitus, fluid retention, GI disturbances.	Inhibition of platelet aggregation may be hazardous to patients on anticoagulant/thrombolytic therapy. For a complete list of NSAID drug interactions, see Chapter 50.
naproxen 🏵 Naprosyn, Naxen, generics	Pediatric: 10 mg/kg PO Q12H Adult: 250 mg PO Q12H	Allergic reactions, tinnitus, rash, GI disturbances.	As for ibuprofen. Prescription required.

* Relatively inexpensive and available over the counter.
🏵 Dosage adjustment may be required in renal impairment – see Appendix I.
† Rectal absorption is delayed and incomplete compared to oral absorption of equal doses.

Therapeutic Choices (Figure 1)

Although the presence of fever may be of theoretical benefit in reducing viral virulence, in most patients it is outweighed by the real advantages of reducing the fever.

Nonpharmacologic Choices

- The patient should be removed from a hot environment.
- Excess clothing and blankets should be removed.
- Conductive heat loss should be increased:
  - water immersion increases conductive heat loss twenty-fold compared to evaporative/radiant loss in normal clothing.
  - sponging with tepid water (not cold) increases heat loss by both conduction and evaporation.
  - alcohol sponging is *not* recommended because dermal absorption may produce systemic toxic effects and, as with all nonpharmacologic approaches, too rapid cooling may stimulate shivering which results in further heat production.
- Fluids should be provided orally or parenterally to replace increased insensible water losses and to allow continued evaporative losses by sweating.

Pharmacologic Choices (Table 1)

Virtually all medications that inhibit prostaglandin synthesis (e.g., **acetaminophen, ASA, all NSAIDs,**[2] **corticosteroids**) will lower the centrally mediated temperature set point.

NB: Acetaminophen is the drug of choice in children due to the association of ASA with Reye's syndrome.

Corticosteroids are *not* recommended as antipyretics unless the fever is caused by an inflammatory (not an infectious) process.

Caution: Do not use more than one antipyretic medication simultaneously, as renal toxicity may be observed.

Therapeutic Tips

- Avoid causing discomfort from too rapid cooling or adverse effects of overly aggressive medication use.

---

[2] *Most NSAIDs are not officially indicated for use as antipyretics.*

Suggested Reading List

Kauffman CA, Jones PG. Diagnosing fever of unknown origin in older patients. *Geriatrics* 1984;39:46–51.

McGravey A, Wise PH. Evaluation of the febrile child under two years of age. *J Emerg Med* 1984;1:299–305.

Mellors JW, Horwitz RI, Harvey MR, et al. A simple index to identify occult bacterial infection in adults with acute unexplained fever. *Arch Intern Med* 1987;147:666–671.

Schmidt BD. Fever in childhood. *Pediatrics* 1984;74:929–936.

CHAPTER 106

Management of Overdose

Milton Tenenbein, MD, FRCPC

Goals of Therapy

- To prevent toxicity after the ingestion of potentially poisonous agents
- To treat toxicity due to the ingestion of toxic agents
- To avoid toxicity of therapeutic interventions
- To prevent future poisoning episodes

Investigations

- History to identify:
  - what was ingested
  - when it was ingested
  - how much was ingested
  - why it was ingested

- Physical examination:
  - assess vital signs and level of consciousness
  - general physical examination for findings consistent with ingestion history and to rule out comorbidities
  - identify specific toxic syndromes that have life-saving interventions (Table 1)

- Laboratory tests:
  - for altered mental status – immediate pulse oximetry, cardiac monitoring and bedside blood glucose determination
  - general laboratory tests guided by history and physical examination
  - as history dictates, laboratory quantification of specific toxins that have therapeutic interventions dependent on laboratory result (Table 2)
  - osmolal and anion gaps – if potential for toxic alcohol ingestion
  - abdominal radiograph if iron has been ingested
  - stat drug screens are of no value in emergency department management; drug screens obtained on a routine turnaround time occasionally are of diagnostic value

- Poison Control Centre:
  - a valuable resource for formulations of consumer products, assessment of the potential for toxicity and treatment advice for all poisonings

Table 1: **Toxic Syndromes with Life-saving Interventions**

Toxin	Findings	Interventions
Opiates	Depressed level of consciousness Depressed respiration Miosis	Naloxone
Cholinesterase inhibiting pesticides	Respiratory distress Bronchoconstriction Apocrine hypersecretion	Atropine
Cyclic antidepressants	Depressed level of consciousness Cardiac arrhythmias Prolonged QRS interval Seizures	Sodium bicarbonate

Therapeutic Choices (Figure 1)

Nonpharmacologic Choices

- Treat life-threatening physiologic disturbances:
  - oxygen for hypoxia.
  - assisted ventilation for respiratory failure.
  - IV crystalloid for hypotension.
  - 50% dextrose in water for hypoglycemia.

- Prevent absorption of poison from the gut:
  - **activated charcoal** for most potentially toxic ingestions presenting within 2 hours of ingestion (25 g in children; 50 to 100 g in adults).
  - **whole bowel irrigation** for iron, lithium and sustained-release pharmaceuticals (2 L/h of polyethylene glycol electrolyte lavage solution by nasogastric tube until rectal effluent is clear).
  - *not recommended:* induced emesis, gastric lavage and cathartics (either alone or in combination with charcoal).[1]

- Enhance elimination:
  - *not recommended:* forced diuresis, because it does not remove a significant amount of a toxin from the body and is associated with significant adverse effects such as pulmonary and cerebral edema, and fluid and electrolyte derangements.
  - *uncertain benefit:* multiple doses of activated charcoal; consider for phenobarbital and theophylline.

---

[1] *J Toxicol Clin Toxicol* 1997;35:695–762.

Table 2: **Interventions for Common Poisonings**

Poison	Intervention	
	Pharmacologic*	**Non-pharmacologic**
acetaminophen[†]	N-acetylcysteine	—
ASA[†]	sodium bicarbonate	hemodialysis
benzodiazepines	flumazenil (not recommended)	—
beta-blockers	glucagon	cardiac pacing
calcium channel blockers	glucagon	cardiac pacing
carbon monoxide[†]	oxygen	—
carbamate insecticides	atropine	—
cyclic antidepressants	sodium bicarbonate	—
digoxin	digoxin Fab antibody fragments	—
dystonia inducers (e.g., haloperidol, metoclopramide)	benztropine or diphenhydramine	—
ethylene glycol[†]	ethanol	hemodialysis
iron[†]	deferoxamine	—
isoniazid	pyridoxine	—
lithium[†]	—	hemodialysis
methanol[†]	ethanol	hemodialysis
organophosphate insecticides	atropine/pralidoxime	—
sulfonylurea hypoglycemics	diazoxide	—
theophylline[†]	—	charcoal hemoperfusion

* It is beyond the scope of this chapter to provide dosing information for the above pharmacologic interventions. The appropriate dose of an antidote is complex and varies with amount of poison absorbed and the therapeutic index of the antidote. Sources to consult include the Compendium of Pharmaceuticals and Specialties from the Canadian Pharmacists Association; the Poison Management Manual 4th ed (1997) of the B.C. Drug and Poison Information Centre [fax (604) 631-5262] or your Regional Poison Control Centre.

[†] These poisonings require rapid serum concentration quantification.

- **urinary alkalinization** with sufficient IV sodium bicarbonate to maintain a urine pH of 7 to 8 for salicylate and phenobarbital poisoning.
- **hemodialysis** for methanol, ethylene glycol, severe salicylate or phenobarbital poisoning.
- **charcoal hemoperfusion** for severe theophylline poisoning.
- Supportive care:
  - continue to support vital functions.
  - correct significant acid/base and fluid/electrolyte abnormalities.
  - treat significant hypothermia.
  - interventions for specific common poisonings (Table 2).

Figure 1: **Management of Overdose**

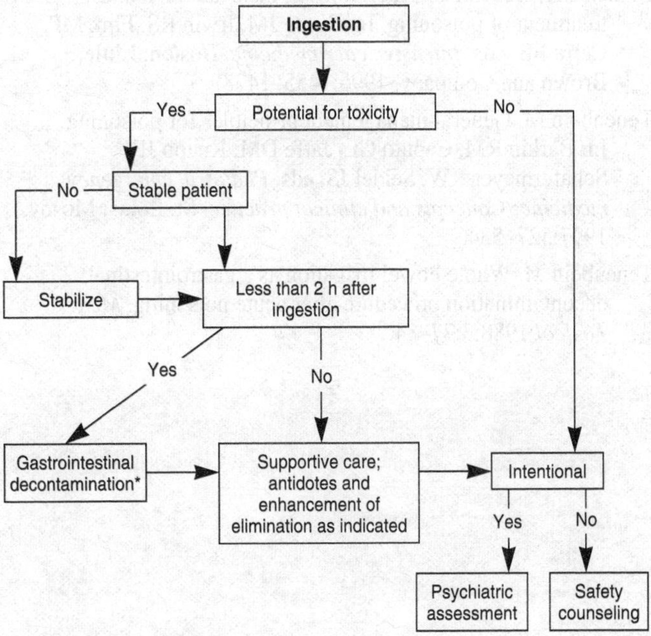

* Usually activated charcoal, occasionally whole bowel irrigation.

Pharmacologic Choices

- Antidotes (Table 2):
  - for specific clinical findings (Table 1).
  - as indicated by laboratory results (Table 2).
  - flumazenil *not* recommended for either known or speculative benzodiazepine ingestion because benzodiazepines are not in themselves fatal. In addition, there is a risk of seizures associated with flumazenil therapy in the presence of coingestants that lower the seizure threshold.

Prevent Future Poisonings

- Safety counseling for nonintentional ingestions by young children and seniors.
- Psychiatric assessment for intentional ingestions by adolescents and adults.

Suggested Reading List

Linden CH. General considerations in the evaluation and treatment of poisoning. In: Rippe JM, Irwin RS, Fink MP, Cerra FB, eds. *Intensive care medicine*. Boston: Little, Brown and Company, 1996:1455–1478.

Tenenbein M. General management principles for poisoning. In: Barkin RM, Caputo GL, Jaffe DM, Knapp JF, Schafermeyer RW, Seidel JS, eds. *Pediatric emergency medicine: Concepts and clinical practice*. St. Louis: Mosby, 1997:527–534.

Tenenbein M. Whole bowel irrigation as a gastrointestinal decontamination procedure after acute poisoning. *Med Toxicol* 1988;3:77–84.

CHAPTER 107

Persistent Hiccoughs

James M. Wright, MD, PhD, FRCPC

Persistent or intractable hiccoughs are unusual but distressing. They may cause insomnia, weight loss or depression and are associated with metabolic causes and abnormalities of the CNS, ear, throat, thorax and abdomen.

Goals of Therapy

- To decrease or stop hiccoughs
- To prevent recurrence

Investigations

- Complete history (including medication and alcohol use) and physical examination to provide clues for further investigations
- If no abnormalities, it is reasonable to do a CBC, electrolytes, creatinine and chest x-ray
- Further investigations depend on findings of the history, physical and baseline investigations: upper GI tract endoscopy, CT brain scan, abdominal ultrasound, etc.

If all investigations are negative or etiological treatment is impossible, a therapeutic trial to stop the hiccoughs is warranted.

Therapeutic Choices

Nonpharmacologic Choices

- Vagal stimulation (e.g., posterior pharyngeal wall stimulation, Valsalva manoeuvre, digital rectal massage, etc.) may be helpful.
- Gastric aspiration is effective in gastric distention.
- Phrenic nerve disruption is reserved for cases where all else has failed.

Pharmacologic Choices

The condition is rare; hence, only two randomized controlled trials were identified. The first was in 51 patients who developed hiccoughs during anesthesia;[1] patients were randomized to

---

[1] *Anesthesiology 1969;31:89–90.*

receive methylphenidate or saline injection in a double-blind protocol. Equal numbers of cures were found in the two groups. The second was a cross-over trial comparing baclofen with placebo (see below). Most of the treatment recommendations are based on case reports/open trials in small numbers of patients.

Dopamine Antagonists

Chlorpromazine historically has been the drug of choice.[2] It has been used IV (25 to 50 mg over 0.5 to 1 hour) in the emergency room. A trial of 50 to 100 mg PO daily for 2 to 3 days is also reasonable. **Haloperidol**, 2 to 5 mg IM or 5 to 15 mg PO, has also been successful in some cases.

Metoclopramide, 10 mg IV or IM followed by 10 to 20 mg QID PO, has been successful. It may act as a dopamine antagonist or by enhancing gastric emptying.

Baclofen

Baclofen has been reported effective in cases of intractable hiccoughs, with maintenance therapy required in at least one half. A randomized double blind cross-over trial in 4 patients with intractable hiccoughs demonstrated that baclofen was unable to eliminate the hiccoughs, but did provide dose related symptomatic relief.[3] Starting with 5 mg BID, the dose is increased gradually every 2 to 3 days to a maximum daily dose of 75 mg. If effective, baclofen should not be discontinued suddenly. The minimum maintenance dose required to control hiccoughs can be determined by gradually reducing the dose over time. Mild side effects (drowsiness, weakness, nausea and fatigue) are relatively frequent.

Nifedipine

Nifedipine (30 to 60 mg daily) was shown to be effective in 4 of 7 patients with persistent hiccoughs[4] and is worth considering if other treatments are unsuccessful.

Many other drugs have been reported effective in a small number of case reports. However, the data are insufficient to recommend any of them.

Therapeutic Tips

- When a drug is effective, hiccoughs generally stop abruptly within a few hours; in some cases the frequency and amplitude may slowly decrease.

[2] JAMA 1955;157:309–310.
[3] Am J Gastroenterol 1992;87:1789–1791.
[4] Neurology 1990;40:531–532.

- Attempts should be made to withdraw treatments gradually; maintenance therapy may be required in some cases.
- Benzodiazepines should be avoided as worsening of hiccoughs has been reported.
- When a drug is ineffective, there is no need to continue treatment for more than 3 days.

Suggested Reading List

Friedman NL. Hiccoughs: A treatment review. *Pharmacotherapy* 1996;16:986–995.

Launois S, Bizec JL, Whitelaw WA, et al. Hiccough in adults: an overview. *Eur Respir* J 1993;6:563–575.

APPENDIX I

Dosage Adjustment in Renal Impairment

*James McCormack, BSc(Pharm), PharmD,
Bruce Carleton, BPharm, PharmD
and Janet Cooper, BSc(Pharm)*

Careful dosage adjustment may reduce the risk of drug toxicity in patients with impaired renal function. The following is an approach to empiric dosage adjustments (dose and/or interval) in adult patients based on an estimate of renal function (Figure 1, Table 1). This approach does not apply to patients on dialysis (consult specialized references).

Patient/Drug Considerations

The following questions should be answered prior to making empiric dosage adjustments. Table 2 provides drug-specific information.

Is the Patient's Renal Function Impaired?

Use the following formula[1] to estimate the weight-corrected creatinine clearance (ClCr) and to guide empiric dosage adjustments:

Males: ClCr (mL/s/70 kg) = $\dfrac{(140-\text{age}) \times 1.5}{\text{serum creatinine } (\mu\text{mol/L})}$

Females: ClCr (mL/s/70 kg) = multiply equation by 0.85

Many clinicians may be more familiar with a ClCr formula which includes weight. When using formulas to estimate ClCr, first identify the reason for the ClCr determination. If an estimate of the patient's true ClCr (in mL/second) is needed, then use a ClCr formula which includes weight. However, if the estimate of the degree of renal impairment is to guide dosage adjustments, use a weight-corrected estimate of ClCr rather than the patient's actual ClCr. This weight-corrected estimate is then compared to a "normal" ClCr for a 72 kg male (1.8 to 2 mL/s) to approximate the degree of renal dysfunction. Charts which suggest empiric dosage adjustments are usually based on the assumption that the baseline or normal ClCr is 1.8 to 2 mL/s. In addition, a weight-corrected ClCr is easier to calculate.

---

[1] *McCormack JP, Cooper J, Carleton B. Simple approach to dosage adjustment in patients with renal impairment. Am J Health-Sys Pharm 1997;54:2505–2509.*

Elderly (older than 65) or malnourished patients may have relatively low muscle mass and therefore produce less creatinine. If the actual serum creatinine for such patients is used, the formula can often overestimate renal function. A rule of thumb in such patients is not to use a serum creatinine < 100 μmol/L in the above formula.

In general, if ClCr estimates are > 1 mL/s/70 kg, empiric dosage adjustments are not required because changes in ClCr from 2 to 1 mL/s/70 kg are associated with relatively small changes in the half-life of a drug or its active metabolite. However, as ClCr falls below 1 mL/s/70 kg, empiric dosage adjustments should be based on the following questions.

Is the Drug Effective/Safe in Patients with Renal Impairment? (Table 2, column 1)

Some drugs are ineffective or potentially toxic in patients with significant renal dysfunction (ClCr < 0.5 mL/s/70 kg) and should be avoided.

Is the Drug Nephrotoxic? (Table 2, column 2)

A number of drugs have the potential to worsen renal function and an alternative non-nephrotoxic agent should be used if possible.

Is an Immediate Clinical Effect Required?

When failure to elicit an immediate response (e.g., life-threatening conditions or severe pain) poses a significant risk of mortality or morbidity, drug dosing should be aimed at obtaining a therapeutic response within minutes or hours irrespective of renal function. In an attempt to achieve a rapid response, usual initial doses should be used, followed by empiric dosage adjustments once the patient has responded.

If an Immediate Effect is Not Required Can the Dose be Titrated? (Table 2, column 3)

Many conditions do not require an immediate or maximal effect and dose titration can often be used to determine the lowest effective dose. To identify the correct dose for any patient, but particularly in patients with renal impairment, start with a low dose (e.g., 1/4 or 1/2 of the typically recommended dose), and titrate up to a clinical effect.

Is the Drug > 50% Renally Eliminated or Does It Have Active or Toxic Metabolites? (Table 2, columns 4–7)

Drugs that are primarily eliminated by the kidney (> 50%) require empiric dosage adjustments based on an estimate of renal function. In addition, some drugs are metabolized to active or toxic metabolites which may be excreted by the kidney and may need dosage adjustments. Some drugs should be avoided in patients with compromised renal function if toxic metabolites can accumulate (e.g., meperidine).

Approach to Empiric Dosage Adjustments

When dose titration is not possible or desired, empiric dosage adjustments should be made on the basis of estimates of renal function.

Interval vs Dose Adjustment

For drugs given intermittently, the dose or the dosing interval can be adjusted based on the desired goal. Often a combination of extending the interval and reducing the dose is effective and convenient. If the aim is to achieve steady-state maximum/peak and minimum/trough concentrations (e.g., aminoglycosides) similar to those seen in patients with normal renal function, the interval between doses can be extended. If a relatively constant steady-state concentration is desired (e.g., antihypertensives), the dose should be reduced.

Drugs Eliminated ≥ 75% by the Kidney (Table 2, column 6)

Guidelines for the dosage of these drugs, based on the usual dosing interval, are provided in Table 1. For frequently administered drugs (e.g., Q4H–Q12H), extending the interval may decrease the cost of administration or compliance problems.

Drugs Eliminated 50–74% by the Kidney (Table 2, column 5)

These drugs have a significant proportion of non-renal clearance and therefore empiric dosage adjustments are generally not required until renal function estimates are < 0.75 mL/s/70 kg (Table 1).

Drugs Eliminated < 50% by the Kidney (Table 2, column 4)

For drugs eliminated < 50% by the kidneys, empiric dosage adjustments are generally not required, assuming the drug has no active or toxic metabolites.

Drugs with Active or Toxic Metabolites (Table 2, column 7)

Empiric dosage adjustments for drugs with active or toxic metabolites which are dependent on renal elimination should be made as if the drug was 75–100% renally eliminated.

Further Dosage Adjustments Based on Clinical Response

All of the above recommendations are for empiric dosage adjustments, and further dosage changes must always be made based on a patient-specific assessment of efficacy and toxicity. Serum drug concentration monitoring may guide dosage adjustments for certain drugs (Table 2, column 8).

Figure 1: **Empiric Dosage Adjustment Based on Renal Function (Adults)**

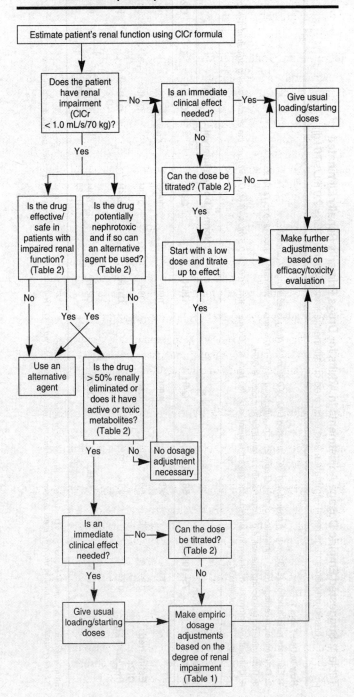

Table 1: **Suggested Empiric Dosage Adjustments in Adults for Drugs Primarily Renally Eliminated**
(based on percentage renal elimination and estimated creatinine clearance [normal ClCr = 2.0 mL/s/70 kg])

How to Use Table 1:

1: Estimate renal function (ClCr), *e.g., a patient with an estimated ClCr of 0.42 mL/s/70 kg is receiving IV ampicillin.*

2: Determine percentage renal elimination of drug (Table 2), *e.g., ampicillin is 75–100% renally eliminated, according to Table 2.*

3: Determine normal dosing interval, *e.g. usual dosing interval for ampicillin is Q6H.*

4: Using above information, determine empiric dosage adjustment, *e.g., the patient's ClCr is between 0.25–0.5 mL/s/70 kg. Therefore, the empiric dosing adjustment is to administer the ampicillin Q12H.*

% Renal Elimination of Drug:	75–100%	50–74%		Normal Dosing Interval					
			Q4H	Q6H	Q8H	Q12H	Q8H	Q12H	Q24H
Estimated ClCr (mL/s/70 kg)	>1.0	>0.75	none	none	none	none	none	none	none
	0.5–1.0	0.33–0.75	Q6H	Q8H	Q12H	Q24H	Q12H	Q24H	↓D 25%*
	0.25–0.5	0.16–0.33	Q8H	Q12H	Q24H	Q24H and ↓D 25%*	Q24H	Q24H and ↓D 25%*	↓D 50%*
	<0.25	<0.16	Q12H	Q24H	Q24H and ↓D 25%*	Q24H and ↓D 50%*	Q24H and ↓D 50%*	Q24H and ↓D 50%*	↓D 75%*

none = no dosage adjustment necessary; ↓**D** = decrease usual dose by indicated percentage.

* For certain drugs, decreasing the dose is not appropriate, or one may need to extend interval > Q24H if available dosage forms do not permit specific dose reductions.

Table 2: **Dosage Adjustment in Renal Impairment—Adults***

Drug	Avoid	Nephro-toxic	Titrate	% Renal Elimination			AM	SDCM
				< 50%	50–74%	≥ 75%		
acarbose			•	•			—	
acebutolol			•		•		■	
acetaminophen			•	•				
acetazolamide	•					•		
acyclovir						•		
alendronate	•			•				
allopurinol			•	•			■	
alprazolam			•	•				
amantadine[1]			•			•		
amikacin		•				•		•
amiloride	•		•		•			
5-aminosalicylic acid				•				
amiodarone			•	•			—	
amitriptyline			•	•			—	
amlodipine			•	•				
amoxapine				•			—	
amoxicillin					•			
amoxicillin/ clavulanate					•			
amphotericin		•		•				
ampicillin						•		
anileridine			•	•				
anistreplase				•			—	
antacids: magnesium/ aluminum[2]	•		•	•				
ASA		•	•	•				
astemizole			•	•				
atenolol			•			•		
atorvastatin			•	•			—	
auranofin	•	•		•				
azathioprine			•	•			■	
azithromycin				•				
aztreonam						•		
bacampicillin						•		
baclofen			•			•		
beclomethasone				•				
benazepril			•	•			■	
benztropine[3]			•					
bezafibrate			•		•			
bismuth subsalicylate				•				
bretylium			•			•	■	
bromocriptine			•					
bumetanide			•	•				
buprenorphine			•	•				
buspirone			•	•			■	

[1] Administer amantadine Q48–72H for ClCr 0.25–1.0 mL/s/70 kg, once weekly for ClCr < 0.25 mL/s/70 kg.

[2] Aluminum and/or magnesium may accumulate in renal impairment.

[3] Route of elimination for benztropine unknown.

Table 2: **Dosage Adjustment in Renal Impairment—Adults*** (cont'd)

Drug	Avoid	Nephro-toxic	Titrate	% Renal Elimination			AM	SDCM
				< 50%	50–74%	≥ 75%		
capreomycin		●			●			
captopril			●		●			
carbamazepine			●	●			—	●
carbidopa			●	●				
carvedilol			●	●			—	
cefaclor					●			
cefadroxil						●		
cefamandole						●		
cefazolin						●		
cefixime					●			
cefoperazone				●				
cefotaxime					●		■	
cefotetan						●		
cefoxitin						●		
cefprozil					●			
ceftazidime						●		
ceftizoxime						●		
ceftriaxone				●				
cefuroxime						●		
cephalexin						●		
cetirizine			●		●			
chloral hydrate	●		●	●			■	
chloramphenicol				●			—	
chlordiazepoxide			●	●			■	
chloroquine					●			
chlorpheniramine			●	●				
chlorpromazine			●	●			—	
chlorpropamide	●		●	●			■	
chlorthalidone	●		●		●			
cholestyramine			●	●				
choline magnesium trisalicylate		●	●	●				
cidofovir	●	●				●	■	
cilazapril			●	●			■	
cimetidine			●		●			
ciprofloxacin					●			
cisapride			●	●				
clarithromycin				●			■	
clindamycin				●				

Avoid = *Avoid drug if ClCr < 0.5 mL/s/70 kg as drug may be ineffective or toxic.*
Nephrotoxic = *Potentially nephrotoxic drug: avoid if possible as may worsen renal function.*
Titrate = *Start with a low dose and titrate to desired effect, regardless of renal function.*
AM = *Drug metabolized to active or toxic metabolites:*
  ■ = *dosage reduction required (calculated as if drug was 75–100% renally eliminated);*
  — = *no dosage reduction required.*
SDCM = *Serum drug concentration monitoring may help guide dosage adjustments.*
*Omission of a drug from this table does not imply that dosage adjustment is NOT required in renal impairment. Refer to specific references for dosing in dialysis.

Table 2: **Dosage Adjustment in Renal Impairment—Adults*** *(cont'd)*

Drug	Avoid	Nephro-toxic	Titrate	% Renal Elimination			AM	SDCM
				< 50%	50–74%	≥ 75%		
clodronate		●				●		
clofibrate	●		●	●				
clonazepam			●	●				
clonidine			●	●				
cloxacillin				●				
clozapine			●	●			—	
codeine			●	●				
colchicine	●		●	●				
co-trimoxazole					●			
cyclosporine		●	●	●			—	●
cyproheptadine			●	●				
delavirdine				●				
desipramine			●	●			—	
dexamethasone				●				
diazepam			●	●			—	
diclofenac		●	●	●				
dicloxacillin				●				
didanosine				●			■	
diflunisal		●	●	●				
digoxin			●			●		●
diltiazem			●	●			—	
dimenhydrinate			●	●				
diphenhydramine			●	●				
disopyramide					●			
dolasetron[4]	●			●			—	
domperidone			●	●				
donepezil			●	●			—	
doxepin			●	●			—	
doxycycline				●				
enalapril			●	●			■	
erythromycin				●				
esmolol				●				
ethacrynic acid	●		●	●				
ethambutol					●			
ethosuximide				●				
etidronate		●			●			
etodolac		●	●	●				
famciclovir				●			■	
famotidine			●			●		
felodipine			●	●				
fenofibrate			●	●			■	
fenoprofen		●	●	●				
fentanyl				●				
fexofenadine[5]			●	●				

[4] *Dolasetron is not recommended in severe renal impairment because of possibility of prolonged QT_c intervals and other cardiac conduction abnormalities due to ↑ hydrodolasetron levels.*

[5] *Clearance of fexofenadine is ↓ in renal impairment; reduce dose to once daily.*

Table 2: **Dosage Adjustment in Renal Impairment—Adults*** *(cont'd)*

Drug	Avoid	Nephro-toxic	Titrate	% Renal Elimination			AM	SDCM
				< 50%	50–74%	≥ 75%		
fluconazole					●			
flucytosine						●		
flunarizine			●	●				
flupenthixol			●	●				
fluphenazine			●	●				
fluoxetine			●	●			—	
flurazepam			●	●			—	
flurbiprofen		●	●	●				
fluvastatin			●	●				
foscarnet	●	●				●		
fosinopril			●	●			—	
furosemide[6]			●		●			
gabapentin			●			●		
ganciclovir						●		
gemfibrozil			●	●			■	
gentamicin		●				●		●
gliclazide			●	●				
glyburide	●		●	●				
gold sodium thiomalate	●	●				●		
granisetron				●				
haloperidol			●	●				
heparin				●				
hydralazine				●				
hydrochlorothiazide	●					●		
hydrocortisone				●				
hydromorphone			●	●				
hydroxyurea		●			●			
hydroxyzine				●			—	
ibuprofen		●	●	●				
imipenem/cilastatin					●			
imipramine			●	●			—	
indapamide	●		●	●				
indinavir				●				
indomethacin		●	●	●				
insulin			●	●				
isoniazid				●				

[6] *In severe renal impairment, larger doses of furosemide than those used in patients with normal renal function may be required.*

Avoid = *Avoid drug if ClCr < 0.5 mL/s/70 kg as drug may be ineffective or toxic.*

Nephrotoxic = *Potentially nephrotoxic drug: avoid if possible as may worsen renal function.*

Titrate = *Start with a low dose and titrate to desired effect, regardless of renal function.*

AM = *Drug metabolized to active or toxic metabolites:*
  ■ = *dosage reduction required (calculated as if drug was 75–100% renally eliminated);*
  — = *no dosage reduction required.*

SDCM = *Serum drug concentration monitoring may help guide dosage adjustments.*

***Omission of a drug from this table does not imply that dosage adjustment is NOT required in renal impairment. Refer to specific references for dosing in dialysis.*

Table 2: **Dosage Adjustment in Renal Impairment—Adults*** *(cont'd)*

Drug	Avoid	Nephro-toxic	Titrate	% Renal Elimination			AM	SDCM
				< 50%	50–74%	≥ 75%		
isosorbide			●	●			—	
itraconazole				●				
kanamycin		●				●		●
ketoconazole				●				
ketoprofen		●	●	●				
ketotifen				●				
labetalol			●	●				
lamivudine					●		■	
lamotrigine			●	●				
lansoprazole			●	●				
levodopa			●	●			—	
levofloxacin						●		
levothyroxine			●	●				
lidocaine			●	●			—	
lisinopril			●			●		
lithium		●				●		●
loratadine			●	●			—	
lorazepam			●	●				
losartan			●	●			—	
lovastatin				●				
loxapine			●	●				
maprotiline			●	●			—	
medroxyprogesterone				●				
mefenamic acid		●		●				
mefloquine				●				
meperidine	●		●	●			■	
mercaptopurine				●			■	
meropenem					●			
mesoridazine			●	●				
metformin	●		●			●		
methadone				●				
methazolamide	●			●				
methotrexate	●	●				●		
methotrimeprazine			●	●			—	
methyldopa			●	●			■	
methylphenidate			●	●				
methylprednisolone				●				
metoclopramide			●		●			
metolazone[7]			●		●			
metoprolol			●	●				
metronidazole				●			—	
mexiletine			●	●			—	
miconazole				●				
midazolam			●	●				
minocycline				●				
minoxidil			●	●				
misoprostol			●	●				

[7] *Dosage reduction of metolazone not necessary in renal impairment.*

Table 2: **Dosage Adjustment in Renal Impairment—Adults*** *(cont'd)*

Drug	Avoid	Nephro-toxic	Titrate	% Renal Elimination			AM	SDCM
				< 50%	50–74%	≥ 75%		
moclobemide			●	●				
morphine			●	●			■	
nabumetone		●	●	●			■	
nadolol			●			●		
nadroparin						●		
nafcillin				●				
nalidixic acid	●			●			■	
naltrexone				●			—	
naproxen		●	●	●				
nelfinavir				●			—	
netilmicin		●				●		●
nevirapine				●				
niacin			●	●				
nicardipine			●	●				
nifedipine			●	●				
nimodipine			●	●				
nitrofurantoin	●			●			■	
nitroglycerin			●	●				
nizatidine			●		●			
norfloxacin						●		
nortriptyline				●			—	
ofloxacin						●		
olanzapine			●	●				
olsalazine			●	●				
omeprazole			●	●				
ondansetron			●	●				
oxaprozin		●	●	●				
oxazepam			●	●				
oxycodone				●				
pamidronate		●			●			
pantoprazole			●	●				
pemoline			●		●			
penicillamine	●	●		●				
penicillin G/V								
pentamidine		●		●				
pentazocine			●	●				
pentoxifylline				●				
pergolide			●	●				

Avoid = *Avoid drug if ClCr < 0.5 mL/s/70 kg as drug may be ineffective or toxic.*
Nephrotoxic = *Potentially nephrotoxic drug: avoid if possible as may worsen renal function.*
Titrate = *Start with a low dose and titrate to desired effect, regardless of renal function.*
AM = *Drug metabolized to active or toxic metabolites:*
■ = *dosage reduction required (calculated as if drug was 75–100% renally eliminated);*
— = *no dosage reduction required.*
SDCM = *Serum drug concentration monitoring may help guide dosage adjustments.*
**Omission of a drug from this table does not imply that dosage adjustment is NOT required in renal impairment. Refer to specific references for dosing in dialysis.*

Table 2: **Dosage Adjustment in Renal Impairment—Adults*** (cont'd)

Drug	Avoid	Nephro-toxic	Titrate	% Renal Elimination			AM	SDCM
				< 50%	50–74%	≥ 75%		
perindopril			●	●			■	
perphenazine			●	●				
phenelzine			●	●				
phenobarbital			●	●			—	
phenylbutazone		●	●	●				
phenytoin			●	●				●
pimozide			●	●				
pindolol			●	●				
piperacillin						●		
piroxicam		●	●	●				
plicamycin		●				●		
pramipexole			●			●		
pravastatin			●	●				
prazosin			●	●				
prednisone			●	●				
primaquine				●				
primidone			●	●			—	
probenecid	●			●				
procainamide					●		■	●
proguanil				●			—	
promethazine			●	●				
propafenone				●				
propantheline				●				
propoxyphene	●		●	●			■	
propranolol			●	●				
propylthiouracil				●				
protriptyline				●			—	
pyrazinamide	●			●				
pyrimethamine				●				
quinapril			●	●			■	
quinidine				●			—	
quinine				●				
ramipril			●	●			■	
ranitidine			●		●			
ranitidine bismuth citrate					●			
reserpine			●	●				
rifampin				●			—	
risperidone			●	●			■	
ritonavir				●			—	
ropinirole			●	●				
salbutamol			●	●				
salsalate		●	●	●			■	
saquinavir				●				
secobarbital				●				
selegiline				●			—	
sertraline			●	●				
simvastatin			●	●				
sodium fluoride						●		

Table 2: Dosage Adjustment in Renal Impairment—Adults* (cont'd)

Drug	Avoid	Nephrotoxic	Titrate	<50%	50–74%	≥75%	AM	SDCM
sotalol			•		•			
spironolactone	•		•	•			■	
stavudine					•		■	
streptomycin		•				•		•
sucralfate[8]				•				
sulfadiazine		•			•			
sulfadoxine/ pyrimethamine[9]						•		
sulfasalazine				•			—	
sulfinpyrazone	•	•	•	•				
sulfisoxazole					•			
sulindac		•	•	•			—	
sumatriptan				•				
teicoplanin		•			•			
temazepam			•	•				
tenoxicam		•	•	•				
terazosin			•	•				
terfenadine				•				
tetracycline		•			•			
theophylline				•				•
thioridazine			•	•			—	
thiothixene			•	•				
tiaprofenic acid		•	•			•		
ticarcillin						•		
ticarcillin/clavulanate					•			
ticlopidine				•				
timolol			•	•				
tobramycin		•				•		•
tolbutamide				•				
tolcapone				•				
tolmetin		•	•	•				
topiramate			•			•		
torsemide			•	•				
trandolapril			•	•			■	
triamterene	•	•	•	•			■	
triazolam			•	•				

[8] Aluminum may accumulate in renal impairment.

[9] Antimalarial prophylaxis with sulfadoxine/pyrimethamine is contraindicated in severe renal insufficiency.

Avoid = Avoid drug if ClCr < 0.5 mL/s/70 kg as drug may be ineffective or toxic.

Nephrotoxic = Potentially nephrotoxic drug: avoid if possible as may worsen renal function.

Titrate = Start with a low dose and titrate to desired effect, regardless of renal function.

AM = Drug metabolized to active or toxic metabolites:
■ = dosage reduction required (calculated as if drug was 75–100% renally eliminated);
— = no dosage reduction required.

SDCM = Serum drug concentration monitoring may help guide dosage adjustments.

*Omission of a drug from this table does not imply that dosage adjustment is NOT required in renal impairment. Refer to specific references for dosing in dialysis.

Table 2: **Dosage Adjustment in Renal Impairment—Adults*** (cont'd)

Drug	Avoid	Nephro-toxic	Titrate	% Renal Elimination			AM	SDCM
				< 50%	50–74%	≥ 75%		
trifluoperazine			●	●				
troglitazone			●	●				
L-tryptophan			●	●				
valacyclovir				●			■	
valproic acid			●	●				
valsartan			●	●				
vancomycin		●				●		●
venlafaxine			●	●			■	
verapamil			●	●			—	
vigabatrin			●			●		
warfarin			●	●				
zafirlukast			●	●				
zalcitabine				●			■	
zidovudine				●				

Avoid = *Avoid drug if ClCr < 0.5 mL/s/70 kg as drug may be ineffective or toxic.*

Nephrotoxic = *Potentially nephrotoxic drug: avoid if possible as may worsen renal function.*

Titrate = *Start with a low dose and titrate to desired effect, regardless of renal function.*

AM = *Drug metabolized to active or toxic metabolites:*
- ■ = *dosage reduction required (calculated as if drug was 75–100% renally eliminated);*
- — = *no dosage reduction required.*

SDCM = *Serum drug concentration monitoring may help guide dosage adjustments.*

*Omission of a drug from this table does not imply that dosage adjustment is NOT required in renal impairment. Refer to specific references for dosing in dialysis.

APPENDIX II

Pharmacoeconomic Considerations

Jeffrey A. Johnson, PhD

The economic impact of the choices made in a therapeutic area is an increasingly important consideration for health care systems and for individual clinicians. **Pharmacoeconomics is the application of economic evaluation techniques in the study of drug therapy.** Increasingly, studies are published incorporating economic evaluations of therapeutic choices for a variety of conditions. Some of the chapters in this edition provide information regarding the pharmacoeconomic considerations for that therapeutic area, where such evidence is available. This Appendix will provide some general guidance when considering the pharmacoeconomic impact of your therapeutic choices.

Pharmacoeconomic evaluations are concerned with comparing the dollars spent on treatment alternatives for the outcomes achieved. It is important to remember that in choosing among many alternatives in a therapeutic area, both sides of the equation must be considered. Drug acquisition costs, while an important component, only provide one side of the cost-outcome story, and, only a part of that story. At the end of most chapters in this edition, a summary table indicates the relative cost of each therapeutic choice. It is also important to consider the relative effectiveness of each choice.

Consider the following hypothetical example. There are three drug choices in a given therapeutic area, Drugs X, Y and Z. Drugs X and Y are older and are less expensive; Drug Z is newer and provides improved clinical outcomes, but is also more expensive.

Drug	Cost	Outcomes
X	$$	+
Y	$$	+
Z	$$$	+++

Although Drug Z costs '$$$', it provides '+++' level of outcomes, whereas Drug X costs '$$' but provides only '+' level of outcomes. This would imply that, in general, Drug Z is more cost effective than Drug X.

However, defining what is a meaningful outcome is often difficult as 'outcomes' have taken on many different forms. For this edition of *Therapeutic Choices*, it was not possible to reconcile all different outcome measures and provide a relative ranking for all therapeutic areas. Instead, we have attempted to draw attention to the issue and remind the reader to consider all possible and relevant treatment costs, not just drug acquisition costs, and also to consider the relative effectiveness of the choices, where such information is available.

Cost Issues

Direct Costs

When considering the cost of drug therapy, it is important to recognize the impact of drug therapy choices on "downstream" costs. Such costs are quite often outside the drug budget, and may include additional laboratory tests required to monitor for adverse side effects, but may also include reduced costs for physician visits or hospitalizations for conditions that were not adequately controlled on previous therapeutic choices. Cost of resources used in the treatment of diseases or conditions is referred to as "direct medical costs."

The following categories of health care resources are all associated with direct medical costs. Any number of these categories may be important considerations when any therapeutic choice is made. That is, when one drug is chosen over another, it is important to consider what impact that treatment may have on any or all of the following:

- Hospitalizations
- Laboratory/radiological tests
- Emergency room/medical center visits
- Drug therapy
- Home care services
- Long-term care

Indirect Costs

Important cost considerations may also include "downstream" costs to society as a result of disease or medical interventions that are outside of the health care system and health care budgets. Such costs include lost or reduced productivity in the workplace due to death or illness. For example, if a drug therapy for migraine headaches is able to reduce the frequency of headaches and consequently reduce the number of days of work missed, this has a positive impact on the overall productivity of the employer and therefore society in general. These costs are referred to as "indirect costs." The impact of health care on indirect costs is often difficult to quantify and may not always be included in economic evaluations, but may be an important consideration in making therapeutic choices.

Perspective on Costs

The perspective used in determining the important and relevant costs is also important. Who would be burdened with what costs? Pharmacoeconomic evaluations may assume the viewpoint of a single provider, an insurer, the provincial health care system, or society as a whole. Depending on the perspective, the total "costs" of a therapeutic choice may differ.

For example, consider a patient who moves through various levels of care from a hospital, to an extended care facility, to home. In the hospital's view, its relevant costs are those incurred during the hospital stay. For instance, the hospital would welcome any therapeutic choice that reduces the length of stay and/or other services during the stay. An earlier discharge, however, may mean that more intensive and more costly nursing home care is required. This is relevant from the perspective of the nursing home and the provincial or regional health care system; it is irrelevant to the hospital. Finally, when the patient is transferred to home, a family member may assume the role of caregiver. From society's perspective, the caregiver's time is a cost; however, this cost is outside the realm of the health care system and outside the coverage of provincial health plans.

Outcomes

The bottom line in pharmacoeconomic considerations is the ratio of net dollars spent per net outcomes achieved. Outcomes, or consequences of drug therapy can be valued in a number of different ways. The choice of which outcome is best depends on the information available and the condition being evaluated. The following are some commonly used approaches in pharmaco-economic evaluations:

Dollars spent per clinical outcome

- Outcomes are some recognized unit of clinical effect (e.g., cost per year of life saved; cost per case of nephrotoxicity avoided).
- Referred to as a **cost-effectiveness analysis**.
- This approach is probably the most commonly used in pharmacoeconomic evaluations.

Dollars spent for dollars saved

- Outcomes given a dollar value.
- Referred to as a **cost-benefit analysis**.
- This approach often requires the economic valuation of a human life, which presents many difficulties, methodological and philosophical.

Dollars spent for quality of life outcomes

- Outcomes are measured as Quality Adjusted Life Years (QALYs) gained.
- Referred to as a **cost-utility analysis**.
- This approach is used when the impact on health-related quality of life is an important outcome of the condition or its treatment.
- Theoretically, the use of a common outcome measure such as QALYs gained, would allow for comparison of cost-outcome relationships across different therapeutic areas (see Laupacis et al., 1992).

Suggested Reading List

Destky AS, Naglie IG. A clinician's guide to cost-effectiveness analysis. *Ann Intern Med* 1990;113:147–154.

Laupacis A, Feeny D, Detsky AS, Tugwell PX. How attractive does a new technology have to be to warrant adoption and utilization? Tentative guidelines for using clinical and economic evaluations. *Can Med Assoc J* 1992;146:473–481.

APPENDIX III

Glossary of Abbreviations

ABG	arterial blood gases
AC	before meals
ACE	angiotensin-converting enzyme
ADD	attention deficit disorder
ADL	activities of daily living
AFB	acid fast bacilli
ALT	alanine transaminase
ANA	antinuclear antibody
Anti HBe	antibody to HBeAg
Anti HCV	antibody to HCV
AOM	acute otitis media
APSAC	anisoylated plasminogen streptokinase activator complex
aPTT	activated partial thromboplastin time
ARDS	acute respiratory distress syndrome
ASA	acetylsalicylic acid
ASOT	antistreptolysin-o titer
AST	aspartate transaminase
BAL	bronchoalveolar lavage
BCC	basal cell carcinoma
BCG	bacillus Calmette-Guérin
BDZ	benzodiazepine
BID	two times per day
BMI	body mass index
BP	blood pressure
BPH	benign prostatic hyperplasia
BSS	bismuth subsalicylate
C&S	culture and sensitivity
CABG	coronary artery bypass graft
CAD	coronary artery disease
CBC	complete blood count
CBT	cognitive behavioral therapy
CCB	calcium channel blocker
cfu/L	colony-forming units/litre
CHF	congestive heart failure
CK	creatine kinase
CMV	cytomegalovirus
CNS	central nervous system
COPD	chronic obstructive pulmonary disease
CPAP	continuous positive airways pressure
CPK	creatine phosphokinase
CSF	cerebrospinal fluid

CT	computed tomography
CTD	connective tissue diseases
CVA	cerebrovascular accident
CVD	cardiovascular disease
CVP	central venous pressure
CXR	chest x-ray
d	day
D-UVA	calcipotriol + psoralen-ultraviolet light
DHE	dihydroergotamine
DIC	disseminated intravascular coagulation
DM	dextromethorphan
DRE	digital rectal examination
DTs	delirium tremens
DVT	deep vein thrombosis
DXA	dual energy x-ray densitometry
ECF	extracellular fluid
ECG	electrocardiogram
ECL	enterochromaffin-like
ECT	electroconvulsive therapy
ED&C	electrodesiccation and curettage
ENT	ear, nose & throat
ERCP	endoscopic retrograde cholangiopancreatography
ESR	erythrocyte sedimentation rate
ESRD	end stage renal disease
FCH	familial combined hyperlipidemia
FEV	forced expiratory volume
FHTG	familial hypertriglyceridemia
FSH	follicle-stimulating hormone
GAD	generalized anxiety disorder
GERD	gastroesophageal reflux disease
GGT	gamma glutamyl transpeptidase
GI	gastrointestinal
GTN	nitroglycerin
GTT	glucose tolerance test
GU	genitourinary
HAV	hepatitis A virus
HBeAg	hepatitis Be antigen
HBIG	hepatitis B immune globulin
HBsAg	hepatitis B surface antigen
HBV	hepatitis B virus
HCV	hepatitis C virus
HDL-C	high-density lipoprotein cholesterol
HDV	hepatitis D (delta) virus
hFH	heterozygous familial hypercholesterolemia
Hgb	hemoglobin
HPN	high-potency neuroleptic

HPV	human papilloma virus
HS	bedtime
HSG	hysterosalpingogram
5HT	5-hydroxytryptamine
IBD	inflammatory bowel disease
IBW	ideal body weight
ICF	intracellular fluid
ICU	intensive care unit
IDDM	insulin-dependent diabetes mellitus
IFNa	interferon alfa
IL-1	interleukin-1
IM	intramuscular
INR	International Normalized Ratio
IOP	intraocular pressure
ISA	intrinsic sympathomimetic activity
ISDN	isosorbide dinitrate
IUCD	intra-uterine contraceptive device
IV	intravenous
IVIG	intravenous immune globulins
IVP	intravenous pyelogram
j	joule
JVP	jugular venous pressure
LBBB	left bundle branch block
LDH	lactic dehydrogenase
LDL-C	low-density lipoprotein cholesterol
LFT	liver function test
LH	luteinizing hormone
LMWH	low-molecular-weight heparins
LP	lumbar puncture
LPN	low-potency neuroleptic
LRTI	lower respiratory tract infection
MAC	mycobacterium avium complex
MAO	monoamine oxidase
MAOI	monoamine oxidase inhibitor
MCV	mean corpuscular volume
MDI	metered-dose inhaler
MDS	myelodysplastic syndrome
MI	myocardial infarction
MMI	methimazole
MMSE	mini-mental state examination
MODY	maturity onset diabetes of the young
MOFS	multiple organ failure syndrome
MRA	magnetic resonance angiography
MRI	magnetic resonance imaging
MSK	musculoskeletal
NE	norepinephrine

NG	nasogastric
NIDDM	non–insulin-dependent diabetes mellitus
NS	normal saline
NSAIDs	nonsteroidal anti-inflammatory drugs
NYHA	New York Heart Association
OA	osteoarthritis
OC	oral contraceptive
OCD	obsessive–compulsive disorder
OCP	oral contraceptive pill
ORT	oral rehydration therapy
PC	after meals
PCP	*Pneumocystis carinii* pneumonia
PCR	polymerase chain reaction
PD	panic disorder
PDA	panic disorder with agoraphobia
PE	pulmonary embolism
PEEP	positive end-expiratory pressure
PEFR	peak expiratory flow rates
PFT	pulmonary function test
PG	prostaglandin
PG inhibitors	prostaglandin synthetase inhibitors
PGE_1	prostaglandin E_1
PID	pelvic inflammatory disease
PMN	polymorphonucleocyte
PO	by mouth
PPD	purified protein derivative (of tuberculin)
PRN	when necessary
PRP	primary Raynaud's phenomenon
PSA	prostate specific antigen
PT	prothrombin time
PTCA	percutaneous transluminal coronary angioplasty
PTH	parathyroid hormone
PTSD	post-traumatic stress disorder
PTT	partial thromboplastin time
PTU	propylthiouracil
PUD	peptic ulcer disease
PUVA	psoralen-ultraviolet light (treatment)
QHS	each bedtime
QID	four times per day
RBC	red blood cell
RE	retinol equivalents
RIMA	reversible inhibitors of monoamine oxidase A
RNA	ribonucleic acid
RNI	recommended nutrient intake
RP	Raynaud's phenomenon

rtPA	recombinant tissue plasminogen activator (alteplase)
SAD	seasonal affective disorder
SAH	subarachnoid hemorrhage
SBT	serum bactericidal titer
SC	subcutaneous
SIADH	syndrome of inappropriate antidiuretic hormone
SK	streptokinase
SL	sublingual
SLE	systemic lupus erythematosus
SMBG	self-monitored blood glucose
SRP	secondary Raynaud's phenomenon
SSRI	selective serotonin reuptake inhibitor
SSSS	staphylococcal scalded skin syndrome
STD	sexually transmitted disease
SVT	supraventricular tachycardia
TCA	tricyclic antidepressant
TD	tardive dyskinesia
TENS	transcutaneous electrical nerve stimulation
TIA	transient ischemic attack
TIBC	total iron binding capacity
TID	three times per day
TIPS	transjugular intrahepatic portosystemic shunt
TNF	tumor necrosis factor
TSH	thyroid-stimulating hormone
TTKG	transtubular K concentration gradient
TUIP	transurethral incision of the prostate
TURP	transurethral resection of the prostate
UK	urokinase
UTI	urinary tract infection
UVA	ultraviolet-A
UVB	ultraviolet-B
VAS	vasoactive substances
VDRL	Venereal Disease Research Laboratories
VF	ventricular fibrillation
VLDL	very low-density lipoprotein
VMO	vastus medialis obliquus
VMS	vasomotor symptoms
VSST	visual sexual stimulation tests
VT	ventricular tachycardia
VTE	venous thromboembolism
WBC	white blood cell

APPENDIX IV

Microorganism Abbreviations Used in *Therapeutic Choices*

Abbreviation	Full Name

Bacteria

Abbreviation	Full Name
B. fragilis	*Bacteroides fragilis*
C. pneumoniae	*Chlamydia pneumoniae*
C. trachomatis	*Chlamydia trachomatis*
C. difficile	*Clostridium difficile*
C. diphtheriae	*Corynebacterium diphtheriae*
E. aerogenes	*Enterobacter aerogenes*
E. cloacae	*Enterobacter cloacae*
E. faecalis	*Enterococcus faecalis*
E. coli	*Escherichia coli*
F. necrophorum	*Fusobacterium necrophorum*
H. influenzae	*Haemophilus influenzae*
K. pneumoniae	*Klebsiella pneumoniae*
L. pneumophila	*Legionella pneumophila*
L. monocytogenes	*Listeria monocytogenes*
M. catarrhalis	*Moraxella catarrhalis*
M. tuberculosis	*Mycobacterium tuberculosis*
M. pneumoniae	*Mycoplasma pneumoniae*
N. gonorrhoeae	*Neisseria gonorrhoeae*
N. meningitidis	*Neisseria meningitidis*
N. asteroides	*Nocardia asteroides*
P. acnes	*Propionibacterium acnes*
P. mirabilis	*Proteus mirabilis*
P. stuartii	*Providencia stuartii*
P. aeruginosa	*Pseudomonas aeruginosa*
S. typhi	*Salmonella typhi*
S. marcescens	*Serratia marcescens*
S. aureus	*Staphylococcus aureus*
S. epidermidis	*Staphylococcus epidermidis*
S. saprophyticus	*Staphylococcus saprophyticus*
S. pneumoniae	*Streptococcus pneumoniae*
S. pyogenes	*Streptococcus pyogenes*
S. viridans	*Streptococcus viridans*

Abbreviation	Full Name

Blood Parasites

P. falciparum	*Plasmodium falciparum*
P. malariae	*Plasmodium malariae*
P. ovale	*Plasmodium ovale*
P. vivax	*Plasmodium vivax*

Fungi

C. albicans	*Candida albicans*
C. neoformans	*Cryptococcus neoformans*

Protozoa/Parasites

E. histolytica	*Entamoeba histolytica*
G. lamblia	*Giardia lamblia*
P. carinii	*Pneumocystis carinii*
T. gondii	*Toxoplasma gondii*
T. vaginalis	*Trichomonas vaginalis*

Viruses

CMV	Cytomegalovirus
HAV	Hepatitis A virus
HBV	Hepatitis B virus
HCV	Hepatitis C virus
HIV	Human immunodeficiency virus
HPV	Human papillomavirus
HSV	Herpes simplex virus

Index

Italic entries indicate a generic drug name. Bold entries indicate that the item receives detailed treatment in the text. An italic *t* beside the page number refers to a table.